A. Gullo (Ed.)

Anaesthesia, Pain, Intensive Care and Emergency Medicine - A.P.I.C.E.

Proceedings of the

17th Postgraduate Course in Critical Care Medicine
Trieste, Italy - November 15-19, 2002

Volume I

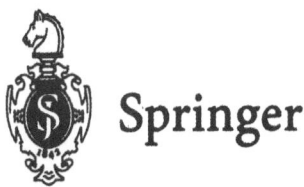 Springer

Prof. ANTONINO GULLO, M.D.
Head, Department of Perioperative Medicine
Intensive Care and Emergency
Trieste University School of Medicine
Trieste, Italy

© Springer-Verlag Italia 2003
Originally published by Springer-Verlag Italia, Milano in 2003

http://www.springer.de

ISBN 978-88-470-0194-7   ISBN 978-88-470-2215-7 (eBook)
DOI 10.1007/978-88-470-2215-7

SPIN 108995326

Springer-Verlag Italia Srl.

Table of Contents

Vol. I

EMERGENCY MEDICINE

Chest pain
F. SCHIRALDI, L. DAMIANO, AND F. PALADINO 3

Advanced Life Support in the management of cardiac arrest: European Resuscitation Council guidelines 2000
L. BOSSAERT, J. NOLAN, AND F. DE LATORRE. 11

Hyperosmolar syndrome
F. SCHIRALDI, G. ESPOSITO, AND G. RUGGIERO 33

Hypertonic solutions: when, how, how long, how much?
J.O.C. AULER JR, L.F. POLI DE FIGUEIREDO, AND M. ROCHA e SILVA 41

Efficacy of non invasive positive pressure ventilation (BIPAP) in acute cardiogenic pulmonary oedema
S. PRAYAG, S TALEKAR, AND S JOG 57

Emergency treatment of acute stroke
P.D. SCHELLINGER, T. STEINER, AND W. HACKE. 69

Early management of severely burned patients
A. LUZZANI, E. POLATI, AND I. SALVETTI 85

SPECIAL CONDITIONS IN CRITICAL CARE

Sedation and analgesia in the critically ill - Principles and practice
S. ANWAR, AND G. PARK 103

Organophosphorus poisoning
S. PRAYAG 113

Physostigmine in the postoperative period
J. RUPREHT 121

Physostigmine use in intensive care
K. LEENDERTSE, AND J. RUPREHT. 129

Blood redistribution during central neural blocks: influence of leg bandaging and other mechanical methods
D. ŠTIFANIC, AND V. PAVER-ERŽEN 137

Management of the post-operative critically ill patient
J. BESSO, E. RIVERO, AND A. BOLIVAR 145

HIV infection in critical care
G. DOMÍNGUEZ-CHERIT, D. BORUNDA, AND J. SIERRA 165

Anaesthesia for TURP: regional vs. general
C. MELLONI, F. SFOGLIAFERRI, AND S. PISTOCCHI 197

BRAIN

GLOBAL AND FOCAL MONITORING IN ACUTE CEREBRAL DAMAGE

The role of jugular O_2 difference
A. BACHER. 223

Intracranial and cerebral perfusion pressure management in traumatic brain injury
J. MYBURGH. 237

Essential cerebral monitoring when resources are limited
W. VIDETTA 253

Therapeutic hypothermia
C.K. SPISS, U.M. ILLIEVICH, AND A. BACHER 263

ADEQUACY OF CEREBRAL PERFUSION IN THE EARLY PHASES AFTER ACUTE DAMAGE

Strategies to maintain cerebral perfusion pressure during rescue and transport
W. VIDETTA, AND G. DOMENICONI 275

The systemic and cerebrovascular effects of inotropes and vasopressors
J. MYBURGH. 283

Awake craniotomy
M. KLIMEK 301

Fast-track neuroanaesthesia
M. KLIMEK 313

LUNG

Interaction between ventilation and pulmonary circulation
G. Hedenstierna 329

Acute Respiratory Distress Syndrome: strategies to improve gas exchange
D. Chiumello, P. Pelosi, and D. D'Onofrio 339

Mechanical ventilation and the kidney
H. Burchardi, and G. Kaczmarczyk 367

Capnography and Pulse oximetry
U. Lucangelo, G. Degrassi, and M.L. Chierego 377

Oximetry spectral analysis and sleep disordered breathing
P.V. Romero, and C. Zamarrón 401

Post-occlusion rapid drop in pressure
W.A. Zin 417

Relaxed expiration
G.L. Chelucci 427

Dynamic hyperinflation
W.A. Zin 439

Bronchodilation in COPD
G.L. Tantucci 449

High Frequency Oscillation in ARDS
R.M. Kacmarek 459

Statics of normal lung
J. Milic-Emili, and A. Koutsoukou 467

Definition of spectrum of ALI
C.S. Valente Barbas, C. Hoelz, and V.L. Capelozzi. 477

Primary and secondary ARDS
P. Rocco 483

Effect of PEEP on gas exchange in ARDS
A. Koutsoukou, CH. Roussos, and J. Milic-Emili 501

Experimental evidence for the use of corticosteroids in ARDS
P. Rocco 513

**Evidence of biological efficacy for prolonged corticosteroid treatment
in unresolving ARDS**
G.U. Meduri, E. Golden, and S. Ratnakant. 531

Effects of nitric oxide in haemodynamics and gas exchange in ARDS
K. Lewandowski, M. Lewandowski, and K.J. Falke. 547

Lung function, dyspnea and exercise tolerance in stable COPD patients
J. Milic-Emili, and C. Tantucci 559

Alveolar recruitment strategy improves arterial oxygenation in severe ARDS patients
A. Gallesio, E. San Roman, and S. Giannasi 569

Ventilator-associated pneumonia
V. Pavoni, G. Gritti, R. Alvisi 585

Surgical treatment of end stage emphysema
E. Cohen. 595

Discontinuing mechanical ventilation: the role of a "Respiratory Acute Care Unit"
L.M. Bigatello, and E. Gettings. 605

Vol. II

PERIOPERATIVE MEDICINE

CARDIOVASCULAR FUNCTION ASSESSMENT

Principles of haemodynamic monitoring
S. MAGDER 619

Cardiovascular integrated monitoring
J.O.C. AULER JR, L.F. POLI DE FIGUEIREDO, AND M. REZENDE LOPES 635

Blood measurements of the oxygen transport in clinical practice
M. GIRARDIS, L. RINALDI, AND S. BUSANI. 649

The importance of information on volemia during the perioperative period: new vs. old technique
M. GIRARDIS, A. ROBERTI, AND A. PASETTO 655

Assessment of pre-load
V. PIRIOU, B. GOSTOLI, AND D. JACQUES 661

Left ventricular dysfunction in complicated CABG
R. SALLUSTI, J.O.C. AULER JR, AND L.M. SÁ MALBOUISSON 679

Reperfusion arrhythmias: prevention and management
J.L. ATLEE. 709

Myocardial ischaemia and cardiac function
P. FOEX 725

Transmural myocardial infarction. Focus on current strategies of myocardial reperfusion
G. SINAGRA, G. SABBADINI, AND A. PERKAN 737

Does technological evolution justify the use of Swan-Ganz catheters in perioperative haemodynamic monitoring?
R. MUCHADA 759

Comparison of haemodynamic monitoring techniques
B. ALLARIA, M. FAVARO, AND M. RESTA 771

Thoracic impedance tracing in perioperative haemodynamic monitoring
M. FAVARO, B. ALLARIA, AND M. RESTA 791

Clinical experience on TED
G. GALIMBERTI, A. AGOSTI, R. MUCHADA. 813

MECHANISMS OF ACTION OF GENERAL ANAESTHETICS

Clinical governance of perioperative medicine
R. ULLRICH, AND M. ZIMPFER 827

Molecular mechanisms of general anaesthesia
N.P. FRANKS, AND W.R. LIEB. 835

2P Domain K+ Channels: Novel Targets for Volatile General Anaesthetics
E. HONORÉ. 843

Sites of anaesthetic action on ligand-gated ion channels
R.A. HARRIS, M.P. MASCIA, AND I.A. LOBO 857

Effects of opioids analgesics on the action of general anaesthetics
P. GIUSTI 863

Mapping cerebral metabolic and blood flow effects of general anaesthetics
U. FREO, and C. ORI 877

Recent advances in mechanisms of action of general anaesthetics from genetically
engineered animal models
G. HOMANICS. 891

POSTOPERATIVE ACUTE PAIN MANAGEMENT

Organization and clinical experience
G. GALIMBERTI, S. NADALIN, AND E. CORSI 903

Techniques
Y. LEYKIN , A.M. MALISANO, AND G. ZANETTE. 919

Recovery room: clinical experience
Y. LEYKIN, S. MILESI, AND S. FURLAN 937

CHALLENGES AND CONTROVERSIES IN OBSTETRIC ANAESTHESIA .

Caudal anaesthesia: does it have a place today?
P. BUSONI. 957

Informed consent in obstetrics
G. CAPOGNA, AND M. CAMORCIA. 965

Anaesthesia in pregnant women with neurological disease
G. Lyons. 971

Cardiac disease in pregnancy
R. Alexander, and T. Thomas. 979

Life-threatening complications in peripartum
G. Capogna, and M. Camorcia. 995

TRAUMA OPERATIVE PROCEDURES (TOP)

Trauma – the integrate system of care
G. Gordini, and M. Menarini 1005

Triage in critical care
K. Hillman, A. Flabouris, and M. Parr 1013

Scoop and run vs. stay and play: strategies in pre-hospital care
C. Deakin 1019

Early assessment of multiple trauma
C. Deakin 1027

Scoring system in trauma
A. Sutcliffe 1037

SEPSIS AND MODS

SIRS, sepsis and MODS
G. Berlot, A. Tomasini, and M. Viviani 1047

Grading severity of sepsis
J-L Vincent, D. Peres-Bota, F. Ferreira. 1057

Sepsis and the role of the human host
M.E. Hartman, and D.C. Angus. 1065

Toll-like receptors in sepsis: where do we stand?
L. Del Sorbo, and H. Zhang. 1075

**Early goal-directed therapy prevents organ failure and mortality
in severe sepsis and septic shock**
E. Rivers, B. Nguyen, and S. Havstad 1089

**The neural and humoral response to acute neurological illness is
the mechanism of consequent new organ failures**
P. Andrews. 1105

Indications of CRRT in sepsis
C. TETTA, V. D'INTINI, AND F. GASTALDON 1119

Advances on membrane biology for CRRT
C. TETTA, A. BRENDOLAN, AND V D'INTINI 1127

Timing of CRRT in sepsis
H. BURCHARDI 1139

Consumption coagulopathy
M.L. CHIEREGO, AND A. GULLO 1147

Step (or leap) into the future. What is new in 2000 and beyond? An emphasis on endocrine failure
A.E. BAUE 1167

CONTINUING MEDICAL EDUCATION IN CRITICAL CARE

Critical care in South Asia
S. PRAYAG 1193

Critical care in South America
J. BESSO, AND A. MARTINELLI 1201

QUANTITATING CAREGIVER WORKLOAD IN THE ICU

Methods of quantifying workload: How ICU nurses' quantitative workload can be studied
A. DE RIJK 1213

QUALITY OF CARE IN THE ICU

Modulation of the innate immune response during respiratory tract infections
M.J. SCHULTZ, T. VAN DER POLL, AND J. KESECIOGLU 1231

Quality management in intensive care
G. WILLIAMS 1239

Auditing
D. REIS MIRANDA 1251

ETHICS AND LAW IN CRITICAL CARE

Withholding and withdrawing treatment
K.D. ROONEY, AND N.A. PACE 1263

Case studies of legal intervention in end-of-life care in the ICU
A. LEFEBVRE 1273

INDEX

Authors Index

Agosti A.
Department of Perioperative Medicine, Intensive Care and Emergency, Trieste University School of Medicine, Trieste (Italy)

Alexander R.
Department of Anaesthesia, Worcestershire Royal Hospital, Worcester (U.K.)

Allaria B.
Department of Intensive Care, National Institute for Cancer Research, Milan (Italy)

Alvisi R.
Department of Surgical Anaesthesiological and Radiological Sciences, Section of Anaesthesiology and Intensive Care, University of Ferrara, Ferrara (Italy)

Andrews P.J.D.
Intensive Care Unit, Western General Hospital, Edinburgh (U.K.)

Angus D.C.
The CRISMA (Clinical Research, Investigation, and Systems Modeling of Acute illness) Laboratory, Department of Critical Care Medicine, University of Pittsburgh, Pittsburgh, Pennsylvania (U.S.A.)

Anwar S.
The John Farman Intensive Care Unit, Addenbrooke's Hospital, Cambridge (U.K.)

Atlee J.L.
Department of Anesthesiology, Medical College of Wisconsin, Froedtert Memorial Lutheran Hospital, Milwaukee, Wisconsin (U.S.A.)

Auler J.O.C. Jr.
Anaesthesia and ICU Department, Heart Institute (InCor), University of Sao Paulo Medical School, Sao Paulo (Brazil)

Bacher A.
Department of Anaesthesiology and General Intensive Care, University of Vienna, Vienna (Austria)

Baue A.E.
Professor of Surgery Emeritus, St. Louis University School of Medicine, Vice-President for the Medical Center Emeritus, St. Louis University Medical Center, Fishers Island, New York (U.S.A.)

Berlot G.
Department of Perioperative Medicine, Intensive Care and Emergency, Trieste University School of Medicine, Trieste (Italy)

Besso J.
ICU and Fellowship Training Program in Critical Care Medicine, Hospital Centro Medico de Caracas, Caracas (Venezuela)

Bigatello L.M.
Department of Anesthesia and Critical Care, Massachusetts General Hospital, Harvard
Medical School, Boston, Massachusetts (U.S.A.)

Bolivar A.
Division of Critical Care Medicine, Hospital Centro Medico de Caracas, Caracas (Venezuela)

Borunda D.
Department of Anaesthesia, National Institute of Medical Sciences and Nutrition "Salvador
Zubiran" (Mexico)

Bossaert L.
European Resuscitation Council Secretariat, Antwerp (Belgium)

Brendolan A.
Department of Nephrology, Dialysis and Transplantation, St Bortolo Hospital, Vicenza (Italy)

Burchardi H.
Centre for Anaesthesiology and Intensive Care, Georg-August University, Gottingen
(Germany)

Busani S.
Department of Anaesthesia and Intensive Care, Modena University General Hospital,
Modena (Italy)

Busoni P.
Department of Anaesthesia and Intensive Care, "A Meyer" Paediatric Hospital, Florence,
(Italy)

Camorcia M.
Department of Anaesthesia, Fatebenefratelli General Hospital, Rome, (Italy)

Capelozzi V.L.
University of Sao Paulo General Hospital, Sao Paulo (Brazil)

Capogna G.
Department of Anaesthesia, Fatebenefratelli General Hospital, Rome, (Italy)

Chelucci G.L.
Department of Respiratory Pathophysiology, Florence University, Florence, (Italy)

Chierego M.L.
Department of Perioperative Medicine, Intensive Care and Emergency, Trieste University
School of Medicine, Trieste (Italy)

Chiumello D.
Department of Anaesthesia and Intensive Care, Milan University General Hospital, Milan
(Italy)

Cohen E.
Thoracic Anesthesia, The Mount Sinai School of Medicine, New York, New York (U.S.A.)

Corsi E.
Department of Perioperative Medicine, Intensive Care and Emergency, Trieste University
School of Medicine, Trieste (Italy)

D'Intini V.
Department of Nephrology, Dialysis and Transplantation, St Bortolo Hospital, Vicenza (Italy)

D'Onofrio D.
Department of Biological Sciences, University of Insubria General Hospital, "Macchi" Foundation, Varese (Italy)

Damiano L.
Department of Emergency, "S. Paolo Hospital", Naples (Italy)

de Latorre F.J.
Department of Intensive Care, University Hospital Vall d'Hebron, Barcelona (Spain)

de Rijk A.
Dept. Health Organisation, Policy and Economics, Faculty of Health Sciences Maastricht University, Maastricht (The Netherlands)

Deakin C.D.
Shackleton Department of Anaesthetics, Southampton General Hospital, Southampton (U.K.)

Degrassi G.
Department of Perioperative Medicine, Intensive Care and Emergency, Trieste University School of Medicine, Trieste (Italy)

Del Sorbo L.
Department of Anaesthesia, University of Toronto, Toronto, Ontario (Canada)

Domeniconi G.
Intensive Care Unit, National Hospital "Prof. A. Posadas", Buenos Aires (Argentina)

Dominguez-Cherit G.
Department of Critical Care, National Institute of Medical Sciences and Nutrition "Salvador Zubiran" (Mexico)

Esposito G.
Department of Emergency, "S. Paolo Hospital", Naples (Italy)

Falke K.J.
Clinic for Anaesthesiology and operative Intensive Care, Rudolf Virchow University Clinic, Berlin (Germany)

Favaro M.
Department of Intensive Care, National Institute for Cancer Research, Milan (Italy)

Ferreira F.
Department of Intensive Care, Erasme University Hospital, Free University of Brussels (Belgium)

Flabouris A.
Intensive Care Unit, University of New South Wales, Liverpool Health Service, Sydney (Australia)

Foëx P.
Department of Anaesthetics, Oxford Radcliffe NHS Trust, Oxford (U.K.)

Franks N.P.
Biophysics Section, Department of Biological Sciences, The Blackett Laboratory, Imperial College of Science, Technology and Medicine, London (U.K.)

Freo U.
Department of Pharmacology and Anaesthesiology, University of Padua, Padua (Italy)

Furlan S.
2nd Department of Anaesthesia and Reanimation, "S. Maria degli Angeli" Hospital, Pordenone (Italy)

Galimberti G.
Department of Perioperative Medicine, Intensive Care and Emergency, Trieste University School of Medicine, Trieste (Italy)

Gallesio A.
Adult Intensive Care Service, Hospital Italiano of Buenos Aires (Argentina)

Gettings E.
Department of Anesthesia and Critical Care, Massachusetts General Hospital, Harvard Medical School, Boston, Massachusetts (U.S.A.)

Giannasi S.
Adult Intensive Care Service, Hospital Italiano of Buenos Aires (Argentina)

Girardis M.
Department of Anaesthesia and Intensive Care, Modena University General Hospital, Modena (Italy)

Giusti P.
Dept. of Pharmacology and Anaesthesiology, University of Padua, Padua (Italy)

Golden E.
Baptist Memorial Hospitals, Memphis, Tennessee (U.S.A.)

Gordini G.
Department of Anaesthesia and Intensive Care, Maggiore Hospital, Bologna (Italy)

Gostoli B.
Department of Anaesthesia and Intensive Care, Louis Pradel Hospital, Lyon (France)

Gritti G.
Department of Anaesthesia and Intensive Care, Padua University Hospital, Padua (Italy)

Gullo A.
Department of Perioperative Medicine, Intensive Care and Emergency, Trieste University School of Medicine, Trieste (Italy)

Hacke W.
Department of Neurology, University Heidelberg, Heidelberg (Germany)

Harris R.A.
Waggoner Center for Alcohol and Addiction Research, Section of Neurobiology and Institute for Cellular and Molecular Biology, University of Texas at Austin, Austin, Texas (U.S.A.)

Hartman M.E.
The CRISMA (Clinical Research, Investigation, and Systems Modeling of Acute illness) Laboratory, Department of Critical Care Medicine, University of Pittsburgh, Pittsburgh, Pennsylvania (U.S.A.)

Havstad S.
Henry Ford Health Systems, Case Western Reserve University, Detroit, Michigan (U.S.A.)

Hedenstierna G.
Department of Medical Sciences, Clinical Physiology, University Hospital, Uppsala (Sweden)

Hillman K.
Department of Intensive Care, University of New South Wales, Sydney (Australia)

Hoelz C.
University of Sao Paulo General Hospital, Sao Paulo (Brazil)

Homanics G.E.
University of Pittsburgh, Departments of Anesthesiology and Pharmacology, Pittsburgh, Pennsylvania (U.S.A.)

Honorè E.
Institute of Molecular and Cellular Pharmacology, CNRS-UMR, Sophia Antipolis, Valbonne (France)

Illievich U.M.
Department of Anaesthesiology and General Intensive Care, University of Vienna (Austria)

Jacques D.
Department of Medical Intensive Care, Lyon Sud Jules Courmont Hospital, Pierre Bénite (France)

Jog S.
Critical Care Centre, Shree Medical Foundation, Prayag Hospital, Deccan Gymkhana, Pune (India)

Kacmarek R.M.
Department of Anesthesia, Harvard Medical School, and Respiratory Care, Massachusetts General Hospital, Boston, Massachusetts (U.S.A.)

Kaczmarczyk G.
Centre for Anaesthesiology and Intensive Care, Georg-August University, Gottingen (Germany)

Kesecioglu J.
Department of Anaesthesiology, University Medical Centre Utrecht, Utrecht (The Netherlands)

Klimek M.
Sub-department "Central location", Department of Anaesthesiology, Erasmus MC, University Medical Centre Rotterdam, Rotterdam (The Netherlands)

Koutsoukou A.
Critical Care Department, Evangelismos General Hospital, Medical School, University of Athens (Greece)

Leendertse K.
Department of Anaesthesiology, Erasmus Medical Centre, Rotterdam (The Netherlands)

Lefebvre A.
Kugler Kandestin, Montreal, Quebec (Canada)

Lewandowski K.
Clinic for Anaesthesiology and operative Intensive Care, Rudolf Virchow University Clinic, Berlin (Germany)

Lewandowski M.
Clinic for Anaesthesiology and operative Intensive Care, Rudolf Virchow University Clinic, Berlin (Germany)

Leykin Y.
2nd Department of Anaesthesia and Reanimation, "S. Maria degli Angeli" Hospital, Pordenone (Italy)

Lieb W.R.
Biophysics Section, Department of Biological Sciences, The Blackett Laboratory, Imperial College of Science, Technology and Medicine, London (U.K.)

Lobo I.A.
Waggoner Center for Alcohol and Addiction Research, Section of Neurobiology and Institute for Cellular and Molecular Biology, University of Texas at Austin, Austin, Texas (U.S.A.)

Lucangelo U.
Department of Perioperative Medicine, Intensive Care and Emergency, Trieste University School of Medicine, Trieste (Italy)

Luzzani A.
Department of Anaesthesia and Intensive Care "A", Borgo Trento City Hospital, Verona (Italy)

Lyons G.
Obstetric Anaesthesia, St. James' University Hospital, Leeds (U.K.)

Magder S.
Division of Critical Care, McGill University Health Centre, Montreal, Quebec (Canada)

Malisano A.M.
2nd Department of Anaesthesia and Reanimation, "S. Maria degli Angeli" Hospital, Pordenone (Italy)

Martinelli A.
Division of Critical Care Medicine, Hospital Centro Medico de Caracas, Caracas (Venezuela)

Mascia M.P.
National Research Centre, Centre of Neuropharmacology, c/o Department of Experimental Biology, University of Cagliari, Cagliari (Italy)

Meduri G.U.
University of Tennessee Health Science Center, Division of Pulmonary and Critical Care Medicine, The Memphis Lung Research Program, Memphis, Tennessee (U.S.A.)

Melloni C.
Department of Anaesthesia and Intensive Care, Faenza Hospital, Faenza (Italy)

Menarini M.
Department of Anaesthesia and Intensive Care, Maggiore Hospital, Bologna (Italy)

Milesi S.
2nd Department of Anaesthesia and Reanimation, "S. Maria degli Angeli" Hospital, Pordenone (Italy)

Milic-Emili J.
Meakins-Christie Laboratories, McGill University, Montreal, Quebec (Canada)

Muchada R.
Department of Anaesthesia and Intensive Care, "Eugène Andre" Hospital, Lyon (France)

Myburgh J.A.
Department of Intensive Care, St George Hospital, Sydney (Australia)

Nadalin S.
Department of Perioperative Medicine, Intensive Care and Emergency, Trieste University School of Medicine, Trieste (Italy)

Nguyen B.
Henry Ford Health Systems, Case Western Reserve University, Detroit, Michigan (U.S.A.)

Nolan J.
Department of Anaesthesia and Intensive Care Medicine, Royal United Hospital, Bath (U.K.)

Ori C.
Department of Pharmacology and Anaesthesiology, University of Padua, Padua (Italy)

Pace N.A.
Consultant Anaesthetist, Western Infirmary, Glasgow, Scotland (U.K.)

Paladino F.
Department of Emergency, "S. Paolo Hospital", Naples (Italy)

Park G.
The John Farman Intensive Care Unit, Addenbrooke's Hospital, Cambridge (U.K.)

Parr M.
Intensive Care Unit, University of New South Wales, Liverpool Health Service, Sydney (Australia)

Pasetto A.
Department of Anaesthesia and Intensive Care, Modena University General Hospital, Modena (Italy)

Paver-Eržen V.
Clinical Department of Anaesthesiology and Intensive Therapy, University Medical Centre, Ljubljana (Slovenia)

Pavoni V.
Department of Anaesthesia and Intensive Care, Padua University Hospital, Padua (Italy)

Pelosi P.
Department of Biological Sciences, University of Insubria General Hospital, "Macchi" Foundation, Varese (Italy)

Peres-Bota D.
Department of Intensive Care, Erasme University Hospital, Free University of Brussels (Belgium)

Perkan A.
Cardiology Unit, "Maggiore" Hospital, Trieste (Italy)

Piriou V.
Department of Anaesthesia and Intensive Care, Louis Pradel Hospital, Lyon (France)

Pistocchi S.
Faenza Hospital, Faenza (Italy)

Polati E.
Department of Anaesthesia and Intensive Care "A", Borgo Trento City Hospital, Verona (Italy)

Poli de Figueiredo L.F.
Department of Cardiopneumology, Heart Institute (InCor), University of Sao Paulo Medical School, Sao Paulo (Brazil)

Prayag S.
Critical Care Centre, Shree Medical Foundation, Prayag Hospital, Deccan Gymkhana, Pune (India)

Ratnakant S.
University of Tennessee Health Science Center, Division of Pulmonary and Critical Care Medicine, The Memphis Lung Research Program, Memphis, Tennessee (U.S.A.)

Reis Miranda D.
Health Services Research Unit, University Hospital of Groningen, Groningen (The Netherlands)

Resta M.
Department of Intensive Care, National Institute for Cancer Research, Milan (Italy)

Rezende Lopes M.
Anaesthesia and ICU Department, Heart Institute (InCor), University of Sao Paulo Medical School, Sao Paulo (Brazil)

Rinaldi L.
Department of Anaesthesia and Intensive Care, Modena University General Hospital, Modena (Italy)

Rivero E.
Division of Critical Care Medicine, Hospital Centro Medico de Caracas, Caracas (Venezuela)

Rivers E.
Henry Ford Health Systems, Case Western Reserve University, Detroit, Michigan (U.S.A.)

Roberti A.
Department of Anaesthesia and Intensive Care, Modena University General Hospital, Modena (Italy)

Rocco P.R.M.
Laboratory of Respiration Physiology, Carlos Chagas Filho Biophysics Institute, Federal University of Rio de Janeiro, Rio de Janeiro (Brazil)

Rocha e Silva M.
Department of Cardiopneumology, Heart Institute (InCor), University of Sao Paulo Medical School, Sao Paulo (Brazil)

Romero P.V.
Lung Function Test Laboratory, Division of Respiratory Medicine, Bellvitge Hospital, Barcelona (Spain)

Ronco C.
Department of Nephrology, Dialysis and Transplantation, St Bortolo Hospital, Vicenza (Italy)

Rooney K.D.
Specialist Registrar in Intensive Care Medicine, Western Infirmary, Glasgow, Scotland (U.K.)

Roussos Ch.
Critical Care Department, Evangelismos General Hospital, Medical School, University of Athens (Greece)

Ruggiero G.
Department of Emergency, "S. Paolo Hospital", Naples (Italy)

Rupreht J.
Department of Anaesthesiology, Erasmus Medical Centre, Rotterdam (The Netherlands)

Sá Malbouisson L.M.
Anaesthesia and ICU Department, Heart Institute (InCor), University of Sao Paulo Medical School, Sao Paulo (Brazil)

Sabbadini G.
Department of Geriatrics, "Maggiore" Hospital, Trieste (Italy)

Sallusti R.
Department of Perioperative Medicine, Intensive Care and Emergency, Trieste University School of Medicine, Trieste (Italy)

Salvetti I.
Department of Anaesthesia and Intensive Care "A", Borgo Trento City Hospital, Verona (Italy)

San Roman E.
Adult Intensive Care Service, Hospital Italiano of Buenos Aires (Argentina)

Schellinger P.D.
Department of Neurology, University Heidelberg, Heidelberg (Germany)

Schiraldi F.
Department of Emergency, "S. Paolo Hospital", Naples (Italy)

Schultz M.J.
Department of Intensive Care Medicine, Academic Medical Centre, Amsterdam (The Netherlands)

Sfogliaferri F.
Parma University, Parma (Italy)

Sierra J.
Department of Infectious Diseases, National Institute of Medical Sciences and Nutrition
"Salvador Zubiran" (Mexico)

Sinagra G.F.
Cardiology Unit, "Maggiore" Hospital, Trieste (Italy)

Spiss C.K.
Department of Anaesthesiology and General Intensive Care, University of Vienna (Austria)

Steiner T.
Department of Neurology, University Heidelberg, Heidelberg (Germany)

Štifanić D.
Clinical Department of Anaesthesiology and Intensive Therapy, University Medical Centre,
Ljubljana (Slovenia)

Sutcliffe A.J.
Department of Anaesthesia and Intensive Care, Queen Elizabeth Hospital, Birmingham (U.K.)

Talekar S.
Critical Care Centre, Shree Medical Foundation, Prayag Hospital, Deccan Gymkhana, Pune
(India)

Tantucci C.
Department of Respiratory Diseases, University of Brescia, Brescia (Italy)

Tetta C.
Clinical and Laboratory Research Department, Bellco SpA, Mirandola (Italy)

Thomas T.
Department of Anaesthesia, Worcestershire Royal Hospital, Worcester (U.K.)

Tomasini A.
Department of Perioperative Medicine, Intensive Care and Emergency, Trieste University
School of Medicine, Trieste (Italy)

Ullrich R.
Department of Anaesthesiology and General Intensive Care, University of Vienna, Vienna
(Austria)

Valente Barbas C.S.
University of Sao Paulo General Hospital, Sao Paulo (Brazil)

van der Poll T.
Department of Infectious Diseases, Tropical Medicine and AIDS, Laboratory of
Experimental Internal Medicine, Academic Medical Center, Amsterdam (The Netherlands)

Videtta W.
Intensive Care Unit, National Hospital "Prof. A. Posadas", Buenos Aires (Argentina)

Vincent J.-L.
Department of Intensive Care, Erasme University Hospital, Free University of Brussels (Belgium)

Viviani M.
Department of Perioperative Medicine, Intensive Care and Emergency, Trieste University School of Medicine, Trieste (Italy)

Williams G.
Nursing Services, Alice Springs Hospital, Alice Springs (Australia)

Zamarrón C.
Sleep Unit, Division of Respiratory Medicine, University Hospital, Santiago de Compostela (Spain)

Zanette G.
2nd Department of Anaesthesia and Reanimation, "S. Maria degli Angeli" Hospital, Pordenone (Italy)

Zhang H.
Critical Care Program, St. Michael's Hospital, Toronto, Ontario (Canada)

Zimpfer M.
Department of Anaesthesiology and General Intensive Care, University of Vienna, Vienna (Austria)

Zin W.A.
Laboratory of Respiration Physiology, Carlos Chagas Filho Biophysics Institute, Federal University of Rio de Janeiro, Rio de Janeiro (Brazil)

Abbreviations

ABG, arterial blood gas
ACE, angiotensin-converting enzyme
ACLS, advanced cardiac life support
ACM, alveolo-capillary membrane
ACTH, adrenocorticotropic hormone
ACV, assist-control ventilation
ADARPEF, Association Des Anésthesistes Réanimateurs Pédiatriques d'Expression Française
ADH, antidiuretic hormone
AFB, atrial fibrillation
AFT, atrial flutter
AHI, apnoea-hypopnoea index
AIS, abbreviated injury score
ALF, advanced life support
ALI, acute lung injury
ALS, amyotrophic lateral sclerosis
AM, alveolar macrophages
AMI, acute myocardial infarction
ANP, atrial natriuretic peptide
AOC, anaesthetic preconditioning
AP, anatomical profile
AP-1, activator protein-1
APACHE, acute physiological and chronic health evaluation
APRV, airway pressure release ventilation
ARDS, acute respiratory distress syndrome
ARF, acute renal failure
ARF, acute respiratory failure
ASA, American Society of Anaesthesiologists
ASCOT, a severity score of trauma
BAL, bronchoalveolar lavage
BiPAP, bilevel positive airway pressure
BMI, body mass index
BOLD, blood oxygenation level-dependent contrast
BOOP, bronchiolitis obliterants organizing pneumonia

BUN, blood urea nitrogen
BV, blood volume
CABG, coronary artery bypass grafting
CAO, chronic airway obstruction
CAS, central anticholinergic syndrome
CBF, cerebral blood flow
CBG, corticosteroid binding globulin
CBP, CREB-binding protein
CBV, central blood volume
CBV, circulating blood volume
CC, closing capacity
Cdyn, dynamic compliance
CFI, cardiac function index
CMRO$_2$, cerebral metabolic rate for oxygen
CMV, conventional mechanic ventilation
CMV, cytomegalovirus
CNS, central nervous system
CO, cardiac output
COLD, chronic obstructive lung disease
COMT, catechol-O-methyltransferase
COPD, chronic obstructive pulmonary disease
COX, cyclooxygenase
CPAP, continuous positive airway pressure
CPB, cardiopulmonary bypass
CPFA, coupled plasma filtration absorption
CPM, central pontine myelinolysis
CPP, cerebral perfusion pressure
CPP, coronary perfusion pressure
CPR, cardiopulmonary resuscitation
CPU, Chest Pain Units
CRH, corticotrophin releasing hormone
CRRT, continuous renal replacement therapy
CT, computed tomography
CVC, central venous catheter
CVP, central venous pressure
CVR, cerebrovascular resistance
CVVH, continuous veno-venous haemofiltration

CVVHDF, continuous veno-venous haemo-diafiltration

DAD, diffuse alveolar damage

DFMO, difluoromethylornithine

DH, dynamic hyperinflation

DIAS, desmoplase in acute ischaemic stroke

DIC, disseminated intravascular coagulation

DNR, do not resuscitate

EDA, end diastolic area

EDAI, end diastolic area indexed

EDRF, endothelium-derived relaxing factor

EDV, end diastolic volume

EELV, end-expiratory lung volume

EF, ejection fraction

EFL, expiratory flow limitation

EL, elastance of the lung

EMD, electromechanical dissociation

EPIC, European prevalence of infection in Intensive Care

ERC, European Resuscitation Council

Est,rs, static elastance of the respiratory system

ET, endotracheal tube

EVLW, extra vascular lung water

EW, elastance of the chest wall

FDA, Food and Drug Administration

FEPIMCTI, Federación Panamericana e Ibérica de Sociedades de Medicina Crítica y Terapía Intensiva

FFT, fast fourier transform

FiO$_2$, fractional concentration of inspired oxygen

FL, flow limitation

fMRI, functional magnetic resonance imaging

FRC, functional residual capacity

FVC, forced vital capacity

GABA, ?-aminobutyric acid

GC, glucocorticoid

GFR, glomerular filtration rate

GI, gastrointestinal

GISIS, Gruppo Italiano di Studio sulle Infezioni Severe

GM-CSF, granulocyte-macrophage colony stimulating factor

GR, glucocorticoid receptor

GREs, glucocorticoid-responsive elements

GRa, glucocorticoid receptor a

HAART, highly active antiretroviral therapy

Hb, haemoglobin concentration

HES, hydroxyethyl starch

HF, haemofiltration

HFJV, high frequency jet ventilation

HFO, high frequency oscillation

HFPPV, high frequency positive pressure ventilation

HIR, host inflammatory response

HIV, human immunodeficiency virus

HMCAS, hyperdense middle cerebral artery sign

HPA, hypothalamic-pituitary-adrenal

HR, heart rate

HRCT, high resolution computed tomography

HRQL, health-related quality o life

HSD, 6% dextran-70 to the 7.5% NaCl solution

HSP 70, heat shock protein 70

HSS, 6% hetastarch to the 7.5% NaCl solution

HVHF, high volume haemofiltration

I/R, ischaemia-reperfusion

IC, index of contractility

IC, inspiratory capacity

ICAM-1, intracellular adhesion molecule-1

ICG, indocyanine green

ICH, intracerebral haemorrhage

ICP, infection control practitioners

ICP, intracranial pressure

ICU, Intensive Care Unit

IDU, injection drug users

IJCCM, Indian Journal of Critical care Medicine

IL-1, interleukin-1

IL-10, interleukin-10

IL-1ra, IL-1 receptor antagonist

ILCOR, International Liaison Committee on Resuscitation

IMV, intermittent mandatory ventilation

iNOS, inducible nitric oxide

IPC, ischaemic preconditioning

ISCCM, Indian Society of Critical Care Medicine

ISS, injury severity score

ITVB, intrathoracic blood volume

IVDG, initial volume of distribution of glucose

IVRT, isovolumic relaxation time

KISS, Krankenhaus – Infection – Surveillance System

LDH, lactate dehydrogenase

LGI, lactate-glucose index

LIS, lung injury score

LOI, lactate-oxygen index

LOS, length of stay

LPS, lipopolysaccharide

LVEDA, left ventricular end-diastolic area

LVEDV, left ventricular end-diastolic volume

LVSW, left ventricular stroke work

MAC, minimum alveolar concentration

MAP, mean arterial pressure

MCA, middle cerebral artery

MD, medical director

MEFV, maximal flow-volume curve

MI, myocardial infarction

MIP, maximum inspiratory pressure

MODS, multiple organ dysfunction syndrome

MOF, multiple organ failure

MP, methylprednisolone

MPT, methylprednisolone treatment

MTS, methanethiosulfonate

MV, mechanical ventilation

NAECC, North American-European Consensus Conference

NEP, negative expiratory pressure

NETT, National Emphysema Treatment Trail

NF-?B, nuclear factor-?B

NICO, non-invasive cardiac output

NIH, National Institutes of Health

NIHSS, National Institutes of Health Stroke Scale

NIPPV, non invasive positive pressure ventilation

NISS, new injury severity score

NMDA, N-methyl-D-aspartate

NNIS, National Nosocomial Infection Surveillance System

NO, nitric oxide

NSAIDs, non-steroidal analgesic drugs

NTE, neurotoxic esterase

ODI, oxygen desaturation indexes

OM, organization and management

OP, organophosphates

OPIM, other potentially infectious materials

OSA, obstructive sleep apnoea

PA, peak amplitude

PAC, pulmonary artery catheter

PAF, platelet activating factor

PAG, periaqueductal grey region

PAI-1, plasminogen activator inhibitor 1

PAOP, pulmonary artery occlusion pressure

Paw, airway pressure

PCA, patient-controlled analgesia

PCCO, pulsed contour cardiac output

PCP, *Pneumocystis carinii* pneumonia

PCR, polymerase chain reaction

PCWP, pulmonary capillary wedge pressure

PDDG, pulse dye densitometry with indocyanine green

PEA, pulseless electrical activity

PEEP, positive end-expiratory pressure

PEEPi, intrinsic positive end-expiratory pressure

PEP, pre-ejection period

PGI₂, aerosolised prostacyclin

PGL, persistens generalized lymphadenopathy

PIRO, predisposing factor, infection, response and organ dysfunction

PKC, protein kinase C

PLA2, phospholipase A2

PLC, phospholipase C

PMN, polymorphonuclear cells

PNMT, phenethanolamine-N-methyltransferase

POCD, postoperative consciousness disturbance

PONV, postoperative nausea and vomiting

PPCM, peripartum cardiomyopathy

Pra, right atrial pressure

PROWESS, protein C worldwide evaluation in severe sepsis

PSG, polysomnography

PSV, pressure support ventilation

PTCA, percutaneous coronary angioplasty

PV, pressure volume

PVF, pulmonary venous flow

PVR, pulmonary vascular resistance

RACU, Respiratory Acute Care Unit

RAP, right atrial pressure

Raw, airway resistance

Rawm, mean airway resistance

rCBF, regional cerebral blood flow

rCMRglc, regional cerebral metabolic rates for glucose

RCV, red cells volume

rhAPC, recombinant human activated protein C

RM, recruitment manoeuvres

ROSC, return of spontaneous circulation

RTS, revised trauma score

RV, residual volume

RVEDV, right ventricular end-diastolic volume

RVEF, right ventricular ejection fraction

RVSW, right ventricular stroke work

SA, surgical auditors

SAB, sub-arachnoid block

SAH, subarachnoid haemorrhage

SBT, spontaneous breathing trials

SG, Swan-Ganz

sICAM-1, soluble intracellular adhesion molecule-1

SICU, surgical ICU

SIRS, systemic inflammatory response score

SLPI, secretory leukocyte protease inhibitor

SPECT, single photon emission computed tomography

SPV, systolic pressure variation

SRC-1, steroid receptor coactivator-1

SSI, surgical site infections

SSS, Scandinavian Score Scale

sTNFR1, soluble TNF receptor 1

SV, stroke volume

SvO₂, mixed venous oxygen saturation

SVR, systemic vascular resistance

SVV, stroke volume variation

TAT, thrombin-antithrombin

TCDB, Traumatic Coma Data Bank

TCP, tri cresyl phosphate

TEE, transesophageal echocardiography

TFPI, tissue factor pathway inhibitor

ThD, thermodilution

TLC, total lung capacity

TLV, total lung volume

TNF a, tumour necrosis factor-a

TOCP, tri orthocresyl phosphate

TP, transpulmonary pressure

t-PA, tissue-type plasminogen activator

TPV, total pulmonary volume

TRISS, trauma and injury severity score

TS, trauma score

TURP, trans urethral resection of prostate
VAP, ventilator associated pneumonia
VF, ventricular fibrillation
VILI, ventilator-induced lung injury
Vr, relaxation volume
Vrec, alveolar recruited volume
V_T, tidal volume
VT, ventricular tachycardia
Vtmax, maximal tidal volume during exercise

WOB, work of breathing
WP, wedge pressure
WUR, work utilization ratio
ZEEP, zero end-expiratory pressure
Δdown, minimal value of systolic pressure
ΔPP, difference between the systolic and the diastolic pressure
Δup, augmentation of LV stroke volume
Δt, time constant

EMERGENCY MEDICINE

Chest pain

F. Schiraldi, L. Damiano, F. Paladino

As recently as 15 years ago, emergency physicians and cardiologists were taught that a diagnosis of myocardial infarction could not be safely ruled out in the emergency department. In particular, serum cardiac enzymes were considered unreliable and could lead to erroneous decisions to discharge patients. So up to 40% of patients admitted to the hospital because of chest pain did not have acute coronary diseases; worse, 2-8% of patients presenting with myocardial infarction were erroneously sent home.

The body of evidence of the benefits of reperfusion therapy strongly supported an evolving strategy aimed at reducing the "door-to-needle" time, allowing at the same time an early risk stratification to perform the best "triage" in the emergency department [1]. The first chest pain units (CPU) were born [2-5].

Nevertheless, despite a growing scientific interest in the field, the optimal protocol for management in the CPU is still unclear and, despite advances in investigative modalities, many scientists agree that a focused history, followed by an accurate clinical examination and ECG interpretation, remain the key tools for the diagnosis. The most powerful features that increase the probability of acute myocardial infarction (AMI), and their associated likelihood ratios (LRs), are new ST segment elevation (LR 5.7 –53.9), new Q wave (LR 5.3-24.8), and chest pain radiating to both left and right arm simultaneously(LR 7.1).The most-powerful features that decrease the probability of AMI are a normal ECG result (LR 0.1-0.3), pleuritic chest pain (LR 0.2), and positional chest pain (LR 0.3) [6].

How to improve diagnostic specificity and sensitivity

A lot of clinical research has been spent looking for the best decision-making aids in the management of acute chest pain or for determining the optimal level of care for those who are admitted. The main problem, because of the beds and resource limitation, is not to mistakenly discharge patients with AMI: these people have short-term mortality rates of about 25 %, at least twice what would be expected if they were admitted [7]. So attention has been focused on the technical resources that could improve the diagnostic strategy:

- ECG secrets
- Bedside multimarkers
- Imaging
- Dynamic assessment

ECG secrets

Some ECG variables are generally accepted as indicating ischaemia or infarction when present in at least two anatomically contiguous leads:

- pathological Q waves ($\geq$ 1 mm in depth and $\geq$ 0.3 s in duration)
- ST segment elevation or depression of 1 mm or more
- elevated or inverted T waves.

The ST segment and T wave abnormalities are not considered diagnostic in case of left ventricular hypertrophy, left or right bundle - branch block (BBB), early re-polarization variant, or an implanted pacemaker [8]. Further suggestions could be added.

In case of BBB, remember that the vectorial sum of the QRS axis and T wave axis should normally stay between –20 and + 80 degrees, otherwise it suggests acute ischaemia.

A positive R wave in V1, not present before, could suggest true posterior infarction.

A negative T pattern in V1-3 is normal only if the negativity in V1 is more than in V3, otherwise it strongly suggests antero-septal ischaemia.

The upward ST trend in acute pericarditis is never linked to any mirror image in the opposite leads.

In persons with implanted pacemakers, acute coronary events could still be suspected when compared with previous ECG recordings.

Similar criteria can be applied in ischaemia or reinfarction affecting a previous necrosed myocardial zone, and in BBB showing any derangement from the usual pattern.

A transient T wave positive pattern in subjects that previous ECG recordings showed stable negative T waves (pseudonormalization) strongly suggests acute ischaemia.

Bedside multimarkers

Some newly identified markers of myocardial injury have permitted new strategies to be used for evaluating patients with acute chest pain. Levels of creatine kinase MB isoenzyme (CK-MB) usually rise above the normal range within 4 hours after the onset of myocardial infarction, and serial sampling of CK-MB over a period of 12-24 h permits the detection of virtually all AMIS. However, CK-MB elevations can result from causes other than myocardial injury [9, 10].

The cardiac troponins, T and I, are encoded by different genes in cardiac muscle, slow skeletal muscle, and fast skeletal muscle; hence these markers are more specific than CK-MB for myocardial injury. After myocardial injury, the levels of cardiac troponins rise after approximately the same amount of time as CK-MB levels (6-12 h) and remain elevated for several days [11-13]. Once elevated, the cardiac troponins are not useful in detecting repeated episodes of myocardial injury, due to the long elimination half-life; nevertheless, they are significantly predictive of death risk in the first 42 days (Fig. 1) [14].

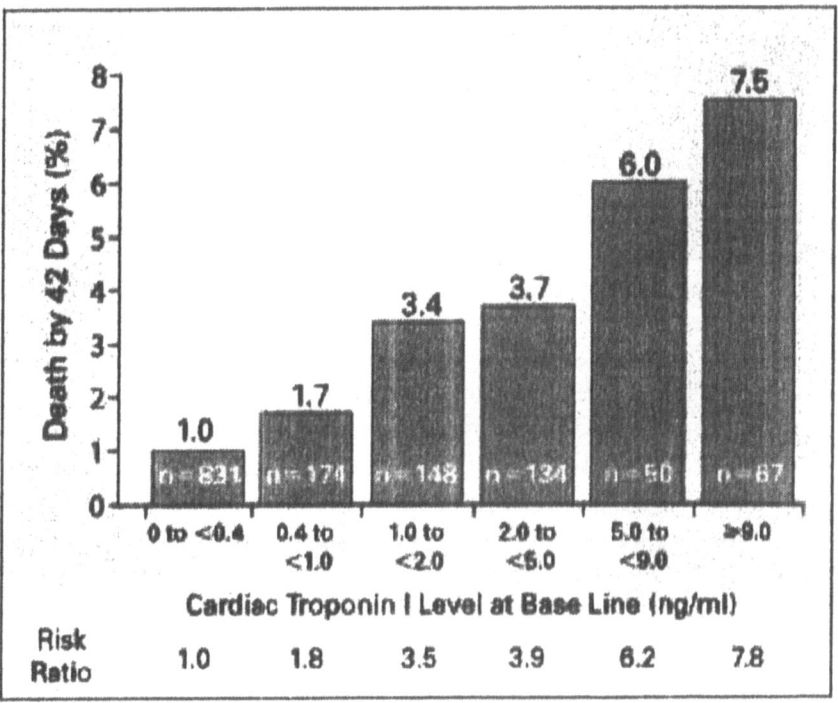

Fig. 1 Quantitative relationship between troponin release and the risk of death within 42 days. Adapted from Antman [14]

Recently a few papers reported spurious troponin elevations, mostly during renal insufficiency [15]. In the first 6 h after myocardial infarction, CK-MB subforms appear to be both more sensitive and more specific than CK-MB mass activity or even the troponins. Myoglobin is a very sensitive, but a poor specific marker of AMI, so its use should be limited to "rule out" the diagnosis, not to "rule in". Its only real advantage is the very good positive timing (90-120 min) [16].

C-reactive protein is a potent predictor of mortality independently of and in combination with troponin T in acute coronary syndromes [17].

Imaging

Echocardiography

There is a growing bulk of evidence supporting the pivotal role of the ultrasonography heart examination (echocardiography) in the emergency departments [18-20].

The positive aspects are:
- High sensitivity and cost-effectiveness to discover wall motion regional abnormalities
- Timely and direct diagnosis of other cardiovascular diseases as a cause of chest pain: aortic dissection, pulmonary embolism, aortic stenosis, pericarditis; moreover it is the golden standard for the early diagnosis of some complications of the AMI (mitral or tricuspid valve acute insufficiency, systolic or diastolic ventricular dysfunction, intracardiac thromboses)
- Reliable monitoring of the therapeutic strategies (successful or unsuccessful reperfusion, beta-blockers effect.)

On the other hand, there is a general agreement about some disadvantages:
- Operator dependency in getting and/or interpreting the US images
- Uncertainty about the age of some kinetic abnormalities (differential diagnosis between previous/recent AMI)
- As it is not continuous monitoring, some temporary ischaemic effects (e.g., myocardial stunning) could be misinterpreted as AMI (false positive)
- Some false-negative results could depend on a very small size of the ischaemic area (so called not critical mass)

The best timing to perform an echocardiogram in patients complaining of chest pain is still controversial; it seems reasonable to submit to the examination:

- patients whose chest pain is ongoing, just resolved, or lasted more than 30 min
- patients with typical chest pain associated with non-diagnostic ECG.

Myocardial scintigraphy

The historical validation of Thallium-201 scintigraphy has been largely supported by many studies confirming a near 100% sensitivity of the "cold spot"(the typical Thallium imaging in true ischaemic patients); moreover it shows good specificity in patients with acute non traumatic chest pain and any suspected coronary syndrome.

Two main related problems could be:
- Suboptimal images if compared with Tecnethium 99
- Suboptimal diagnostic reliability when there is any delay in getting the imaging after the tracer injection

On the other hand, acute positive rest Tc-99m sestamibi perfusion imaging accurately identifies patient at high risk for adverse cardiac outcomes, whereas negative perfusion imaging identifies a low-risk patient group [21, 22]

So, depending on the institutional facilities, myocardial scintigraphy may be a useful, additional diagnostic tool, which is better performed with Technetium 99. Further investigation is necessary to determine if such a routine approach results in reduced costs compared with current standard practice.

Magnetic resonance

Despite a great reliability, it still seems too-sophisticated a diagnostic aid to be suggested in the emergency department. Nevertheless some room exists for magnetic resonance imaging in the so-called X syndrome subgroup, usually affecting women, whose ECG, echocardiogram and myocardial scintigraphy could be normal or puzzling, even during acute chest pain crisis [23, 24]. There is consistent evidence in patients with syndrome X of an abnormality of myocardial perfusion limited to the subendocardium. This happens because transmural resolution is higher with cardiovascular magnetic resonance imaging than with other techniques. A possible explanation could rely on the inherent capability of uncovering subendocardial ischemic areas.

Dynamic assessment

The first American guideline for unstable angina (including myocardial infarction without ST-segment elevation), published in 1994, emphasized early
risk stratification as the pivotal process that drives initial treatment and decision
about triage in the emergency department [25]. Until then, there had been great
concern about the safety of the patient, whilst undergoing exercise testing for
detecting ischaemic myocardium. However, studies have shown that patients
who have a low clinical risk of complications can safely undergo exercise testing
within 6-12 h of presentation at the hospital or even immediately [26-28].

Radionuclide imaging, stress echocardiography, and prompt coronary angiography may all be useful for diagnosing coronary artery disease in some
subgroups of patients [29-31]. Nevertheless it should always be remembered
that, for example, studies with stress echocardiography demonstrated that,
despite the provocation of chest pain, there were patients showing no impairment in contractility. To complicate matters further, it has been shown that the
typical chest pain reported by patients with normal coronary angiograms can
be evoked by electrical stimulation of the right ventricle, which does not cause
myocardial ischaemia. Positron-emission tomographic scanning of the brain
has demonstrated an abnormally sensitive perception of cardiac pain in at least
some of these patients [32].

Conclusions

Multivariate algorithms have been developed and prospectively validated with
the goal of improving the stratification of risk in patients with possible acute
ischaemic heart disease [33, 34]. Nevertheless, despite the availability of
different diagnostic techniques, such as early monitoring of cardiac enzymes,
non-invasive cardiac imaging, dynamic evaluation, and "chest pain programs"
[35, 36], how to reduce the number of missed diagnoses of myocardial infarction or unstable angina is still an unanswered question. However, a trial
examining the effect of any new diagnostic strategies that could yield a
reduction of the missed diagnosis from the current 2% to only 1% would
require tens of thousands of patients.

References

1. Newby KL, Mark DB (1998) The chest pain unit – ready for prime time? N Engl J Med 339:1930-1932
2. Garber MA, Solomon NA (1999) Cost-effectiveness of alternative test strategies for the diagnosis of coronary artery disease. Ann Intern Med 130:719-728
3. Kuntz MK, Fleischmann KE, Hunink GM, et al (1999) Cost-effectiveness of diagnostic strategies for patients with chest pain. Ann Intern Med 130:709-718
4. Meuwissen M, Piek JJ, Wal AC van der, et al (2001) Recurrent unstable angina after directional coronary atherectomy is related to the extent of initial coronary plaque inflammation. J Am Coll Cardiol 37:1271-1276
5. Panju AA, Hemmelgarn BR, Giyatt GH, et al (1998) The rational clinical examination. Is this patient having a myocardial infarction? JAMA 280:1256-1263
6. Gaspoz JM, Lee TH, Weinstein MC, et al (1994) Cost-effectiveness of a new short-stay unit to "rule out" acute myocardial infarction in low risk patients. J Am Coll Cardiol 24:1249-1259
7. Lee TH, Goldman L (2000) Evaluation of the patient with acute chest pain. N Engl J Med 342:1187-1195
8. Pope JH, Ruthazer R, Beshansky JR, et al (1998) The clinical presentation of patients with acute cardiac ischemia in the emergency department: a multicenter controlled clinical trial. J Thromb Thromb 6:63-74
9. Zimmerman J, Fromm R, Meyer D, et al (1999) Diagnostic marker cooperative study for the diagnosis of myocardial infarction. Circulation 99:1671-1677
10. Adams JE III, Abendschein DR, Jaffe AS (1993) Biochemical markers of myocardial injury: is MB creatine kinase the choice for the 1990s? Circulation 88:750-763
11. Newby LK, Storrow AB, Gibler WB, et al (2001) Bedside multimarker testing for risk stratification in chest pain units. Circulation 103:1832
12. Polanczyk CA, Lee TH, Cook EF, et al (1998) Cardiac troponin I as a predictor of major cardiac events in emergency department patients with acute chest pain. J Am Coll Cardiol 32:8-14
13. Ravkilde J, Nissen H, Horder M, et al (1995) Independent prognostic value of serum creatine kinase isoenzyme mb mass, cardiac troponin t and myosin light chain levels in suspected acute myocardial infarction. J Am Coll Cardiol 25:574-581
14. Antman EM (2002) Decision making with cardiac troponin tests. N Engl J Med 346:2079-2082
15. Aviles RJ, Askari AT, Lindahl B, et al (2002) Troponin T levels in patients with acute coronary syndromes, with or without renal dysfunction. N Engl J Med 346:2047-2052
16. Sonel A, Sasseen MB, Fineberg N, et al (2000) Prospective study correlating fibrinopeptide a, troponin i, myoglobin, and myosin light chain levels with early and late ischemic events in consecutive patients presenting to the emergency department with chest pain. Circulation 102:1107
17. Roberts R, Fromm RE (1998) Management of acute coronary syndromes based on risk stratification. An idea whose time has come. Circulation 98:1831-1833
18. Morrow DA, Rifai N, Antman EM, et al (1998) C-reactive protein is a potent predictor of mortality independently of and in combination with troponin T: a TIMI 11A substudy. J Am Coll Cardiol 31:1460-1465
19. Zalenski RJ, Rydman RY, Mc Careen M, et al (1997) Feasibility of a rapid diagnostic protocol for an emergency department chest pain unit. Ann Emerg Med 29:99-108
20. Farkouh ME, Smars PA, Reeder GS, et al (1998) A clinical trial of a chest-pain observation unit for patients with unstable angina. N Engl J Med 339:1882-1888
21. Theroux P, Fuster V (1998) Acute coronary syndromes: unstable angina and non-Q-wave myocardial infarction. Circulation 1195-1206
22. Kontos MC, Jesse RL, Schimdt KL, et al (1997) Value of acute rest sestamibi perfusion imaging for evaluation of patients admitted to the emergency department with chest pain. J Am Coll Cardiol 30:976-982

23. Hilton TC, Thompson RC, Williams HJ, et al (1994) Technetium-99m sestamibi myocardial perfusion imaging in the emergency room evaluation of chest pain. J Am Coll Cardiol 23:1016--1022
24. Cannon RO, Balaban RS (2000) Chest pain in women with normal coronary angiograms N Engl J Med 342:885-887
25. Panting JR, Gatehouse PD, Yang GZ ,et al (2002) Abnormal subendocardial perfusion in cardiac syndrome X detected by cardiovascular magnetic resonance imaging N Engl J Med 346:1948--1953
26. Braunwald E, Mark DB, Jones RH, et al (1994) Unstable angina: diagnosis and management. Clinical practice guideline n°10. Department of Health and Human Services, Rockville
27. Polanczyk CA, Johnson PA, Hartley LH, et al (1998) Clinical correlates and prognostic significance of early negative exercise tolerance test in patients with acute chest pain seen in the hospital emergency department. Am J Cardiol 81:288-292
28. Roberts RR, Zalenski RJ, Mensah EK, et al (1997) Cost of an emergency department-based accelerated diagnostic protocol vs. hospitalization in patients with chest pain: a randomized controlled trial. JAMA 278:1670-1676
29. Lewis WR, Amsterdam EA, Turnipseed S, et al (1999) Immediate exercise testing of low risk patients with known coronary artery disease presenting to the emergency department with chest pain. J Am Coll Cardiol 33:1843-1847
30. Nichol G, Walls R, Goldman L, et al (1997) A critical pathway for management of patients with acute chest pain who are at low risk for myocardial ischemia: recommendations and potential impact. Ann Intern Med 127:996-1005
31. Colon PJ III, Mobarek SK, Milahi RV, et al (1998) Prognostic value of stress echocardiography in the evaluation of atypical chest pain in patients without known coronary artery disease. Am J Cardiol 81:545-551
32. Kuntz KM, Fleishmann KE, Hunink MG, et al (1999) Cost-effectiveness of diagnostic strategies for patients with chest pain. Ann Intern Med 130:709-718
33. Panza JA (2002) Myocardial ischemia and the pains of the heart. N Engl J Med 346:1934-1935
34. Salker HP, Griffith JL, Dorey FJ, et al (1987) How do physicians adapt when the coronary care unit is full? A prospective multicenter study. JAMA 257:1181-1185
35. Platt SO (2000) The acute chest syndrome of sickle cell disease. N Engl J Med 342:1904-1907
36. Pope JH, Aufderheide TP, Ruthazer R, et al (2000) Missed diagnoses of acute cardiac ischemia in the emergency department. N Engl J Med 342:1163-1170

Advanced life support in the management of cardiac arrest: European Resuscitation Council Guidelines 2000

L. Bossaert, J. Nolan, F. de Latorre

There are only two interventions that have been shown to improve survival unequivocally. The first of these is competent basic life support and the second is prompt defibrillation for patients in ventricular fibrillation (VF) or pulseless ventricular tachycardia (VT). Several drugs are advocated as adjuvants to treat cardiac arrest, but their impact on long-term survival is uncertain. The present review will focus on recent experimental and clinical data concerning the use of drugs during advanced life support (ALS).

The publication of Guidelines for Advanced Life Support (ALS) by the European Resuscitation Council (ERC) in 1998 and 2000 was a landmark in international co-operation and co-ordination. These guidelines were based on the 1997 International Liaison Committee on Resuscitation (ILCOR) advisory statements. Previously, individual countries or groups had produced guidelines but for the first time an international group of experts produced consensus views based on the best available information. Since 1992, there has been wide international collaboration and support. In particular, the establishment of the ILCOR has facilitated global co-operation and discussion between representatives from North America, Europe, Southern Africa, Australia and New Zealand, and South America.

The 1992-98-2000 ERC Guideline documents indicated that review would occur on a regular basis. Change is not advocated for its own sake, and is not warranted without convincing scientific or educational reasons. Education and its organization is a process with a long latency, and it can be confusing and distracting for trainers and trainees if the message lacks consistency.

Changes in guidelines are only the first step in the process of care. Their implementation necessitates considerable effort. Training materials and methods may require modification, information must be disseminated and, perhaps most importantly, evaluation of efficacy is needed. For these purposes, reporting and publication of out-of-hospital and in-hospital cardiac arrest events using the

Utstein templates is strongly advised to provide objective outcome assessment.

The limitations of guidelines must be recognized. As always in the practice of medicine, words and flow charts must be interpreted with common sense and an appreciation of their intent. While much is known about the theory and practice of resuscitation, in many areas our ignorance is profound. Resuscitation practice remains as much an art as a science. Further, the interpretation of guidelines may differ according to the environment in which they are employed. We acknowledge that individual resuscitation councils may wish to customize the details while accepting that the guiding principles are universal. Any such changes must be approved by the ERC if they are to be regarded by this organization as their official guidelines.

Specific ALS interventions and their use in the ALS algorithm

Defibrillation

In adults, the commonest primary arrhythmia at the onset of cardiac arrest is VF or pulseless VT. The overwhelming majority of eventual survivors come from this group. If the definitive therapy for these arrhythmias - defibrillation - can be implemented promptly, a perfusing cardiac rhythm may be restored and lead to ultimate survival. The *only* interventions that have been shown unequivocally to improve long-term survival are basic life support and defibrillation. VF is an eminently treatable rhythm, but the chances of successful defibrillation decline substantially with the passage of each minute. The amplitude and waveform of VF deteriorate rapidly, reflecting the depletion of myocardial high-energy phosphate stores. The rate of decline in success depends in part upon the provision and adequacy of basic life support (BLS). As a result, the priority is to minimize any delay between the onset of cardiac arrest and the administration of defibrillating shocks.

At present, the most commonly used transthoracic defibrillation waveform has a damped sinusoidal pattern. Newer techniques such as biphasic waveforms, or sequentially overlapping shocks producing a rapidly shifting electrical vector during a multi-pulse shock, may reduce the energy requirements for successful defibrillation. Automated defibrillators, which can deliver a current--based shock appropriate to the measured transthoracic impedance, are now available. Their use may increase the efficacy of individual shocks, while reducing myocardial injury in patients with unusually high, or low, transthoracic impedance.

The use of groups of three shocks is retained, the initial sequence having energies of 200 J, 200 J, and 360 J. The reasons for choosing 200 J as the energy for the first two shocks of conventional waveform defibrillation have been presented. Subsequent shocks, if required, should have energies of 360 J. If a co-ordinated rhythm has supervened for a limited interval, there is no strong scientific basis for deciding whether one should revert to 200 J or continue at 360 J. There is evidence that myocardial injury, both functionally and morphologically, is greater with increasing energies, but the comparative success rates for defibrillation attempts at this point with 200 J versus 360 J are unknown. Both strategies are therefore acceptable. Most AED's have an algorithm that does not revert to 200 J after a short period of non-VF/VT. In this case, defibrillation should continue with 360 J instead of restarting the AED to allow a 200 J shock to be given.

Alternative waveforms and energy levels are acceptable if demonstrated to be of equal or greater net clinical benefit in terms of safety and efficacy. A pulse check is required after a shock (and should be prompted by an AED), only if a change in waveform to one compatible with cardiac output is produced. Thus if VF, or VT with an identical waveform, persists after the first 200 J shock, the second shock at 200 J is given without a pulse check being performed. If, in turn, this shock is unsuccessful, the third shock – this time at 360 J – is given. With modern defibrillators, charging times are sufficiently short for three shocks to be administered within 1 min.

Only a very small proportion of the delivered electrical energy traverses the myocardium during transthoracic defibrillation and efforts to maximize this proportion are important. The commonest defects are inadequate contact with the chest wall, failure or poor use of couplants to aid the passage of current at the interface between the paddles and the chest wall, and faulty paddle positioning or size. One paddle should be placed below the right clavicle in the mid-clavicular line and the other over the lower left ribs in the mid/anterior axillary line (just outside the position of the normal cardiac apex). In female patients the second pad/paddle should be placed firmly on the chest wall just outside the position of the normal cardiac apex avoiding the breast tissue.

If unsuccessful, other positions such as apex-posterior can be considered. Although the polarity of the electrodes affects success with internal techniques such as implantable defibrillators, during transthoracic defibrillation the polarity of the paddles seems to be unimportant.

Drugs and drug delivery

Drug delivery

The venous route remains the optimal method of drug administration during cardiopulmonary resuscitation (CPR). The previous guidance with regard to venous cannulation is unchanged. If already in situ, central venous cannulae can deliver agents rapidly to the central circulation. If a central line is not present, the risks associated with the technique – which can themselves be life threatening – mean that for an individual patient the decision as to peripheral versus central cannulation will depend upon the skill of the operator, the nature of the surrounding events, and available equipment. If a decision is made to attempt central venous cannulation, this must not delay defibrillation attempts, CPR, or airway security. When peripheral venous cannulation and drug delivery is performed, a flush of 20 ml of 0.9% saline is advised to expedite entry to the circulation.

The administration of drugs via a tracheal tube remains only a second line approach because of impaired absorption and unpredictable pharmacodynamics. The agents, which can be given by this route, are limited to adrenaline, lidocaine, and atropine. Doses of 2-3 times the standard IV dose diluted up to a total volume of at least 10 ml of 0.9% saline are currently recommended. Following administration, five ventilations are given to increase dispersion to the distal bronchial tree thus maximizing absorption.

Specific drug therapy

Vasopressors

During CPR the pressure gradient between the aorta and the right atrium during the decompression phase, the coronary perfusion pressure (CPP), correlates positively with return of spontaneous circulation (ROSC) and survival. A vasopressor is given during cardiac arrest to increase this perfusion pressure and thereby enhance both myocardial and cerebral blood flow, in the belief that this will improve survival.

Adrenaline

Despite a lack of robust data demonstrating improved long-term outcome, adrenaline, in a "standard" dose of 1 mg every 3 min, continues to be advocated during resuscitation. Its α-adrenergic receptor-stimulating properties should result in improved CPP, but the β-adrenergic effects of adrenaline are potentially harmful. These include increased myocardial oxygen consumption, ventricular arrhythmias, and increased intrapulmonary shunting caused by reduced hypoxic pulmonary vasoconstriction. High-dose (up to 0.2 mg/kg) adrenaline may further enhance CPP, but does not seem to improve long-term survival after out-of-hospital or in-hospital cardiac arrest. Its use is therefore no longer recommended.

Vasopressin

During cardiac arrest, plasma concentrations of several endogenous vasopressors increase greatly but there are important differences. In successfully resuscitated patients levels of vasopressin are higher, and adrenaline and noradrenaline levels lower, compared with concentrations in those who die. These findings, along with the disadvantages of adrenaline, have encouraged extensive investigation of vasopressin as a therapy during CPR.

Endogenous arginine vasopressin, also called antidiuretic hormone (ADH), is released from the posterior pituitary in response to increased serum osmolality or reduced plasma volume. Under normal circumstances, it has a major role in water regulation, but even high circulating levels do not produce hypertension. However, in shock states the pressor action of vasopressin is enhanced greatly. Vasopressin acts via specific renal (V-2) and vascular (V-1) receptors. It produces vasoconstriction in "non-vital" circulations, such as the skin, skeletal muscle, and small bowel, thereby diverting blood to the brain, heart and kidneys. The vasopressin analogue desmopressin (DDAVP) is mainly a V-2 agonist and has only 0.4% of the pressor activity of arginine vasopressin. Vasopressin has a plasma half-life of 24 min and approximately two-thirds is metabolized by the kidneys.

Animal studies

Three different doses of vasopressin (0.2 U/kg, 0.4 U/kg, and 0.8 U/kg) were compared with adrenaline 0.2 mg/kg in 28 pigs after 4 min of VF and 3 min of closed-chest CPR. Vasopressin 0.8 U/kg produced significantly higher CPP and myocardial and cerebral blood flow than adrenaline, and the effects of vasopressin lasted significantly longer than adrenaline. The same group has shown that after prolonged cardiac arrest, in comparison with adrenaline, vasopressin produces better vital organ blood flow, improved neurological recovery, and higher mean frequency and amplitude of ventricular fibrillation waveform. Another group has compared repeated doses of either 0.045 mg/kg adrenaline or 0.4 U/kg vasopressin in 22 piglets. Although the onset and peak effects were slower in the vasopressin group, the overall effect on blood pressure and cerebral perfusion did not differ significantly during CPR. However, vasopressin produced greater cerebral cortical flow after ROSC.

In comparison with placebo, the administration of vasopressin during CPR results in significantly lower plasma levels of endogenous adrenaline and noradrenaline. For this reason, the effect of combinations of adrenaline and vasopressin has been studied in animal models of asphyxial cardiac arrest. In one of these studies, the addition of adrenaline to vasopressin improved left ventricular myocardial blood flow. In this asphyxia model, vasopressin alone resulted in worse myocardial blood flow and reduced ROSC compared with adrenaline alone. In another study of asphyxial cardiac arrest, the combination of vasopressin and adrenaline resulted in higher CPP and survival than either of the drugs given alone. In contrast, compared with vasopressin alone, the combination of adrenaline and vasopressin caused reduced cerebral perfusion.

In comparison with adrenaline, vasopressin produced better vital organ perfusion in an animal model of hypovolaemic cardiac arrest, and less systemic acidosis in cardiac arrest during epidural anaesthesia. Endobronchial or intraosseous administration of vasopressin during CPR achieves similar systemic effects as the same dose given intravenously.

If the vascular effects of endogenous vasopressin are blocked with a selective V-1 receptor antagonist during CPR in a porcine model, CPP, left ventricular blood flow, and survival are lower in comparison with pigs given placebo or exogenous vasopressin. It is likely that during cardiac arrest endogenous vasopressin enhances the vasopressor effects of adrenaline.

Among all the apparent benefits of exogenous vasopressin during CPR there are some concerns. Some animal data suggest that vasopressin may be less beneficial than adrenaline after asphyxial cardiac arrest. Vasopressin improves vital organ blood flow at the expense of considerably reduced splanchnic blood flow. This may be inconsequential in animals with normal blood vessels, but is likely to be detrimental to humans. After ROSC, prolonged vasoconstriction in other vascular beds may also be harmful.

Human studies

It has often proven difficult to convert promising results achieved with ALS drugs in animals to improved outcome after cardiac arrest in humans. On the basis of the animal data, vasopressin 40 U was given to eight adults with in-hospital cardiac arrest refractory to standard therapies, including intravenous adrenaline. A spontaneous circulation was restored in all eight patients and three survived, neurologically intact, to hospital discharge. In another case series, 4 of 19 patients failing to respond to at least 40 min of ALS had a mean increase in CPP of 28 mmHg after vasopressin 1 U/kg. In a prospective, randomized study 40 patients with out-of-hospital VF resistant to shocks were given either adrenaline 1 mg or vasopressin 40 U. Significantly more patients receiving vasopressin were alive at 24 h, but this very small study lacked the power to demonstrate any significant differences in long-term survival. Following the encouraging results in this study, two further prospective, randomized studies have been undertaken. The first of these involved 200 patients with in-hospital cardiac arrest (all rhythms) who were given either vasopressin 40 U or adrenaline 1 mg as the initial vasopressor. The study was powered to allow detection of a 20% absolute difference in survival to 1 h, assuming the baseline survival at 1 h to be 30%. Forty (39%) of the vasopressin group survived to 1 h versus 34 (35%) of the adrenaline group ($P=0.66$). The difference in the findings between these two studies is not readily explained at present. The response times were much shorter in the in-hospital study and it could be postulated that vasopressin may be more beneficial than adrenaline in the presence of severe acidosis. A European multicenter study to determine the effect of vasopressin 40 U versus adrenaline 1 mg on short-term survival after out-of-hospital cardiac arrest (all rhythms) has finished. Results will be presented in October 2002 (personal communication, Volker Wenzel).

Vasopressin and current CPR guidelines

The International Guidelines 2000 for Cardiopulmonary Resuscitation and Emergency Cardiovascular Care was the culmination of a series of detailed evidence-based reviews and discussions amongst experts from around the world. The role of vasopressin in CPR was debated intensely. The lack of data from large-scale human studies was a concern to many experts. The final decision mandated a class IIb recommendation (acceptable, safe, and useful – an optional or alternative intervention) for vasopressin to be used as an alternative to adrenaline for shock refractory VF. There were inadequate data to support the use of vasopressin in patients with asystole or pulseless electrical activity (class indeterminate) or in infants and children (class indeterminate). In addition, logistical problems have to be solved relating to the availability of the drug for clinical use. Not all experts agree with the decision to recommend vasopressin for shock refractory VF and the Advanced Life Support Working Group of the ERC did not include vasopressin in the ERC Guidelines 2000 for adult ALS.

Antiarrhythmics

Survival from VF cardiac arrest is dependent primarily on the prompt delivery of an electric shock. Shock-refractory VF is conventionally described as the persistence of VF despite the delivery of three or more shocks. It seems logical that antiarrhythmic drugs should increase the likelihood of successful defibrillation, as they are clearly effective in suppressing a variety of potentially malignant arrhythmias. Although the benefits of antiarrhythmic drugs in the patient with a spontaneous circulation are clear, it has proved very difficult to show that they improve survival when given for refractory VF.

Lidocaine

Lidocaine given prophylactically to patients with acute myocardial infarction (AMI) probably reduces the incidence of VF, but mortality rates are unchanged or possibly higher. Lidocaine has featured in the guidelines of the ERC and the American Heart Association for the past 2 decades, but the lack of evidence supporting its clinical efficacy in refractory VF led to an indeterminate class recommendation in the International Guidelines 2000. Amiodarone has now replaced lidocaine as the drug of choice for patients who remain in VF/pulseless VT after three shocks.

Amiodarone

Amiodarone is a Vaughan Williams class III drug and, as such, it blocks potassium channels and prolongs the duration of the action potential. It has additional electrophysiological properties typical of the other three classes, such as sodium and calcium channel blockade, and alpha and beta-adrenergic blocking actions. The use of amiodarone for the prevention of arrhythmic death in high-risk patients is contentious. In some parts of the world it has now largely been superseded by cardioverter defibrillators. Amiodarone is effective in treating the majority of ventricular and supraventricular tachyarrhythmias. There are anecdotal reports of the effectiveness of amiodarone in ventricular fibrillation and it is at least as effective as bretylium in treating refractory ventricular arrhythmias.

The efficacy of amiodarone in out-of-hospital VF cardiac arrest has been evaluated in a randomized, double-blind, placebo-controlled study. Patients remaining in VF or pulseless VT after three shocks were given an intravenous bolus of amiodarone 300 mg or placebo. More patients in the amiodarone group survived to hospital admission [108/246 (44%) vs. 89/258 (34%), $P = 0.03$], but survival to hospital discharge was similar (13.4% vs. 13.2%). Hypotension (the need for vasopressor infusions) and bradycardia (the need for chronotropic therapy) were significantly more common in the amiodarone group (59% vs. 48% and 41% vs. 25%, respectively). There are some limitations to the wider applicability of this study. It took place in Seattle and King County, Washington, where response times are extraordinarily short (dispatch to arrival of first responder was 4.3 min). Many would argue that an intervention that has been shown to improve survival to hospital admission, but not to hospital discharge neurologically intact, should not be adopted without data on long-term outcome. This study was not powered to detect a difference in survival to hospital discharge, but the increased incidence of hypotension and bradycardia might partly explain the higher mortality after hospital admission among the amiodarone group. However, on the grounds that the short-term benefit of amiodarone was the best evidence yet for the efficacy of an antiarrhythmic drug, experts at the Evidence Evaluation and Guidelines 2000 conferences made a class IIb recommendation for amiodarone in the treatment of shock-refractory cardiac arrest due to VF or pulseless VT. Amiodarone 300 mg can be given as an intravenous bolus after the third shock, but it should not delay delivery of the fourth shock.

Data from the Amiodarone versus Lidocaine in pre-hospital refractory Ventricular Fibrillation Evaluation (ALIVE) study have been published recently. Drugs were given by the paramedics in the Toronto EMS system. Following amiodarone 5 mg/kg, 41 (22.7%) of 179 patients survived to hospital admission versus 18 (11.0%) of patients given lidocaine 1.5 mg/kg ($P<0.0043$). In comparison with the Seattle study, the mean interval to first defibrillation was 2.5 min longer and the interval to study drug administration was 4 min longer. The results of this study support the choice of amiodarone instead of lidocaine for shock-refractory VF, but the uncertainty of the impact of amiodarone on long--term outcome remains.

Magnesium

The antiarrhythmic action of magnesium is through activation of membrane sodium-potassium adenosine triphosphatase and blocking of slow calcium channels. Despite being supported by only two uncontrolled case series, magnesium is a universally accepted therapy for torsades de pointes. Magnesium sulphate 2 g (8 mmol) is also recommended for shock-refractory VF when hypomagnesemia is suspected. However, its routine use in cardiac arrest is contentious. There are anecdotal reports of the successful use of magnesium in shock-refractory VF, but a randomized, double-blind, placebo-controlled trial of 2 g (8 mmol) magnesium sulfate in 116 patients with out-of-hospital VF arrest failed to show any benefit. Other small, prospective, randomized trials of magnesium after in-hospital and out-of-hospital cardiac arrest have also failed to show any survival benefit. On the basis of these data, magnesium is not recommended for routine use in cardiac arrest.

Fibrinolytics

At least 80% of patients who experience sudden cardiac death have coronary artery disease. At postmortem examination, more than 50% of sudden cardiac death victims have acute changes in coronary plaque morphology, such as thrombus or plaque disruption, and in hearts with myocardial scars and no acute infarction, active coronary lesions are identified in 46% of cases. It is possible that a proportion of these patients might benefit from a fibrinolytic given during CPR. In addition to its activity in coronary arteries, a fibrinolytic may improve cerebral and coronary reperfusion after cardiac arrest. In the past, because of the fear of severe bleeding complications, the need for CPR has been a relative contraindication to fibrinolysis. However, there are several case series documenting the safety of fibrinolysis in patients with AMI who have undergone CPR. Most clinicians would now consider that fibrinolysis is frequently appropriate after CPR, based on the relative risks and benefits in individual patients.

There are several reports on the use of fibrinolysis during CPR in patients with massive pulmonary embolism. Of the 80 patients reported, 42 (53%) survived to hospital discharge, and only 1 of these patients died from intracerebral haemorrhage after ROSC. Inevitably, there is a considerable reporting bias and the true chances of survival after the use of fibrinolysis during CPR for pulmonary embolism are less than this. A prospective randomized trial would provide an indication of the true efficacy of fibrinolysis for cardiac arrest after pulmonary embolism but, following these case series, few clinicians would be prepared to withhold fibrinolysis during CPR if there is good evidence of pulmonary embolism. Recombinant tissue plasminogen activator (rt-PA) given as two 100-mg bolus doses 30 min apart is a simple fibrinolytic technique to use during CPR.

Fibrinolysis has also been used successfully during CPR in patients with AMI. Of 23 such patients, 12 (52%) survived to hospital discharge. The successful use of fibrinolysis in hospital during and after CPR has led to studies of its efficacy during CPR after out-of-hospital cardiac arrest. In the first of these studies, 40 patients with out-of-hospital cardiac arrest, and with no ROSC after 15 min of CPR, were given rt-PA 50 mg over 2 min. In comparison with an historical control group of 50 patients, patients receiving rt-PA were more likely to achieve ROSC (68% vs. 44%, $P=0.026$) and to be admitted to an intensive care unit (58% vs. 30%, $P=0.009$). There was no CPR-related bleeding, but upper gastrointestinal haemorrhage occurred in 2 patients in the rt-PA group. The second study retrospectively compared 108 patients who were given rt-PA during out-of-hospital CPR with 216 matched controls. Patients given rt-PA were more likely to achieve ROSC (70.4% vs. 51%, $P=0.001$) and to survive to hospital discharge (25.0% vs. 15.3%, $P= 0.048$). Massive intracranial haemorrhage occurred in 1 patient who had received rt-PA and in 2 controls. The small number of patients, lack of randomization, and historical controls makes it very difficult to draw firm conclusions on the routine use of fibrinolysis in out-of-hospital cardiac arrest from these studies. A randomized trial is essential and is now being planned. Four percent of out-of-hospital cardiac arrests are caused by spontaneous subarachnoid haemorrhage, which would be exacerbated by fibrinolysis. However, even in the absence of fibrinolysis, the chances of long-term survival under these circumstances are very poor.

Using the Universal Algorithm

Each step that follows in the ALS algorithm (Fig. 1) assumes that the preceding one has been unsuccessful. A single precordial thump may be performed by professional healthcare providers, in a witnessed or monitored arrest before the defibrillator is attached and is therefore incorporated into the ERC ALS Universal algorithm. It is unlikely to be successful after more than 30 s of arrest.

ECG monitoring then provides the link between BLS and ALS procedures. ECG rhythm assessment must be always interpreted within the clinical context as movement artefact, lead disconnection, and electrical interference can mimic rhythms associated with cardiac arrest. Following this assessment, the algorithm splits into two pathways - VF/VT and other rhythms.

Ventricular fibrillation / pulseless ventricular tachycardia

The first defibrillating shock must be given without any delay. If unsuccessful it is repeated once and if necessary, twice. This initial group of three shocks should occur with successive energies of 200 J, 200 J, and 360 J. If VF/VT persists, further shocks are given with 360 J energies or the biphasic equivalent. A pulse check is performed, and should be prompted by an AED if, following a defibrillating shock a change in waveform is produced that is compatible with output. If the monitor/defibrillator indicates that VF/VT persists, then further DC shocks are administered without a further pulse check.

It is important to note that after a shock the ECG monitor screen will often show an isoelectric line for several seconds. This is commonly due to a transient period of electrical and/or myocardial 'stunning', and does not necessarily mean that the rhythm has converted to asystole, as a co-ordinated rhythm or return of VF/VT may supervene subsequently. If the monitor screen of a manual defibrillator shows a 'straight' line for more than one sweep immediately after a shock, 1 min of CPR should be given without a new dose of adrenaline, and the patient reassessed. Only if the result of this reassessment is a non-VF/VT rhythm without a pulse should a new dose of adrenaline be administered and

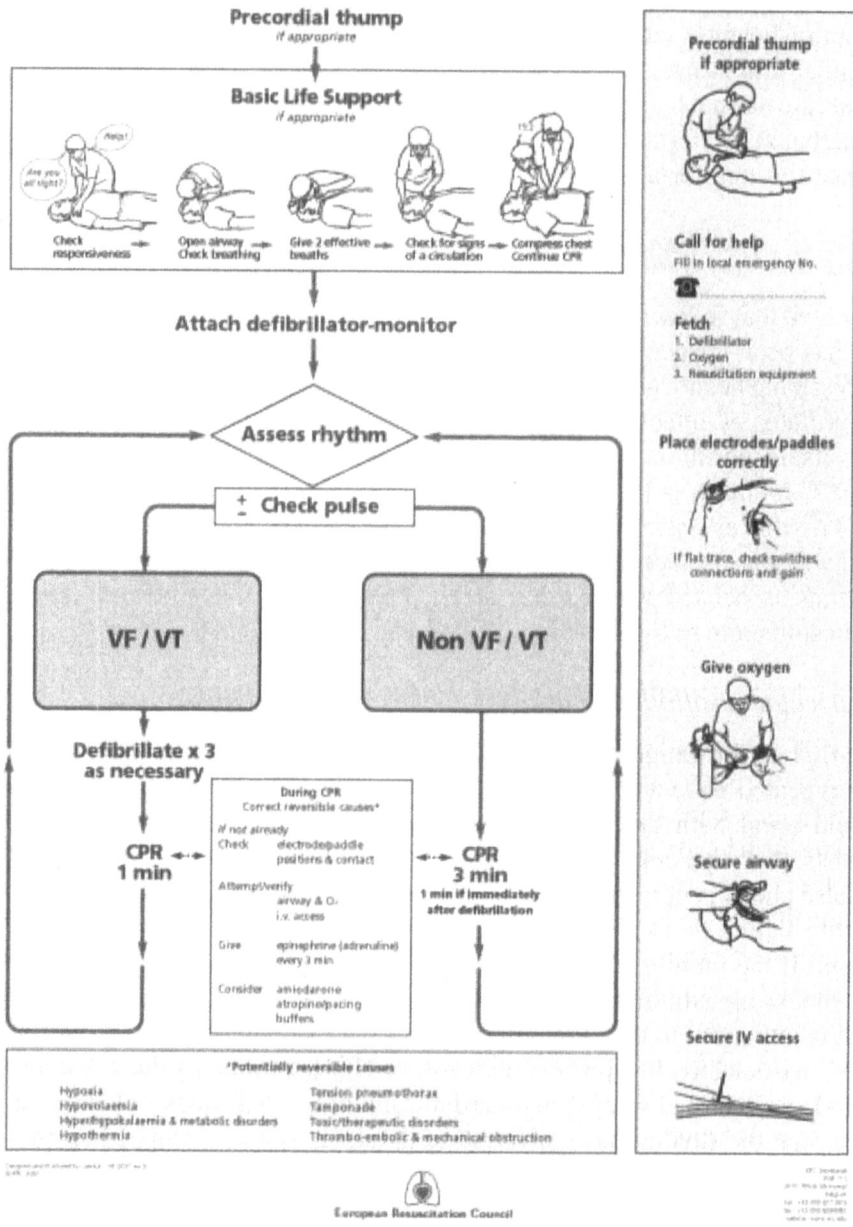

Fig. 1 Universal algorithms for the advanced management of cardiac arrest (copyright ERC 2001, with permission)

CPR given for a further 2 min before the patient is assessed again. Algorithms of AEDs should also take account of this phenomenon.

Emphasis must be placed on the correct performance of defibrillation, including the use of couplants. The safety of the resuscitation team is paramount. During defibrillation, no-one must be in contact with the patient. Liquids, wet clothing, or the spreading of excess electrode gel can cause problems. Transdermal patches should be removed to prevent the possibility of electrical arcing. Paddle/pads should be kept 12-15 cm away from implanted pacemakers. During manual defibrillation, the operator must give a command e.g., 'Stand clear!' and check that this is obeyed before the shock is given. With automated systems an audio command is given, and all team members must comply with this command.

Over 80% of individuals who will be successfully defibrillated have this achieved by one of the first three shocks. Subsequently, the best prospects for restoring a perfusing rhythm still remain with defibrillation, but at this stage the search for and correction of potentially reversible causes or aggravating factors is indicated, together with an opportunity to maintain myocardial and cerebral viability with chest compressions and ventilation. During CPR attempts can be made to institute advanced airway management and ventilation, venous access, and to administer drugs if appropriate.

The time interval between the third and fourth shocks should not exceed 2 min. Although the interventions, which can be performed during this period, may improve the prospects for successful defibrillation, this is unproven, while it is well established that with the passage of time the chances of success for defibrillating shocks lessen.

Adrenaline is given in a dose of 1 mg intravenously or 2-3 mg via the tracheal tube. Adrenaline has not yet been shown to improve outcome (Class indeterminate). High-dose adrenaline is no longer recommended.

Vasopressin, in a single dose of 40 U, has been proposed as an alternative to adrenaline in VF/pulseless VT refractory to three initial shocks (class IIb), but further evidence is required before this agent can be firmly recommended.

The evidence supporting the use of antiarrhythmic drugs in VF/pulseless VT is weak, and no agent has been found that improves survival to hospital discharge. However, amiodarone should be considered, following adrenaline, to treat shock refractory VF/pulseless VT as early as after the third shock, provided it does not delay further shock delivery (class IIb). Amiodarone 300 mg (made up to 20 ml with dextrose or from a prefilled syringe) may be given into a peripheral vein. A further dose of 150 mg may be required in refractory cases, followed by an infusion of 1 mg/min for 6 h and then 0.5 mg/min, to a maximum of 2 g (note that this maximum dose is larger than the current European datasheet recommendation of 1.2 g).

Magnesium (8 mmol) is recommended for refractory VF if there is a suspicion of hypomagnesaemia, e.g., patients on potassium-losing diuretics (class IIb).

Lidocaine and procainamide (class IIb) are alternatives if amiodarone is not available, but should not be given in addition to amiodarone. Procainamide is given at 30 mg/mm to a total dose of 17 mg/kg. The necessity for this relatively slow rate of infusion makes it a less-favoured option. Bretylium is no longer recommended.

Non-VF/VT rhythms

If VF/VT can be positively excluded, defibrillation is not indicated as a primary intervention (although it may be required later if VF develops), and the right-sided path of the algorithm is followed.

For patients in cardiac arrest with non-VF/VT rhythms, the prognosis is in general much less favourable. The overall survival rate with these rhythms is approximately 10%-15% of the survival rate with VF/VT rhythms, but the possibility of survival should not be disregarded. In some series, approximately 20% of eventual survivors present with a non-VF/VT rhythm.

With the passage of time, all electrical rhythms associated with cardiac arrest deteriorate with the eventual production of asystole. The abysmal prognosis of this degenerated rhythm is well justified. There are, nevertheless, some situations where a non-VF/VT rhythm may be caused or aggravated by remediable conditions, especially if this was the primary rhythm. As a consequence the detection and treatment of reversible causes (referred to as the four 'Hs' and the four 'Ts') become relatively more important.

The four 'Hs'
- Hypoxia
- Hypovolaemia
- Hyper-/ hypokalaemia, hypocalcaemia, acidaemia
- Hypothermia

The four 'Ts'
- Tension pneumothorax
- Cardiac tamponade
- Thromboembolic or mechanical obstruction (e.g. pulmonary embolism)
- Toxic or therapeutic substances in overdose

During the search for and correction of these causes, CPR together with advanced airway management, oxygenation, and ventilation, and any necessary attempts to secure venous access should occur, with adrenaline administered every 3 min.

The use of atropine for asystole has been discussed above. Atropine 3 mg intravenously is given once, along with adrenaline 1 mg for asystole on the first loop. Pacing may play a valuable role in patients with extreme bradyarrhythmias, but its value in asystole is questionable, except in cases of trifascicular block where P waves are seen. In patients where pacing is to be performed, but a delay occurs before it can be achieved, external cardiac percussion (as known as 'fist' or 'thump' pacing) may generate QRS complexes with an effective cardiac output, particularly in cases where myocardial contractility is not critically compromised. External cardiac percussion is performed with blows at a rate of 100/min, given with less force than a precordial thump and delivered over the heart, not the sternum. Conventional CPR should be substituted immediately if QRS complexes with a discernable output are not being achieved.

After 3 min of CPR, the patient's electrical rhythm is reassessed. If VF/VT has supervened, the left-sided path of the algorithm is followed, otherwise loops of the right-sided path of the algorithm will continue for as long as it is considered appropriate for resuscitation to continue. Resuscitation should generally continue for at least 20-30 min from the time of collapse unless there are overwhelming reasons to believe that resuscitation is likely to be futile.

Pulseless electrical activity / electromechanical dissociation

If pulseless electrical activity is associated with a bradycardia (<60/min) atropine, 3 mg intravenously or 6 mg via the tracheal tube, should be given. High-dose adrenaline is no longer recommended.

Asystole

No significant changes in treatment. There is emphasis on careful confirmation of asystole before and after delivery of a shock. Guidance is given on the criteria to be satisfied and the timing before resuscitation is abandoned. High-dose adrenaline is no longer recommended.

Rhythms preceding or following cardiac arrest

- Bradycardias (Fig. 2)

The sequence of the ERC bradycardia algorithm has been modified slightly. Isoprenaline is no longer recommended; if external pacing is unavailable, a low--dose adrenaline infusion is recommended instead.

- Tachycardias

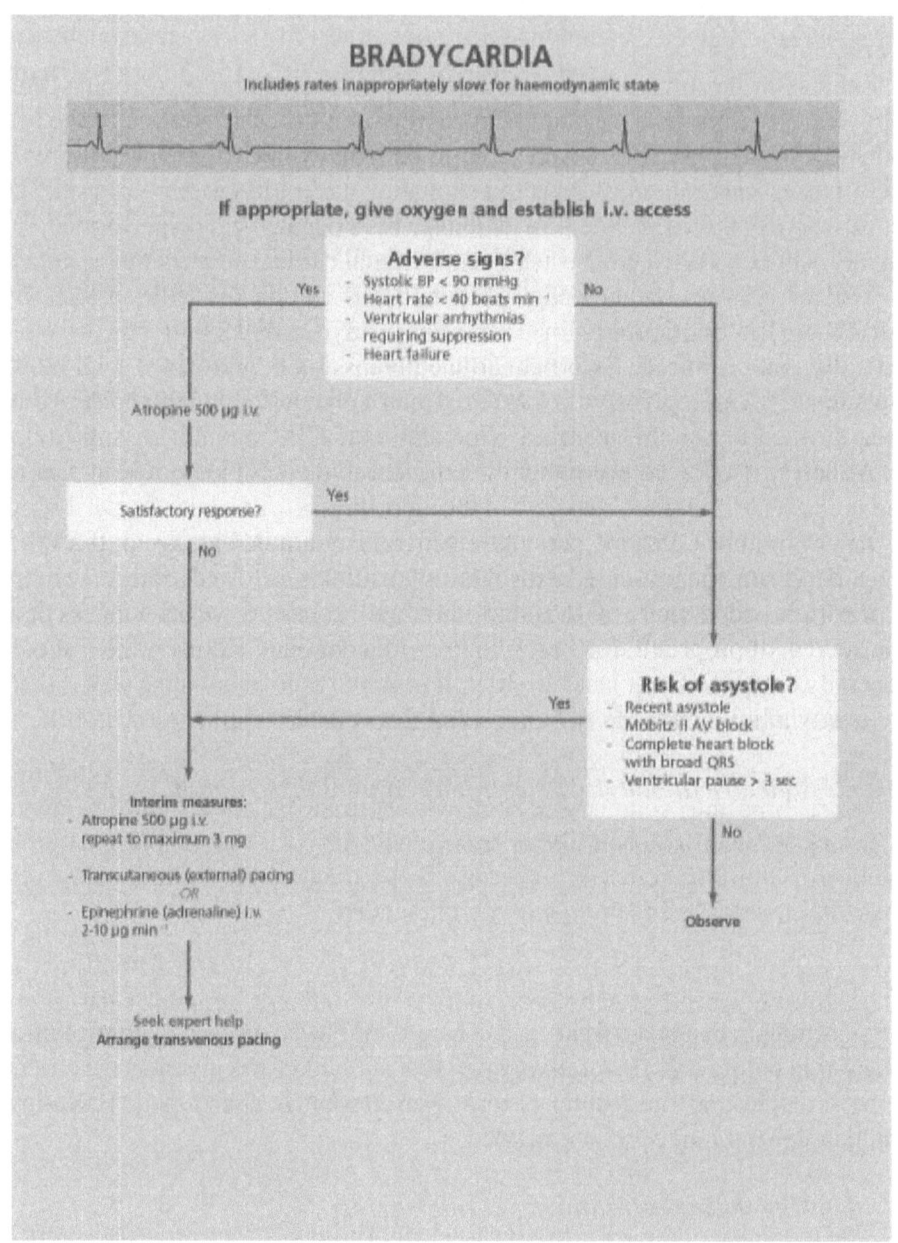

Fig. 2 Algorithm for the management of life-threatening bradycardia (copyright ERC 2001, with permission)

Certain basic principles apply:

1. Immediate treatment will depend on whether the patient is stable or unstable (displays adverse signs).
2. Cardioversion is preferred when the patient is unstable.
3. All antiarrhythmic drugs have proarrhythmic properties.
4. The use of more than one antiarrhythmic drug is undesirable.
5. If a drug does not work, cardioversion should be considered the second antiarrhythmic.
6. If the patient has impaired myocardial function, most antiarrhythmic drugs will cause further impairment.

Atrial fibrillation and flutter (Fig. 3)

The patient is placed into one of three risk groups on the basis of heart rate and the presence of additional signs and symptoms. If the patient is in the high-risk group attempt electoral cardioversion after heparinization. The treatment options for patients at intermediate risk depend on the presence or absence of impaired haemodynamics or structural heart disease and whether the onset of the atrial fibrillation is known to be within the last 24 h.

Attempted cardioversion can be undertaken also in those patients in the low--risk group where the onset of the atrial fibrillation is known to be within the last 24 h. In fibrillation of more than 24 h duration cardioversion should not be attempted until the patient has been anticoagulated for 3-4 weeks.

Narrow complex supraventricular tachycardia (Fig. 4)

If the patient is pulseless in association with a narrow complex tachycardia with a rate greater than 250/min, attempted electrical cardioversion should be undertaken. Otherwise, vagal manoeuvres should be tried first (Valsava manoeuvre, carotid massage). Adenosine is the first-choice drug (class IIa).

If the patient displays adverse signs, attempt electrical cardioversion, supplemented, if necessary, with amiodarone. In the absence of adverse signs, choose one drug from esmolol, verapamil, amiodarone, or digoxin.

Broad complex tachycardia (Fig. 5)

If there is no pulse, follow the VF/VT algorithm. If the patient displays adverse signs or the rhythm is unresponsive to drugs (amiodarone or lidocaine), attempt electrical cardioversion.

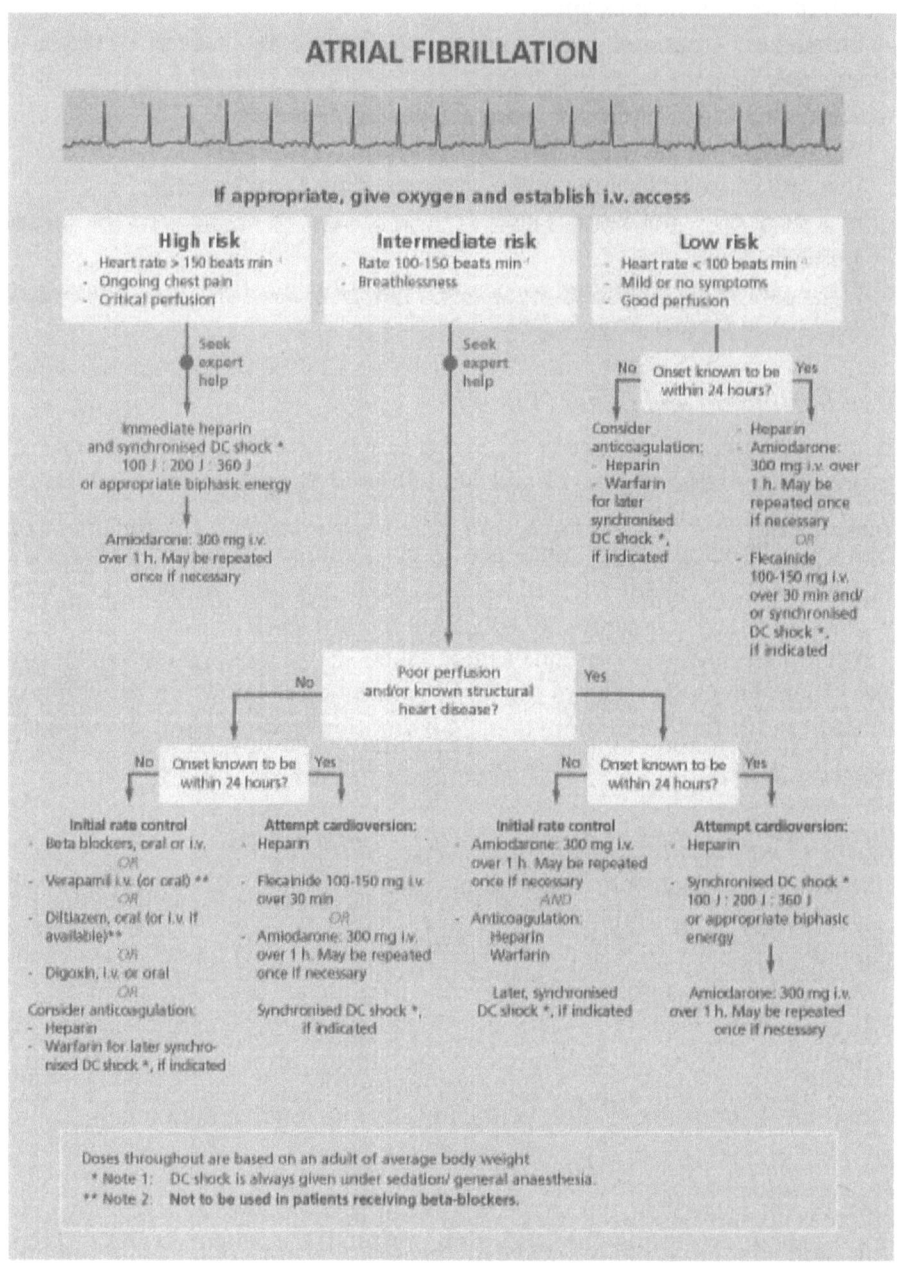

Fig. 3 Algorithm for the management of atrial fibrillation (copyright ERC 2001, with permission)

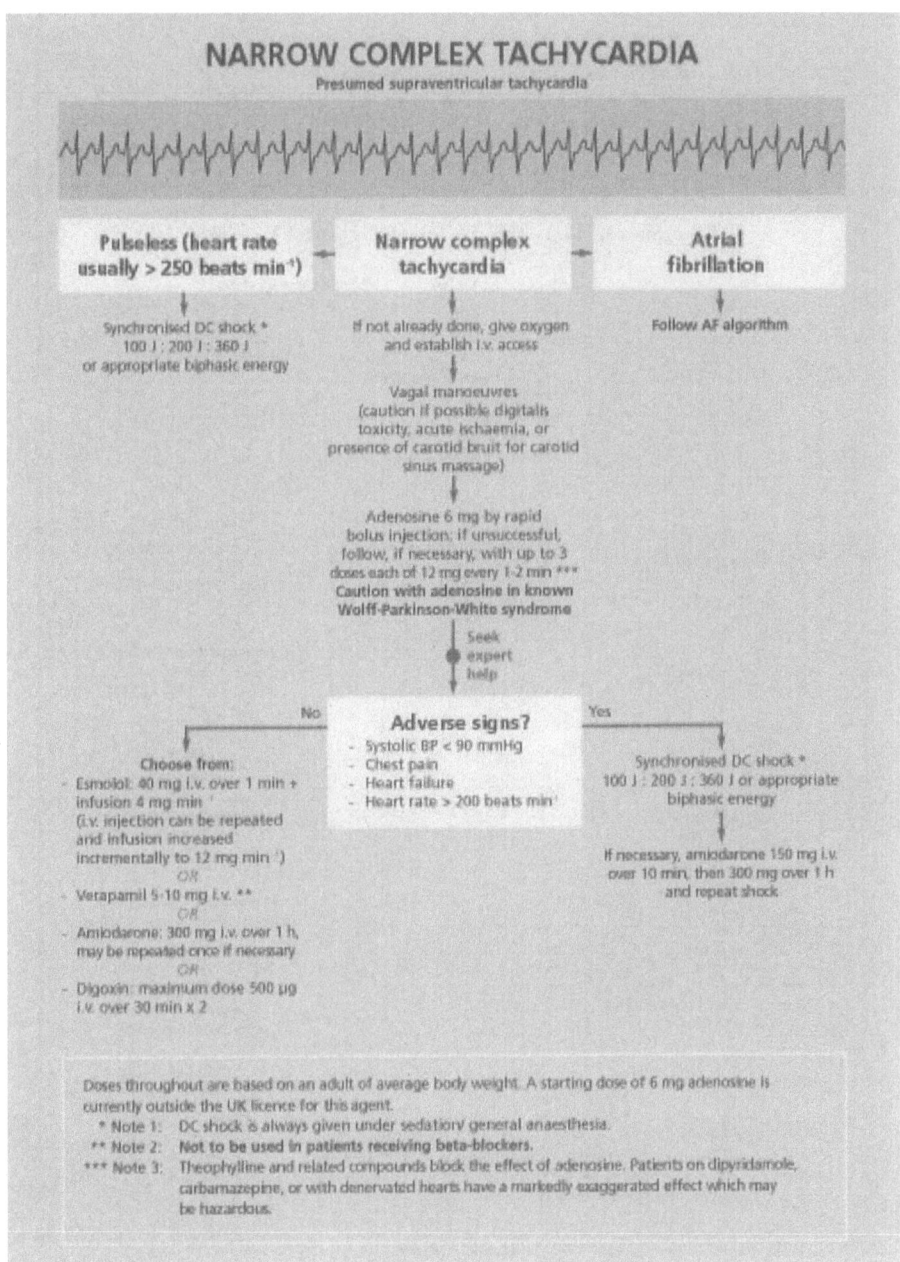

Fig. 4 Algorithm for the management of narrow complex tachycardia (copyright ERC 2001, with permission)

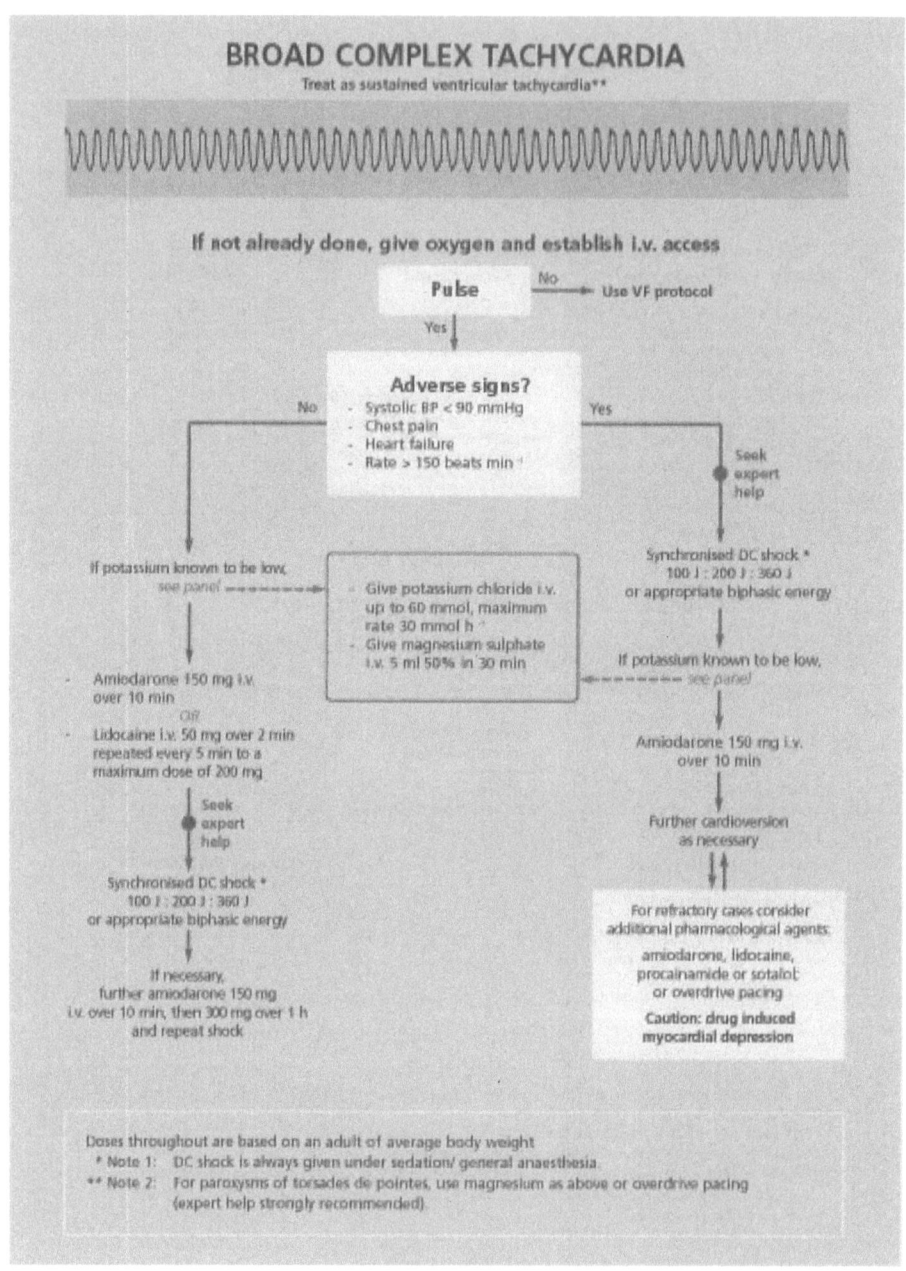

Fig. 5 Algorithm for the management of broad complex tachycardia (copyright ERC 2001, with permission)

Post-resuscitation care

There are no changes in the recommendations for post-resuscitation care. The most-vulnerable organ for the ischaemic/hypoxic damage occurring in association with cardiac arrest is the central nervous system (CNS). Approximately one-third of the patients who have return of spontaneous circulation die a neurological death, with one-third of long-term survivors having recognizable motor or cognitive deficits. Fortunately, only 1%-2% of these individuals do not achieve an independent existence.

Intensive research efforts are rapidly increasing our knowledge about the pathophysiology of CNS ischaemia/hypoxia, but there are no new clinically validated treatment strategies for the cerebral damage sustained with cardiac arrest. Efforts should be directed to the avoidance and/or correction of hypotension, hypoxia, hypercarbia, electrolyte imbalance, and hypo- or hyperglycaemia.

Many victims of cardiac arrest have features indicating that the event was precipitated by acute myocardial infarction. In these patients, there is an urgent need for appropriate management, including such aspects as thrombolysis or other methods for obtaining coronary reperfusion and maintaining electrical stability to reduce the chances of further episodes of cardiac arrest and to improve the overall prognosis. These aspects are covered by the publications on the Management of Acute Myocardial Infarction of the European Society of Cardiology and the ESC/ERC Task force on the Prehospital Management of Myocardial Infarction.

Conclusions

Despite very encouraging animal data, no drug has been reliably proven to increase survival to hospital discharge after cardiac arrest. Data from two prospective, randomized trials suggest that amiodarone may improve short--term survival after out-of-hospital VF cardiac arrest. Further data on the efficacy of vasopressin after cardiac arrest are awaited. In the absence of data from large studies demonstrating even a short-term survival advantage, we do not recommend the routine use of vasopressin for shock-refractory VF cardiac arrest. We anticipate that the role of fibrinolysis during CPR will be defined by a prospective, randomized trial. In the meantime, if there is good evidence that pulmonary embolism is the cause of cardiac arrest it is appropriate to give a fibrinolytic during CPR.

References

A comprehensive list of references can be found in
1. Nolan J, De Latorre F, Steen P et al (2002) Advanced life support drugs: do they really work? Curr Opin Crit Care 8:212-218
2. American Heart Association in collaboration with the International Liaison Committee on Resuscitation (ILCOR). International Guidelines 2000 for Cardiopulmonary Resuscitation and Emergency Cardiovascular Care – A Consensus on Science. Resuscitation 2000; 46:1-448 and Circulation 102:I1-384
3. De Latorre F, Nolan J, Robertson C et al (2001) European Resuscitation Council Guidelines 2000 for Adult Advanced Life Support. A statement from the Advanced Life Support Working Group and approved by the Executive Committee of the European Resuscitation Council. Resuscitation 48:211-221

Hyperosmolar syndrome

F. SCHIRALDI, G. ESPOSITO, G. RUGGIERO

Basic principles

The osmotic pressure is a negative force, resulting in movement of water from compartments with high concentration of water (low concentration of solutes) to compartments of low concentration of water (high concentration of solutes). The process is fundamental in the control of volume and concentration of the intracellular, interstitial and plasma water compartments.

The driving force for osmotic water movement is the difference in concentration of solutes between two compartments divided by a permeable membrane. This osmotic pressure can be calculated from the van't Hoff's law:

π = IRTc

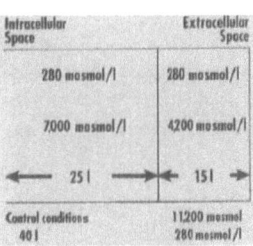

in which,

π = osmotic pressure (in atmospheres)
I = number of particles dissociated
R = ideal gas constant (22.4 l/mol)
T = Kelvin temperature
C = the molar concentration of the solute.

Fig.1 Normal composition of intra- and extracellular water compartments and changes (*right panel*) following addition of 500 mosmol of NaCl

A quick look at the formula reveals the paramount importance of the molecular weight (molwt) of the substances infused or ingested due to the inverse relationship between the molwt and the particles number (i.e., 23 g sodium exerts the same osmotic pressure as 180 g glucose).

The measurement of the osmolar concentration of a solution is based on physical properties of solvents and solutions, particularly the so-called colligative properties. When a solute is added to a solvent, the solution differs from the pure solvent in that:

- the osmotic pressure increases,
- the boiling point increases,
- the vapor pressure decreases,
- the freezing point decreases.

Usually the osmometers employ this last phenomenon: the normal freezing point of water, 0°C, is depressed by 1.86°C for each mole of a non-ionized solute in an aqueous solution; for ionic solvents, each dissociated ion contributes to the osmotic concentration and, consequently, to the lowering of the freezing point [1].

Although the distribution of ion species differs across the plasma membrane, the osmotic concentration (the molar concentration of all dissolved particles) of the body fluids is always equal in intra- and extracellular spaces [2].

As a consequence, any alteration of the osmotic concentration in the extracellular spaces alters the concentration in the intracellular spaces. Moreover, since changes across the cellular membrane involve the movement of water rather than solute, they necessarily effect changes in cellular volume (Fig. 1) [3].

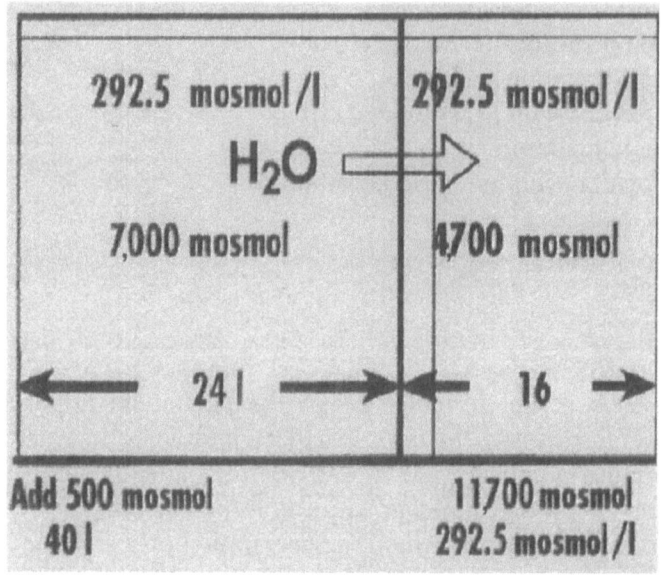

Fig. 2

Putting it another way, extra- and intracellular fluids (ICF) have different compositions, but almost equal solute concentrations. Because water diffuses from the compartment with lower concentrations to the other, what makes the water move across the membranes is a "temporary" difference between solute concentrations, this is the osmotic gradient. Moreover, the solutes should be divided into osmotically active (mostly confined to the extracellular or intracellular spaces) and osmotically inactive (urea, ethanol), which are free to cross the cellular membranes [4].

From a clinical point of view, the accumulation of osmotically active solutes in extracellular fluid (ECF) is hypertonicity, which is responsible for the hyperosmolar syndromes; while if urea (freely crossing membranes) accumulates in blood due to renal insufficiency, osmolality may increase, but tonicity could still be normal [5].

Pathophysiology

The body tonicity regulation is finely tuned and strictly linked to the control of extracellular sodium concentration, which is mainly determined by:
- salt and water intake
- antidiuretic hormone secretion
- aldosterone release
- atrial natriuretic peptides
- intrarenal hemodynamics

The key receptors are firstly the osmotically sensitive ones, sometimes associated with the volume receptors, if circulating volume depletion is superimposed. There is an intimate relationship between osmotic sensors and water balance, clearly underlined by the following mathematical coupling:

$$\Delta Uosm = 95\Delta Posm,$$

which indicates how a 1 mosmol/l change in plasma osmolality (Posm) is able to produce a 95 mosmol/l in urine osmolality (Uosm), if renal function is normal.

Not to be forgotten, stretch receptors in the atria and baroreceptors in the great vessels are the "haemodynamic modulators" of similar responses.

Such a sophisticated interplay between receptors and effectors is linked to the paramount relevance of preserving the intravascular circulating volume.

Provided a normal access to (and intestinal absorption of) water, even subjects affected by diabetes insipidus should be able to preserve the total body water (TBW).

So the diagnostic approach should firstly exclude any causes impairing such a finely tuned autoregulatory mechanism; among elderly patients affected by hyperosmolar syndrome at the time of hospital admission, over 70% are women, nearly half of whom have a febrile illness associated with stroke, decompensated diabetes mellitus, or diuretics abuse [6-8]. It is always mandatory to correlate the urinalysis (osmolarity included) with the corresponding Posm, and think about the derangement of the Uosm from the so-called expected response, to exclude a renal/endocrine mechanism for the syndrome. As a useful simple remind, and a rough rule of thumb, remember the following:

π (Density)	Osmolality
1,010	< 350 mosmol/l
1,020	700
1,030	1,050

Whatever the causes of hypertonicity, there is a common cellular and metabolic response to the hyperosmolar syndromes [9]. As the water tends to diffuse down its concentration gradient from the ICF to the ECF, a decrease in cell volume will ensue with cell shrinkage and possibly metabolic derangements. The brain is very susceptible to alterations in cell volume. Decreases in brain volume can lead to disruption of bridging blood vessels and likelihood of intracranial haemorrhage. Obviously there are some adaptive mechanisms. Following exposure to hyperosmolar solutions, neurons undergo rapid changes in their cytoplasmic make up in order to minimize osmotically induced cell dehydration [10-12]. The quite complex compensatory mechanisms are due to:

- the increased flow of cerebrospinal fluid into the cerebral interstitium;
- the selective increase in potassium transporters, followed by chloride and sodium, which could counteract nearly two-thirds of the cellular water losses;
- the generation of the so-called idiogenic osmoles (amino acids, methylamines, polyols), which tentatively lead the cellular volume to normal.

These are key processes that should always be taken into account whatever therapeutic strategy is to be planned. A safe approach should always take account of the various "timings" (when the disturbance arose, which level the compensating mechanisms reached, what speed the salt/water therapeutic handling should have) [13-15].

A small help from the laboratory

Applying these principles to a urine sample collected over a period of time, one can calculate the volume of plasma from which all osmoles of solute have been removed during that time, obtaining the osmolal clearance (Cosmol), numerically expressed as milliliters per minute:

$$(Cosmol) = Urinary\ flow\ (ml/min)\ x\ Uosm/\ Posm.$$

The further step is the evaluation of the "free water" clearance (C H_2O):

$$C\ H_2O = Urinary\ flow - Cosmol.$$

It is obvious that the more negative the C H_2O, the best work is being performed by the kidney in a hyperosmolar setting (so one could virtually exclude any renal/endocrine responsibility) [16].

Due to the frequent association of hyperosmolar syndromes with dehydration and underfilling of the intravascular compartment, another associated value to obtain as soon as possible is the central venous pressure (CVP), which – a few well-known conditions excluded – could be a useful guide to the therapy.

As Adrogué and Madias very precisely described [17, 18], within minutes after the development of hypertonicity, loss of water from brain cells causes shrinkage of the brain and an increase in osmolality. Partial restitution of brain volume occurs within a few hours as electrolytes enter the brain cells (rapid adaptation). The normalization of brain volume is completed within several days as a result of the intracellular accumulation of organic osmolytes (slow adaptation). The high osmolality persists despite the normalization of brain volume. So, the more the therapeutic approach takes into account these adaptive mechanisms, the better results should be achieved.

Therapeutic problems

Whatever approach the intensivist takes to the therapy of a subject with a hyperosmolar syndrome, he should take into account the physiological priorities. As the vast majority of cases are due to TBW reduction, it is safe – to buy time- to firstly provide a correction of the circulating volume, if needed, particularly if the CVP is very low. The goal could be possibly achieved by tailoring the fluid therapy with regard to as much information on CNS and cardiovascular responses as possible [19-21].

Slow correction of the hypertonic state re-establishes normal brain osmolality without inducing cerebral oedema, as the dissipation of accumulated electrolytes and organic osmolytes keeps pace with water repletion. In contrast, rapid correction may result in cerebral oedema as water uptake by brain cells outpaces the dissipation of accumulated electrolytes and organic osmolytes. Such overly aggressive therapy carries the risk of serious neurological impairment due to cerebral oedema. Moreover, a slight hyperosmolarity could have positive effects on some cellular functions, which confirms the choice not to correct overzealously whatever form of hyperosmolarity [22-25].

Based on current knowledge, a few steps could be safely followed:

1. Correct hypoperfusion and stabilize the circulation
2. Estimate the fluid deficit on the basis of serum sodium, urinary indexes and TBW; use Posm if measured, calculating the water deficit as :
$$\text{Water Deficit} = \text{TBW} \times (285 - \text{Posm}) / \text{Posm}$$
3. Give the calculated deficit as isotonic or half tonic sodium chloride, avoiding, if possible, solutions containing glucose, in almost 48 h
4. Try to correct the Posm aiming for a decrement ≤ 1 mosmol/l per hour
5. Check plasma electrolytes every 2 h
6. As many patients with hypernatremia have serious underlying systemic illness, pay close attention to the treatment of associated medical conditions.

Conclusions

Hyperosmolar syndromes are still a difficult challenge to the intensivist, as they usually carry around 40% mortality, mostly in elderly people. A very close clinical monitoring and intensive nursing are mandatory and could improve the prognosis, especially if the treatment of the underlying disorders (stroke, infections, diabetes...) is timely and effective. Advanced invasive monitoring is rarely requested.

References

1. Edelman IS, Leibman J (1959) Anatomy of body water and electrolytes. Am J Med 27: 256-277
2. Maxwell MH, Kleeman CR (eds) (1998) Clinical disorders of fluid and electrolyte metabolism, 5th edn. McGraw-Hill, New York
3. Lang F, Ritter M, Volkl M (1993) The biological significance of cell volume. Renal Physiol Biochem 16:48-56
4. Daugirdas JT, Kronfol NO (1989) Hyperosmolar coma: cellular dehydration and the serum sodium concentration. Ann Intern Med 110:855-857
5. Lewis SA, Donaldson P (1990) Ion channels and cell volume regulation:chaos in an organized system. News Physiol Sci 5:112-118

6. Long CA, Marin P, Bayer AJ et al (1991) Hypernatremia in an adult in-patient population. Postgrad Med J 67:643-645
7. Palevsky PM, Bhagrath R, Greenberg A (1996) Hypernatremia in hospitalised patients. Ann Intern Med 124:197-203
8. Snyder NA, Feigal DW, Arieff AI (1987) Hypernatremia in elderly patients. A heterogeneous, morbid and iatrogenic entity. Ann Intern Med 107:309-319
9. Lang F, Busch GL, Ritter M et al (1998) Functional significance of cell volume regulatory mechanisms. Physiol Rev 78:247-306
10. Lien YHH, Shapiro JI, Chan L (1990) Effects of hypernatremia on organic brain osmoles. J Clin Invest 85:1427-1433
11. Elisaf M, Litou H, Siamopoulos KC (1989) Survival after severe iatrogenic hypernatremia. Am J Kidney Dis 14:230-234
12. Cserr HF, De Pasquale F, Patlak CS (1987) Regulation of water and electrolytes during acute hyperosmolarity in rats . Am J Physiol 253: F522-F526
13. Snyder NA, Feigal DW, Arieff AI (1987) Hypernatremia in elderly patients: a heterogeneous, morbid and iatrogenic entity. Ann Intern Med 107:309-314
14. Vin-Christian K, Arieff AI (1993) Diabetes insipidus, massive polyuria and hypernatremia leading to a permanent brain damage. Am J Med 94:341-345
15. Oh MS, Carroll HJ (1992) Disorders of sodium metabolism: hypernatremia and hyponatremia. Crit Care Med 20 1:94-103
16. Schiraldi F (1993) Acqua, elettroliti, equilibrio acido-base:l'essenziale. Idelson, Naples, pp182--184
17. Adrogué H, Madias NE (2000) Hypernatremia. N Engl J Med 342:1493-1499
18. Adrogué H, Madias NE (2000) Hyponatremia. N Engl J Med 342:1581-1589
19. Levine SN, Sanson TH (1989) Treatment of hyperglycaemic hyperosmolar non-ketotic syndrome. Drugs 38: 462-472
20. Schierhout G, Roberts I (1998) Fluid resuscitation with colloid or crystalloid solutions in critically ill patients: a systematic review of randomised trials. BMJ 316:961-964
21. Neumann P (1999) Extravascular lung water and intrathoracic blood volume: double versus single indicator dilution technique. Intensive Care Med 25:216-219
22. Lang F, Busch GL, Ritter M et al (1995) Interplay of pH and cell volume in the regulation of metabolism, cell proliferation and cell death. In: De Santo NG, Capasso G. Acid base and electrolyte bilance. Iiss, Naples, pp 111-118
23. Oreopoulos GD, Hamilton J, Rizoli SB et al (2000) In vivo and in vitro modulation of intercellular adhesion molecule expression by hypertonicity . Shock 14:409-414
24. Rizoli SB, Rotstein OD, Parodo J et al (2000) Hypertonic inhibition of exocytosis in neutrophils: central role for osmotic actin skeleton remodelling. Am J Physiol 279:C619-C633
25. Dmitrieva N, Kultz D, Michea L (2000) Protection of renal inner medullary epithelial cells from apoptosis by hypertonic stress-induced p53 activation. J Biol Chem 275:18243-18249

Hypertonic solutions: when, how, how long, how much?

J. O. C. AULER, L. F. POLI de FIGUEIREDO, M.ROCHA e SILVA

The current interest for the use of hypertonic solutions was triggered by our institution in 1980. It was shown that a bolus injections of 7.5% NaCl, 4 ml/kg, a volume equivalent to only 10% of the volume of shed blood, rapidly restored arterial pressure and cardiac output in a severely hemorrhaged dog, resulting in long-term survival. Control animals, which received the same volume of isotonic saline, did not respond with hemodynamic improvement or survival [1].

Human use of 7.5% NaCl solutions began with Fellipe et al. [2], treating patients with refractory shock in a critical care unit and showing hemodynamic benefits. Both studies were the basis for hundreds of subsequent experimental studies and more than 60 clinical trials with 7.5% NaCl in the treatment of several conditions, such as hemorrhagic, cardiogenic, and septic shock, as well as a volume-supporting solution during major surgical procedural studies. We address the questions regarding when, how, how long, and how much based on the available clinical data for efficacy and safety in several emergency and elective conditions [3].

Mechanisms for hypertonic resuscitation

Small volumes of 7.5% NaCl, rapidly restored arterial pressure, cardiac output and vital organs blood flows in animals that have bled 40%-50% their blood volumes [4-8]. The cardiovascular improvement following is instantaneous and has been attributed to plasma volume expansion, vasodilatation in several vascular beds, and to a direct cardiac inotropic effect [9-11].

Volume expansion

A purely physical component causes the initial effect of a 4 ml/kg bolus injection of 7.5% NaCl (2,400 mosmol/l), which is volume expansion as a result of the osmotic gradient created, shifting fluid to the intravascular compartment. The infusion of 250 ml of 7.5% NaCl solutions to adult patients, the most commonly used dose, usually takes more than 2 min. The respective reflection coefficients of the endothelial barrier and cellular membrane must be considered in the determination of the osmotic force generated by the sodium gradient established after the use of hypertonic saline solution. The endothelial layer has a coefficient of 0.1, while the cell membrane coefficient is 1. Immediately after injection of 7.5% NaCl, a gradient of 25 mosmol/l exerts an osmotic pressure of about 500 mmHg through the cellular membrane and of only 50 mmHg through the endothelial membrane. Thus, the equilibrium across the endothelial membrane will be reached in seconds, while the equilibrium process across the cellular membrane will require longer periods.

Thus, the plasma expansion induced by hypertonic resuscitation is maximum during the administration of the solution. It occurs from the intracellular compartment and not from the interstitial compartment, which is also expanded. This fluid shift from the intracellular to the extracellular compartment may be regarded as beneficial, since during shock states, ischemia-reperfusion, extracorporeal circulation and sepsis, among other conditions, there is cellular edema, due to the action of inflammatory mediators and because of sodium/potassium pump dysfunction in the cellular membranes [11, 12].

Using plasma volume measurements and hematocrit changes after 7.5% NaCl, we detected an increment in plasma volume of 11 ml/kg, which disappeared after 6 h. The initial volume expansion represents about 2.75 ml of plasma for each milliliter of the injected solution, while with standard isotonic solutions, an expansion ratio of 0.33 ml is observed for each milliliter injected, as a consequence of the distribution of the isotonic solution into the extravascular compartment [1].

Association with colloids

The addition of 6% dextran-70 to the 7.5% NaCl solution (HSD) does not add to the initial plasma expansion; however, it does contributes to the maintenance of the fluid in the intravascular compartment for longer periods, thus prolonging the hemodynamic and metabolic benefits of the hypertonic solutions [5, 6, 13]. The dextran-70 exerts a colloidosmotic pressure two to three times greater than that observed with a similar concentration of human albumin, being therefore hyperoncotic. Similar results with HSD have been demonstrated with the addition of 6% hetastarch to the 7.5% NaCl solution (HSS) [14, 15].

In all clinical studies performed to date with the use of 7.5% NaCl, isotonic fluids have been injected after the hypertonic solution, correcting an eventual loss of cellular volume. Clinical manifestations of cellular dehydration would be apparent first in the central nervous system; however, there is no report of seizures or neurological dysfunction in any of the more than 1,700 patients that received hypertonic solutions.

Microcirculatory blood flow improvement

The main sources for the observed plasma expansion after 7.5% NaCl injection are the red blood cells and the endothelium, which are in close contact with the hypertonicity, losing about 8% of their volumes directly to the intravascular compartment. Apart from the volume expansion, these events result in important hemodynamic effects on the microcirculation, since the edema in the red blood cells and endothelium, as observed in shock and ischemia-reperfusion, are of critical importance in terms of viscosity and hydraulic resistance in the microcirculation, where the ratio between the vascular lumen and the red blood cell approaches unity. Under these circumstances, cellular edema compromises the microcirculatory blood flow. Hypertonic solutions, but not isotonic, contribute to hemodynamic improvement at the microcirculatory level [16].

These microcirculatory disturbances have been implicated in the origin of sepsis and multiple organ dysfunction that have been observed after an initially successful resuscitation of post-traumatic shock [17]. The resulting sustained splanchnic vasoconstriction may cause gut mucosal ischemia and consequent compromise of its integrity and predisposition to bacterial and toxin penetration from the intestinal lumen into the systemic circulation. The changes in the gut mucosa may be even more severe during the reperfusion period, mediated by oxygen free radicals, which also results in capillary lumen narrowing, leukocyte adhesion and activation, stimulation of several inflammatory mediators and cytokines, which may cause local tissue and remote organ injuries [17-19].

Under these conditions, hypertonic solutions may produce several beneficial effects through the rapid hemodynamic restoration at the macro- and microcirculatory levels. Based on these observed effects in post-traumatic shock, studies with 7.5% NaCl solutions, with and without dextran or hetastarch, have been performed using several models of sepsis and septic shock, and transient similar benefits have been observed in global and regional hemodynamics [20-22].

The hypertonicity induced by the 7.5% NaCl injection is responsible for the increased blood flow in the peripheral circulation and in the microcirculation as a consequence of a reduced vascular resistance, primarily by arteriolar vasodilatation. This response is caused by a direct relaxant effect of hypertonicity on vascular smooth muscle.

The reduction in blood viscosity, by the hemodilution rapidly induced by the hypertonic solution, also contributes to the reduction in vascular resistance and vasodilatation. The use of 7.5% NaCl in shock produces vasodilatation and increased regional blood flow to coronary [23], renal [24], intestinal [8, 9, 25] and skeletal muscle [8] circulations.

Cardiac effects

The hemodynamic benefits observed after 7.5% NaCl have been partially attributed to a direct cardiac inotropic effect induced by hypertonicity [26,27]. However, an evaluation of left ventricular contractility after 7.2% NaCl/6% hetastarch in anaesthetized, stable patients without cardiovascular disease did not demonstrate any clinically relevant positive inotropic effect. All hemodynamic benefits were therefore attributed to the combination of volume expansion and decreased afterload [28].

Some authors showed no direct inotropic effect with hypertonic solutions in the treatment of hemorrhagic shock [29], while others showed negative inotropic effects in normovolemic dogs [30]. Thus, whether hypertonic solutions have a direct positive inotropic effect by the hypertonicity contributing to the hemodynamic benefits remains controversial.

Renal effects

Improvements in renal function have been observed after HSD infusion to animals in shock. This benefit is probably multifactorial, resulting from volume expansion, general hemodynamic improvement, and increased renal blood flow [31].

Cerebral effects

A great benefit with hypertonic resuscitation has been observed on cerebral hemodynamics during hemorrhagic shock, particularly in the presence of intracranial hypertension and systemic hypotension [32-34]. The rapid restoration of the arterial pressure associated with a reduction in intracranial hypertension induced by hypertonic solutions suggests a potential clinical application of these solutions for trauma victims with head injury and associated lesions with hypotension, a subset of trauma victims with poor prognosis. In the clinical trials, patients with low Glasgow Coma Score and hypotension after trauma benefited from an initial infusion of hypertonic solutions [35].

Oxygen free radicals scavenging

The role of the dextran component as an oxygen free radicals scavenger and the role of HSD as an inhibitor of leukocyte activation have been recognized [36]. More recently, a series of experiments by Coimbra et al. has shown that hypertonic saline solution, even without dextran, significantly interferes with the immune responses, both in vitro and in vivo [37-41].

Immunological effects

The addition of hypertonic saline solution to lymphocyte culture media, in concentrations similar to those obtained with the infusion of 4 ml/kg of 7.5% NaCl in humans, determined a significant increase in lymphocyte proliferation [37]. The addition of prostaglandin E_2 (PGE$_2$) to the culture media, in the absence of hypertonic saline, caused a reduction in T-cell proliferation compared with control cultures. On the other hand, when hypertonic saline was added to the culture media containing PGE$_2$, there was a complete reversal on the PGE$_2$-induced immunosupression [40]. These in vitro findings were confirmed in vivo using a hemorrhagic shock model in mice, in which the infusion of 7.5% NaCl revesed the cellular immune function depression that occurs after hemorrhage. Plasma levels of several cytokines were determined, and the authors concluded that hypertonic saline solution prevents immunosupression probably by decreasing plasma levels of interleukin-4 and PGE$_2$ [39]. Using a hemorrhagic shock model in mice, followed by cecal puncture 24 h later, these authors have shown that with the use of 7.5% NaCl there was a significant decrease in mortality 72 h after peritonitis induction compared with conventional isotonic resuscitation. Moreover, a significant reduction in pulmonary and hepatic changes after hypertonic solutions was observed [40]. Recently, we have described a significant reduction in bacterial translocation and pulmonary lesions in rats with hemorrhagic shock that were treated with hypertonic saline solution [41].

Based on this evidence, it has been suggested that resuscitation with hypertonic saline solutions presents significant potential as an immunomodulator agent for trauma victims [42]. However, all this evidence requires additional research and careful evaluation in clinical trials using these solutions.

Experimental data on septic shock

Despite extensive documentation regarding efficacy of hypertonic saline solutions used alone or in combination with colloids for the treatment of hemorrhagic shock, a consensus regarding use of these solutions to treat animals and human beings with shock septic has not been established. Our group investigated prospectively the use of hypertonic saline (7.5%) with 6% dextran 70 (HSSD) (1.82 ml/kg) or isotonic saline (0.9%) solution (ISS) (32 ml/kg) in dogs with septic shock secondary to uterine infection (pyometra). The data were obtained 5 and 20 min after fluid infusion; mean arterial pressure (MAP) increased significantly after administration of HSSD, whereas ISS did not affect MAP. However cardiac output and oxygen delivery increased, and hematocrit decreased after both treatments. Oxygen consumption and extraction rate and degree of acidosis did not improve after either treatment. It is important to note that only MAP increased significantly after HSSD, and cardiac output in both, whereas a volume of ISS 8 times higher than HSSD was necessary to produce the same effect. Our data allowed us to conclude that in this model of septic shock a small amount of HSSD was able to re-establish hemodynamic parameters in dogs compared with ISS, which required 8 times more [42].

Human use of hypertonic solutions

A substantial clinical experience has been accumulated regarding the use of 7.5% NaCl solutions (Table 1). A majority of patients received these solutions as the initial treatment for post-traumatic hypotension followed by standard-of-care isotonic crystalloid solutions, both in pre-hospital or in the emergency room environment, including several prospective and double blind studies [44-52].

These patients have been submitted to extensive clinical and laboratory evaluation, demonstrating their remarkable safety, even when infused to trauma victims, with immediate risk of death from hypovolemia, hemodynamic instability and severe associated lesions. These same studies have provided valuable insights regarding the efficacy of these hypertonic saline solutions. Studies performed in patients undergoing cardiovascular surgeries and in critically ill patients in intensive care units provide data regarding the effects of hypertonic saline solutions in patients presenting associated pre-existing diseases and organs and systems with limited reserve [53-63].

Table 1 Published clinical experience with 7.5 % Na Cl solutions (*HS*, 7.5% NaCl, *HSD* 7.5% NaCl/6% dextran-70, *HSS* 7.5% NaCl/6% hetastarch)

Setting	Studies (n)	HS	HSD	HSS	Total
Pre-hospital	9	202	495	16	713
Emergency room	8	138	326		464
Intraoperative	21	34	58	175	267
Intensive care unit	18	91	65	116	272
Clinical	4	18	19	4	41
Total	**60**	**483**	**963**	**311**	**1,757**

Studies on trauma

The ultimate test of efficacy for treatment of trauma with shock is enhanced survival. Secondary, but equally important, endpoints are reduced complications, and lower treatment costs. A number of reports have demonstrated significantly increased efficacy in patients treated with hypertonic saline followed by standard-of-care, when compared with equivalent patients receiving standard-of-care.

In the first performed trial, which included 105 patients in hypovolemic shock, patients treated with hypertonic saline showed a significant initial improvement of arterial pressure, and reduced intravenous fluid requirements. No significant difference in mortality was detected [44]. In a subsequent study, in which 212 hypotensive patients were enrolled, Younes et al. [49] showed that hypertonic saline as initial treatment caused a significant decrease in long-term mortality rate for the subpopulation with an entry MAP below 70 mmHg.

The United States multicenter trial, which included 422 patients, showed a significant increase in survival for the HSD-treated patients in the subpopulation requiring surgery. It also showed a greater incidence of adult respiratory distress syndrome, renal failure, and coagulopathy in the standard-of-care alone treatment group [53].

Hypotensive patients sustaining head injury with Glasgow Coma Scale scores of 8 or less that received hypertonic saline treatment presented higher survival to hospital discharge. This was demonstrated in a multicenter trial [51], as well as in a meta-analysis of individual patients from all the known clinical trials [64]. A meta-analysis conducted on the individual patient records from controlled clinical studies on trauma demonstrated a significant increase in survival favoring HSD versus standard of care [52].

Safety based on human data

Bleeding

Since hypertonic saline resuscitation induces an immediate restoration of both cardiac output and arterial pressure, vasodilatation, and hemodilution, several investigators raised concerns that these effects could overcome homeostatic mechanisms, such as vasoconstriction and local tamponade, or even hypotension. They would therefore represent a potential risk for increased internal bleeding [53, 54].

These concerns were highlighted by a controversial study, which challenged the guidelines recommended by the Advanced Trauma Life Support Course [55] for the resuscitation of penetrating trauma victims and hypotension with large volumes of isotonic crystalloid solutions [56]. This study suggested that standard-of-care pre-hospital and emergency room fluid infusion for these patients resulted in higher mortality and morbidity than observed for patients in whom fluid resuscitation was delayed, i.e., after operative bleeding control [61].

On the other hand, the United States multicenter trial, which compared standard-of-care fluid infusion with HSD followed by standard-of-care in the pre-hospital treatment of post-traumatic hypotension, demonstrated that penetrating trauma victims with hypotension that received HSD presented higher arterial blood pressure and trends toward higher survival and less complications, when compared with standard-of-care fluid treatment alone [48]. Similar results were observed in other studies, recently presented as a meta-analysis [52]. These data suggest that the negative effects of large volume infusion of crystalloid solutions are not related to increased arterial pressure but to factors related to the isotonic solution itself. A trial comparing standard-of-care, HSD and delayed resuscitation is needed to establish the best means to treat post--traumatic hypotension.

Patients receiving hypertonic solutions in these studies on post-traumatic hypotension underwent extensive laboratory investigation, which showed that the amount of dextran 70 in the HSD formulation did not alter the coagulation profile. Additionally, none of the studies with trauma victims or those testing the intraoperative use of HSD demonstrated any association between hypertonic solutions and blood loss or with increased requirements of blood products. In all studies so far performed, blood product requirements have always been associated with the severity and mechanism of injury, and not with the solution used. In fact, a reduction in subsequent fluid requirements is a common finding after the use of HSD [52].

Neither was the use of HSD during complex cardiovascular surgical procedures, in which hemostasis alterations are common [57], associated with increased blood loss or increased blood product requirement. Moreover, the use hypertonic solutions in cardiac and aortic surgery has been frequently associated with hemodynamic stability and less, rather than more postoperative fluid requirements [58-61].

Overall, the common observation of less fluid requirements, no increase in blood product requirements, and trends toward less morbidity and mortality with the use of hypertonic solutions suggests that there is no increase in bleeding associated with its use, even in patients sustaining penetrating trauma or during complex cardiovascular surgeries.

Hypernatremia

A frequent concern with hypertonic resuscitation is that it might possibly induce significant hypernatremia of potentially deleterious consequences. Such hypernatremia would of course result from cellular dehydration produced by the osmotic mechanisms already described. In severe hypernatremia, evidence of cellular dehydration is manifest much earlier in the central nervous system than in other organs or systems. Symptoms of hypernatremia include lethargy, tremors, weakness, irritability, delirium, mental confusion, seizures, coma, and death. They occur in severe cases and, particularly, in small children and in the elderly.

The use of hypertonic sodium solutions to rapidly correct hyponatremia in patients with severe malnutrition or alcoholism may result in central pontine myelinolysis, which is manifest through dysarthria, paraparesis, or paraplegia [62]. Another described complication with hypertonic sodium solutions for the correction of hyponatremia in neonates is the rupture of cerebral veins and intracranial hemorrhage, caused by the retraction of the cerebral tissue [63].

With these questions in the forefront of all clinical trials, patients receiving 7.5% NaCl were carefully evaluated for signs and symptoms of hypernatremia, particularly for the associated neurological alterations. This was especially true for patients at highest risk for neurological dysfunction and intracranial hypertension, i.e., those sustaining head trauma and systemic hypotension.

Despite the fact that moderate hypernatremia and hyperosmolarity have been detected in the overwhelming majority of patients receiving 7.5% NaCl solutions, there was not a single case, among more than 1,700 patients, of seizures, intracranial bleeding, or neurological deterioration induced by the hypertonic solution [55, 67]. Necropsies and careful anatopathological studies of the brain tissues were performed in trauma victims, and produced no evidence of central pontine desmyelinization or of focal intracranial bleeding that could be attributed to the use of 7.5% NaCl [52, 64].

The short duration of the moderate hypernatremia, the absence of pre-existing hyponatremia, and the exclusion of children and patients with chronic disabling diseases may have contributed to the lack of hypernatremia-related undesirable effects. On the other hand, hypotensive patients with head trauma and low Glasgow Coma Scale were one of the subgroups that most benefited from 7.5% NaCl solutions as the initial treatment, presenting better neurological outcome and a significant increase in survival [64]. Thus, 7.5% NaCl-induced hypernatremia and hyperosmolarity were actually associated with neurological benefits, not with neurological dysfunction.

Although we cannot exclude that higher doses of hypertonic saline might induce hypernatremia-related side effects, it is also true that the prescribed dose cannot result in such effects. However, it does seem prudent to avoid these solutions for patients with the highest risk for severe neurological disturbances induced by hypernatremia, i.e., patients with chronic debilitating diseases and children.

Hemodynamic instability

Experiments with anaesthetized animals in shock have shown that a rapid injection of 7.5% NaCl may cause hypotension and arrhythmia, caused by hypertonicity induced vasodilatation and reduction in peripheral vascular resistance [65]. These events may be particularly dangerous when the arterial pressure is very low before the infusion of the solution. This hemodynamic instability is directly dependent on the speed with which the solution is being infused and may be avoided with infusion times greater than 2 min.

Most trials with intraoperative use of 7.5% NaCl has demonstrated physiological benefits and no side-effects [58-61]. However, there is one study in patients with myocardial dysfunction undergoing coronary artery bypass in which pre-operative volume expansion with 250 ml of HSS caused hypotension and transient left ventricular failure [66]. This study showed that 7.5% NaCl solutions could be deleterious if rapidly infused in patients with ventricular dysfunction, in whom a fixed dose may be inadequate [67]. In a similar study, in patients with cardiac dysfunction, in which the volume of 7.5% NaCl solution was titrated to a target cardiac filling pressure, it was found that a lower dosage was enough to achieve the desired hemodynamic profile, with no haemodynamic instability [67].

In a separate study, a fixed dose of HSD (250 ml) was used during extracorporeal circulation in Jehovah witness patients, with no hemodynamic changes and reduced fluid requirements in the postoperative period [61]. A similar dose was used in surgical procedures for correction of thoracic and abdominal aortic aneurysms [58,59,68]. These procedures are normally associated with sudden hemodynamic changes, marked fluid loss to the third space, and a high incidence of postoperative complication [69]. The use of hypertonic saline solutions resulted in hemodynamic stability and fluid sparing in the postoperative period in these procedures.

The administration of 7.5% NaCl solution to patients with cardiogenic shock after right ventricular infarction also produced sustained hemodynamic benefits [70].

When the whole population of 1,700 patients in which 7.5% NaCl solutions were used is examined, there were no cases of cardiac death. However, it seems prudent to recommend caution with the use of hypertonic solutions in patients with heart diseases. Rigorous monitoring is mandatory and gradual and slower infusions should be employed.

Hyperchloremic acidosis

There is a significant increase in chloride plasma levels after 7.5% NaCl injection and this could predispose to hyperchloremic acidosis. Clinically relevant acidosis was observed in trauma victims that were moribund on arrival, and the acidosis was associated with pre-existing conditions such as cardiac arrest or severe hypothermia [46]. Despite hemodynamic and metabolic improvement after 7.5% NaCl solutions in the majority of patients, based on the clinical evidence we suggest that these solutions should be avoided in patients with pre-existing severe acidosis, probably developed during longer periods.

Anaphylaxis

There is a low incidence of side effects associated with all colloids, including dextran, with an incidence of anaphylactic reaction (pre-formed antibodies) or more common anaphylactoid reaction (no pre-formed antibodies) of 1:2,500 [70]. Thus, even though HSD and HSS solutions contain a very limited amount of colloid, the use of hapten-dextran 1 (molecular weight 1,000) is recommended preceding the elective use of HSD, in order to reduce the risk of allergic reactions to levels similar to those observed with human albumin solution. On the other hand, amongst the hundreds of trauma patients receiving HSD without hapten-dextran-1, there was no report of allergic reactions.

When, how, how long, how much?

Based on the available clinical experience with 7.5% NaCl solutions, we can conclude that the use of hypertonic solutions is safe, but it is prudent to avoid their use for a well-defined patient population, i.e., acute renal failure, children, moribund, or chronic debilitating diseases.

The most-striking benefits with the use of hypertonic solutions have been achieved as the first treatment for post-traumatic hypotension, particularly for penetrating trauma victims requiring surgery and for those sustaining head trauma. A single 250-ml infusion of HSD, preceding standard-of-care fluid crystalloid infusion and definitive trauma care, is the recommended dosage for most hypotensive trauma patients.

For elective intraoperative use, particularly for major cardiovascular procedures, 250 ml of HSD has been associated with hemodynamic stability and fluid sparing. However, in those with cardiac failure, titrated dosage and careful monitoring are required.

Although safety has been well established, it does appear that larger prospective, multicenter trials are essential to show superiority over standard-of-care and to better define the patient population to maximally benefit from hypertonic saline solutions.

References

1. Velasco IT, Pontieri V, Rocha e Silva M, et al (1980) Hyperosmotic NaCl and severe hemorrhagic shock. Am J Physiol 239:H664-H673
2. De Fellipe J Jr, Timoner J, Velasco IT, et al (1980) Treatment of refractory hypovolaemic shock by 7.5% sodium chloride injections. Lancet II:1002-1004
3. Poli de Figueiredo LF, Kramer GC. Safety concerns and contraindications of hyperosmolar small-volume resuscitation. In: Kreimeier U, Christ F, Messmer K, editors. Small-volume hyperosmolar volume resuscitation. Springer-Verlag, Heidelberg Berlin New York (in press)
4. Nakayama S, Sibley L, Gunther R, et al (1984) Small volume resuscitation with hypertonic saline resuscitation (2400 mOsm/l) during hemorrhagic shock. Circ Shock 13:149-159
5. Smith GJ, Kramer GC, Perron P, et al (1985) A comparison of several hypertonic solutions for resuscitation of bled sheep. J Surg Res 39:517-528
6. Kramer GC, Perron PR, Lindsey DC, et al (1986) Small-volume resuscitation with hypertonic saline dextran solution. Surgery 100:239-247
7. Poli de Figueiredo LF, Peres CA, Attalah AN, et al (1995) Hemodynamic improvement in hemorrhagic shock by aortic balloon occlusion and hypertonic saline solutions. Cardiovasc Surg 3:679-686
8. Rocha e Silva M, Negraes G, Soares A, et al (1986) Hypertonic resuscitation from severe hemorrhagic shock: patterns of regional circulation. Circ Shock 19:165-75
9. Kreimeier U, Bruckner U, Niemczyk S, et al (1990) Hyperosmotic saline dextran for resuscitation from traumatic-hemorrhagic hypotension: effect on regional blood flow. Circ Shock 32:83-99
10. Rocha e Silva, M, Velasco IT, Nogueira da Silva RI, et al (1987) Hyperosmotic sodium salts reverse severe hemorrhagic shock: other solutes do not. Am J Physiol 253:H751-H762
11. Auler Jr JOC, Rocha e Silva M (1993) Hyperosmolar and hypoosmolar states. In: Gullo A (ed) Anaesthesia pain intensive care and emergency: APICE. Trieste, Tipografia Moderna, pp 49-56
12. Rocha e Silva M. Evolving concepts in small volume resuscitation: the experimental basis. In: Kreimeier U, Christ F, Messmer K (eds) Small-volume hyperosmolar volume resuscitation. Springer-Verlag, Heidelberg Berlin New York (in press)
13. Velasco I, Rocha e Silva M, Oliveira M, et al (1989) Hypertonic and hyperoncotic resuscitation from severe hemorrhagic shock in dogs: a comparative study. Crit Care Med 17:261-264.
14. Kramer GC, Elgjo GI, Poli de Figueiredo LF, et al (1997) Hyperosmotic-hyperoncotic solutions. Ballieres Clin Anaesthesiol 11:143-161
15. Matteucci MJ, Wisner DH, Gunther RA, et al (1993) Effects of hypertonic and isotonic fluid infusion on the flash evoked potential in rats: hemorrhage, resuscitation, and hypernatremia. J Trauma 34:1-7
16. Mazzoni M, Borgstrom P, Intaglietta M, et al (1990) Capillary narrowing in hemorrhagic shock is rectified by hyperosmotic saline-dextran reinfusion. Circ Shock 31:407-418
17. Border JR, Hassett J, LaDuca J, et al (1987) The gut origins septic states in blunt multiple trauma (ISS=40) in the ICU. Ann Surg 206:427-448
18. Carrico CJ, Meakins JL, Marshall JC, et al (1986) Multiple organ failure syndrome. Arch Surg 121:196-208

19. Deitch EA, Bridges W, Ma L, et al (1990) Hemorrhagic shock-induced bacterial translocation: the role of neutrophils and hydroxyl radicals. J Trauma 30:942-952
20. Mullins RJ, Hudgens RW (1987) Hypertonic saline resuscitates dogs in endotoxin shock. J Surg Res 43:37-44.
21. Armistead CW, Vincent JL, Preiser JC, et al (1989) Hypertonic saline solution-hetastarch for fluid resuscitation in experimental septic shock. Anesth Analg 69:714-720
22. Kreimeier U, Frey L, Dentz J, et al (1991) Hypertonic saline dextran resuscitation during the initial phase of acute endotoxemia: effect on regional blood flow. Crit Care Med 19:801-809
23. Crystal GJ, Gurevicius J, Kim SJ, et al (1994) Effects of hypertonic saline solutions in the coronary circulation. Circ Shock 42:27-38
24. Maningas PA (1987) Resuscitation with 7.5% NaCl in 6% dextran-70 during hemorrhagic shock in swine: effects on organ blood flow. Crit Care Med 15:1121-1126
25. Kreimeier U, Bruckner U, Schmidt J, et al (1990) Instantaneous restoration of regional organ blood flow after severe hemorrhage: effect of small-volume resuscitation with hypertonic-hyperoncotic solution. J Surg Res 49:493-503
26. Ing RD, Nazeeri MN, Zelds S, et al (1994) Hypertonic saline/dextran improves septic myocardial performance. Am Surg 60:507-508
27. Kien ND, Kramer GC (1989) Cardiac performance following hypertonic saline. Braz J Med Biol Res 22:2245-2248.
28. Goertz AW, Mehl T, Lindner KH, et al (1995) Effect of 7.2% hypertonic saline/6% hetastarch on left ventricular contractility in anesthetized humans. Anesthesiology 82:1389-1395.
29. Welte M, Goresch T, Frey L, et al (1995) Hypertonic saline dextran does not increase cardiac contractile function during small volume resuscitation from hemorrhagic shock in anesthetized pigs. Anesth Analg 80:1099-1107
30. Constable PD, Muir WW, Binkley PF (1994) Hypertonic saline is negative inotropic agent in normovolemic dogs. Am J Physiol 267:H667-H677
31. Sondeen JL, Gonzaludo GA, Loveday JA, et al (1990) Hypertonic saline/dextran improves renal function after hemorrhage in conscious swine. Resuscitation 20:231-241
32. Prough DS, Johnson JC, Poole GV, et al (1985) Effects on intracranial pressure of resuscitation from hemorrhagic shock with hypertonic saline versus lactated Ringer's solution. Crit Care Med 13:407-411
33. Prough DS, Johnson JC, Stump DA, et al (1986) Effects of hypertonic saline versus lactated Ringer's solution on cerebral oxygen transport during resuscitation from hemorrhagic shock. J Neurosurg 64:627-632
34. Walsh JC, Zhuang J, Shackford SR (1991) A comparison of hypertonic to isotonic fluid in the resuscitation of brain injury and hemorrhagic shock. J Surg Res 50:284-287
35. Wade CE, Grady J, Kramer GC, et al (1997) Individual cohort analysis of the efficacy of hypertonic saline/dextran in patients with traumatic brain injury and hypotension. J Trauma 42:S61-S65
36. Bayer M, Nolte D, Lehr HA, et al (1991) Hypertonic-hyperoncotic dextran solution reduces post-ischemic leukocyte adherence in post-capillary vessels. Langenbecks Arch Chir [Suppl 1]:375-378
37. Coimbra R, Junger WG, Hoyt DB, et al (1995) Immunosuppression following hemorrhage is reduced by hypertonic saline resuscitation. Surg Forum 46:84-87
38. Coimbra R, Junger WG, Liu FC, et al (1995) Hypertonic/hyperoncotic fluids reverse prostaglandin E2 (PGE2) induced T-cell suppression. Shock 3:45-49
39. Coimbra R, Junger WG, Hoyt DB, et al (1996) Hypertonic saline resuscitation restores hemorrhage-induced immunosuppression by decreasing prostaglandin E2 and interleukin-4 production. J Surg Res 64:203-209
40. Coimbra R, Hoyt DB, Junger WG, et al (1997) Hypertonic saline resuscitation decreases susceptibility to sepsis after hemorrhagic shock. J Trauma 42:602-607
41. Yada-Langui MM, Coimbra R, Lancellotti C et al (2000) Hypertonic saline and pentoxifylline

prevent lung injury and bacterial translocation after hemorrhagic shock. Shock 14:594-598

42. Junger WG, Coimbra R, Liu FC, et al (1997) Hypertonic saline resuscitation. A tool to modulate immune function in trauma patients. Shock 8:235-241

43. Fantoni. DD, Auler Jr JOC, Futema F, et al (1999) Intravenous administration of hypertonic sodium chloride with dextran solution or isotonic sodium chloride solution for treatment of septic shock secondary to pyometra in dogs. J Am Vet Med Assoc 215:1283-1287

44. Younes RN, Aun F, Accioly CQ, et al (1992) Hypertonic solutions in the treatment of hypovolemic shock: A prospective, randomized study in patients admitted to the emergency room. Surgery 111:380-385

45. Maningas PA, Mattox KL, Pepe PE, et al (1989) Hypertonic saline-dextran solutions for the prehospital management of traumatic hypotension. Am Surg 157:528-534

46. Vassar MJ, Perry CA, Holcroft JW (1990) Analysis of potential risks associated with 7.5% sodium chloride resuscitation of traumatic shock. Arch Surg 125:1309-1315

47. Vassar MJ, Perry CA, Gannaway WL, et al (1991) 7.5% sodium chloride/dextran for resuscitation of trauma patients undergoing helicopter transport. Arch Surg 126:1065-1072

48. Mattox KL, Maningas PA, Moore EE, et al (1991) Prehospital hypertonic saline/dextran infusion for post-traumatic hypotension - The USA multicenter trial. Ann Surg 213:482-491

49. Younes RN, Aun F, Ching CT, et al (1997) Prognostic factors to predict outcome following the administration of hypertonic/hyperoncotic solution in hypovolemic patients. Shock 7:79-83

50. Vassar MJ, Perry CA, Holcroft JW (1993) Prehospital resuscitation of hypotensive trauma patients with 7.5% NaCl versus 7.5% NaCl with added dextran: a controlled trial. J Trauma 34:622-632

51. Vassar MJ, Fisher RP, O'Brien PE, et al (1993) A multicentre trial for resuscitation of injured patients with 7.5% sodium chloride. The multicenter group for the study of hypertonic saline in trauma patients. Arch Surg 128:1003-1011

52. Wade CE, Kramer GC, Grady JJ, et al (1997) Efficacy of hypertonic 7.5% saline and 6% dextran-70 in treating trauma: a meta-analysis of controlled clinical studies. Surgery 122:609-616

53. Gross D, Landau EH, Klin B, et al (1988) Is hypertonic saline resuscitation safe in "uncontrolled" hemorrhagic shock? J Trauma 28:751-756

54. Bickell WH, Bruttig SP, Wade CE (1989) Hemodynamic responses to abdominal aortotomy in the anesthetized swine. Circ Shock 28:321-232

55. American College of Surgeons, Committee on Trauma. (1993) Advanced Trauma Life Support Program for Physicians, 5th edn. American College of Surgeons, Chicago

56. Bickell WH, Wall MJ, Pepe PE, et al (1994) Immediate versus delayed fluid resuscitation for hypotensive patients with penetrating torso injuries. N Engl J Med 331:1105-1109

57. Poli de Figueiredo LF, Coselli JS (1997) Individual strategies of hemostasis for thoracic aortic surgery. J Card Surg 12:222-228

58. Younes RN, Bechara MJ, Langer B, et al (1987) Emprego da solução hipertônica de NaCl 7.5% na prevenção da hipotensão pós-desclampeamento da aorta abdominal. Rev Ass Med Brasil 34:150-154

59. Auler JOC, Pereira MH, Gomide-Amaral RV et al (1987) Hemodynamic effects of hypertonic sodium chloride during surgical treatment of aortic aneurysms. Surgery 101:594-601

60. Boldt J, Zickmann B, Ballesteros M, et al (1991) Cardiorespiratory responses to hypertonic saline solution in cardiac operations. Ann Thorac Surg 51:610-615

61. Oliveira SA, Bueno RM, Souza JM, et al (1995) Effects of hypertonic saline dextran on the postoperative evolution of Jehovah's Witness patients submitted to cardiac surgery with cardiopulmonary bypass. Shock 3:391-394

62. Sterns RH, Riggs JE, Schochet SS Jr (1986) Osmotic demyelination syndrome following rapid correction of hyponatremia. N Engl J Med 314:1535-1541

63. Finberg L, Luttrell E, Redd H (1959) Pathogenesis of lesions in the nervous system in hypernatremic states. II. Experimental studies of gross anatomic changes and alterations of chemical composition of the tissues. Pediatrics 23:46-66

64. Wade CE, Grady JJ, Kramer GC, et al (1997) Individual patient cohort analysis of the efficacy of hypertonic saline/dextran in patients with traumatic brain injury and hypotension. J Trauma 42:S61-S65
65. Kien ND, Kramer GC, White DA (1991) Acute hypotension caused by rapid saline infusion in anesthetized dogs. Anesth Analg 73:597-602
66. Prien T, Thulig B, Wuasten R, et al (1993) Effects of hypertonic saline hyperoncotic hydroxyethyl starch infusion prior to coronary artery bypass grafting (CABG) Zentralbl Chir 118:257- -266
67. Ellinger K, Fahnle M, Schroth M, et al (1995) Optimal preoperative titrated dosage of hyperto-nic-hyperoncotic solutions in cardiac risk patients. Shock 3:167-172
68. Christ F, Niklas M, Kreimeier U, et al (1997) Hyperosmotic-hyperoncotic solutions during abdominal aortic aneurysm (AAA) resection. Acta Anaesthesiol Scand 41:62-70
69. Coselli JS, Poli de Figueiredo LF, LaMarie SA (1997) Impact of a previous thoracic aneurysm repair on the management of thoracoabdominal aortic aneurysm. Ann Thorac Surg 64:639-650
70. Ramires JAF, Serrano CV, César LAM, et al (1992) Acute hemodynamic effects of hypertonic (7.5%) saline infusion in patients with cardiogenic shock due to right ventricular infarction. Circ Shock 37:220-225
71. Ring J, Messmer K (1977) Incidence and severity of anaphylactoid reactions to colloid volume substitutes. Lancet I:466-469

Efficacy of non-invasive positive pressure ventilation in acute cardiogenic pulmonary oedema

S. Prayag, S. Talekar, S. Jog

Non-invasive positive pressure ventilation (NIPPV), administered via a nasal or full-face mask, is now a well-documented modality of ventilatory assistance to avoid endotracheal intubation in selected patients with acute respiratory failure (ARF) [1-9]. Preservation of airway defence mechanisms and speech, complete avoidance of trauma to oropharynx, larynx, and trachea, reduction in ventilator-associated pneumonia (VAP) [4], and reduction in length of stay (LOS) [4, 7] are the main advantages over conventional invasive ventilation. However NIPPV has potential limitations, including the lack of direct access to the airway for removal of secretions, facial trauma related to a mask, and need for patient co-operation. NIPPV using bilevel positive airway pressure (BiPAP), via nasal or full-face mask, has been shown to improve arterial blood gas (ABG), decrease intensive care unit (ICU) LOS and complication rates, and improve patient survival [8, 9]. In majority of trials with BiPAP, the major patient group enrolled was ARF due to exacerbation of chronic obstructive pulmonary disease (COPD) [7, 10, 11]. Many researchers, such as Meduri et al. [5] Kramer et al. [7], and Popnick et al. [10] have included a few patients with acute cardiogenic pulmonary edema (ACPE) presenting as ARF in their studies, and have reported improvement in clinical and ABG status of this subset of patients. Although a few studies on the utility of continuous positive airway pressure (CPAP) in ACPE have been performed in the past, very few studies have been published on the efficacy of BiPAP in ACPE [12-15]. Mehta et al. [16] compared BiPAP and CPAP in their trial, and concluded that BiPAP improves ventilation and vital signs more rapidly than CPAP in patients with ACPE. One of the largest studies is by Hoffman and Welte [12] from Germany. In an open, prospective, uncontrolled trial in patients with ACPE in ARF, they reported successful avoidance of intubation in 28 of 29 patients, with significant improvement in PCO_2, pH, and oxygen saturation.

We conducted a trial to study the efficacy of BiPAP in the treatment of ARF due to ACPE with special reference to:

1. Clinical and ABG improvement
2. Successful avoidance of endotracheal intubation
3. Comparison of Responders and non-responders to BiPAP

Materials and methods

This single centre, prospective, uncontrolled study was carried out between April 1999 and October 2000 at the Critical Care Center, Prayag Hospital, Pune, India. All the patients admitted with ARF due to ACPE were admitted to our ICU during the study period. On admission to the ICU, a detailed clinical examination, baseline ABG analysis, electrocardiogram, and a chest X-ray were obtained, to judge the patient's need for mechanical ventilation (MV). Appropriate medical management in the form of diuretics, vasodilators, angio-tensin converting enzyme (ACE) inhibitors, and inotropes was instituted im-mediately. Patients having severe respiratory distress evidenced by

- NYHA grade IV dyspnea,
- accessory muscle over activity,
- paradoxical breathing,
- respiratory rate 30/min

or ABG showing evidence of ARF (pH 7.30 or PCO_2 40 mmHg) were imme-diately considered for MV.

   Of these patients who were ventilated, those who showed evidence of any of the following signs

- cardiac or respiratory arrest,
- systolic BP 90 mmHg,
- uncontrolled arrhythmia,
- excessive respiratory secretions
- encephalopathy

were ventilated invasively after endotracheal intubation. Remaining patients who did not fulfil any of the above-mentioned criteria were ventilated non--invasively with BiPAP. After stabilization of the patient, a careful search was made for the cause of ACPE. Other etiological factors in the decompensation of these patients were also looked for. At the earliest, a bedside two-dimensional echocardiography was performed by an experienced cardiologist. Patients who were ventilated with BiPAP and found to have any concomitant medical problems contributing to the development of ARF (e.g., COPD, bronchial asthma, pneumonia, septicemia, neuromuscular disorders, etc.) were excluded from this study. Continuous clinical and pulse oximetric monitoring was performed by an experienced ICU physician and nursing staff to detect the need for intubation at the earliest. Clinical parameters and ABG were documented over 3 h duration. Patients who met any of the following predetermined intubation criteria were intubated and mechanically ventilated.

Pre-determined criteria for intubation of NIPPV patients

Major criteria

1. Cardiac/respiratory arrest
2. Deteriorating levels of consciousness
3. Hemodynamic instability
   a) Hypotension ≤ 90 mmHg
   b) Uncontrolled arrhythmias

Minor criteria

1. Respiratory rate (RR) ≥ 35/min or respiratory fatigue
2. Persistent respiratory acidosis
3. Drop in PO_2 below 60 mmHg despite NIPPV
4. Encephalopathy appearing on NIPPV

Monitoring during NIPPV

A ventilatory support system with monitoring facility (BiPAP-VISION model S/T by Respironics, USA) was used for our trial. Thus our trial tested the efficacy of BiPAP as a modality of NIPPV. This ventilator measures the following patient parameters on per-breath basis.
- Actual inspiratory positive airway pressure (IPAP) delivered;
- Actual expiratory positive airway pressure (EPAP) delivered;
- Estimated tidal volume (V_T)
- Estimated leak

A consultant was present at the bedside for the initial instrument set up and subsequent titration of IPAP, EPAP, rise time, and FIO_2. Initial IPAP setting was 15 cmH$_2$O and was titrated with patient comfort, hemodynamic parameters, and pulse oximetry. Initial EPAP setting of 5 cmH$_2$O was used. Initial FIO_2 setting was 1, but was later altered by the attending consultant as per the response. A tight fitting full-face mask was fitted to the patient's face with Velcro straps and its position was adjusted as per the leak shown and the patient comfort. All the patients were repeatedly reassured by the nursing staff and ICU physician. Tidal volume and minute ventilation were noted continuously.

The patients were closely monitored for changing levels of consciousness, signs of hypoxia or hypercarbia, and also for possible complications of NIPPV, i.e., facial skin necrosis, gastric distension, eye congestion, hypotension, or any other.

Discontinuation of BiPAP

- Avoidance of endotracheal intubation for ventilatory assistance throughout the trial was considered as "success" of BiPAP.
- The need to intubate and invasively ventilate the patient at any point of time during NIPPV was taken as a "failure" of BiPAP.

In patients who were treated successfully with BiPAP, weaning was attempted once clinical stability was achieved, as seen by any of the following signs:
- reduction in heart rate by 25% or more,
- respiratory rate 25/min,
- absence of respiratory distress,
- $SaO_2 > 90$ % with $FIO_2 < 0.5$.

During weaning, IPAP and FIO_2 were gradually reduced and then discontinued. When BiPAP was discontinued, oxygen was provided with face mask.

Statistical analysis was carried out after noting the results in various groups and subgroups.

Results

During the period of our trial, 60 patients with ARF due to ACPE were admitted to our ICU. Of these, 45 needed ventilatory support. Of these 45 ventilated patients, 15 patients were intubated directly and ventilated invasively, as they fulfilled one of the criteria for intubation and ventilation; 30 patients were thus ventilated with BiPAP mode of NIPPV; 7 of these 30 patients were found to have one of the associated medical disorders (such as COPD, bronchial asthma, pneumonia, septicemia, neuromuscular disorders, etc.) that could have contributed to the ARF. These 7 patients were excluded from the study as our aim was to study efficacy of BiPAP in patients with ARF exclusively due to ACPE, without any other concomitant disease contributing to ARF. Thus, finally 23 patients with ARF purely due to ACPE were included in our study.

There were 12 males and 11 females. Mean age of patients was 66.2±12.3 years (range 33-87 years). Table 1 shows the various causes for ACPE in our patients. Most common underlying etiologies were acute myocardial infarction (AMI) in 9 patients, ischemic heart disease without acute MI (ischemia) in 9 patients, valvular heart disease (VHD) in 3, myocarditis in 1, and accelerated hypertension (AH) in 1.

Table 1 Etiological diagnosis and outcome

Etiology	Number	Percentage	Weaned	Intubated
AMI	9	39.13	5	4
VHD	3	13.04	2	1
Myocarditis	1	4.34	1	0
AH	1	4.34	1	0
Ischemia	9	39.13	9	0
Total	23	100	18 (78.26%)	5 (21.74%)

Table 2 shows the comparison of pre-trial and post-trial values of important hemodynamic and biochemical parameters. Mean heart rate (HR) reduced from 113.7 ± 14.84 to 99.3 ± 17.38 and RR decreased from 33 ± 4.8 to 22.2 ± 2.7 at the end of 3 h. Post-trial pH and PO_2 improved significantly. Mean pH increased from 7.29 ± 0.07 to 7.36 ± 0.01 and mean PO_2 increased from 72.61 ± 18.8 to 151.08 ± 65.52. Mean PCO_2 reduced from 36.91 ± 16.8 to 30.32 ± 8.62.

Table 2 Comparison of pre-trial and post-trial parameters (*MAP* mean arterial pressure)

Parameter	Pre-trial values (mean±SD)	Post-trial values (mean ± SD)
HR (per min)	113.7±14.84	99.3±17.38
RR (per min)	33±5.8	22.2±2.7
MAP (mmHg)	102±24.7	86.26±17.43
PH	7.29±0.07	7.36±0.01
PO_2 (mmHg)	72.61±18.8	151.08±65.52
PCO_2 (mm Hg)	36.91±16.8	30.32±8.62

In all patients, EPAP was kept at 5 cm and mean IPAP used was 21.5cm±3.8, i.e., mean pressure support was 16.5±3.8cm. Mean FIO_2 used was 0.76 ±0.11. Eighteen patients (78.26%) were weaned off BiPAP in a mean duration of 36.27±24.82 h (range 6-120 h). Five patients (21.74%) were intubated as they met one or more pre-defined intubation criteria, in a mean duration of 17.6±14.21 h (range: 3-45 h).All these 5 patients expired later; 4 of them died of persistent cardiac failure and 1 succumbed to resistant ventricular tachycardia. There was no mortality in the successfully weaned patients and all of them were discharged from the hospital.

Table 3 shows a comparison of the pre-trial hemodynamic and ABG parameters between success and failure groups.

Table 3 Comparison of various parameters in success and failure group of patients

Pre-trial parameters	Weaned (success) group 18 patients	Intubated (failure) group 5 patients	P value
HR (per min)	104.4 ± 20.75	117.9 ± 18.86	> 0.05 NS
RR (per min)	33.66 ± 5.15	31.2 ± 9.01	> 0.05 NS
MAP (mmHg)	100.48 ± 26.65	91.4 ± 27.32	> 0.05 NS
pH	7.29 ± 0.07	7.33 ± 0.09	> 0.05 NS
PO$_2$ (mmHg)	71.73 ± 21.26	75.8±7.50	> 0.05 NS
PCO$_2$ (mmHg)	37.12 ±13.32	36.34 ± 9.51	> 0.05 NS
2-D Echo (LVEF %)[a]	**37.11± 10.15**	**25 ±7.07**	**<0.05 S***

[a] 2 D echo examination was not performed before starting BiPAP, but at some point during first 3 h of BiPAP ventilation)
* Statistically significant

Unpaired t-test was applied to the two groups. Success group and failure group matched well for their pre-trial hemodynamic and ABG status (P > 0.05) and their difference was not statistically significant. However, two-dimensional echocardiographic ejection fraction (LVEF) of the success group was 37.11 ± 10.5 % and that of the failure group 25 ± 7.07 %. This difference was statistically significant (P< 0.05).

The patients were also analyzed for success rate according to etiology of ACPE. Table 4 shows that the success rate of NIPPV was significantly high in the non-AMI group compared with the AMI group.

Table 4 Comparison of outcome in two subgroups

	AMI	Non-AMI	Total
Success	5	13	18
Failure	4	1	5
Total	9	14	23

Table 5 shows the comparison of AMI and non-AMI groups regarding the pre-trial hemodynamic and biochemical parameters. These were well matched in both groups and statistically not significant (P > 0.05).

Table 5 Comparison of various parameters in AMI and non-AMI groups

Pre-trial parameter	AMI (9 patients) (mean±SD)	Non-AMI (14 patients) (mean±SD)	P value
HR (per min)	108.66 ± 21.2	1118.61 ± 18.19	> 0.05
MAP (mmHg)	98.77 ± 25.38	104 ± 28.05	> 0.05
RR (per min)	31.55 ± 5.81	34 ± 3.81	> 0.05
I PAP (cmH$_2$O)	20.66 ± 3.08	22.14 ± 4.25	> 0.05
pH	7.32 ± 0.08	7.28 ± 0.07	> 0.05
PCO$_2$ (mmHg)	34.68 ± 10.90	38.35 ± 13.46	> 0.05
PO$_2$ (mmHg)	72.45± 24.21	76.87 ± 20.45	> 0.05

Table 6 shows the results of the subgroup analysis of the AMI patients and the non-AMI patients who were successfully ventilated or otherwise by their LVEF. All 9 patients with LVEF > 35% were in the success group. Of the 14 patients with LVEF < 35%, 9 (64%) were successfully weaned, whereas 5 (36%) required intubation and invasive MV. These failures were more common in the AMI group than the non-AMI group.

Table 6 Comparison of AMI and non-AMI with respect to ejection fraction and outcome

Outcome	AMI		Non-AMI	
	LVEF ≤ 35 %	LVEF > 35 %	LVEF ≤ 35 %	LVEF >35 %
Weaned	2	3	7	6
Intubated	4	0	1	0
Total	6	3	8	6

Of the 23 patients, 4 developed facial erosion at the mask/skin interface; 2 patients had abdominal distension that needed nasogastric decompression; 1 patient had eye congestion due to air blast leaking through the mask/face interface. Besides these minor complications, all patients tolerated NIPPV very well. No patient needed to be intubated because of intolerance to NIPPV.

Discussion

We conducted this study to evaluate the outcome of patients with severe cardiogenic pulmonary oedema treated with BiPAP and to identify the determinants of success and failure of treatment with BiPAP, if any. Patients with ACPE who had developed ARF were screened for suitability for NIPPV or invasive MV at the outset. Amongst those who were ventilated with the BiPAP mode of NIPPV, we excluded all patients in whom concomitant medical disorders could have affected or contributed to the ARF. The effect of BiPAP in ARF "purely" or "exclusively" due to ACPE could thus be studied.

In this study we evaluated the patients for two end points: (1) short-term (3-h) improvement with BiPAP and (2) efficacy of BiPAP in avoiding endotracheal intubation.

One of the most-important mechanisms by which NIPPV relieves respiratory distress is by reducing work of breathing [1, 11, 17]. This was apparent in our study. Mean pre-trial HR of 113.7 ± 14.84/min settled to 99.3 ± 17.38/min. and mean RR decreased from 33 ± 5.8/min to 22.2 ± 2.7/min. Studies in the past have shown that NIPPV relieves distress and improves oxygenation within 30-45 min [4, 10]. But we chose a longer duration of 3 h, as we found that in some of our patients the initial period was taken up with adjustment of face mask, reassuring the patient, titration, and achieving the most comfortable and effective level of IPAP and FIO_2. Thus we evaluated the post-trial hemodynamic and ABG parameters at the end of 3 h. Respiratory distress that was evident before starting BiPAP was much relieved in all patients at the end of 3 h. Pre-trial pH increased remarkably from 7.29 ± 0.07 to 7.36 ± 0.01 and PO_2 increased from 72.61 ± 18.8 to 151.08 ± 65.52. NIPPV recruits atelectatic lung units and reduces intrapulmonary shunting, resulting in minimizing ventilation/perfusion mismatch and better oxygenation of blood [10, 18]. Reduction in PCO_2 from 36.91 ± 16.8 to 30.32 ± 8.62 was not as impressive as seen by Brochard et al. [4] and Meduri et al. [5]. This was perhaps because we used more-strict exclusion criteria, and excluded patients who had overlapping medical problems like COPD. This meant that the ARF was caused purely by ACPE and not contributed to by any other co-existing medical problems. The other reason could be a lower threshold of the staff to use NIPPV before fatigue had set in. Thus all our patients had mainly hypoxic ARF and not hypercapnic ARF, as in the other studies. Our study indicates that BiPAP does improve oxygenation status in addition to its well-documented role in hypercapnoeic ARF.

In 70-90% of ARF patients of mixed etiology in various studies, NIPPV has been shown to contribute to the avoidance of endotracheal intubation [4, 5, 7]. NIPPV not only improves short-term oxygenation but also helps in reversing ACPE by reducing pre-load and afterload [19], augmenting left ventricular ejection fraction and cardiac output [20], and reducing pulmonary artery pressure [21]. In our study, 18 of 23 patients (78.26%) with ACPE were successfully treated with BiPAP, obviating the need for endotracheal intubation.

It is noteworthy that despite this being a group of patients with only cardiac etiology of ARF and no overlapping or co-existing medical conditions, the success rate was similar to the previous studies of ARF due to ACPE where such strict exclusions were not applied [12-15].

In our study, pre-trial hemodynamic and ABG parameters were statistically well matched in success and failure groups, as shown in Table 3. The only variable that was different was LVEF on two-dimensional echocardiography. (25 ± 7.07% in failure group and 37.11±10.15% in success group). This difference was statistically significant (P <0.05). We could not find any analysis of the efficacy of NIPPV based on LVEF variability in any of the previous studies. Thus this is an important observation, which could indicate not only the overall outcome, but also the success of NIPPV as a modality. Interestingly 4 of the 5 patients in the failure group died of resistant cardiac failure despite intubation, invasive MV, and other treatment for heart failure. Thus, they were probably cases of irreversible or resistant cardiac failure, as also indicated by their low LVEF. None of the other variables, i.e., pH, PO_2, PCO_2, or hemodynamic parameters, assessed before the trial could predict the success or failure of NIPPV.

Mehta et al. [16] compared CPAP and BiPAP in the treatment of ACPE. ABG improvement and avoidance of endotracheal intubation was well documented in both groups. Their trial was terminated prematurely as 10 of 14 patients developed AMI in the BiPAP group. But there was no clear explanation of whether AMI was present on admission, caused the ACPE in the first place and was only diagnosed later, or whether it occurred during/due to BiPAP ventilation. Moreover, the diagnosis of AMI was made purely on the basis of raised cardiac enzymes. The link between AMI and NIPPV has left some unanswered questions. Rusterholtz et al. [13] also reported that 4 of the 5 patients in the BiPAP failure group had AMI as a cause of ACPE versus only 2 of the 21 in the BiPAP success group. In his editorial comment on the use of NIPPV in ACPE, Wysocki [6] therefore suggested that ACPE due to AMI is probably not a good indication for NIPPV. Conversely, ACPE due to other cardiac etiologies reverses rapidly on NIPPV and these are good indications for NIPPV. We therefore analyzed the two subgroups in our study, i.e., ACPE due to AMI and ACPE due to non-AMI etiologies. Of 9 patients with AMI, 4 failed the NIPPV trial and had to be intubated, while only 1 of 14 patients in the non--AMI group failed NIPPV and required intubation and invasive ventilation. These results clearly showed a higher failure rate in the AMI group.

When we further stratified these groups using a LVEF ≤35% cutoff limit, it was observed that all the 3 patients in AMI group with LVEF >35% were treated successfully with BiPAP. However, of the 6 patients in AMI group who had

LVEF < 35%, 4 patients needed intubation and only 2 patients were weaned successfully. The lone failure in the non-AMI group was the patient who had LVEF < 35%. These results indicate that even in the AMI group, patients with LVEF < 35% had poorer outcome than patients with AMI with LVEF > 35%.

Although this is an uncontrolled study with a relatively small patient cohort, we raise the possibility of using LVEF, assessed by two-dimensional echocardiography, as a parameter to predict the success or failure of NIPPV in patients with ARF due to ACPE, especially due to AMI. In our study the subgroup of AMI as a cause of ACPE with LVEF < 35% had a success rate of 33.33% (2 of 6 patients), while the AMI subgroup with LVEF > 35% had a success rate of 100% (3 of 3 patients). Thus we agree with the suggestion of Wysocki [6] that ACPE due to AMI is not a good indication for NIPPV, but we feel that an echocardiographic evaluation for LVEF should be performed before deciding the ventilatory modality (invasive or NIPPV). This is due to the observations that a subgroup of ACPE due to AMI with low LVEF is unlikely to respond to NIPPV and probably should be intubated and conventionally ventilated. In contrast, in the subgroup of ACPE due to AMI with higher LVEF; a cautious NIPPV trial may be worthwhile. All patients with AMI may thus not be rejected from receiving NIPPV. As recommended by the consensus conference, a randomized, well-controlled trial with a larger patient population is needed to clarify these issues [22].

Conclusions

- NIPPV with BiPAP was a safe and effective ventilatory modality in avoiding endotracheal intubation in patients with ARF due to ACPE, if chosen in appropriate patients.
- The subgroup of ACPE due to AMI had higher incidence of failure of BiPAP.
- Patients with LVEF < 35% had a significantly poorer outcome and higher rate of failure of NIPPV compared with those having LVEF >35%.
- ACPE patients with AMI as an etiology and especially with low LVEF need to be studied further to define the benefits and risks of NIPPV with BiPAP.

References

1. Brochard L, Esabey D, Piquet J, et al (1990) Reversal of acute exacerbation of COPD by inspiratory assistance with a face mask. N Engl J Med 323:1523-1530
2. Meduri GU, Conoscenti CC, Menashe P, et al (1991) Noninvasive face mask mechanical ventilation in patients with acute hypercapnic respiratory failure. Chest 100:445-454
3. Wysocki M, Tric L, Wolff MA, et al (1993) Noninvasive pressure support ventilation in patients with acute respiratory failure. Chest 103:907-913
4. Brochard L, Mancebo J, Wysocki M, et al (1995) Noninvasive ventilation for acute exacerbation of COPD. N Engl J Med 333:817-822
5. Meduri GU, Turner R, Abou-Shala N, et al (1996) Noninvasive positive pressure ventilation via face mask. Chest 109:179-193
6. Wysocki M (1999) Noninvasive ventilation in acute cardiogenic pulmonary oedema: better than continuous positive airway pressure? Intensive Care Med 25:1-2
7. Kramer N, Meyer T, Mehrang J, et al (1995) Randomised prospective trial of NIPPV in acute respiratory failure. Am J Respir Crit Care Med 151:1799-1806
8. Abou-Shala N, Meduri GU (1996) Noninvasive mechanical ventilation in patients with acute respiratory failure. Crit Care Med 24:705-715
9. Hillberg RE, Johnson DC (1997) Noninvasive ventilation. N Engl J Med 337:1746-1752
10. Popnick J, Renston J, Bennet R, et al (1999) Use of ventilatory support system (BIPAP) for acute respiratory failure in the emergency department. Chest 116:166-171
11. Renston, DiMarco, Supinski (1994) Respiratory muscle rest using BIPAP ventilation in patients with stable severe COPD. Chest 105:1053-1060
12. Hoffman B, Welte T (1999) The use of noninvasive pressure support ventilation for severe respiratory insufficiency due to pulmonary oedema. Intensive Care Med 25:15-20
13. Rusterholtz T, Kempf J, Berton C, et al (1999) Noninvasive pressure support ventilation with face mask in patients with acute cardiogenic pulmonary oedema. Intensive Care Med 25:21-28
14. Bersten AD, Holt AW, Vedig AE, et al (1991) Treatment of severe cardiogenic pulmonary oedema with continuous positive airway pressure delivered by face mask. N Engl J Med 325: 1825-1830
15. Räsänen J, Heikkila J, Downs J, et al (1985) Continuous positive airway pressure by face mask in acute cardiogenic pulmonary oedema Am J Cardiol 55:296-300
16. Mehta S, Jay GD, Woolard RH, et al (1997) Randomised prospective trial of bilevel versus continuous positive air way pressure in acute pulmonary oedema. Crit Care Med 25:620-628
17. Katz JA, Marks JD, et al (1985) Inspiratory work with and without continuous positive airway pressure in patients with acute respiratory failure. Anesthesiology 63:598-607
18. Räsänen J, Vaisanen I, Heikkila J, et al (1985) Acute myocardial infarction complicated by left ventricular dysfunction and respiratory failure. The effects of continuous positive airway pressure. Chest 87:159-162
19. Bradley D, Holloway RM, McLaughlin PR, et al (1992) Cardiac output response to continuous positive airway pressure in congestive heart failure. Am Rev Respir Dis 145:377-382
20. Acosta B, Morrow L, Acosta F, et al (1999) Hemodynamic effects of BIPAP on patients with chronic congestive heart failure with systolic dysfunction. Chest 116:271s
21. Thorens JB, Ritz M, Reynard C, et al (1997) Hemodynamic and endocrinological effects of noninvasive mechanical ventilation in respiratory failure. Eur Respir J 10:2553-2559
22. Evans TW (2001) International consensus conferences in intensive care medicine: Non invasive positive pressure ventilation in acute respiratory failure. Intensive Care Med 27: 166-178

Emergency treatment of acute stroke

P.D. SCHELLINGER, T. STEINER, W. HACKE

Stroke is the third most-common cause of death in the industrialized nations, after myocardial infarction and cancer, and the single most-common reason for permanent disability [1]. Up to 85% of all strokes are of ischemic origin and mostly due to blockage of a cerebral artery by a blood clot [2]. Emergency brain resuscitation in acute cerebrovascular disease (CVD), as well as the initial clinical and neurological evaluation, in general take place in the emergency room setting. The definitive discrimination between ischemic stroke, intracerebral hemorrhage (ICH), and subarachnoid haemorrhage (SAH) is made by neuroradiological examinations. Once ICH has been ruled out, the etiology of ischemic stroke can be determined by several ancillary tests that are described in detail elsewhere [3].

The therapeutic nihilism concerning ischemic stroke is definitely not justified. Every acute stroke patient has to be recognized as severely ill, irrespective of severity of symptoms [4]. Of course, only a minority of patients are in a life--threatening condition, here more frequently patients with ICH. Nevertheless there are often underlying conditions such as cardiac disease (infarction, insufficiency, arrhythmias), hypo- or hypertension, renal disease, diabetes, electrolyte imbalances, dehydration, and the possibility of impending intracranial hypertension, and progression of infarct. Time is of uttermost importance in brain resuscitation and diagnosis of ischemic stroke, as the time window for causal treatment of patients with acute brain infarction, i.e., systemic/intravenous or local/intraarterial thrombolysis with rt-PA (rsp prourokinase or urokinase) is as narrow as 3-6 h, rarely more in individual patients [5-7]. Accordingly, a new urgency for immediate treatment has developed during the past years – the decade of the brain – so that all initial measures taken, including clinical examination, information about patient history, and the organization of further diagnostic procedures and consecutive specific treatment should happen simultaneously rather than in sequence. The selection of special treatment strategies may already be ongoing before the final decision for therapy of the subtype of stroke has been made. Speed and rapid decision making are essential.

Initial evaluation in the emergency room

All of the following may also be implemented into the preclinical stage if feasible. The initial assessment of a patient with presumed stroke includes pulmonary function, heart rate (HR), and blood pressure (BP), pupillary reaction, and vigilance. Minimum monitoring consists of pulse oximetry, continuous recording of electroencephalogram (at least one lead), and repeated measurements of BP. Simultaneously two peripheral venous lines are inserted. A central venous catheter (CVC) or the femoral vein route only are indicated when antebrachial veins are not accessible. Introduction of a CVC is time consuming and risky if applied in a hurry or by an inexperienced physician [8]. Moreover, one has to take into account that in an emergency situation all drugs can be given via a large-bore cubital vein cannula. With insertion of a venous line, blood samples for an instant blood glucose test, clinical chemistry, coagulation assays, and hematology studies are drawn. Until the arrival of the laboratory results, standard electrolyte solutions (isotonic saline, Ringer's lactate, etc.) are given. Several stopcocks should be applied to the venous cannulas to give direct access for not only infusions but also i.v. injections and "flush in injections" with normotonic saline. If deemed necessary, an arterial blood gas sample is taken. Easiest and therefore fastest access is the femoral artery.

After having approached the stroke patient with the ABC rule, a closer evaluation of airways, breathing, and pulmonary function may become necessary. Pulse oximetry is a useful and fast applicable tool to detect ventilatory distress. In ischemic stroke, however, unstable airways and breathing abnormalities are rare. Exceptions are large hemispheric infarctions middle cerebral artery [(MCA) or MCA/arterior cerebral artery (ACA)], vertebrobasilar territory infarctions, sustained seizure activity, and of course ICH, which has not been ruled out at this point of the patient management. Some patients with acute MCA or inferior cerebral artery (ICA) infarction may have breathing abnormalities due to neurogenic ventilatory dysfunction, loss of protective reflexes with danger of aspiration or neurogenic pulmonary edema [2, 9]. One has to take into account that there are also pre-existing extracerebral conditions, such as chronic obstructive lung disease (COLD), cardiac insufficiency, asthma etc., that predispose to ventilatory distress and may exacerbate during acute stroke. Furthermore, it is known that oxygen saturations slightly above 90%, which are in general considered to be sufficient, do not necessarily reflect the situation in the brain, where especially in the deep white matter there may be profound hypercarbia and hypoxemia [10]. Therefore we recommend the application of a nasal tube with 4–6 l oxygen per minute, which generally suffices to keep oxygen saturation within 95-100% and is an easy way to improve oxygenation without any side effects. With a pathological breathing pattern, severe hypoxemia or hypercarbia, danger of aspiration, or progressive loss of vigilance, early endotracheal intubation is recommended. The decision whether to intubate and ventilate a patient should take into consideration his age, medical condition before stroke, extent of brain injury, deficits to be expected on survival, and of course the presumed will of the patient. Many neurologists have never considered stroke patients to be candidates for intubation and ventilation, except for those electively intubated for angiography or operation [11], our own data show a 1-year survival rate of almost one-third of the intubated patients as well as an improved Barthel and Rankin score in the survivors [12].

Blood glucose levels must be measured in every patient with suspected stroke [13, 14]. Hyperglycemia in stroke leads to increased formation of lactic acid, drop in pH, accumulation of other metabolites, and worsens neuronal damage, although hypoglycemia also seems to worsen stroke [15, 16]. The aim therefore should be to normalize blood glucose into a range of 100 mg/dl – 200 mg/dl, high-osmolarity glucose solutions (40%) should be avoided in acute stroke [17]. It should be borne in mind that glucocorticoids and catecholamines, whether endogenous or exogenous also raise blood glucose levels via increased glucose formation and increased peripheral insulin resistance [18]. Fever commonly is present in acute stroke, whether of infectious origin, altered cerebral mechanisms of temperature control, dehydration, or for other reasons. Experimental [19] as well as clinical data show that a raised temperature of even 0.5°C is associated with poor outcome in ischemic stroke [20-22]. Azzimondi et al. [23] found in 78 patients with stroke and fever that a rise in body temperature of equal to or higher than 37.9° C was an independent risk factor for a worse prognosis in stroke, with an odds ratio of 3.4. Patients who have fever in acute stroke should be treated with antipyretics like acetaminophen or metamizole (beware drop in BP). Also in the first few days after stroke, the body temperature should be kept within a normal range, either by physical measures, e.g., cooling blankets, intravascular cooling devices, or causal therapy, e.g., antibiotics in infection.

After the emergency assessment, a targeted neurological examination has to be performed. Cardiovascular risk factors, prothrombotic premedications, such as birth control pills, and history of trauma or migraine, as well as antithrombotics such as warfarin, aspirin, or clopidogrel may give important clues. Rare causative factors like drug use, multi-system disease (vasculitis), or postpartum state should be considered. Auscultation and palpation of heart and peripheral pulses, with special regard to subclavian and carotid bruits, orientating check of all other organ systems, and BPs of *both* arms in suspected vertebrobasilar disease are assessed. Funduscopic examination may reveal signs of general

vascular disease, like hyaline plaques, cholesterol, or other emboli. Pharmacological pupil dilation should never be used in acute stroke, as the early signs of
brainstem compromise, like loss of pupillary reaction or mydriasis, cannot be
seen. The extent and nature of the neurological examination varies between
patients. The unconscious patient may be assessed using the Glasgow Coma
Scale (GCS), primitive reflexes (Babinski), and brain stem reflexes/cranial
nerve function (pupillary light reaction, corneal reflex, deviation of gaze,
oculocephalic reflex) [24]. Noxious stimuli like pinching the skin of the
proximal arm and vigorous pressure to the nailbeds, as well as other verbal or
tactile stimulation, are used [24]. By attending carefully to the patient's responses, the presence of a hemiparesis or hemisensory loss may be elicited. Abnormal posturing gives a clue to the extent of brainstem compromise. Meningism
can be tested the same way as in the wake patient, and an increase in neck
muscle tone evaluated by placing a hand under the occipit and flexing the head
forward. The National Institutes of Health Stroke Scale (NIHSS) is a useful
tool for the neurological evaluation of the awake patient [25]. The examination
can be performed rapidly within 5 to 10 min, is easy to perform for non-neuro-
logists, and has a good inter-rater reliability [26]. At this point it still has to be
kept in mind that it is impossible to differentiate between ICH and ischemic
stroke. No treatment that might be of potential hazard to either disease, i.e., ICH
and ischemia, should be initiated before a computed tomography (CT) scan or
stroke magnatic resonance imaging (MRI) has been performed.

Stroke imaging

In spite of discouraging reports that CT cannot demonstrate ischemic tissue
changes during the first 12 h after symptom onset [27, 28], it has been generally
accepted in the academic stroke community that CT can demonstrate early
infarct signs within the first 2-6 h after stroke. The reported sensitivity of early
CT findings ranges from 12% to 92%, depending on the infarct signs, the exact
time window of the investigated population, and on the authors. The most-
-common early infarct sign is a frequently subtle grey matter and/or cortical
hypodensity [29-32]. Other early infarct signs include the loss of the insular
ribbon [33], sulcal effacement due to early edema in 12-41% of stroke patients
[29-31, 34], and the hyperdense MCA sign (HMCAS) in 40-60% of patients
with angiographically proven MCA occlusion [26, 35-37]. More-recent studies
have reported incidences of early CT signs of infarction between 53% and 92%
within the first 6 h for all acute stroke patients [29-31, 34, 35, 38]. There is an
association between the size of early hypodensities and the risk of a secondary

hemorrhage [39] and clinical outcome, as early parenchymal hypodensity of more than 50% of the MCA territory is associated with a mortality of up to 85% [35]. ECASS I and II showed that in patients with a small area of hypoattenuation (<33% of the MCA territory), treatment increased the chance of a good clinical outcome, while rt-PA in patients with a large area of hypoattenuation (>33% of the MCA territory) had no benefit but increased the risk for a fatal brain haemorrhage [30]. While several studies have shown the usefulness of early CT findings in selecting patients before intravenous thrombolytic therapy, other studies demonstrated that physicians, including general radiologists and neurologists, do not uniformly achieve a sufficient level of sensitivity for identifying CT contraindications for thrombolytic therapy [40]. However, radiologists can be trained to recognize early infarct signs on CT, and the positive effect of being trained to read CT scans of hyperacute stroke patients has recently been demonstrated in a large trial [31]. CT angiography (CTA) can provide additional information on stenoses or occlusions in the basal arteries of the brain [41], as non-ionic contrast material does not affect infarction volume or worsen the symptoms of cerebral ischaemia [42]. In addition to the assessment of a major vessel occlusion, CTA has the potential to deliver information about the quality of the collateral circulation, as contrast enhancement in arterial branches beyond the occlusion occurs in those patients [41, 43]. Volume CT scanners may produce images that can be used to construct functional maps of cerebral blood volume, cerebral blood flow, or time to peak enhancement, utilizing a first-pass curve of a contrast bolus [44]. However, at present only one slice and not images of the whole brain can be obtained.

The need for an all-round diagnostic tool with which all the important pathophysiological aspects of hyperacute stroke can be investigated is evident. Such a method must answer five decisive questions: (1) Where and how large is the actual area of irreversible ischaemic brain damage? (2) How old is the infarction? (3) Is there tissue at risk and how much tissue is at risk? (4) Is there a vessel occlusion and where is it? (5) Is an ICH or another underlying, non-ischemic disease present? Currently, the decision to initiate i.v. rt-PA treatment is based on clinical findings and CT scanning. The reported diagnostic yield of CT within 3 h after symptom onset does not adequately meet these criteria [45]. The advent of new MRI techniques such as perfusion- (PWI) and diffusion- (DWI) weighted imaging has revolutionized diagnostic imaging in stroke [46, 47]. DWI may delineate infarcted brain tissue in less than 1 h after symptom onset, probably within minutes [48], although there is cumulating evidence that in the very early stage of stroke there may be reversible DWI changes [49, 50], while PWI defines the area of cerebral hypoperfusion. The absolute volume difference or ratio of PWI and DWI reveals the ischemic tissue potentially at risk of irreversible infarction [51, 52]. MRA can reliably assess the cerebral vessel status [53]. Stroke MRI further allows a definitive diagnosis of ICH within the first hours of stroke [54-56] and possibly also that of SAH [57]. Several studies have reported early findings of stroke MRI within the first 6-12 h, demonstrating the feasibility and practicality of this method in the setting of acute stroke and thrombolytic therapy [47, 51, 58-63]. In essence, the presence of a vessel occlusion according to MRA is associated with a PWI/DWI mismatch, the stroke MRI setting that defines the ideal candidate for thrombolysis [61, 64]. In addition, there are five studies that clearly demonstrate that early recanalization achieved by thrombolysis results in significantly smaller infarcts and a significantly better clinical outcome [50, 51, 61, 63, 65]. Although presently limited by a low availability, the utility of stroke MRI is likely to lie in the early identification of those patients in whom outcome and final infarct size, ultimately the patient's fate, have not yet been determined. Furthermore, cost effectiveness is likely as there is no need for CT or Doppler ultrasonography in the hyperacute stage of stroke. With an increasing distribution and "around the clock" availability of stroke MRI, the identification of patients more suitable for thrombolytic therapy, and those who are not, may lead to an increased benefit and a reduction in complications in patients receiving thrombolytic therapy [61]. Furthermore, the rather strictly defined therapeutic window may be qualified and individualized according to the findings in each individual patient.

Thrombolytic therapy

After introduction of thrombolytic therapy for the treatment of acute myocardial infarction in the early 1990s, The GUSTO Angiographic Investigators major trials for the evaluation of this new therapeutic approach to ischemic stroke were initiated. Occlusion of a brain vessel leads to a critical reduction in cerebral perfusion and, within minutes, to ischemic infarction with a central infarct core of irreversibly damaged brain tissue and a more or less large area of hypoperfused but still vital brain tissue (the ischemic penumbra), which can be salvaged by rapid restoration of blood flow. Therefore, the underlying rationale for the introduction and application of thrombolytic agents is the lysis of an obliterating thrombus and subsequent re-establishment of cerebral blood flow by cerebrovascular recanalization [66]. Proof of an occluded vessel by Doppler ultrasonography, CT, MR or digital subtraction angiography should be established, at least when i.v. thrombolysis is performed later than 3 h after symptom onset; however, it is not required yet for the indication of thrombolytic therapy.

Overall, the proverb "time is brain" holds true; therefore, a rapid workup of the patient who is a potential candidate for thrombolytic therapy is mandatory. The delivery of thrombolytic agents locally, at or within the occluding thrombus, has the advantage of providing a higher concentration of the particular thrombolytic agent where it is needed, while minimizing the concentration systemically. Hence, local intra-arterial thrombolysis has the potential for greater efficacy with regard to arterial recanalization rates and greater safety with regard to lower risk of hemorrhage. The technique involves performing a cerebral arteriogram, localizing the occluding clot, navigating a microcatheter to the site of the clot, and administering the lytic agent at or inside the clot with or without mechanical dissolution of the thrombus.

Meta-analyses of the ECASS I and II, NINDS, ATLANTIS trials [67, 68] assessed the benefit of rt-PA. In the first meta-analysis by Hacke et al. [67] ICH, the most-relevant complication of thrombolytic therapy, occurred significantly more often in patients receiving rt-PA (144/1,034 versus 43/1,010, OR 3.23, CI 2.39 – 4.37), and was slightly less increased in the 3-h time window than at the lower dosage (41/393 versus 15/389, OR 2.68, CI 1.56 – 4.62). There was no significant difference in mortality between rt-PA and placebo (OR 1.07, CI 0.84 – 1.36), but a slight trend towards a lower mortality in the 0.9 mg/kg and 3-h group (OR 0.91, 0.63 – 1.32). rt-PA, on the other hand, led to a 37% reduction in death and dependence, regardless of dose and time window (OR 0.63, CI 0.53 – 0.76). If treated with the lower dose and within 3 h, the chance of an unfavorable outcome was reduced by 45% (OR 0.55, CI 0.41 – 0.72). For every 1,000 patients treated with either dose there are 90 fewer patients who are dead or disabled but 96 hemorrhages more than expected with placebo. Conversely, for 1000 patients treated with 0.9 mg/kg and within 3 h, there are 65 additional ICH and 140 fewer patients dead or disabled. The NNT for all doses and time windows is 11; for the 3-hour and 0.9 mg/kg group it is 7. These numbers are far better than the NNT for thrombolysis in myocardial infarctions, which is 30 – 40 [67]. Wardlaw et al. [68] included in their Cochrane Library meta-analysis all 17 randomized trials of thrombolysis with a total of 5,216 patients (2,889 of which were from rt-PA trials), regardless of time window, dosage, administration route, and substance. The main objectives were to show that thrombolytic therapy reduces the risk of late death, increases the risk of early and fatal ICH, and that the benefit at outcome (reduction of death and dependence) offsets any early hazard. Symptomatic and fatal ICH were significantly more common as a result of thrombolytic therapy (symptomatic ICH OR 3.53, CI 2.79 – 4.45, P < 0.000001; fatal ICH OR 4.15, CI 2.96 – 5.84). This translates into 70 additional instances of symptomatic ICH for patients receiving thrombolysis and 29 of 1,000 (OR 3.2) additional instances of fatal ICH in rt-PA patients, but

92 of 1,000 (OR 6.03) additional ICH in those patients receiving streptokinase as opposed to placebo. Despite this, thrombolytic therapy, administered up to 6 h after ischemic stroke, significantly reduced death or dependence at the end of follow-up (55.2% versus 59.7%, OR 0.83, CI 0.73-0.94, $P=0.0015$), which is equivalent to 44 fewer patients being dead or dependent per 1,000 treated (CI 15 – 73). For patients treated with rt-PA only, the OR was 0.79 (CI 0.68 – 0.92, $P=0.001$) or 57 deaths/dependence prevented per 1,000 patients treated (CI 20 – 93). An alternative endpoint analysis yields similar results for favorable versus unfavorable outcome (OR 0.79 for all patients and 0.76 for rt-PA patients). When treatment was given within 3 h after stroke onset, there was an even better risk reduction for dependency or death (55.2% versus 68.3%, OR 0.58, CI 0.46-0.74, $P=0.00001$) or 126 fewer dead or dependent patients per 1000 treated. The difference of benefit of rt-PA in the 0- to 3-h window or 3- to 6-h window was non-significant, but showed a trend towards better improvement with early therapy (OR 0.7 versus 0.76). The authors concluded that the significant increase in early death and fatal and non-fatal symptomatic ICH are offset by the significant reduction of disability in survivors. Therapy with rt-PA is associated with less risk and more benefit than with other substances.

Intra-arterial thrombolytic therapy of acute M1 and M2 occlusion with 9 mg /2 h significantly improves outcome if administered within 6 h after stroke onset. Seven patients need to be treated in order to prevent 1 patient from death or dependence. The higher rate of symptomatic ICH (10.2% in PROACT II versus 8.8% in ECASS II, 6.4% in NINDS and 7.2% in ATLANTIS) is very well explained by the far larger baseline severity of stroke in PROACT II (NIHSS of 17 in PROACT II versus 11 in ECASS II and ATLANTIS, and 14 in NINDS). According to the Cochrane meta-analysis, combining PROACT I and II data (34), there is a 0.55 OR (CI 0.31 – 1.00) for death or disability, an OR of 2.39 (CI 0.88 – 6.47) for early symptomatic ICH (7-10 days), and an OR of 0.75 (CI 0.4 – 1.42) for death from all causes at follow-up. Although recanalization rates may be superior with intra-arterial (66%) than with i.v. ($\approx$55%) thrombolysis, and may even be increased by careful mechanical disruption of a thrombus, in addition to the lytic effect of the drug, a limited availability of centers with 24 h a day / 7 days a week interventional neuroradiology service may restrict the use of this therapy. On the other hand, the clinically more-severe strokes may benefit even more from an intra-arterial than an i.v. approach. Furthermore, the time to eventual recanalization may be substantially shorter with intra-arterial thrombolysis. Another intra-arterial rpro-UK trial (PROACT III), which is partly stroke MRI based, to reduce the rate of screening angiography and optimize patient selection is underway.

Overall, thrombolysis with 0.9 mg/kg rt-PA for acute ischemic stroke within

6 h leads to an overall clinically significant effect in favor of treated patients, but is associated with an excess rate of symptomatic ICH, which does, however, not take effect on mortality. i.v. rt-PA (0.9 mg/kg, maximum of 90 mg) is therefore the recommended treatment within 3 h after onset of stroke symptoms. Thrombolytic therapy should be performed in centers experienced with the procedure. The benefit from the use of i.v. rt-PA for acute ischemic stroke beyond 3 h from onset of symptoms is lower, but definitely present in selected patients. The adjunctive use (and also the optimal time-point of use) of anti-thrombotic agents is still controversial, and at present no recommendation can be given with regard to concomitant administration of heparin or antiplatelet agents in the setting of thrombolytic therapy. i.v. rt-PA is not recommended when the time of onset of stroke cannot be ascertained reliably; this includes patients in whom strokes are recognized upon awakening. Intravenous administration of streptokinase for acute ischemic stroke is dangerous and not indicated. Data on the efficacy of any other i.v. thrombolytic drugs are not available such that a recommendation could be provided. A stroke MRI-based study on the efficacy of recombinant desmoteplase (DSPA, derived from saliva of the vampire bat *Desmodus rotundus*) for treatment of stroke in the 3- to 6-h time window is underway (DIAS=desmoplase in acute ischemic stroke). Finally, the benefits of arterial recanalization may be supplemented by neuronal protection (first protocol drafts underway), particularly when the two strategies are used simultaneously, and if they can be used very early following symptom onset. At present thrombolytic therapy is still underutilized. Among the major problems are that relatively few candidates meet the clinical and time criteria. Educating the general public to regard stroke as a treatable emergency and training emergency caregivers in the use of thrombolysis may decrease these problems. Healthcare institutions should be made aware of the potential in long-term cost savings, once stroke management is optimized and thrombolysis is more widely available. Patients and their relatives should be informed not only about the hazards of thrombolytic therapy, but also about its potential benefit and thus the risk of **not** being treated.

Malignant or space occupying MCA infarction

Patients with acute, nearly complete MCA or panhemispheric infarction may develop massive concomitant edema with significant midline shift or compression of the basal cisterns resulting in clinical signs of uncal herniation, a condition called "malignant" MCA infarction [69]. This syndrome is defined clinically and by means of CT scanning criteria. The patients are somewhat younger (about 10 years in average) than other stroke patients. Standard anti-edema treatment often fails to prevent herniation and brain death, which may occur in up to 80% of the cases [69].

It is quite uncommon that a patient with acute ischaemic stroke shows signs of raised intracarnial pressure (ICP) within the first 24 h, as the maximum of edema formation is reached around day 3 and 5 [17, 24, 70-72]. However complete MCA infarctions in young patients with small outer cerebraspinal fluid (CSF) spaces, an acute carotid T-occlusion, or extensive ICH may cause profound swelling and midline shift [2]. Initial clinical signs of elevated ICP are reduced vigilance, vomiting, and hiccups, and in the further course unilaterally or bilaterally dilated pupils with loss of pupillary response to light and loss of corneal reflex. If those signs are present, acute actions taken are intubation, if possible with thiopental for induction of anaesthesia, hyperventilation (PCO_2 28-32 mmHg), i.v. boluses of 20% mannitol 125 ml or Hyper Haes (NaCl 10% plus hydroxyethyl starch), or if not successful 10 ml TRIS buffer and as a last effort 250-500 mg thiopental. [73] If those immediate measures do not lead to normalization of pupillary reaction and corneal reflexes go on with resuscitation and try to perform a CCT scan as fast as possible to obtain information on the etiology of the stroke [2]. Usually these patients show a rapid decline in consciousness and develop the signs of herniation 2-4 days after onset of symptoms. Most patients require intubation and artificial ventilation. During the further clinical course, failure of medical treatment for elevated ICP occurs. Once the ICP has moved into critical values (20 mmHg or beyond), both clinical appearance and CT already show signs of herniation. Brain death usually occurs between days 2 and 5 after onset of stroke.

Moderate hypothermia (33 - 36°C) has been shown to reduce secondary brain injury and infarction size and to improve neurological outcome in animal models with both focal and global ischemia [74]. Most of the studies used a narrow time-window between 60 and 90 min. However, there are several clinical trials in head-injured patients that showed a significant reduction in ICP and cerebral blood flow, better neurological outcome, and limited secondary brain injury, although the time window varied between 6 and 16 h. The duration of hypothermia varied from 24 to 48 h, while neither the optimal duration of hypothermia nor the optimal time after the trauma for therapy in these patients could be identified [75]. Recently the first clinical trial on the use of moderate hypothermia in severe MCA infarction was published [76]. Hypothermia was induced with a mean of 14 h after the ischemic injury. Hypothermia was maintained over 72 h to overcome the maximum brain swelling, which is known to occur between days 2 and 5 after ischemia. All patients in this study fulfilled the criteria for diagnosis of a "malignant" MCA infarction. The mortality was only 44% and the survivors reached a favorable outcome with Barthel indices ranging from 60 to 85. Hypothermia significantly reduced the ICP. However, rewarming the patients constantly led to a secondary rise of ICP, which required additional ICP therapy with mannitol. In some cases it even exaggerated the initial ICP levels. This rebound after rewarming might be due to a proposed hypermetabolic response after induced hypothermia, as was described after cardiopulmonary bypass. A new series of patients indicates that a modified rewarming protocol seems to reduce ICP elevation, which occurs during and after rewarming. [77] Ventricular ectopy and fibrillation limit the extent of hypothermia, but this is known to occur only at temperatures below 30°C. In this study, pneumonia was the only severe side effect of moderate hypothermia. Other side effects of hypothermia, which have been shown in animal studies, are clotting abnormalities and coagulopathy. In men the enzymatic reactions of the coagulation cascade were shown to be strongly inhibited by hypothermia. Although an elevation of high serum amylase and lipase levels is frequently observed, the association between hypothermia and pancreatitis is poorly understood.

Although case series impressively show a dramatic reduction of mortality in patients with both cerebellar and hemispheric space-occupying infarction if decompressive surgery is performed, there are no controlled data to support its superiority. The rationale of decompressive surgery is to allow expansion of the edematous tissue away from the lateral ventricle, the diencephalon, and the mesencephalon to reduce ICP, to increase perfusion pressure, and to preserve cerebral blood flow by preventing further compression of the collateral vessels. These factors may help to increase cerebral blood flow in areas surrounding ischemic regions, thereby preventing further brain tissue necrosis. The hypothesis is supported by a recent experimental stroke study on the value of decompressive surgery [78, 79]. In human space-occupying hemispheric infarction, surgical treatment has been reported to lower mortality and improve the unfavorable outcome [80, 81]. It has been shown in a spherical model that the diameter of the craniectomy has to be at least 12 cm or more. The temporal bone should the resected to the skull base. The dura is opened and an adjusted, biconvex-shaped dural patch (lyophilized dura or homologous temporal fascia) is placed into the incision. In surviving patients an artificial bone flap is re--implanted 6-12 weeks after surgery. There is some controversy about whether infarcted tissue should be resected or not. There are some reports with positive results in outcome and neurological function [82]. However, since in acute stroke the margins of the infarction are poorly defined and the differentiation between definitely damaged tissue and the ischemic penumbra is not possible, we do not remove the ischemic tissue. Surgical complications include infections, subdural or epidural hematoma, space-occupying subdural CSF hygroma, and paradoxical herniation after the swelling period. Close clinical follow-up, including palpation of the trepanation site, ICP monitoring, and daily B-mode scanning of the affected hemisphere for detection of epidural or subdural blood and space-occupying effect on the lateral ventricle, may detect these events in time and prevent unfavorable outcome in these patients.

In the first Heidelberg trial, space-occupying MCA infarction was defined as massive supratentorial infarction involving the territory of the MCA or both MCA and ACA. The definition also included the dynamic aspect of the syndrome by including reversible signs of herniation: increasing space-occupying oedema with a midline shift of more than 10 mm at the septum pellucidum level documented on serial CT; 32 patients underwent surgery. The control group consisted of 21 patients with left hemispheric malignant MCA infarcts or of patients whose relatives did not give informed consent to perform the operation. Without surgery, 76% patients (16/21) with space-occupying hemispheric infarction died from herniation despite maximal conservative treatment. Only 5 patients survived, all of them moderately disabled. Mortality of the surgically treated group was significantly lower (32%, 11/32); 21 patients survived. Seven of the survivors were rated as severely disabled and dependent, while 14 of the surviving patients were independent and only mildly or moderately disabled. More than 80% reached a Barthel index of 60 or above. Of the left hemispheric patients, few only stayed with a complete global aphasia, all others have a severe Broca aphasia [80]. During the evaluation of the pilot study we realized that in some patients the intervention seemed to come too late. Furthermore, by looking at the CT scan, and the clinical course of the patients it seemed feasible to identify patients likely to develop malignant MCA infarct within the next 24-36 h. We therefore changed the protocol. We do not wait anymore for signs of reversible herniation. Surgery is performed as soon as the CT scan shows a complete MCA infarction leading to significant mass-effect with displacement of the lateral ventricle and midline shift, and if the patient's consciousness level is deteriorating. Using these entry criteria, the medium time of stroke onset to intervention dropped from 39 h to 21 h in the second part of the study. We included 31 patients in that trial. This approach lead to a further decrease of mortality to 16% (5/31). The number of independent or moderately disabled patients was 17 [81]. Both trials taken together, we observed 8 hemorrhages within the infarcted area, which did not require surgical intervention. Eight epidural bleedings occurred. They were all detected by daily B-mode ultrasound monitoring and easily evacuated. We did not have any deaths related to surgery in decompression for MCA infarction. Decompressive surgery should be performed early enough to prevent irreversible damage to adjacent brain structures. On the other hand, the procedure should not be performed too early to avoid the inclusion of patients who probably would not need decompressive surgery for survival. Early CT signs of infarction, initial clinical presentation, and angiographical or other information (TCD, MRA) about arterial occlusion site and state of collateral blood flow should be obtained. In Heidelberg we increasingly use dynamic MRI studies for early patient selection. The next prospective case series started in late 1998. Eleven patients are now included. New results will be available after 25 patients have been included. In the United States a NINDS-funded phase II trial (HEADDFIRST) will be launched in the near future. This trial will be a randomized controlled clinical trial.

References

1. WHO Task Force (1989) Stroke--1989. Recommendations on stroke prevention, diagnosis, and therapy. Report of the WHO Task Force on Stroke and other Cerebrovascular Disorders. Stroke 20:1407-1431
2. Hacke W, Steiner T, Schwab S (1996) Critical management of the acute stroke: medical and surgical therapy. In: Batjer HH, Caplan LR, Freiberg L, Greenlee RG Jr, Kopitnik TH, Jr, Young WL (eds) Cerebrovascular disease. Lippincott-Raven, Hagerstown, pp 523-533
3. Schellinger P, Steiner T (1998) Emergency and intensive-care treatment after a stroke. Recommendations of the European Consensus Group. Nervenarzt 69:530-539
4. Hacke W, Kaste M, Olsen TS, et al (2000) European Stroke Initiative (EUSI) recommendations for stroke management. Cerebrovasc Dis (in press)
5. Albers GW, Amarenco P, Easton JD, et al (2001) Anthithrombotic and thrombolytic therapy for ischemic stroke. Chest 119:300S-320S
6. Schellinger PD, Fiebach JB, Mohr A et al (2001) Thrombolytic therapy for ischemic stroke-A review. I. Intravenous thrombolysis. Crit Care Med 29:1812-1818
7. Schellinger PD, Fiebach JB, Mohr A, et al (2001) Thrombolytic therapy for ischemic stroke-A review. II. Intra-arterial thrombolysis, vertebrobasilar stroke, phase IV trials, and stroke imaging. Crit Care Med 29:1819-1825
8. Mansfield PF, Hohn DC, Fornage BD, et al (1994) Complications and failures of subclavian-vein catheterization. N Engl J Med 331:1735-1738
9. Schwarz S, Schwab S, Keller E, et al (1997) Neurogenic impairment of cardiopulmonary function in acute cerebral lesions. Nervenarzt 68:956-962
10. Kennealy JA, McLennan JE, Loudon RG, et al (1980) Hyperventilation induced cerebral hypoxia. Am Rev Respir Dis 122:407-412
11. Burtin P, Bollaert Pe, Feldmann L, et al (1994) Prognosis of stroke patients undergoing mechanical ventilation. Intensive Care Med 20:32-36
12. Steiner T, Mendoza G, De Georgia M, et al (1997) Prognosis of stroke patients requiring mechanical ventilation in a neurological critical care unit. Stroke 28:711-715
13. Pulsinelli WA, Waldman S, Sigsbee B (1980) Experimental hyperglycemia and diabetes mellitus worsen stroke outcome. Trans Am Neurol Assoc 105:21-24
14. Pulsinelli WA, Levy DE, Sigsbee B, et al (1983) Increased damage after ischemic stroke in patients with hyperglycemia with or without established diabetes mellitus. Am J Med 74: 540-544
15. Wagner KR, Kleinholz M, Courten Myers GM de, et al (1992) Hyperglycemic versus normoglycemic stroke: topography of brain metabolites, intracellular pH, and infarct size. J Cereb Blood Flow Metab 12:213-222

16. Hacke W, Stingele R, Steiner T, et al (1995) Critical care of acute ischemic stroke. Intensive Care Med 21:856-862
17. Ringleb P, Dörfler A, Hacke W (1996) Intensivmedizinische Behandlung der akuten zerebralen Ischämie. Intensivmedizin Notfallmedizin 33:307-315
18. Toni D, De Michele M, Fiorelli M et al (1994) Influence of hyperglycaemia on infarct size and clinical outcome of acute ischemic stroke patients with intracranial arterial occlusion. J Neurol Sci 123:129-133
19. Busto R, Dietrich WD, Globus MY-T, et al (1987) Small differences in intraischemic brain temperature critically determine the extent of ischemic injury. J Cereb Blood Flow Metab 7:729-738
20. Terent A, Andersson B (1981) The prognosis for patients with cerebrovascular stroke and transient ischemic attacks. Ups J Med Sci 86:63-74
21. Hindfelt B (1976) The prognostic significance of subfebrility and fever in ischaemic cerebral infarction. Acta Neurol Scand 53:72-79
22. Reith J, Jorgensen HS, Pedersen PM, et al (1996) Body temperature in acute stroke: relation to stroke severity, infarct size, mortality, and outcome. Lancet 347:422-425
23. Azzimondi G, Bassein L, Nonino F, et al (1995) Fever in acute stroke worsens prognosis. A prospective study. Stroke 26:2040-2043
24. Jannett B, Teasdale D, Braakmarz R (1979) Prognosis of patients with severe head injury. Neurosurgery 4:283-289
25. The National Institute of Neurological Disorders and Stroke rt-PA Stroke Study Group (1995) Tissue plasminogen activator for acute ischemic stroke. N Engl J Med 333:1581-1587
26. Tomsick T, Brott T, Barsan W, et al (1996) Prognostic value of the hyperdense middle cerebral artery sign and stroke scale score before ultraearly thrombolytic therapy. AJNR 17:1-7
27. Gilman S (1998) Imaging the brain. First of two parts. N Engl J Med 338:812-820
28. Gilman S (1998) Imaging the brain. Second of two parts. N Engl J Med 338:889-896
29. Kummer R von, Nolte PN, Schnittger H, et al (1996) Detectability of cerebral hemisphere ischaemic infarcts by CT within 6 h of stroke. Neuroradiology 38:31-33
30. Kummer R von, Allen KL, Holle R, et al (1997) Acute stroke: usefulness of early CT findings before thrombolytic therapy. Radiology 205:327-333
31. Kummer R von (1998) Effect of training in reading CT scans on patient selection for ECASS II. Neurology 51:S50-S52
32. Bozzao L, Bastianello S, Fantozzi LM, et al (1989) Correlation of angiographic and sequential CT findings in patients with evolving cerebral infarction. AJNR 10:1215-1222
33. Truwit CL, Barkovich AJ, Gean-Marton A, et al (1990) Loss of the insular ribbon: another early CT sign of acute middle cerebral artery infarction. Radiology 176:801-806
34. Horowitz SH, Zito JL, Donnarumma R, et al (1991) Computed tomographic-angiographic findings within the first five hours of cerebral infarction. Stroke 22:1245-1253
35. Kummer R von, Meyding-Lamade U, Forsting M, et al (1994) Sensitivity and prognostic value of early CT in occlusion of the middle cerebral artery trunk. Am J Neuroradiol 15:9-15
36. Tomsick TA, Brott TG, Chambers AA, et al (1990) Hyperdense middle cerebral artery sign on CT: efficacy in detecting middle cerebral artery thrombosis. AJNR 11:473-477
37. Leys D, Pruvo JP, Godefroy O, et al (1992) Prevalence and significance of hyperdense middle cerebral artery in acute stroke. Stroke 23:317-324
38. Tomura N, Uemura K, Inugami A, et al (1988) Early CT finding in cerebral infarction: obscuration of the lentiform nucleus. Radiology 168:463-467
39. Bozzao L, Angeloni U, Bastianello S, et al (1991) Early angiographic and CT findings in patients with hemorrhagic infarction in the distribution of the middle cerebral artery. AJNR 12:1115-1121
40. Schriger DL, Kalafut M, Starkman S, et al (1998) Cranial computed tomography interpretation in acute stroke: physician accuracy in determining eligibility for thrombolytic therapy. JAMA 279:1293-1297
41. Knauth M, Kummer R, Jansen O et al (1997) Potential of CT angiography in acute ischemic stroke. AJNR 18:1001-1010
42. Doerfler A, Engelhorn T, Kummer R von, et al (1998) Are iodinated contrast agents detrimental

in acute cerebral ischemia? An experimental study in rats. Radiology 206:211-217

43. Wildermuth S, Knauth M, Brandt T, et al (1998) Role of CT angiography in patient selection for thrombolytic therapy in acute hemispheric stroke. Stroke 29:935-938

44. Hamberg LM, Hunter GJ, Halpern EF, et al (1996) Quantitative high-resolution measurement of cerebrovascular physiology with slip-ring CT. AJNR 17:639-650

45. Hacke W, Kaste M, Fieschi C, et al (1998) Randomised double-blind placebo-controlled trial of thrombolytic therapy with intravenous alteplase in acute ischaemic stroke (ECASS II). Lancet 352:1245-1251

46. Warach S, Dashe JF, Edelman RR (1996) Clinical outcome in ischemic stroke predicted by early diffusion-weighted and perfusion magnetic resonance imaging: a preliminary analysis. J Cereb Blood Flow Metab 16:53-59

47. Barber PA, Darby DG, Desmond PM, et al (1998) Prediction of stroke outcome with echoplanar perfusion- and diffusion-weighted MRI. Neurology 51:418-426

48. Conturo TE, McKinstry RC, Aronovitz JA, et al (1995) Diffusion MRI: precision, accuracy and flow effects. NMR Biomed 8:307-332

49. Kidwell CS, Alger JR, Di Salle F, et al (1999) Diffusion MRI in patients with transient ischemic attacks. Stroke 30:1174-1180

50. Kidwell CS, Saver JL, Mattiello J, et al (2000) Thrombolytic reversal of acute human cerebral ischemic injury shown by diffusion/perfusion magnetic resonance imaging. Ann Neurol 47: 462-469

51. Jansen O, Schellinger PD, Fiebach JB, et al (1999) Early recanalization in acute ischemic stroke saves tissue at risk defined by MRI. Lancet 353:2036-2037

52. Schlaug G, Benfield A, Baird AE, et al (1999) The ischemic penumbra: operationally defined by diffusion and perfusion MRI. Neurology 53:1528-1537

53. Jansen O, Heiland S, Schellinger P (1998) Neuroradiological diagnosis in acute ischemic stroke. Value of modern techniques. Nervenarzt 69:465-471

54. Linfante I, Llinas RH, Caplan LR, et al (1999) MRI features of intracerebral hemorrhage within 2 hours from symptom onset. Stroke 30:2263-2267

55. Patel MR, Edelman RR, Warach S (1996) Detection of hyperacute primary intraparenchymal hemorrhage by magnetic resonance imaging. Stroke 27:2321-2324

56. Schellinger PD, Jansen O, Fiebach JB, et al (1999) A standardized MRI stroke protocol: comparison with CT in hyperacute intracerebral hemorrhage. Stroke 30:765-768

57. Wiesmann M, Mayer T, Yousri I, et al (1999) Comparison of FLAIR and fast spin-echo MR imaging at 1.5T for detection of acute subarachnoid hemorrhage. Joint Annual Meeting of the American Society of Neuroradiology. 22-28 May, San Diego, Calif., USA

58. Tong DC, Yenari MA, Albers GW et al (1998) Correlation of perfusion- and diffusion-weighted MRI with NIHSS score in acute (.5 hour) ischemic stroke. Neurology 50:864-870

59. Baird AE, Warach S (1999) Imaging developing brain infarction. Curr Opin Neurol 12:65-71

60. Beaulieu C, Crespigny A de, Tong DC, et al (1999) Longitudinal magnetic resonance imaging study of perfusion and diffusion in stroke: evolution of lesion volume and correlation with clinical outcome. Ann Neurol 46:568-578

61. Schellinger PD, Jansen O, Fiebach JB, et al (2000) Monitoring intravenous recombinant tissue plasminogen activator thrombolysis for acute ischemic stroke with diffusion and perfusion MRI. Stroke 31:1318-1328

62. Schellinger PD, Jansen O, Fiebach JB, et al (2000) Feasibility and practicality of MR imaging of stroke in the management of hyperacute cerebral ischemia. AJNR 21:1184-1189

63. Schellinger PD, Fiebach JB, Jansen O, et al (2001) Stroke magnetic resonance imaging within 6 hours after onset of hyperacute cerebral ischemia. Ann Neurol 49:460-469

64. Rordorf G, Koroshetz WJ, Copen WA, et al (1998) Regional ischemia and ischemic injury in patients with acute middle cerebral artery stroke as defined by early diffusion-weighted and perfusion-weighted MRI. Stroke 29:939-943

65. Marks MP, Tong D, Beaulieu C, et al (1999) Evaluation of early reperfusion and IV rt-PA therapy using diffusion- and perfusion-weighted MRI. Neurology 52:1792-1798

66. Hacke W, Willig V, Steiner T (1997) Update on thrombolytic therapy in ischemic stroke. Fibrinolysis Proteolysis 11:1-4
67. Hacke W, Brott T, Caplan L, et al (1999) Thrombolysis in acute ischemic stroke: controlled trials and clinical experience. Neurology 53:S3-S14
68. Wardlaw JM, Zoppo G del, Yamaguchi T (2002) Thrombolysis for acute ischaemic stroke (Cochrane Review). In The Cochrane Library
69. Hacke W, Schwab S, Horn M, et al (1996) 'Malignant' middle cerebral artery territory infarction: clinical course and prognostic signs. Arch Neurol 53:309-315
70. Schwab S, Aschoff A, Spranger M, et al (1996) The value of intracranial pressure monitoring in acute hemispheric stroke. Neurology 47:393-398
71. Frank JI (1995) Large hemispheric infarction, deterioration, and intracranial pressure. Neurology 45:1286-1290
72. Raichle ME (1983) The pathophysiology of brain ischemia. Ann Neurol 13:2-10
73. Schwarz S, Schwab S, Bertram M. et al (1998) Effects of hypertomic saline hydroxyethyl starch solution and mannitol in patients with increased intracranial pressure after stroke. Stroke 29: 1550-1555
74. Karibe H, Chen J, Zarow GJ et al (1994) Delayed induction of mild hypothermie to reduce infarct volume after temporary middle cerebral artery occlusion in rats. Neurosurgery 80:112-119
75. Clifton GL, Miller ER, Choi SC, et al (2001) Lack of effect of induction of hypothermia after acute brain injury. N Engl J Med 344:556-563
76. Schwab S, Schwarz S, Spranger M, et al (1998) Moderate hypothermia in the treatment of patients with severe middle cerebral artery infarction. Stroke 29:2461-2466
77. Steiner T, Friede T, Aschoff A, et al (2001) Effect and feasibility of controlled rewarming after moderate hypothermia in stroke patients with malignant infarction of the middle cerebral artery. Stroke 32: (in press)
78. Doerfler A, Forsting M, Reith W, et al (1996) Decompressive Surgery in a rat model of "malignant" cerebral hemispherical stroke: experimental support for an aggressive therapeutic approach. J Neurosurg 85:853-859
79. Forsting M, Reith W, Schabitz WR, et al (1995) Decompressive craniectomy for cerebral infarction. An experimental study in rats. Stroke 26:259-264
80. Rieke K, Schwab S, Krieger D, et al (1995) Decompressive surgery in space-occupying hemispheric infarction: results of an open, prospective trial. Crit Care Med 23:1576-1587
81. Schwab S, Steiner T, Aschoff A, et al (1998) Early hemicraniectomy in patients with complete middle cerebral artery infarction. Stroke 29:1888-1893
82. Nussbaum E, Wolf A, Sebring L (1991) Complete temporal lobectomy for surgical resuscitation of patients with transtentorial herniation secondary to unilateral hemisperic swelling. Neurosurgery 29:62-66

Early management of severely burned patients

A. Luzzani, E. Polati, I. Salvetti

Burn injury is very common [1]. It is estimated that it affects approximately 1% of the population each year [1]. The accidents occur mostly at home (60%-70%) and, to a smaller extent, at work (10%-20%). The burn victims are often children (1-3 years) and the elderly (> 60 years) [2].

In 1993, the American Burn Association established guide-lines to identify patients requiring medical care in specialized burn centers [3]:
- Greater than 10% total body surface area (TBSA) burns in patients less than 10 or greater than 50 years of age
- Greater than 20% TBSA burns in patients 10-50 years of age
- Significant burns of the face, hands, feet, genitalia, perineum, or skin overlying major joints
- Full-thickness burns greater than 5% TBSA
- Significant electric injury, lightning injury, and chemical burns
- Inhalation injury
- Burns associated with significant preexisting illness
- Burns associated with a need for special social or emotional support, rehabilitation, and cases involving child abuse or neglect

These guidelines were then reproposed by the Committee on Trauma of the College of Surgeons in 1999 [4]. Improvements in the management of severely burned patients, leading to a decreased mortality and morbidity, have occurred in the last 2 decades. In particular, the reduced incidence of hypovolemic shock and renal failure makes infections the most-important cause of morbidity and mortality in burned patients [5, 6].

The outcome of burned patients is essentially affected by two factors: percentage of TBSA burned and patient's age.

Many indices were proposed to establish the probability of deaths. Actually, the most used index is the Abbreviated Burn Severity Index (ABSI), by Tobiasen et al. (Table 1) [7].

Table 1 Tobiasen's abbreviated burn severity index [7] (*TBSA* total body surface area)

		Score
Sex	Female	1
	Male	0
Age (years)	0-20	1
	21-40	2
	41-60	3
	61-80	4
	81-100	5
Inhalation injury		1
Third-degree injury		1
Extent of burn injury (% TBSA)	1-10	1
	11-20	2
	21-30	3
	31-40	4
	41-50	5
	51-60	6
	61-70	7
	71-80	8
	81-90	9
	91-100	10

Score 4, survival probability is 0.99
Score 4-5, survival probability is 0.98
Score 6-7, survival probability is 0.8-0.9
Score 8-9, survival probability is 0.5-0.7
Score 10-11, survival probability is 0.2-0.4
Score > 11, survival probability is ≤ 0.1

Pathophysiology

Early response to serious thermal injury is inflammation. The main characteristic of this inflammatory response is massive development of edema, in both
burned and unburned tissue [8, 9]. The edema develops rapidly, within 8 h after
burn injury. It follows vasodilatation, increased vascular permeability, and
alterations in extracellular matrix. The severity of edema is such that a severe
hypovolemia (depletion of intravascular volume) and hypotension occur if an
adequate fluid resuscitation is not rapidly established. The occurrence of
hypovolemia and hypotension is due to the presence of numerous vasoactive
substances, systemic cytokinemia, and myocardial depression factors from the
systemic inflammatory response syndrome [9-11].

This systemic inflammatory response syndrome involves the pulmonary
vascular bed. In the absence of an inhalation injury, there is no significant
increase in pulmonary microvascular permeability, although transvascular fluid
flux in the lungs is increased. On the other hand, in the presence of an inhalation

injury, the flogosis causes damages in the alveolus capillary membrane (cellular necrosis and inactivation of the surfactant) with occlusion of small, distal airways by inflammatory exudates and sloughed debris [3, 8].

Prehospital care

At the scene, the patient should be removed from the source of heat or flame. It is important to ascertain the airway patency, to consider respiratory and cardiocirculatory conditions (ABC) and, if necessary, to start with adequate resuscitation treatments [8].

Early care of the burn wounds is summarized as 5 "Cs": clothing (removing clothing), cooling (application of cool or cold water or cold towels), cleaning (lavage with water or saline solution), covering (with a clean dry sheet), comforting (pain relief) [12].

It is necessary to organize the transport of the victim to the burn center. If it is impossible within 1 h, it is necessary to go to a near by hospital to make an accurate evaluation of the patient, to insert a venous access and bladder catheter. Later it is possible to go to a specialized center [8]. Early management includes tetanus prophylaxis. In the presence of deep burns or circumferential full-thickness thermal injury, with impaired tissue perfusion (and subsequent tissue ischaemia and muscle necrosis) and neurological changes, escharotomy is needed. Sometimes a fasciotomy may also be indicated [2, 8, 12].

Airway management

It is always necessary to ascertain airway patency. Then it is important to consider the need for oxygen therapy and/or mechanical ventilation with (high) positive end-expiratory pressure [3, 10]. Initially the airway may be normal. Unfortunately, supraglottic and glottic edema can rapidly develop even in absence of severe burns involving the head and the neck, and/or in the absence of inhalation injury. This may be due to the systemic inflammatory response syndrome, or, subsequently, to an over-resuscitation, with an excessive fluid therapy. In these patients orotracheal or nasotracheal tracheobronchoscopic guided intubation may be required, or emergency cricothyrotomy or tracheostomy in cases of failure of endotracheal intubation [3, 6, 8]. Early tracheostomy should be considered for all severely burned children and an anticipated need for prolonged intubation, especially those with severe facial burns and in the presence of inhalation injury [13]. In the absence of inhalation injury, respirator9 failure may occur as a consequence of deep thermal injuries involving the chest and the abdomen and impairing chest wall excursions [3, 6, 8].

In 20%-40% of severely burned patients, airway damages occur, after a few hours of latency, as a consequence of inhalation of warm air or the entry of products of incomplete combustion. These injuries induce flogosis and edema. They require timely treatment and increase the mortality rate of 20% [8]. The inhalation injury causes pulmonary edema, acute respiratory distress syndrome (2%-7%), and, in case of absorption, systemic intoxication. The edema supports the development of atelectases that predispose burn patients to pulmonary complications (38%) [3, 8, 14].

Carbon monoxide poisoning is also to be considered. Diagnosis is made by direct measurement of carboxyhemoglobin (COHb) levels [3, 8, 15]. Fundamental aims of therapy are management of cardiac and neurological impairment (if they are present) and rapid removal of carbon monoxide from hemoglobin. To remove carbon monoxide, the first measure is administration of 100% oxygen (by mask in conscious patients with spontaneous breathing with COHb ≤30%), by mechanical ventilation in unconscious patients with COHb >30%. In these latter patients it is generally necessary to use hyperbaric oxygen therapy. If a hyperbaric chamber is not available, exsanguinotransfusion may be useful in patients with very high levels of COHb [15]. Rapid reduction of carbon monoxide is the main mechanism by which hypoxic injury may be avoided, and treatment should be continued until the COHb level decreases to less than 10% [15]. Finally, it is important to consider the pulmonary damage due to blast, which consists of pressure alveolar damage with injury to the alveolus capillary membrane and hemorrhage [8].

Cardiovascular resuscitation

Patient size and the extent of the burn injury are the most-important determinants of the volume of resuscitation fluid requirement, i.e., administration of a sufficient volume to produce adequate tissue perfusion [3]. It is necessary to rapidly assess the severity of burn injuries: site, extent, depth, associated damages.

The extent is estimated as percentage of total body surface area. Usually the rule of nines guides estimations: the head and each of the upper extremities represent 9% TBSA; anterior trunk, posterior trunk and each of the lower extremities represent 18% TBSA; the perineum represent the remaining 1% (Fig. 1) [2, 3, 6, 8, 11, 16, 17]. Lund and Browder chart, a surface area diagram, offers more-exact determination, because it considers patient's age and ac-

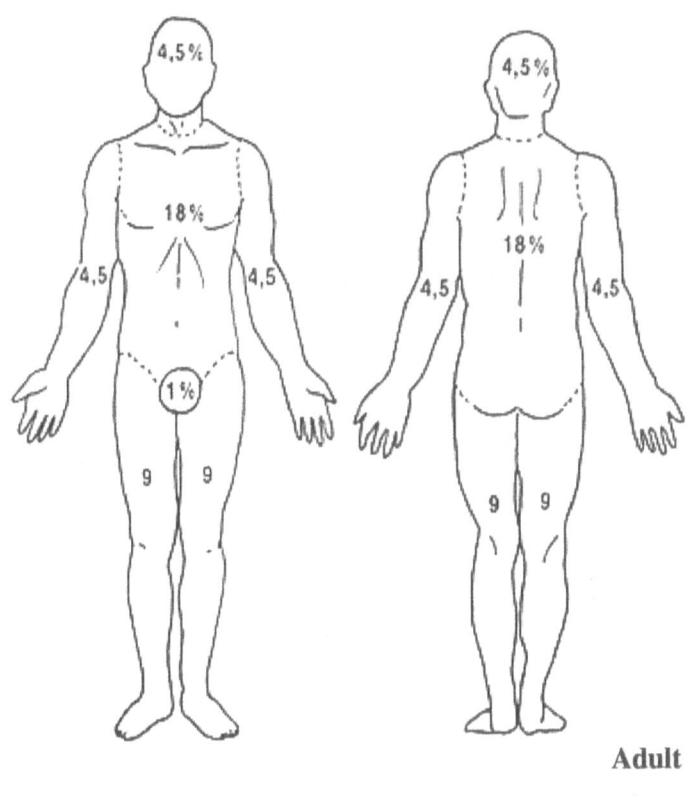

Adult

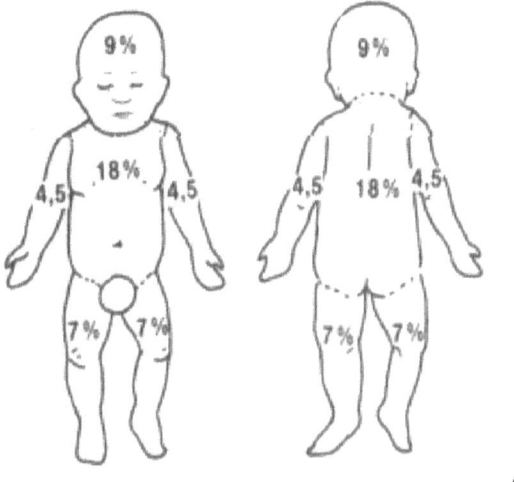

Child

Fig. 1 The rule of nine (Modified from: Sheridan RL (2000) The burned patient [6]

counts for the different anatomical relationships in pediatric patients. Thus it is very useful for infants or children (Table 2 and Fig. 2) [18]. Another practical method to estimate percentage TBSA is that the area of the patient's palm covers about 1% TBSA.

Table 2 Lund and Browder chart [18]

	Newborn	1 year	5 years	10 years	15 years	Adult
Head	19	17	13	11	9	7
Neck	2	2	2	2	2	2
Trunk (anterior)	13	13	13	13	13	13
Trunk (posterior)	13	13	13	13	13	13
Arms	8	8	8	8	8	8
Forearms	6	6	6	6	6	6
Hands	5	5	5	5	5	5
Buttocks	5	5	5	5	5	5
Genitalia	1	1	1	1	1	1
Thighs	11	13	16	17	18	19
Legs	10	10	11	12	13	14
Feet	7	7	7	7	7	7

According to the depth, the burn injuries are classified as: first degree (erythema and epidermal damage), second degree (involving the entire epidermal layer and part of the underlying dermis, with development of flittens), and third degree or full thickness (destruction of all epidermal and dermal elements, with appearance of eschars). When calculating the extent of a burn, only second- and third-degree injuries are included; epidermal injury alone is not considered [8, 19]. Accurate determination of the extent of the burn wound is essential for properly estimating the initial resuscitation fluid needs.

Many burn resuscitation formulae are used to provide an estimation of fluid requirements in severely burned patients [3, 8]. Parkland's formula and Brooke's modified formula [3, 8]:

1. (0.25 ml/kg)/(%TBSA)/h in 8 h, then (0.125 ml/kg)/(%TBSA)/h in 16 h, with dextrose (0.8 ml/kg)/(%TBSA)/h, with 5% albumin (0.015 ml/kg)/(%TBSA)/h in 24 h
2. see Table 3

Table 3 Brooke's modified formula [3]

First 24 h post burn
Adults and children >20-30 kg
Lactated Ringer's solution: 2-4 ml/kg per % TBSA per 24 h (half during the first 8 h, half in remaining 16 h)
Colloids: nothing
Children <20kg
Lactated Ringer's solution: 2-3 ml/Kg per % TBSA per 24h (half during the first 8 h; half in remaining 16 h)
Lactated Ringer's solution + 5% dextrose: maintenance of an adequate urine output (0.5-1.5 ml/kg per hour)
Colloids: nothing
Second 24 h post burn
All patients:
Crystalloids:
Maintenance of an adequate urine output (children 0.5-1.5 ml/kg per hour; adults 30-50 ml/kg per hour)
Colloids: (albumin 5% in lactated Ringer's solution):
0-30% TBSA: nothing
30-50% TBSA: 0.3 ml/kg per % TBSA per 24 h
50-70% TBSA: 0.4 ml/kg per % TBSA per 24h
>70% TBSA : 0.5 ml/kg per % TBSA per 24h

However, it is very important to make some considerations.

First of all, an adequate cardiopulmonary resuscitation cannot be based on simple application of formulae: they are simply a guide, but it is necessary to make adjustments according to a single patient's needs [7, 20, 21]. Many authors say that this aim is realized by careful clinical evaluation and with not too-invasive monitoring system (heart rate, blood pressure, urine output, eventually central venous pressure) [3, 8, 10, 22, 23]. The goal is preserving organ perfusion, and the urine output is the most clinically useful and readily available means of judging the volemia, the cardiovascular function, and the adequacy of resuscitation [3, 8, 10, 22, 23].

Other authors stress the importance but, unfortunately, the inaccuracy of these standard criteria, and suggest using data obtainable by more-invasive monitoring systems [10, 20, 22, 24]. In such a way, we are able to evaluate more accurately a single patient's needs. Indeed, only invasive monitoring may provide the true hemodynamic status of these patients and resuscitation guided by means of invasive hemodynamic monitoring is associated with a substantially higher volume administration than with empirical resuscitation formulae and clinical evaluation. We would like to stress that the most-important goals are to avoid sub-optimal resuscitation, and to guarantee a fluid administration sufficient to maintain an adequate organ perfusion, to repay oxygen debt, to eliminate tissue acidosis, and to restore aerobic metabolism [20-22, 25].

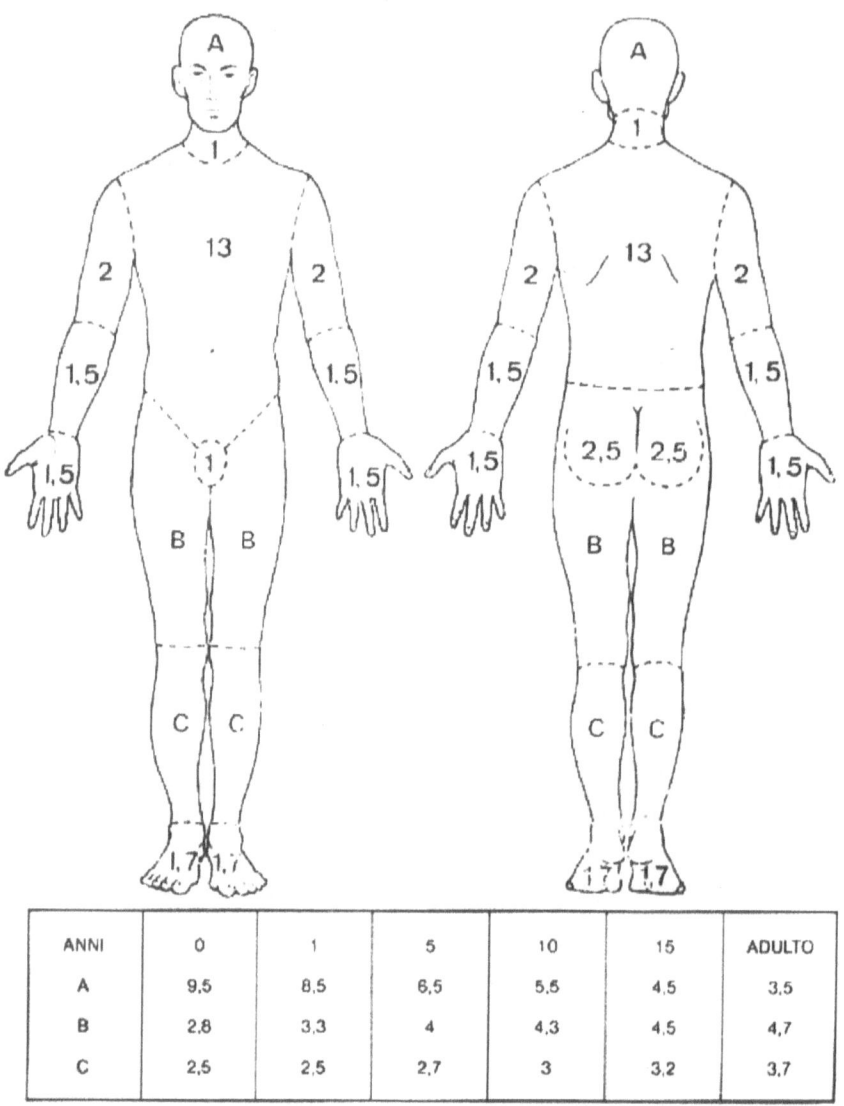

ANNI	0	1	5	10	15	ADULTO
A	9,5	8,5	6,5	5,5	4,5	3,5
B	2,8	3,3	4	4,3	4,5	4,7
C	2,5	2,5	2,7	3	3,2	3,7

Fig. 2 Lund and Browder chart. Modified from: Manelli JC, Badetti C (1997) Rèanimation et anesthèsie du brûlè [8]

For this purpose, measurement of cardiac output (CO), pulmonary capillary wedge pressure (PCWP), systemic vascular resistance (SVR), oxygen delivery rate (DO_2), intrathoracic blood volume (ITVB), base deficit, and serum lactate level are useful [20, 23, 26]. The clinical utility of CO, PCWP, SVR, DO_2, and ITVB as end-points variables for fluid resuscitation has been evaluated, and they were demonstrated to be of predictive value for survival in this group of patients. They are used as preload indicators to guide volume therapy and, after restoration of filling pressures, for a more-precise application of inotropic support [20, 23]. Serum lactate level is an indirect measure of the oxygen debt and therefore it is an approximation of the magnitude of the hypoperfusion and the severity of shock; base deficit is also an approximation of global tissue acidosis. Serum lactate levels and the amount of base deficit but, in particular, the time in which they are normalized appear to be suitable end-points for resuscitation [20, 23, 26].

Gastric intramucosal PCO_2 ($PiCO_2$) changes or, better, the difference between arterial and tonometer PCO_2 ($P[i\text{-}a]CO_2$), is thought to indicate the state of oxygen supply relative to oxygen demand in the splanchnic district [9, 27]. PHi values are also associated with outcome and with the development of organ failure in critically ill patients. In fact, a burn trauma is associated with gastric intramucosal acidosis because there is a splanchnic vasoconstriction [9, 27].

Venkatesh et al. [22] observed that, despite fluid resuscitation leading to adequate global indices of tissue perfusion, tissue monitoring indicated significant deterioration in the splanchnic circulation and in normal and burnt skin. The most-likely explanation for this is a selective gastrointestinal vasoconstriction in severely burned patients, combined with the development of tissue edema (that is exacerbated by fluid administration and hypoproteinemia) [22].

Thus, the cardiovascular function of severely burned patients seems to be highly responsive to volume loading. Interestingly, the extravascular lung water (EVLW) does not increase beyond normal, despite a massive fluid infusion; fluid accumulation in the lung seems to be a result of inadequate resuscitation with worsening of the lung capillary permeability rather than infusion of too-large fluid volumes [20, 22, 23].

All the authors agree about the inadequacy of the Parkland formula in predicting the amount of fluid requirements for inhalation injured patients [9, 20, 21, 25]. It is clear that these patients need fluid volumes in excess of those required in noninhalation injured cases (up to 50% more fluid than predicted). Moreover, patients with inhalation injuries also require a significantly longer time to be completely resuscitated from burn-induced shock. Fluid restriction will not protect the lung with an inhalation injury; instead, by decreasing perfusion, fluid restriction will increase the degree of shunt [9, 20, 21, 25].

Debate continues over the most-appropriate type of fluid therapy. In fact there is a dilemma: "crystalloid solutions or colloid solutions?" Most authors agree: the use of human albumin and/or plasma during the first 24 h is not only barely useful but also harmful, because there is an increased microvascular permeability [2, 6, 8, 11, 16, 17, 19, 28]. According to a recent American Consensus Conference [28], in early fluid resuscitation we must use crystalloids; only after 24 h, or in burns greater 50% TBSA, or if the crystalloids alone are unable to correct hypovolemia do we need to use colloids or human albumin [8]. However, the debate is still open. Cochrane Injuries Group Albumin Reviewers published in 1998 a meta-analysis that demonstrated that the use of albumin as plasma-expander is not safe nor effective. In 1,419 hypovolemic, burned, or hypoalbuminemic patients, human albumin was not able to reduce the mortality. Moreover, it is possible that its use may be responsible for 6 deaths in every 100 patients treated [29]. In contrast, a recent meta-analysis reiterated the importance and the safety of human albumin in critically ill patients. In this study the authors showed the unreliability of the conclusions of the Cochrane Group (much bias invalidated the results) and demonstrated that albumin is able to improve survival and that side effects are rare [30, 31].

Lactated Ringer's solution is the fluid of choice during initial resuscitation [3, 8, 10, 11, 17, 22, 25]. Guha et al. [32] showed that, to re-establish normal cardiovascular function, minimizing edema, hypertonic saline dextran, and hetastarch appear to be superior to lactated Ringer's solution, and hypertonic saline dextran superior to hetastarch, at least for early resuscitation [32,33]. Although net volume through 8 h is reduced by 48% with hetastarch and by 74% with hypertonic saline dextran compared with lactated Ringer's solution, the interstitial entry of large amounts of colloid may result in delayed pulmonary edema. The edema post colloid resuscitation resolves more slowly than after crystalloid resuscitation. Furthermore, colloids (hetastarch and hypertonic saline dextran) can have initial volume-sparing effects, even in the presence of increased permeability after burns, but such effects, not sustained, must be tested and confirmed in longer-term studies before being considered clinically important [32, 33]. Berger et al. [34] tested the impact of a bicarbonated saline solution on early resuscitation after major burns. The use of this solution does not reduce the amount of fluid infused for resuscitation, and does not decrease the probability of the development of dilutional acidosis.

When volume replacement is adequate and perfusion pressure well maintained, overall outcome in severely burned patients is not improved by using inotropic and vasoactive supports (dobutamine or adrenaline in the presence of adequate filling pressures and low CO, norepinephrine in the presence of low mean arterial pressure and low systemic vascular resistances) in an attempt to achieve target values for oxygen delivery and consumption [35, 36]. Of greater interest is the fact that mortality is increased in patients who attain the goals with, for example, dobutamine. Larger doses exacerbate maldistribution of blood flow within the microcirculation, resulting in impaired perfusion of vital organs, and thereby contributing to the higher incidence of multiple-organ failure [35, 36]. Only if fluid replacement alone fails to achieve the therapeutic goals, are catecholamines added in cases of hypotension or oliguria [20, 23]. Patients with delayed or inadequate resuscitation often require more fluid than would be anticipated by most formulae.

Finally, we must also consider that the volume of fluid infused may be related to the development of intra-abdominal hypertension (IAH), associated with malperfusion of the gut, liver, and kidneys, as well as with cardiac and pulmonary dysfunction. IAH can lead to abdominal compartment syndrome (ACS), defined as IAH combined with a decreased pulmonary compliance or oliguria, despite adequate filling pressure and cardiac output. Open decompression is often mandatory for patients with ACS, whereas conservative therapy should be considered for patients with isolated IAH [37].

Renal complications

Acute renal failure is a complication that affects 1%-30% of thermally and electrically burned patients. Its pathogenesis is not well known, but it is known that its incidence is related to the severity of burn damage [38, 39]. There are two different forms of acute renal failure in the severely burned patient.

Early acute renal failure appears during the first 5 days, as a consequence of severe hypovolemia, acidosis, and myoglobinuria-induced tubular injury [38, 39]. The damage, i.e., ischaemic damage, involves tubular cells and, if the shock persists and exaggerated production of catecholamines continues, can lead to tubular necrosis. To avoid this form of acute renal failure, we must provide an adequate fluid resuscitation during the first hours post burn; fluid load improves cardiovascular performance and reduces plasma and urinary levels of myoglobin. It could be useful to alkalize the urine and use iron-chelating substances. The therapy can include hydration associated with diuretics. The diuretic of choice is mannitol. In fact, this drug, with osmotic properties, acts without modifying urinary pH and works as plasma expanders, reducing plasma viscosity; it has vasodilating renal activity and is a scavenger for free radicals [40, 41].

Late acute renal failure appears after 5 days and is frequently associated with sepsis or multi-organ dysfunction. It is often fatal and it seems to involve patients with concurrent inhalation injury. Other frequent causes of renal failure, especially of the late form are severe lasting hypovolemia, hypertonic dehydration, aggressive diuretic therapy, the use of nephrotoxic drugs (such as antibiotics, non-steroidal anti-inflammatory drugs), and the use of dye for radiological diagnostic techniques [20, 38, 39].

Infectious complications

The burn injury patient is particularly exposed to infectious diseases and to their diffusion. The main causes are the serious injury or the complete loss of skin and mucosa barrier, the presence of necrotic tissues, and the depression of both cell-mediated and humoural immunity (the mechanisms responsible for the depression of immunity are not known). Other important factors to be considered are the depth and extent of the burn, the general condition of the patients, the bacterial load, the intrinsic pathogenicity of microbes and their resistance to antimicrobial therapy [8, 42].

Immediately after thermal injury, burned skin is sterilized. If we do not provide the correct topical antimicrobial therapy within 48 h after injury, there is the risk of bacterial colonization [19]. The incidence of sepsis may be reduced by using temporary biological dressings, allografts, or xenografts. The use of systemic antibiotics is controversial. Systemic antimicrobial therapy is limited to treatment of documented generalized infections and to prophylaxis before surgical procedures, because it may promote the selection of more-resistant microbes even if it may avoid cross colonization [6]. Perhaps systemic antibiotic drugs are the cause of increased fungal and viral infectious diseases. There is only one condition in which the prophylaxis with systemic antimicrobial therapy is justified: the presence of deep and dirty burns, that are at high risk of infection by Gram-positive organisms [8, 42].

If the burn injuries become infected, the best strategy is early excision and grafting of full-thickness burns and deep partial-thickness burns; antimicrobial drugs, topical or systemic, have only a supportive role [3, 6]. It is important doing these maneuvers that the patient is hemodynamically stable, because they may worsen cardiovascular balance and may often be associated with massive blood loss (more than 100 ml per percentage of body surface excised, depending on the anatomical location and the maturity of the wound). Excision and grafting of the burns are the main reasons for surgery. As a rule, no drug for anaesthesia is contraindicated in burns patients [8]. It is very important to use depolarising muscle-relaxant drugs, such as succinylcholine. When using 24 h after the trauma, an important increase in serum potassium levels occurs, with possible consequent disorders in cardiac rhythm and sometimes cardiac arrest.

These effects do not a correlate with the dosage of drugs, or the depth or the extent of burn damage. Moreover, it is not known, because this phenomenon happens after and not before 24 h, how much time should pass before the use of this muscle-relaxant drug is safe [6, 8, 43]. When muscle relaxation is required, nondepolarising relaxants are used. Burn patients show a "resistance" to these drugs, in some cases requiring three- to fivefold higher doses than unburned persons [6, 43]. The burned patient needs a large amount of analgesic and opioid drugs. The drug of choice is morphine or its analogues [6, 8]. It is important to remember that intraoperatory hypothermia is inevitable and that normothermia must be restored before the awakening of the patient [8].

Metabolism and nutrition

Following serious thermal injury a generalized metabolic response develops, with consequent increase and alteration of the metabolism, and potential profound deterioration of the nutritional state [6]. Schematically, the hypermetabolic response consists of two phases: the ebb phase (hypometabolism and decrease in cardiac output) that develops within a few hours and the flow phase (hypermetabolism and two- to threefold increase in cardiac output) that develops after 3-5 days and persists for weeks to months [6]. Early enteral feeding (not parenteral) may attenuate the hypermetabolic response. The barrier function of the intestinal mucosa is lost immediately after a burn injury. Early enteral nutrition has been shown to be safe and effective in patients with serious thermal injuries. It preserves the intestinal mucosal barrier and thereby prevents the translocation of bacteria and endotoxin from the gut to the systemic circulation [9]. Many formulae have been proposed to calculate basal energy expenditure in burned patients (Table 4), but only indirect calorimetry, measured in the single patient, can offer an exact estimate [8]. It is important to pay attention to other factors that may blunt this hypermetabolic state: maintenance of an adequate patient room temperature (28-32°C) and humidity (88-92%), the performance of effective physiotherapy and the patient moving, and the control of pain [2, 8, 20].

Table 4 Estimate of caloric requirements in burn patients (*BEE* basal energetic expenditure (Harris-Bene-dict's formula); *CC* caloric contribution; *T* temperature (Celsius's scale); *J* days postburn. Modified from Manelli JC, Badetti C (1997) Rèanimation et anesthèsie du brûlè [8]

	Adults		
Curreri	25 kcal/kg + 40 kcal/% TBSA		
Wolfe	BEE x 2		
Allard	-4.343 + (0.84 x BEE) + (0.23 x CC) + (10.5 x TBSA) + (114 x T) – (4.5 x J)		
Deitch	15-30% TBSA:	31-45% TBSA:	>46% TBSA:
Calories	1.5 x BEE	1.5-1.8 x BEE	1.8-2.2 x BEE
Proteins (g/kg)	1.5	1.5-2.0	2.0-2.3
	Children		
Curreri	0-1 years		BEE + 15 kcal/% TBSA
	1-3 years		BEE + 25 kcal/% TBSA
	4-15 years		BEE + 40 kcal/% TBSA
Grotte	kcal/kg	g N/kg	
	Burn <20% TBSA Burn >20% TBSA	Burn <20% TBSA Burn >20% TBSA	
0-1 years	125 150	0.45 0.5	
1-8 years	100 125	0.3 0.45	
9-15 years	75 100	0.23 0.3	

Gastrointestinal complications

In two of three severely burned patients (burns > 30%) the mucosa of the esophagus, stomach, and gut develops widespread superficial lesions due to hypotension and microvascular alterations. Deep lesions (Curling's ulcers) are not frequent (about 6%) and their bleeding is rare [44]. Although acid hyper-secretion is not the main cause of the development of these ulcers, in burned patients prophylaxis with drugs that decrease acid secretion (ranitidine or omeprazole) or increase the protection of the cells (sucralfate) is recommended [45-47].

Acknowledgements

We would like to thank Dr. Alberto Merlini for his support in this work.

References

1. Muller MJ, Pegg SP, Rule MR (2001) Determinants of death following burn injury. Br J Surg 88:583-587
2. Donati L (1997) Le ustioni e il loro trattamento. Bi and Gi Editori, Verona
3. Martin RR, Becker WK, Cioffi WG, et al (1996) Thermal injuries. In: Wilson RF, Walt AJ (eds) Management of trauma. Pitfalls and practice. Williams and Wilkins, Baltimore, pp 760-771
4. http://www.ameriburn.org/
5. Pruitt BA, McManus AT (1992) The changing epidemiology of infection in burn patient. World J Surg 16:57-67
6. Sheridan RL (2000) The burned patient. In: Hurford WE, Bigatello LM, Haspel KL, Hess D, Warren RL (eds) Critical care handbook of the Massachusetts General Hospital. Lippincott Williams and Wilkins, Philadelphia, pp 584-609
7. Tobiasen J, Hiebert JH, Edlich RF (1982) Prediction of burn mortality. Surg Gynecol Obstet 154: 711-714
8. Manelli JC, Badetti C (1997) Rèanimation et anesthèsie du brûlè. In: Encycl Mèd Chir, Anesthèsie-Rèanimation. Elsevier, Paris, pp 1-20
9. Edwin AD (1990) The management of burns. N Engl J Med 323:1249-1253
10. Sherwood ER, Woodson LC (2002) Perioperative management of the severely burned patients. In: Vincent JL (ed) Yearbook of Intensive Care and Medicine. Springer-Verlag, Berlin, Heidelberg New York, pp 853-862
11. Deitch EA (1996) Burn management. In: Rippe JM, Irwin RS, Fink MP, Cerra FB (eds) Intensive care medicine. Little Brown, Boston, pp 1957-1965
12. http/www.aafp.org/afp/
13. Palmieri TL, Jackson W, Greenhalgh DG (2002) Benefits of early tracheostomy in severely burned children. Crit Care Med 30:922-924
14. Hollingsed TC, Saffle JR, Barton RG, et al (1993) Etiology and consequences of respiratory failure in thermally injured patients. Am J Surg 166:592-597
15. Bozza Marrubini ML, Ghezzi Laurenzi R, Uccelli P (1989) Tossici che interferiscono con il metabolismo energetico e con l'omeostasi del mezzo interno. In: Bozza Marrubini ML, Grezzi Laurenzi R, Uccelli P Intossicazioni acute. Meccanismi, diagnosi e terapia. OEMF, Milan, pp 495-502
16. Carter C, Baker K (1998) Anesthesia for trauma and burns. In: Hurford WE, Bailin MT, Davison JK, Haspel KL, Rosow C (eds) Clinical anesthesia procedures of the Massachusetts General Hospital, Lippincott Williams and Wilkins, Philadelphia, pp 574-582
17. Peck MD, Ward CG (1997) Burn injury. In: Civetta JM, Taylor RW, Kirby RR (eds) Critical care Lippincott Raven, Philadelphia, pp 1265-1275
18. Lund CC, Browder JR (1944) An estimation of areas of burns. Surg Gynecol Obstet 79:351-352
19. Barisoni D (1984) Le ustioni e il loro trattamento. Piccin Nuova Libraria Italia, Padova
20. Holm C, Melcer B, Horbrand F, et al (2000) Haemodynamic and oxygen transport responses in survivors and non-survivors following thermal injury. Burns 26:25-33
21. Navar PD, Saffle JR, Warden GD (1985) Effect of inhalation injury on fluid resuscitation requirements after thermal injury. Am J Surg 150:716-720
22. Venkatesh B, Meacher R, Muller MJ, et al (2001) Monitoring tissue oxygenation during resuscitation of major burns. J Trauma 50:485-494
23. Holm C, Melcer B, Horbrand F, et al (2000) Intrathoracic blood volume as an end point in resuscitation of the severely burned: an observational study of 24 patients. J Trauma 48:728-734
24. Dries DJ, Waxman K (1991) Adequate resuscitation of burn patients may not be measured by urine output and vital signs. Crit Care Med 19:327-329
25. Dai NT, Chen TM, Cheng TY (1998) The comparision of early fluid therapy in extensive flame burns between inhalation and noninhalation injuries. Burns 24:671-675
26. Porter JM, Ivatury RR (1998) In search of the optimal end points of resuscitation in trauma patients: a review. J Trauma 44:908-914

27. Lorente JA, Ezpeleta A, Esteban A, et al (2000) Systemic haemodynamics, gastric intramucosal PCO2 changes, and outcome in critically ill burn patients. Crit Care Med 28:1728-1735

28. Vermeulen LC, Ratko TA, Erstad BL, et al (1995) A paradigm for consensus: the university hospital consortium guidelines for the use of albumin, non protein colloid and crystalloid solutions. Arch Intern Med 155:373-379

29. Cochrane Injuries Group Albumin Reviewers (1998) Human albumin administration in critically ill patients: systematic review of randomised controlled trials. BMJ 317:235-240

30. Wilkes MM, Navickis RJ (2002) Does albumin infusion affect survival? Review of meta-analytic findings. In: Vincent JL (ed) Yearbook of Intensive Care and Medicine. Springer-Verlag, Berlin Heidelberg New York, pp 454-464

31. Wilkes MM, Navickis RJ (2001) Patient survival after human albumin administration. A meta-analysis of randomized, controlled trials. Ann Intern Med 135:149-164

32. Guha SC, Kinsky MP, Button B, et al (1996) Burn resuscitation: crystalloid versus colloid versus hypertonic saline hyperoncotic colloid in sheep. Crit Care Med 24:1849-1857

33. Elgjo GI, Poli de Figueiredo LF, Schenarts PJ, et al (2000) Hypertonic saline dextran early (8-12 hrs) fluid sparing in burn resuscitation: a 24-hr prospective, double-blind study in sheep. Crit Care Med 28:163-171

34. Berger MM, Pictet A, Revelly J-P, et al (2000) Impact of a bicarbonated saline solution on early resuscitation after major burns. Intensive Care Med 26:1382-1385

35. Durham RM, Neunaber K, Mazuski JE, et al (1996) The use of oxygen consumption and delivery as endpoints for resuscitation in critically ill patients. J Trauma 41:32-40

36. Hayes MA, Timmins AC, Yau HS, et al (1994) Elevation of systemic oxygen delivery in the treatment of critically ill patients. N Engl J Med 330:1717-1722

37. Ivy ME, Atweh NA, Palmer J, et al (2000) Intra-abdominal hypertension and abdominal compartment syndrome in burn patients. J Trauma 49:387-391

38. Holm C, Horbrand F, Henckel von Donnersmark G, et al (1999) Acute renal failure in severely burned patients. Burns 25:171-178

39. Muther RS (1997) Acute renal failure. In: Civetta JM, Taylor RW, Kirby RR (eds) Critical care. Lippincott Raven, Philadelphia, pp 2081-2093

40. Lucas CE, Ledgerwood AM (1996) Renal response to severe injury and hypovolemic shock. In: Wilson RF, Walt AJ (eds) Management of trauma: pitfalls and practice. Williams and Wilkins, Baltimore, pp 945-965

41. Slater MS, Mullins R (1998) Rhabdomyolysis and myoglobinuric renal failure in trauma and surgical patients: a review. J Am Coll Surg 186:693-716

42. Yurt RW (1995) Burns. In: Mandell GL, Douglas RG, Bennett JE (eds) Principles and practice of infectious diseases. Churchill Livingstone, New York, pp 2761-2765

43. Savarese JJ, Caldwell JE, Lien CA, et al (2000) Pharmacology of muscle relaxants and their antagonists. In: Miller RD (ed) Anesthesia. Churchill Livingstone, Philadelphia, p 472

44. American Society of Health-System Pharmacist (1999) ASHP therapeutic guidelines on stress ulcer prophylaxis. Am J Health Syst Pharm 56:347-379

45. Cook DJ, Reeve BK, Guyatt GH, et al (1996) Stress ulcer prophylaxis in critically ill patients: resolving discordant meta-analysis. JAMA 275:308-314

46. Abraham E (2002) Acid suppression in a critical care environment: state of the art and beyond. Crit Care Med 30 [Suppl]: S349-S350

47. Fennerty MB (2002) Pathophysiology of the upper gastrointestinal tract in the critically ill patient: rationale for the therapeutic benefits of acid suppression. Crit Care Med 30 [Suppl]: S351-S355

SPECIAL CONDITIONS IN CRITICAL CARE

Sedation and analgesia in the critically ill – principles and practice

S. Anwar, G. Park

Sedation and analgesia is one of the commonest procedures carried out in the critically ill. There are several components, including analgesia, hypnosis, and sleep. Recently some of the old concepts have been challenged. Using opioids has questioned the widespread use of hypnotics such as propofol and midazolam. Having patients awake and pain free may be the best option of all. However, better monitoring of hypnotic drugs using sedation scales and the BIS may also reduce adverse effects when they are needed. A further, simple way of monitoring their effects is just to stop them each day and let the patient recover from them, although there are still no data on what is best.

Another area that has been challenged is the influence of drugs on memory. Amnesia was thought to be desirable, but we now realise "tinkering" with the memory of patients may have the potential for long-term psychological sequelae.

Above all else patient carers must not forget that a kind word, an unrumpled bed, and a room that is dark and quiet at night may be worth several syringes of hypnotics and analgesics.

Over the last 2 decades there has been a shift in intensive care unit (ICU) practice from routinely deeply sedating patients to an approach that is characterized by addressing specific indications and titrating sedation and analgesia appropriately [1]. In this article we review the principles behind this move and how current practice is changing.

Indications

The relief of pain is a fundamental aim for any clinician. Sedation encompasses the relief of a number of different causes of discomfort, including a decreased level of consciousness (hypnosis). This may be to decrease awareness of the unfamiliar, confusing, and somewhat hostile environment of the ICU, anxiolysis, and the facilitation of sleep. Together they provide a means of reducing physical and psychological stress and their complications in the critically ill.

The patient's response to distress

Sedative and analgesic agents play an important role in ICU patients. Physical comfort is clearly a humane and essential end in itself. However, it also has a number of other beneficial effects. It enables tolerance of unpleasant, but necessary, interventions such as tracheal suctioning and physiotherapy, cooperation with invasive procedures, and improved synchronization with mechanical ventilation, particularly when uncomfortable regimens such as inverse ratio ventilation are used. This not only enables maximum benefit to be derived from therapeutic interventions, but also helps to limit the unwanted physiological responses to distress, including hypertension, tachycardia, and peripheral vasoconstriction, predisposing to myocardial ischaemia in vulnerable patients. It also prevents respiratory compromise as a consequence of hypo- or hyper-ventilation resulting in impaired gas exchange, atelectasis, and bronchopneumonia. Thus, adequate analgesia may decrease the time to tracheal extubation and hence shorten the duration of ICU stay. Other physical effects of uncontrolled pain include gastric stasis, with resultant enteral feeding difficulties, urinary retention, hypercoagulable states and consequences of immobility, such as muscle wasting and venous thrombosis. The incidence of such complications is reduced in patients with appropriate analgesia [2]. As well as providing preventative measures such drugs have a therapeutic function, particularly in those patients with critical oxygen requirements.

Sedatives also play a role in modulating the stress response in critically ill patients. The stress response occurs at times of illness, trauma, or surgery. It leads to a number of neuro-endocrine changes. These include increased levels of circulating catecholamines, cortisol, and antidiuretic hormone in association with a catabolic state resulting in salt and water retention, insulin resistance, and sympathetic hyperactivity. Notably these effects are further compounded by fear and anxiety. Although in certain groups of patients this may be a beneficial reaction to noxious stimuli, in many others it may result in further embarrassment of physiological reserves, by increasing metabolism and oxygen consumption and suppressing the immune response. Additionally, recent work has shown poorer outcomes in association with impaired glycaemic control [3]. By attenuating the stress response, adequate sedation contributes to the limitation of these potentially detrimental effects.

Recent work has revealed the effect of ICU stay on the mental and psychological well-being of patients. Many find the environment frightening and bewildering, with unfamiliar faces, machines, alarms sounding, and feelings of loss of control. ICU agitation syndromes and ICU psychosis are not infrequent and, thus, part of the rationale behind the use of sedative agents has been to provide anxiolysis and decreased awareness of the environment. Traditionally it has been thought that the induction of amnesia is beneficial by limiting unpleasant recollections of the ICU environment. However, some authors have suggested that it is delusional memories that promote the development of ICU syndromes [4] and some factual memory may protect patients from such psychological sequelae. A comfortable, but aware patient may be at less risk of developing these complications.

The issue of sleep is contentious. Some research has suggested that disruption of the sleep wake cycle and cumulative sleep deprivation is associated with poorer outcomes in terms of psychiatric disturbance and increased pain perception [5]. There may be a beneficial role for sedative agents by virtue of their hypnotic properties. It is also known that sleep promotes an anabolic state [6], which may aid in the healing process. However, the effects of sleep disturbance on ICU patient morbidity are unclear and it is unknown what benefit, if any, may be derived from restoring sleep quality or quantity. It is also noteworthy that sedation is not synonymous with sleep, and therefore rendering a patient unconscious overnight may not provide the anticipated benefits of natural sleep.

The clinician's response to distress: pharmacological and non--pharmacological

Techniques employed to relieve patient distress include non-pharmacological as well as pharmacological means. These are of critical importance and include human interaction and soothing. They provide repeated reassurance and explanation in addition to human touch, which serve to decrease the perception of a hostile and alien environment. Reduction of noise levels and the presence of natural light may aid orientation.

Given the difficulty in recognizing pain in patients with limited abilities to communicate, analgesic drugs should be used if the patient may have pain. This ought not to detract, however, from seeking the cause of distress and starting specific therapy. In most ICUs, opioids are the mainstay of analgesia and provide an excellent means of pain control, as well as having anxiolytic and sedative properties. Commonly used agents include morphine, pethidine, fentanyl, and alfentanil delivered by the intravenous or epidural route. All opioids have side effects, most important of which is respiratory depression, which may be exacerbated by metabolite accumulation and unpredictable recovery in critically ill patients.

Should additional sedative agents be needed, benzodiazepines, such as midazolam, are frequently the drugs of choice with the advantage of providing anxiolysis, hypnosis, and amnesia. Alternatively propofol is often used, particularly when a shorter-acting drug is needed, although this has to be offset against its tendency to provoke haemodynamic instability. Factors determining drug selection include drug properties, patient group, clinician opinion, and cost. For example, drug properties such as onset and duration of action, side effect profile, pharmacokinetics, and pharmacodynamics are important. The characteristics of the individual patient and the specific indication for treatment need close attention. Many of these drugs are metabolized by liver enzymes and undergo renal excretion, therefore, when there is organ failure and polypharmacy, the choice, dose, and length of therapy require greater scrutiny by the clinician. In the absence of strong evidence to support a particular practice, the onus is on the clinician to consider the relative merits of differing regimens in each individual patient.

New agents

Promising new agents are finding their way into current practice. Remifentanil is a recently introduced opioid with potent sedative and analgesic properties [7, 8]. It is a μ receptor agonist that, uniquely, is metabolized by non-specific blood and tissue esterases to remifentanil acid, an essentially inactive product. Hence its metabolism is unaffected by organ failure and there is no drug accumulation, even when no liver is present [9]. This is of great importance in a critically ill patient with multiple organ failure. It has a very rapid onset and offset of action that is independent of the dose of drug used and the duration of infusion. These key, predictable features make it a very easy drug to titrate and control, in contrast to other opioids. It is usually given as a continuous intravenous infusion because of its rapid offset. However, it may be given by boluses for a short--acting effect before an intervention such as insertion of a chest tube. Although it is still new, initial research has been very encouraging with one study revealing that at least two-third of mechanically ventilated patients sedated with remifentanil could be extubated within 15 min of stopping the infusion. By facilitating early tracheal extubation, remifentanil may also relieve some of the demand for ICU beds [10]. Furthermore 60%–75% of patients when given an analgesia-based sedative regimen did not need a hypnotic agent such as midazolam or propofol [7, 8].

Dexmedetomidine is a centrally acting α_2-receptor agonist eight times more potent than clonidine [11]. It is a short-acting drug causing sedation, anxiolysis, and sympatholysis. Crucially, when given by continuous infusion it achieves a state of sedation where a high degree of rousability is maintained without compromising patient comfort. In addition, it has the advantage of causing minimal respiratory depression. The main limitations of dexmedetomidine are adverse haemodynamic effects resulting in bradycardia and hypotension. Its full role in ICU practice is yet to be established.

Optimal sedation

The need for sedation is well recognised and as a consequence undersedation is a less-frequent problem than oversedation. Once the purpose of sedation has been achieved, further increments are unnecessary and indeed may be detrimental. There are many hazards of oversedation [12]. Effects include hypotension, gastroparesis, immunosuppression, and respiratory depression. The process of weaning from artificial ventilation is protracted and there is an increased incidence of ventilator-associated pneumonia. The consequences of prolonged immobility such as venous thromboses and severe muscle wasting are further complications. Additionally, unnecessarily large amounts of sedative agents results in increased side effects, drug tolerance, and withdrawal phenomena. Cumulatively, these iatrogenic complications result in increased patient morbidity and delay in subsequent discharge from ICU [13, 14]. Despite increasing awareness of these problems, patients may remain oversedated owing to difficulty in recognizing this, poor appreciation of the consequences, and for ease of nursing. Also it may be difficult to manipulate the degree of sedation owing to drug properties and their altered metabolism in the critically ill resulting in unpredictability [15].

Defining the optimal level of sedation is itself problematic. This will depend on the needs of different patient groups, the specific indications and will vary from one patient to another. It is also subject to change within the same patient as his/her condition and stage of illness alters. Certain patient groups such as those with critical oxygenation or cerebral insults require deep sedation and paralysis as an increase in oxygen demand or intracranial pressure may be catastrophic. However, most medical or surgical patients require comfort alone, so the abolition of responsiveness is unnecessary. Although there is currently a shortage of good evidence comparing differing degrees of sedation with outcome in matched patient groups, it is logical for the delivery of sedative to be determined by the clinical indication. Thus, drug administration should be titrated against the desired effect rather than blindly accepting deep sedation in all patients. This more-refined method has a number of advantages. It is a rational approach that avoids the attendant risks of oversedation, minimizes drug side effects, and maximizes cost-effectiveness. Significantly, it maintains a degree of rousability that enables patients to communicate effectively and facilitates patient cooperation with therapeutic interventions.

Assessment of sedation and analgesia

If sedation and analgesia are to be titrated effectively, their effects must be readily assessable and quantifiable. This enables appropriate increments or decrements in drug delivery to be made in response to the prevailing level of sedation. Establishing objective measures of sedation and analgesia has proved difficult. Assessment of adequacy of analgesia may be relatively easy in patients who are able to communicate distress, but critically ill patients may be unable to do so, due to sedation or mechanical ventilation for example. In this case medical staff rely on non-verbal cues, such as grimacing or autonomic responses such as tachycardia and hypertension. These features are, however, unreliable and non-specific indicators of distress, and as yet no good measure of pain is available in such patients. While it is hoped that most patients are left sufficiently rousable to be able to answer simple questions about the presence or absence of pain, perhaps the most-important point is to have a high index of suspicion.

The clinical assessment and measurement of sedation is a recent practice following recognition of the benefits of light sedation. Traditionally the subjective assessment of the patient's attendants provided the only means of qualitatively assessing rousability. In an attempt to make this process more objective, sedation scales have been established. These enable more-precise descriptions of the degree of sedation by documenting patient response to given stimuli such as voice. Although they remain qualitative assessments, they provide a means of stereotyped assessment of the patient, reducing interobserver variability and providing standardized descriptions. Without such a measure the process of titration is impossible, since it relies on the principle of aiming at a target clinical end-point, in most cases a comfortable but rousable patient. The precise target end-point will vary according to patient group, clinician preference, and possibly staffing levels. However, the fundamental principle of measuring the response to a therapeutic intervention remains. Depending on the level of sedation, the sedative agent can be adjusted appropriately and the patient reassessed regularly when the process is repeated. This system is well established in other areas, for example, the insulin sliding scale, where there is an easy-to-measure number to titrate the drug to. Different institutions have devised their own sedation scales. Examples include the Ramsay scale [16], the most commonly used, the Brussels scale [17] and the Addenbrooke's sedation scale [18], shown below. Although there is good evidence to support the premise that the use of such scales can avoid excessive sedation in ICU patients, many establishments fail to institute this essential practice.

	0100	0200	0300	0400	0500
Agitated					
Awake					
Roused by voice					
Roused by tracheal suction					
Unrousable					
Paralyzed					
Asleep					

Fig. 1 The Addenbrooke's sedation scale

Use of the bispectral index (a derivative of the EEG) is starting to show promise as a measure of hypnosis, but not analgesia [19]. Its major advantage is that it generates a single number that shows the depth of sedation. However, the electromyogram of the facial and especially the frontalis muscle can interfere with it.

Clinical practice and optimal sedation

"These are my drowsy days: in vain do I now awake – to sleep again" Sir Thomas Browne, Religio Medici

A recent European survey [20] revealed wide variation in the clinical use of sedative agents. Although the particular sedative regimen used is dependent upon the characteristics of the individual patient, a number of measures may be employed to achieve controlled sedation. Frequently the choice of agent is influenced by the expected duration of ventilatory support. Thus if a long period of mechanical ventilation is anticipated, midazolam is often used. As the patient successfully weans from artificial ventilation they may benefit from changing to a shorter-acting agent, allowing elimination of accumulated metabolites and preventing delayed emergence. The risks of oversedation can also be minimized by addressing the dosing strategy. For example, boluses rather than infusions of drugs are more likely to result in lighter sedation with a rousable, communicative patient without drug accumulation, a shorter period of mechanical ventilation, length of stay in the ICU and hospital, and a reduction in organ dysfunction [21]. This also makes assessment of neurological status easier. However, intermittent administration may provoke haemodynamic instability and breakthrough discomfort. Additionally this method may be impractical if boluses are required very frequently, since it relies heavily on nursing staff availability.

Allowing patients to recover from sedation on a daily basis by stopping the drug infusion [22] until the patient emerges from sedation also reduces the period of mechanical ventilation, rate of brain computed tomographic scan, and length of ICU stay [14]. This ensures that the minimal dose of drug is administered for the shortest period of time to achieve the aims of sedation.

Despite increasing recognition that many patients have pain during their stay in the ICU, our treatment is not based on this. Current practice uses a hypnotic-based technique where the sedative agent is titrated against rousability and a fixed dose of opioid analgesic given [23]. Since it is difficult to assess pain in a sedated patient, pain control may be suboptimal. An analgesia-based technique also uses hypnotics in conjunction with analgesic agents, but it is the opioid that is titrated first against pain in a patient who is awake. A hypnotic agent is only added if necessary once adequate pain control has been achieved. There may be reluctance to use opioids in this way due to the problems of respiratory depression, the unpredictability of the drugs and fear of promoting addiction. However, recent studies have shown that using an analgesia-based technique decreases the need for hypnotic drugs significantly [7, 8]. The influence this has on physical and psychological morbidity is not yet established.

Conclusion

Over recent years deep sedation has been reserved for specific patient groups and the concept of controlled sedation has become widely accepted. The principle of titrating to desired effect is not novel (it is used with many drugs such as catecholamines), but its application to sedation is. Defining optimal sedation and quantifying measures of change are more difficult for sedative agents than other drugs. Although there are no established guidelines for current best practice the process of monitoring sedation in all patients is an essential first step towards a rational approach and needs to be pursued with zeal. Clearly, there is no universal regimen suitable for all patients, but establishing the principles of controlled sedation is fundamental to improving patient care and addressing the problems of increasing demand for intensive care by reducing morbidity and unnecessary periods of ventilation and ICU stay.

References

1. Bion JF, Oh TE (1997) Sedation in intensive care. In: Oh TE (ed) Intensive care manual, Butterworth Heineman, Oxford:, pp 672-678
2. Lewis KS, Whipple JK, Michael KA, Quebbeman EJ (1994) Effect of analgesic treatment on the physiological consequences of acute pain. Am J Hosp Pharm 51:1539-1554
3. BG van den, Wouters P, Weekers F et al (2001) Intensive insulin therapy in the critically ill patients. N Engl J Med 345:1359-1367
4. Jones C, Griffiths RD, Humphris G, Skirrow PM (2001) Memory, delusions, and the development of acute posttraumatic stress disorder-related symptoms after intensive care. Crit Care Med 29:573-580
5. Onen SH, Alloui A, Gross A et al (2001) The effects of total sleep deprivation, selective sleep interruption and sleep recovery on pain tolerance thresholds in healthy subjects. J Sleep Res 10:35-42
6. Krachman SL, D'Alonzo GE, Criner GJ (1995) Sleep in the intensive care unit. Chest 107:1713--1720
7. Kessler P, Chinachoni T, Berg P van der et al (2001) Remifentanil versus morphine for the provision of optimal sedation in ICU patients. Intensive Care Med 27 [Suppl 2]:S239-S406
8. Lopez A, Muellejans B, Cross MH et al (2001) The safety and efficacy of remifentanil for the provision of optimal sedation in ICU patients. Intensive Care Med 27 [Suppl 2]:S239-S407
9. Navapurkar VU, Archer S, Gupta SK et al (1998) Metabolism of remifentanil during liver transplantation. Br J Anaesth 81:881-886
10. Wilhelm W, Dorscheid E, Schlaich N et al (1999) The use of remifentanil in critically ill patients. Clinical findings and early experience. Anaesthesist 48:625-629
11. Bhana N, Goa KL, McClellan KJ (2000) Dexmedetomidine. Drugs 59:263-268
12. Park GR, Gempeler F (1993) The hazards of sedation and analgesia. Sedation and Analgesia, Saunders, London, pp 20-40
13. Brook AD, Ahrens TS, Schaiff R et al (1999) Effect of a nursing-implemented sedation protocol on the duration of mechanical ventilation. Crit Care Med 27:2609-2615
14. Kress JP, Pohlman AS, O'Connor MF, Hall JB (2000) Daily interruption of sedative infusions in critically ill patients undergoing mechanical ventilation. N Engl J Med 342:1471-1477
15. Shelly MP, Park GR, Mendel L (1987) Failure of critically ill patients to metabolise midazolam. Anaesthesia 42:619-626
16. Ramsay MAE, Savege TM, Simpson BJR, Goodwin R (1974) Controlled sedation with alphaxalone- alphadolone. B M J 2:656-659
17. Detriche O, Berre J, Massaut J, Vincent JL (1999) The Brussels sedation scale: use of a simple clinical sedation scale can avoid excessive sedation in patients undergoing mechanical ventilation in the intensive care unit. Br J Anaesth 83:698-701
18. O'Sullivan G, Park GR (1990) The assessment of sedation. Clin Intensive Care 1:116-122
19. Simmons LE, Riker RR, Prato BS, Fraser GL (1999) Assessing sedation during intensive care unit mechanical ventilation with the Bispectral Index and the Sedation-Agitation Scale. Crit Care Med 27:1499-504
20. Soliman HM, Mélot M, Vincent J-L (2001) Sedative and analgesic practice in the intensive care unit: the results of a European survey. Br J Anaesth 87:186-192
21. Kollef MH, Levy NT, Ahrens TS et al (1998) The use of continuous i.v. sedation is associated with prolongation of mechanical ventilation. Chest 114:541-548

22. Bodenham A, Shelly MP, Park GR (1988) The altered pharmacokinetics and pharmacodynamics of drugs commonly used in critically ill patients. Clin Pharmacokinet 14:347-373
23. Aitkenhead AR, Pepperman ML, Willatts SM et al (1989) Comparison of propofol and midazo-lam for sedation in critically ill patients. Lancet II:704-709

Organophosphorus poisoning

S. Prayag

Organophosphates (OP) represent a class of poisons that are highly toxic compounds used as insecticides, pesticides, and as nerve gas. An estimated 3 million cases of pesticide poisoning with 2,000 deaths occur all over the world every year [1].

Amongst the agents that cause pesticide poisoning, OP poisoning ranks foremost. Although the agents were known for a long time, interest in them has increased only since 1930s. Today about 50,000 compounds have been developed for potential use as pesticides. [2]. Although the Geneva Convention in 1974 banned the use of OP as part of a larger ban on chemical warfare, use still continues in chemical warfare, particularly in terrorist crime [3, 4].

Epidemiology

OP poisoning exists all over the world. As a suicidal agent, it has reached an epidemic proportion in India and some other developing countries. The reason for its commonness is the ease of availability and inexpensive nature. Although ingestion is the commonest route of entry, inhalation can also occur in patients who are accidental victims of OP poisoning. This is common in India in agricultural workers while spraying the crop.

Biochemical basis of clinical features

Acetylcholine is a common neurotransmitter released at the terminal nerve ending. This happens at all post-ganglionic parasympathetic nerve endings. It is also released in sympathetic and parasympathetic ganglia, the central nervous system (CNS), and skeletal muscle myoneural junction. The main action of OP compounds is to irreversibly inhibit the enzyme acetylcholinesterase [1]. This enzyme is functionally important at three sites of the human nerve endings:

muscarinic, nicotinic, and CNS synapses. As a result of the inhibition of acetylcholinesterase enzymes, there is a continued and prolonged excess of acetylcholine in the autonomic, neuromuscular, and CNS synapses. Recovery from OP poisoning depends therefore on the reactivation of the acetylcholine-sterase enzyme. Spontaneous reactivation occurs very slowly, while pharma-cological agents like oximes, which function as acetylcholinesterase reactiva-tors, can cause rapid activation. The action of oximes is limited by a time--dependent process known as the aging reaction. Generally, the aging reaction occurs after 48 – 72 h. In reality, different OP compounds have different aging half lives, as a result of which the duration and the efficacy of oximes varies considerably. Nicotinic transmission failure requires inhibition of at least 80% of acetylcholinesterase, and thus is seen in severe poisoning only. [5]

The main cholinesterase, acetylcholinesterase, also exists at functionally inert sites, like red blood cells (RBCs). Pseudocholinesterases also exist in the serum and, because of the ease of estimation, these enzymes are measured as a marker of the diagnosis and severity of OP poisoning. In the absence an antidote, the acetylcholinesterase is irreversibly destroyed and the enzyme resynthesis may take weeks. With appropriate support, the recovery in these patients may take weeks.

Clinical features

The time from exposure to the onset of toxicity varies from minutes to hours but is usually between 30 min and 2 h. The clinical features can be grouped as muscarinic, nicotinic, and central, according to the site of excessive acetylcholine.

Table 1 Various clinical features of organophosphorus (OP) poisoning

Muscarinic	• Sweating
	• Constricted pupil
	• Excessive lacrimation
	• Excessive salivation
	• Bronchorrhea
	• Wheezing
	• Vomiting
	• Diarrhea
	• Abdominal cramps
	• Bradycardia
	• Fall in blood pressure
	• Blurred vision
	• Urinary incontinence
Nicotinic	• Fasciculations
	• Cramps
	• Muscle weakness

	• Twitching
	• Respiratory distress
Central	• Coma
	• Cogwheeling
	• Convulsions
	• Respiratory depression
	• Circulatory depression
	• Cheyne Stokes respiration
	• Anxiety
	• Bilateral pyramidal signs (hyperreflexia, extensor plantars)

All these are called type I signs [6].

While bradycardia and miosis are the rule, tachycardia and mydriasis can rarely occur due to hyperstimulation at the preganglionic sympathetic nerve endings [1, 2, 6]. The muscarinic syndrome occurs immediately after exposure and may last for a few days, depending on the severity of intoxication. The threat to life in this early phase can come from various sources as seen in Table 2.

Table 2 How critical care units are useful for the specific disorders in OP poisoning (*ARDS* acute respiratory distress syndrome)

Respiratory failure	• Pulmonary edema
	• Central respiratory depression
	• Paralysis of respiratory muscles
	• Bulbar weakness causing aspirations
	• Drowning in secretions
	• Bronchoconstriction
	• Unconsciousness
	• ARDS [14]
Cardiac failure	• Central depression
	• Disturbances of cardiac conduction (multiple ectopics, junctional rhythm, AV blocks)

Nicotinic signs, which are initially commonly seen, are muscle twitching and fasciculations; 24 – 48 h later, neurological deficits lasting 2-18 days are seen [7-9]. Ocular, bulbar, neck, proximal limb, and respiratory muscles are involved, usually in that order.

Some OP compounds, particularly triorthocresyl phosphate (TOCP) and tricresyl phosphate (TCP), produce what is called delayed neurotoxicity. On ingestion, these do not produce significant signs of acetylcholine excess, but 7-20 days later they show a pure motor axonal neuropathy without any sensory loss. This phenomenon is due to depression of a different esterase, called neurotoxic esterase (NTE), in the nervous system [10].

Dual neurotoxicity, consisting of an early stage of neurological signs due to cholinesterase deficiency followed by delayed neurotoxicity, is also seen rarely [10].

Nerve gases used in warfare work via OP poisoning. They are powerful irreversible inhibitors of cholinesterases. The infamous Tokyo subway disaster is believed to be due to these.

Variation amongst the OP may also be seen, due to differences in chemical structure and actions. Carbamates produce fulminant early muscarinic signs with few nicotinic signs. Fenthion causes fewer muscarinic signs but neuroparalysis is more frequently observed than with the others.

Investigations

The initial diagnosis is mostly clinical with the history, typical signs, and the smell of the gastric aspirate raising the suspicion of OP poisoning. Cholinesterase studies are helpful. Besides causing the depression of the enzymes at the myoneural junction, OP poisons depress both the true cholinesterase enzyme of RBC and the pseudocholinesterase in the plasma. The latter is easier to measure. A reduction in RBC cholinesterase is more specific but less readily available and some OP poisons may reduce only one type of cholinesterase. A reduction in plasma or RBC enzyme levels to less than 50 % of their basal levels confirms the diagnosis [11]. Reports of correlation of the levels with the severity and thus prognosis have limited value in view of the compounding effects of various signs. The levels may stay low for days, but treatment should be adjusted according to the clinical picture and not the cholinesterase levels. With carbamates, the depression in the levels is usually transient. Specific tests may identify these poisons in the urine.

Electrophysiology studies show typical features, consisting of repetitive motor unit activity, normal nerve conduction velocity, reduced amplitude of motor action potentials, and decrement on repetitive stimulation [10]. The administration of antidotes is associated with abolition of decremental response, and some have used this as a guide to decisions regarding duration and dose of oximes [9, 12].

Treatment

General measures

Removal of the source of poisons has to be done by change of contaminated clothing, washing the skin with soap and water, and removal from the site of inhalational exposure. If ingestion is the route of entry, gastrointestinal decontamination with use of nasogastric tube lavage and activated charcoal should be performed.

Patients should be admitted to the intesive care unit if the toxicity is severe and if there is need for hemodynamic support, or respiratory support and for monitoring for organ failure. Airway protection by endotracheal intubation is necessary in patients with obtunded levels of consciousness or increased oral or broncheal secretions. Mechanical ventilatory support is needed for all patients who have developed frank respiratory failure or who are on the verge of it. Since the most-common cause of death is respiratory failure, it is obvious that mechanical ventilation should be able to reduce the mortality in OP poisoning. In fact the availability of mechanical ventilation even in peripheral areas and the understanding of the concepts of respiratory care has significantly and favorably altered the course of OP poisoning.

Atropine

Atropine is the physiological antidote of OP poisoning and therefore remains the mainstay of treatment along with oximes. A trial dose of atropine becomes justified in all cases in which OP poisoning is even suspected [13, 14]. The ability to tolerate large doses of atropine without any significant side effects is virtually diagnostic of OP poisoning [13]. Initial doses need to be given under cardiac monitoring and with the close supervision of a physician. Initial dose should be consistent with the severity of clinical signs of OP poisoning; 2 mg IV is usually recommended as the initial dose. However, it is not unusual to require 3 – 10 mg as the initial dose [10]. Depending on the clinical response, repeat doses are given in same or increasing amount at 15- to 60-min intervals, until signs of atropinization occur. Continuous infusions are used by some as a substitute for repeat doses. Signs of atropinization include dry mouth, flushing, dilated pupils, tachycardia, increased body temperature, and irritability. The duration of use of atropine on average is believed to be 4 – 7 days, but depends on the clinical response and rate of recovery and metabolism of OP poisons. Close observation is necessary during the period of reduction and omission of atropine. Delayed signs of cholinergic excess in the form of pulmonary edema or cardiac effects or other muscarinic effects of OP poisoning are seen in some patients due to gradual release of lipophilic OP compounds like fenthion from the fat depots. The duration of necessity of atropine may thus be much more prolonged than clinically thought. Signs of excessive atropinization include fever, delirium, tachycardia, cardiac arrhythmia, and muscular twitching.

Glycopyrrolate, a quaternary ammonium compound, is like atropine and gives better control of secretions, less tachycardia, and does not cross the blood brain barrier.

Atropine has no action on the nicotinic signs or muscle weakness [15-17].

Oximes

Oximes are the treatment agents of choice for OP poisoning and should be used for nearly all patients with clinically significant OP poisoning, particularly those with nicotinic signs like weakness or fasciculations. This class of agents has the capacity to reactivate the cholinesterases.

The oximes used include pralidoxime chloride, pralidoxime iodide, pralidoxime methylsulfate, pralidoxime mesylate, obidoxime chloride, trimedoxime, BI 6, HI 6, HiO 7, etc. Amongst these, pralidoxime is the most commonly used.

The actions of oximes are [18]:
1. Primary effect of cleaving the phosporylation–acetylcholinesterase bond, thus freeing and reactivating cholinesterases
2. Directly acting with and detoxifying the OP compounds
3. Having an anti-cholinergic "atropine-like" effect

Pralidoxime is used in doses of 1 g IV given over 15 –30 min, followed by 4- to 6-hourly doses. The effect or reversal of neurological signs is often dramatic.

The frequency and duration of the oxime use has been an issue that has been under considerable debate. This is compounded by the experience of it being ineffective against certain OP compounds. The use of oximes in human OP poisoning is derived from their protective influences in experimental nerve gas poisoning [19]. Over the years its use has been largely empirical. An occasional study has shown that oximes may have no benefit [20]. A randomized controlled trial in India between placebo and oximes showed no benefit of oximes [21] and no difference in one single dose versus continuous infusion [22]. Despite such observations, it is conventional practice to administer oximes in patients with OP poisoning. The discrepancies between its rationale and its clinical benefit can be understood better if one understands its actions. Half-life of oximes is 1.5-3.5 h. Thus a single dose is likely to be ineffective. Certain OP compounds do not respond to certain oximes [23]. It was also reported that if the blood levels of OP were above a certain level, they may not respond to oximes [24]. Oximes also produce an "aging reaction" that determines the time for which the oximes may continue to be useful [1]. The beneficial effect of oximes is also limited by the observations that patients sometimes may worsen while on oximes [25, 26], a phenomenon that has not been properly explained.

Given these limitations, it is quite rational to expect uncertainty with the response to oximes, thus requiring close observations, monitoring, and titration rather than fixed doses for a pre-determined period.

Other agents

A new drug Gacyclidine (GK 11) has recently been found to be useful for the CNS effects of OP poisons. Other agents like A 1 receptor antagonists have shown promising results in animals [27].

Outcome

All previous reports have shown a significant mortality with respiratory failure as the predominant cause of death [10, 27]. It is this author's experience that with the current expertise in ventilation, such respiratory failures should be none too difficult to manage and cases of OP poisoning who reach such good centers should have very little mortality.

References

1. WHO (1986) Organophosphate insecticides: a general introduction. Environmental Health Criteria no. 63, World Health Organization, Geneva
2. Besser R, Gutmann L (1994) Intoxication with organophosphate compounds. In: Vinken PJ, Bruyn GW (eds) Handbook of clinical neurology, vol 64. Intoxications of the nervous system. Elsevier, Amsterdam, pp 151-182
3. Nozaki M, Aikawa N (1995) Sarin poisoning in Tokyo subway (letter). Lancet 245:1446
4. Schaler SN (1996) CIA studying nerve gas exposure. Indianapolis Star, Indianapolis, A3
5. Awasthi G, Singh G (2002) Serial neuro electrophysiological studies in acute organophosphate poisoning (OPP). Correlation with serum cholinesterase levels and atropine dosages. J Assoc Physicians India (in press)
6. Wadia RS, Chitra S, Amin RB, et al (1987) Electrophysiological studies in acute organophosphate poisoning. J Neurol Neurosurg Psychiatry 50:1442-1448
7. Senanayake N, Karalidde L (1987) Neurotoxic effects of organophosphate insecticide. An intermediate syndrome. N Engl J Med 316:761-763
8. Singh G, Khurana D, Awasthi G, et al (1998) The spectrum and clinical correlates of electrodiagnostic abnormalities in acute organophosphate poisoning. A study of 55 patients. Neurol India 45:28-35
9. Singh G Mahajan R, Whig J (1998) The importance of electrodiagnostic studies in acute organophosphate poisoning. J Neurol Sci 157:191-200
10. Wadia RS (1999) Organophosphate poisoning. In: Sainani GS (ed) API textbook of medicine. Association of Physicians of India, Mumbai, pp 1306-1308
11. Linden CH, Lovejoy FH Jr (1998) Poisoning and drug overdose. In: Fauci AS, Braunwald E, Isselbacher KJ, et al (eds) Harrison's principles of internal medicine. McGraw Hill, New York, p 2539
12. Singh G, Awasthi G, Khurana D et al (1998) Neurophysiological monitoring of pharmacological manipulation in acute organophosphate (OP) poisoning. The effects of pralidoxime, pancuronium and magnesium sulphate. Electroencephal Clin Neurophysiol 107:140-148
13. Namba T, Nolte CT, Jackrel J, et al (1971) Poisoning due to organophosphate insecticides. Am J Med 5:475-490

14. Haddad LM (1983) Organophosphorus poisoning. In: Haddad LM, Winchester JF (eds) Clinical management of poisoning and drug overdose. Saunders, Philadelphia, pp 704-710
15. Arena JM (1970) Poisoning: toxicology, symptoms, treatment, 2nd edn, Thomas, Springfield
16. Gleason MN, Gosselin RE, Hodge HC, et al (1976) Clinical toxicology of commercial products, 3rd edn Williams and Wilkins, Baltimore
17. Gilman AG, Goodman LS, Gilman A (1985) The pharmacologic basis of therapeutics, 7th edn MacMillan, New York
18. Hayes WJ (1975) Toxicology of pesticides. Williams and Wilkins, Baltimore
19. Dultz L, Epstein MA, Freeman G, et al (1957) Studies on a group of oximes as therapeutic compounds in sarin poisoning J Pharmacol Exp Ther 119:522-531
20. DeSilva HJ, Wijewickrema R, Senanayake N (1992) Does pralidoxime affect outcome of management in acute organophosphorus poisoning? Lancet 339:1136-1138
21. Cherian AM, Peter JV, Johnson S, et al (1997) Effectiveness of P2AM (PAM – pralidoxime) in the treatment of organophosphorus poisoning. A randomized double blind placebo controlled trial. J Assoc Physicians India 45:22-24
22. Johnson S, Peter JV, Thomas K, et al (1996) Evaluation of two treatment regimens of pralidoxime (1 gm single bolus vs. 12 gm infusion) in the management of organophosphorus poisoning. J Assoc Physicians India 44:529-531
23. Worek F, Dieplod C, Eyer P (1999) Dimethyl phosphoryl inhibited human cholinesterases inhibition, reactivation, and aging kinetics. Arch Toxicol 73:7-14
24. Willems JL, De Bisschop HC, Verstraete AG, et al (1993) Cholinesterase reactivation in organophosphate poisoned patients depends on the plasma concentrations of oximes, pralidoxime methylsulphate and of organophosphate. Arch Toxicol. 67:79-84
25. Eyer F, Eyer P (1998) Enzyme based assay for quantification of paroxan in blood of parathion poisoned patients. Hum Exp Toxicol 17:645-651
26. Du Pont PW, Muller FO, Van Tonder WN, et al (1981) Experience with the intensive care management of organophosphate insecticide poisoning. S Afr Med J 60:227-229
27. Awasthi G, Mahajan R, Avasthi R (2001) Organophosphorus poisoning – present status. In: Panja M (ed) Medicine update, vol. 11. The Association of Physicians of India, Calcutta, pp 792-798

Physostigmine in the postoperative period

J. RUPREHT

Physostigmine improves recovery from anaesthesia in several distinct ways

Recovery from the anaesthetic effect of drugs has by large remained a spontaneous biological process that depends on the capacity of the body to exhale, excrete or metabolize general anaesthetic agents. There are no drugs in sight for reversal of general anaesthetic action, which, apparently, is not receptor bound to any significant degree. However, during the general anaesthetic effect of drugs, the central nervous system (CNS) neurotransmitter functioning is considerably affected and may be either depressed or excited. The effect of anaesthetics on CNS neurotransmission may be direct or indirect and, depending on functional connections of different transmitter systems, may result in either augmentation or depression of activity of a specific transmission system. Neurotransmitters function in a feed-back interdependent manner: excitation of inhibitory systems will prevail over normal functioning of excitatory systems, and vice versa, until functional equilibrium is re-established. Furthermore, functional exhaustion of a certain transmitter system results in behavioural and functional depression of its normal functioning.

Acetylcholine (ACh) is widely present in the CNS and subserves transmission at the muscarinic and nicotinic receptors. The CNS-muscarinic cholinergic transmission has been explored to a far greater degree than the nicotinic one [1]. The reason for this lies in the fact that until recently no specific antagonists were available for the CNS-nicotinic receptors. In contrast, specific antagonists to the CNS-muscarinic receptors have been around since time immemorial, examples being atropine or scopolamine. Therefore, effects of these drugs on the functioning of the brain are well known [2], as well as the functions of the brain subserved by the action of ACh on the CNS-muscarinic receptors (Table 1) [3].

Table 1 Functions subserved by the central nervous system (CNS)-muscarinic (cholinergic) transmission

Auditory input	Transfer to memory store
Olfactory input	Attention, alertness
Cardiovascular control	Vigilance
Respiratory control	Antinociception
Drinking	Thermoregulation
Grooming	Muscle coordination
Affective behaviour	Reflex coordination
Complex behaviours	REM sleep
Learning (initial stage)	Process of adaptation
Working (short-term) memory	Addiction

Anaesthesia, local or general, may profoundly diminish normal functioning of the CNS-muscarinic transmission. Elevation of the CNS-ACh can easily be achieved by physostigmine, which can pass the blood-brain barrier and inhibit the ACh esterase (AChE). Recovery from anaesthesia can be smoothened and shortened as a whole, motor unrest controlled, and coordination of protective reflexes normalized. Physostigmine clearly improves breathing, enhances analgesia, controls shivering, sustains process of vigilance, memory, alertness, and thermoregulation. In specific settings, physostigmine may help fast tracking in anaesthesia for day case surgery.

Physostigmine improves postoperative consciousness and vigilance

Weinstock et al. [4] in 1982 evaluated the beneficial effect of physostigmine on postoperative morphine-induced respiratory depression and somnolence and found that the analgesic effect of morphine was increased [4]. Excitement following conscious sedation was successfully reversed by physostigmine [5], and somnolence following epidural morphine was successfully treated [6]. Transient confusion and amnesia caused by electroconvulsive therapy were improved by physostigmine [7] and diminished postoperative vigilance disappeared quickly and fully, without significant unwanted side effects [8]. Level of consciousness on arrival in the recovery room is of paramount importance in prevention of early respiratory complications. In an audit of 16,065 patients, a significant relationship was found between diminished consciousness and the incidence of respiratory complications, regardless of the ASA risk grade or age [9]. Adjustment of anaesthetic techniques and more-frequent use of physostigmine would result in reduction of early postoperative complications. The fact is that physostigmine results in early return and normal coordination of protective reflexes, and the shortening of recovery of full consciousness is of lesser importance in this regard. Aminophylline can also significantly shorten recovery of consciousness after nitrous oxide/enflurane anaesthesia, but results in more pain and increased restlessness [10]. In contrast, physostigmine produced a calm patient with well-functioning protective reflexes, thus improving greatly the quality of recovery. The time from stopping the anaesthetic mixture to awakening was 12±3 min for aminophylline and 18±9 min for physostigmine. The control time was 18±5 min. This clearly shows that aminophylline is a specific CNS excitatory agent, called an analeptic, whereas physostigmine specifically normalized ACh-dependent CNS functions without antagonizing the anaesthetic action of enflurane.

Physostigmine improves breathing postoperatively

It has been established that physostigmine can reverse the respiratory depressant effect of opiates [11] and the accompanying somnolence, leaving analgesia unaffected. In clinical practice, the patients become more alert during the recovery, after administration of physostigmine, restlessness disappears and symptoms or complaints of pain subside. One mechanism of opioid respiratory depressant effect is decreased release of ACh in the medulla oblongata, which is easily corrected by the centrally acting AChE inhibitor physostigmine. Breathing is thus improved because of increased vigilance, improved memory functioning, and normalization of ACh in the respiratory center. Clinical experience with physostigmine post anaesthetic shows that physostigmine indeed greatly reduces indications for opiate antagonists postoperatively, but cannot resolve respiratory depression of gross opiate overdose. In such cases, it is good clinical practice to continue mechanical ventilation and refrain from short- -acting opiate antagonists. Experimental analysis of improved breathing following physostigmine, during morphine respiratory depression, was performed by Berkenbosch et al. [12] in Leiden, on cats in which extracorporeal circulation enabled separation of peripheral chemoreceptors from the activity of the respiratory center. It was shown that physostigmine certainly stimulates ventilation, due to a decrease in apnoeic threshold.

Physostigmine enhances postoperative analgesia

There are several analgesia mechanisms based on the ACh transmitter system in the CNS. Physostigmine causes threefold analgesia, firstly by its intrinsic analgesic action through the serotonin system [2], secondly through increase of ACh in the brain and the spinal cord. These two analgesic effects cannot be reversed by opiate antagonists. Furthermore, the metabolites of physostigmine, eserolin and eserolinol are morphine-like substances capable of considerable cholinesterase inhibition. They produce ACh-dependent and opiate-like analgesia, but with moderate respiratory depression. These substances have not yet been developed for clinical use, but neostigmine has already been added to cocktails injected into the liquor space. Achieving a degree of systemic analgesia with physostigmine is obviously more practical, as this drug can be administered intravenously for its CNS effect. Petersson et al. [13] in Uppsala established that in postoperative patients 2 mg physostigmine produces the same analgesia as 50 mg pethidine for 15 min and gradually subsides within 30 min. In short, physostigmine greatly improves postoperative analgesia through its own analgesic actions, leaves the existing opiate analgesia intact, but decreases the residual opiate-induced respiratory depression. According to Eisenach [14], muscarinic cholinergic agonists and cholinesterase inhibitors hold promise as non-opiate agents for the treatment of moderate-to-severe acute and chronic pain, and of all such agents physostigmine has already firmly established its place in clinical practice and is by far most studied. Knowledge of physostigmine has become a part of standard international textbooks [2].

Physostigmine improves thermoregulation

It has long been known that normal functioning of muscarinic receptors in the thermoregulatory center of the hypothalamus is essential for thermoregulation [15]. Many anaesthetic drugs possess a degree of affinity for muscarinic receptors or may completely block them [2], inducing a tendency to increased body temperature. This is obvious in intoxication with anticholinergics where centrally induced hyperpyrexia is worsened by the inhibited sweating, caused by direct effect of anticholinergics on sweat glands. It was also found that increased cholinergic activity in the hypothalamus results in down-regulation of body temperature [20]. Whenever cooling of the patient is indicated, it is wise to include physostigmine in the treatment protocol. In cases of hyperthermia in head injuries or CNS infection and anticholinergic poisoning, clearing of mental status after physostigmine may save the patient from direct computed tomography, magnetic resonance imaging, or lumbar puncture [16]. A normal dose of atropine sulphate or scopolamine may induce extreme central hyperpyrexia. This is very likely to occur in an already febrile patient [17], either perioperatively or in the intensive care unit. Central hyperpyrexia should be treated with physostigmine in all patients who are already febrile from other causes. This may be life saving in the very young or very old patients suffering from fever, when they present for surgery and anaesthesia. We have observed postoperatively that administration of physostigmine lowers febrile temperatures, which had been blamed only on the infection. Whole-body hyperthermia used in the treatment of cancer, causes serious depression of the patient's sensorium, but this was readily relieved with physostigmine [18].

Physostigmine decreases postoperative shivering

Postoperative shivering is caused by a multitude of factors, decreased body temperature being most known. Acute withdrawal from nitrous oxide or propofol may cause rhythmic, spontaneous, but intermittent motor unrest. Shivering certainly is not a reliable sign of body hypothermia, and may be a sign of dangerously rapid increase of fever in sepsis. Therefore, before warming of the patient is started, one must measure the core temperature. In undercooled patients, pethidine is very useful to decrease shivering and accompanying consumption of oxygen, while increasing the patient's comfort [28]. Physostigmine is also very useful in this situation, at the same time increasing vigilance, improving analgesia, and breathing [2]. Its effect is based on down-regulation of the central thermostat [15] and on better inhibitory control of non-hypothermia shivering in cases of acute withdrawal of anaesthetic agents. Physostigmine reliably prevents the overshoot of core temperature often occurring during postoperative rewarming.

Physostigmine prevents or treats the central anticholinergic syndrome

The clinical picture caused by anticholinergic action in the brain and periphery is called the central anticholinergic syndrome (CAS), consisting of many signs and symptoms [2]. Consciousness may be unduly suppressed following anaesthesia, the patient may be amnesic and restless, extremely agitated, or comatose. Experienced anaesthetists recognize the syndrome readily, and it resolves within 1-5 min following administration of physostigmine [2]. The CAS has also been called physostigmine responsive syndrome by the Edinburgh anaesthetists [26]. In practice, physostigmine can be administered 15-10 min before the end of anaesthesia in order to prevent unwanted central anticholinergic symptoms during the recovery [2, 10]. Knowledge of CAS is comprehensive and the reader is advised to consult standard textbooks [2].

Postoperative physostigmine: dosage and administration

Whatever the perioperative indication for physostigmine, about 0.03 mg kg^{-1} is required to achieve a satisfactory effect [2]. This dosage is sufficient for the necessary plasma concentration to cause an analeptic effect in the CNS, which lies between 3 and 5 ng ml^{-1} [19]. Physostigmine is preferably injected slowly intravenously, but can also be administered intramuscularly or subcutaneously. Less than 2 mg may be sufficient in postoperative patients in cases of mild CNS anticholinergic toxicity. One administration is usually sufficient postoperatively once the CAS symptomatology has been resolved. In contrast, cases of severe anticholinergic poisonings require repeat administration of physostigmine approximately every 90-120 min or, only in selected cases, a continuous infusion of about 2 mg physostigmine per hour [21]. The affinity of physostigmine for plasma cholinesterases is lower than for the CNS cholinesterase, which means that the drug is readily taken up by the brain and the levels in blood are seldom high enough to cause considerable salivation or bradycardia. The predominant cardiovascular effect of physostigmine is centrally increased sympathetic tone, resulting in increase of blood pressure and heart rate [2].

Physostigmine as differential diagnostic agent in recovery

Postoperative consciousness disturbance (POCD) is often not caused by anticholinergic drugs and may result from CNS haemorrhage, pre-existent psychiatric disorders, metabolic disorders, CNS trauma, extreme temperature deviations, or microgravitational brain oedema. The latter may occur during operations lasting more than 10 h. In all these cases, physostigmine should be indicated – when the POCD does not clear up following physostigmine one must promptly search for a non-pharmacological cause of failed consciousness [2]. An absolute prerequisite before administration of physostigmine is adequate muscle power, as it is otherwise impossible to judge the patient's reactions to internal or external stimuli [2]. Signs of residual muscle relaxation or of muscle weakness caused by some antibiotics are upper airway obstruction, rise in blood pressure and heart rate, and agitation. Such signs are very similar to those of CAS. Neostigmine should, therefore, be administered first in doubtful cases, preferably along with a peripherally acting anticholinergic, like methylatropine or glycopyrrolate [29].

Physostigmine improves fast tracking in anaesthesia

Rapid, complete, and reliable recovery from anaesthesia is an important demand for the contemporary anaesthetist. Fast tracking has been made easier by the advent of controllable, short-acting anaesthetic drugs. Nevertheless, serious disturbances of recovery have been reported for propofol [22], ranging from delayed recovery to prolonged amnesia or hallucinations. Treatment of these symptoms with physostigmine resolved all disturbances promptly [23], indicating that these were caused by central anticholinergic action of propofol. In military trauma anaesthesia, the improved recovery profile from physostigmine following ketamine enabled earlier transfer of patients [27].

Availability of physostigmine

It is not uncommon that anaesthetists do not learn to recognize the CAS and may consider its occurrence as a failure, to the detriment of their patients and anaesthetic performance. CAS occurs during anaesthesia as a pharmacological rule, but it is not always necessary to treat it. The underlying cause for such professional behaviour is the lack of knowledge of the effect of drugs on complex behavioural functioning of the brain. In some places physostigmine is not available, obviously the consequence of inadequate demand for it [24, 25]. Ries [25] recommended that physostigmine should be re-stocked in all emergency, intensive care, and postanaesthetic areas. Any major hospital pharmacy can produce ampules of 1 mg/ml physostigmine. Alternatively, Anticholium (Köhler, Germany) is the classical standard formulation of commercially available physostigmine in Europe.

References

1. Karczmar AG (1990) Physiological cholinergic functions in the CNS. Prog Brain Res 84: 437-442
2. Rupreht J, Dworacek B (1996) The central anticholinergic syndrome in the postoperative period. In: Prys-Roberts C, et al (eds). International practice of anaesthesia, vol. 2. Butterworth-Heinemann, Oxford, pp 132:1-11
3. Van Delft AML, Hagan JJ, Tonnaer JADM (1988) Muscarinic receptors in the central nervous system. Prog Pharmacol 7:93-117
4. Weinstock M, Roll D, Erez E (1982) Effect of physostigmine on morfine-induced postoperative pain and somnolence. Br J Anaesth 54:429-434
5. Milam SB, Bennett CR (1987) Physostigmine reversal of drug-induced paradoxical excitement. Int J Oral Maxillofac Surg 16:190-193
6. Shulman MS, Sandler A, Brebner J (1984) The reversal of epidural morphine induced somnolence with physostigmine. Can Anaesth Soc J 31:678-680

7. Levyn Y, Elizur A, Korczyn AD (1987) Physostigmine improves ECT-induced memory disturbances. Neurology 37:871-875
8. Schneck HJ, Tempel G, Hundelshausen B von (1985) Zur Beeinflussung der Vigilanz in der
   postnarkotischen Phase durch Physostigmin. Anaesthesist 34:465-471
9. Parr SM, Robinson BJ, Glover PW, et al (1991) Level of consciousness on arrival in the recovery
   room and the development of early respiratory morbidity. Anaesth Intensive Care 19:369-372
10. Kesecioglu J, Rupreht J, Telci L, et al (1991) Effect of aminophylline or physostigmine on
    recovery from nitrous oxide-enflurane anaesthesia. Acta Anaesthesiol Scand 35:616-620
11. Snir-Mor I, Weinstok M, Davidson JT, et al (1983) Physostigmine antagonises morphine-induced
    respiratory depression in human subjects. Anesthesiology 59:6-9
12. Berkenbosch A, Rupreht J, De Goede J, et al (1993) Effect of eserine on the ventilatory response
    to CO_2. Eur J Pharmacol 232:21-28
13. Petersson J, Gordh TE, Hartvig P, et al (1986) A double-blind trial of the analgesic properties of
    physostigmine in postoperative patients. Acta Anesthesiol Scand 30:283-288
14. Eisenach JC (1999) Muscarinic-mediated analgesia. Life Sci 64:549-554
15. Varagic VM, Zugic M, Roll D (1971) The hypothermic effect of eserine in the rat. Naunyn
    Schmiedebergs Arch Pharmacol 270:407-418
16. Smilkstein MJ (1991) Editorial. J Emerg Med 9:275-277
17. Torline RL (1992) Extreme hyperpyrexia associated with central anticholinergic syndrome.
    Anesthesiology 76:470-471
18. Versteegh PMR (1980) Gegeneraliseerde hyperthermie: een klinische methode. Thesis. Univer-
    sity of Leiden, pp 88-90
19. Hartvig P, Wiklund L, Lindström B (1986) Pharmacokinetics of physostigmine after intravenous,
    intramuscular and subcutaneous administration in surgical patients. Acta Anaesthesiol Scand 30:
    177-182
20. Maickel RP, Kinney DR, Ryker DL et al (1991) Antagonism of physostigmine induced hypot-
    hermia and neuroendocrine changes following exposure to different environmental temperatu-
    res. Prog Neuropsychoparmacol Biol Psychiatry 15:873-884
21. Stern TA (1983) Continuous infusion of physostigmine in anticholinergic delirium: a case report.
    J Clin Psychiatry 44:463-464
22. Anaesthesia Correspondence Hallucinations after propofol (1988) 43:170-171
23. Dworacek B, Rupreht J, Erdmann W, et al (1989) Das Auftreten eines zentralen anticholinergen
    Syndroms nach Propofol und seine Therapie mit Physostigmin. In: Tempel G (ed) Physostigmin
    und postnarkotische Vigilanz. Gustav Fischer Verlag, Stuttgart, pp 23-29
24. Martin B, Howell PR (1997) Physostigmine: going…going…gone? Eur J Anaesth 14: 476-470
25. Ries CR (1999) Physostigmine in 1999; tolerability, indications and availability. Can J Anaesth
    46:707-707
26. Cook B, Spence AA (1997) Postoperative central anticholinergic syndrome. Editorial. Eur J
    Anaesth 14: 1-2
27. Hamilton-Davies C, Bailie R, Restall J, et al (1995) Physostigmine in recovery from anaesthesia.
    Anaesthesia 50:456-458
28. Horn E-P, Standl T, Sessler D, et al (1998) Physostigmine prevents postanesthetic shivering as
    does meperidine or clonidine. Anesthesiology 88:108-113
29. Viby-Mogensen J (2000) Central anticholinergic syndrome or postoperative residual block?
    Correspondence. Eur J Anesth 17:466-467

Physostigmine use in intensive care

K. LEENDERTSE, J. RUPREHT

Full recovery of patients in the intensive care (IC) unit after anaesthesia or long-term sedation is not always predictable and uneventful. Patients may fail to regain consciousness or be agitated and uncooperative. Other patients are admitted to the IC unit unconscious due to intended drug overdose, intoxication, or poisoning. Central anticholinergic syndrome (CAS), first described by Longo in 1966 [1] is an important diagnosis in these patients. Many drugs frequently used in anaesthesia and IC may induce impairment of central cholinergic transmission [2-4] and are responsible for this clinical picture, but many other clinical conditions with identical symptoms may challenge the intensivist. The differential diagnosis in IC patients is much more complicated [3, 5, 6], and includes a prolonged action of anaesthetic drugs, neurological problems like cerebral trauma, oedema, haemorrhage, ischaemia, or embolism, metabolic derangements such as hyper- or hypoglycaemia, hepatic or renal encephalopathy, acid-base disturbances, electrolyte abnormalities, endocrinopathies like thyrotoxicosis, hypo- and hyperadrenalcorticism, body temperature dysregulation, respiratory problems causing hypo- or hypercapnia or hypoxia, and psychiatric pathology like organic psycho-syndrome or acute psychosis. Administration of physostigmine, a centrally active cholinesterase inhibitor, can be useful in those patients where central acetylcholine deficit may be a problem.

Indications for physostigmine in IC

CAS in IC

The reported incidence of CAS following general anaesthesia varies between 1% and 40 % [2, 7, 8].The reason for this great difference in incidence is the lack of strict criteria to diagnose CAS. In IC the incidence is not well known, because it is underdiagnosed frequently and confused with prolonged drug action. Schneck [9] and Brede and Dennhardt [10] reported an incidence of 4% and Rathgeber et al. [11] and incidence of 5% in patients after cardiothoracic surgery.

Many centrally acting drugs with anticholinergic properties, opioids, and sedative drugs cause an impairment of central cholinergic transmission (see Table 1), as described by Wise and Cassem in 1992 [12], and are frequently used in IC.

Table 1 Drugs with central anticholinergic activity

Antidepressants	Sympathomimetics
Antihistamines	Tranquillizers (benzodiazepines)
Antipsychotics	Anticonvulsants
Antispasmodics	Anti-inflammatory drugs
Anti-Parkinson agents	Anti-neoplastic drugs
Belladonna-alkaloids	Antihypertensive and cardiac drugs
Analgesics	Hallucinogens (LSD, ketamine, mescaline)
Anaesthetic gases	Contrast agents
Opioids	

CAS or the central physostigmine responsive syndrome, as mentioned by Cook and Spence in 1997 [13], may be an underlying problem in IC patients. The symptoms are numerous and unpredictable, in combinations as well as in varying degrees of severity. They result from disturbances of cerebral functions dependent on acetylcholine muscarinic transmission in the central nervous system (Table 2). Undiagnosed CAS may be dangerous for patients because they may harm themselves and the surgical results. The risk of aspiration, unnecessary tracheal intubation, and mechanical ventilation may prolong the stay in the IC unit [2, 6]. The differential diagnosis is complicated and many

Table 2 Central and peripheral symptoms of the central anticholinergic syndrome

Central symptoms	Peripheral symptoms
Agitation	Dry mouth, thirst
Amnesia	Disturbed speech
Confusion	Dry, red skin
Hallucinations	Mydriasis, blurred vision
Ataxia	Tachycardia
Nausea	Decreased gastrointestinal motility
Hyperalgesia	Photophobia
Hyperpyrexia	Heart dysrhythmias
Disorientation	Impairment of micturition
Convulsions	Hyperpyrexia (peripheral origin)
Somnolence	
Coma	
Respiratory insufficiency	
Delirium	

other causes of abnormal neurological behavior must be excluded before diagnosing CAS. Once the CAS is suspected, treatment with physostigmine is indicated and patients may recover in a matter of minutes.

Acute poisoning

In anticholinergic intoxication, patients present classical symptoms of central and peripheral anticholinergic blockade, including tachycardia, hyperpyrexia, dry red skin, drying of mucous membranes and secretions, mydriasis, urinary retention, paralytic ileus, hallucinations, restlessness, disorientation, delirium, convulsions, and coma [14, 15].

A variety of drugs, like tricyclic and tetracyclic antidepressants (amitriptyline, imipramine, and maprotiline) antihistamines, phenothiazines, anti-Parkinson agents, butyrophenones, belladonna alkaloids [16], plant extracts [14], and herbal tea, may cause this clinical picture.

The differential diagnosis of anticholinergic poisoning includes:
- delirium tremens
- amphetamine or cocaine overdose
- acute psychosis
- encephalitis
- accidental hyperpyrexia

The management of anticholinergic overdose is mainly supportive and consists of intubation and mechanical ventilation, gastric emptying, aggressive cooling if indicated, fluid administration to restore hypotension, anticonvulsive therapy in case of seizures, and treatment of cardiac failure. Diagnosis of suspected anticholinergic overdose is made clinically and physostigmine must be administered to confirm the differential diagnosis and for the specific therapeutic effect, which is restoration of consciousness and resolution of hyperpyrexia [2, 17]. Treatment of these patients with physostigmine will readily reverse symptoms of anticholinergic toxicity like agitation, delirium, or coma, and will facilitate cooling in cases of hyperpyrexia [18]. Otherwise, in cases of mixed intoxication, the clinical picture may improve markedly. Especially in cases of overdose with tricyclic antidepressants, there is a serious risk for ventricular tachydysrhythmias, disturbed cardiac conductivity, and bradyarrhythmias. Cardiac arrest may occur and cardiac pacing might be necessary [19]. Sophisticated cardiac monitoring in such cases is recommended, sometimes for several days, regardless of the state of consciousness [20]. It is a general rule that the patient should have normal blood gas values before administration of physostigmine, because cholinesterase inhibitors may otherwise result in bradyarrhythmias or heart standstill [21]. Physostigmine has also been used, with some success, in patients with heroin intoxication [22].

Hyperpyrexia

Fever is very common in IC patients and is commonly due to infection, but may result from other causes, especially when consciousness is disturbed and either agitation or depression and coma are present. The intensivist must always be aware that hyperpyrexia that cannot be resolved with antibiotic therapy may be caused by anticholinergic poisoning. CAS may cause central hyperpyrexia in addition to diminished heat loss [23].

Treatment with physostigmine and antipyretics will readily improve this clinical picture and will facilitate active cooling. The neuroleptic malignant syndrome may occur following administration of some antipsychotic drugs, like phenothiazines or butyrophenones. This syndrome is also characterized by hyperthermia, extrapyramidal symptoms, and delirium. If unrecognized, the malignant neuroleptic syndrome may lead to pulmonary complications and can be fatal. Neuroleptic drugs must be discontinued and supportive therapy started: antipyretics, cooling of the body and administration of bromocriptine or dantrolene sodium may be useful [24]. The differential diagnosis of neuroleptic malignant syndrome includes malignant hyperthermia, thyrotoxicosis, anticholinergic overdose, and overdose of cocaine, amphetamine, or ecstasy.

Other uses of physostigmine

Physostigmine has been successfully used in acute alcohol intoxication and can reverse withdrawal symptoms of delirium tremens, partly as described by Daunderer in 1985 [25].

In patients with brain injury in the chronic phase, more than 4 weeks after the initial trauma, physostigmine can be administered to diagnose a possible recovery due to restore previously disturbed central cholinergic transmission, as described by van Woerkom et al. in 1982 [26].

Physostigmine: pharmacokinetics, dosage, and administration

Pharmacokinetics and dosage

Physostigmine is a selective and reversible cholinesterase inhibitor. A lipid--soluble, tertiary amine can easily penetrate into the cerebrospinal fluid and is thus suitable for increasing the level of acetylcholine in the brain [2, 4]. Quaternary cholinesterase inhibitors like neostigmine and pyridostigmine do not cross the blood-brain barrier.

Physostigmine can be administered orally, intravenously, or intramuscularly. It is rapidly hydrolyzed and the duration of its effect is 90-120 min. The onset of action may be rapid after intravenous administration, within 0.5-5 min, but may take 20 min after intramuscular injection. Slow injection of physostigmine will prevent gastrointestinal hypermotility or short-lived bradycardia. The distribution half-life is 2-3 min. The initial dosage of physostigmine is 0.03-0.04 mg/kg body weight [2, 3, 27]. This dosage may need to be higher in cases of severe intoxication with anticholinergics and depends on severity of symptoms. For differential diagnostic purposes, one administration of physostigmine is usually sufficient. However, in cases of severe intoxication repeated administration is necessary after about 90 min or when the symptoms return. Continuous administration has been practised for several days in selected cases [28]. In a patient with anticholinergic poisoning a dosage of 3 mg physostigmine per hour was administered in a continuous drip for more than 2 days. Some authors prefer repeat administration of physostigmine in order to establish the time when the intoxication has subsided and the treatment can be discontinued. In some mixed intoxications, only symptoms of CAS are reversed by physostigmine and underlying effects of other depressant drugs may remain unchanged. The recovery in such cases will be partial [10].

Side effects of physostigmine

In a volunteer, physostigmine may provoke salivation, intestinal hypermotility, and transient bradycardia. These effects are far less obvious in patients suffering from effects of anticholinergic drugs. Furthermore, side effects of physostigmine depend on dosage and infusion rate. Slow injection of 0.03mg/kg may cause symptoms of para-sympathetic stimulation: salivation, nausea, sweating, and bradycardia. Prevention of peripheral side effects can easily be achieved by administration of glycopyrrolate [29]. Hypertension and tachycardia may occur due to a direct central, acetylcholine-dependent pressor response to physostigmine. Caution has been advocated in patients with hypertension or coronary artery disease [30]. As a rule, in the absence of bradycardia, hypoxaemia, and hypercapnia, administration of physostigmine is safe [3, 21].

Contraindications to physostigmine

Physostigmine may cause increased intracranial pressure and should therefore not be used in patients with already elevated intracranial pressure, such as cases of acute cerebral trauma or haemorrhage, or in barbiturate intoxication. Caution is necessary in patients with Parkinson's disease, gastrointestinal or urinary mechanical obstruction. Physostigmine is absolutely contraindicated in cases of severe myotonia dystrophica and intoxication with cholinesterase inhibitors in clinical practice. Pulmonary hyperreactivity has never proved to be a contraindication to physostigmine. Moreover, when a bronchospasm might be a problem, it can easily be resolved by pre-treatment with a selective peripherally acting anticholinergic agent, like ipratropium (Atrovent). An overdose of physostigmine might cause convulsions and caution has therefore been advocated in epileptic patients. Again, most epileptics are well treated nowadays and no untoward effects of physostigmine have been observed in such cases [3].

Envoi

Physostigmine is a valuable prognostic, diagnostic, and therapeutic agent, which should be available in every IC and emergency department. It should be used more freely in IC patients in whom the central anticholinergic syndrome is suspected and in serious poisonings with centrally acting anticholinergics. Physostigmine may be a crucial centrally acting agent in the differential diagnostic evaluation of postoperative delayed awakening [5, 31], in cases of suspected permanent brain damage, and in mixed intoxications. In cases of nonanticholinergic drug poisonings, physostigmine produces negligible haemodynamic and neurological changes. In anticholinergic poisoning, physostigmine produces improved consciousness, significantly increased blood pressure, cardiac work and output, without significantly affecting systemic vascular resistance [32]. In comparison with many other drugs used in IC, physostigmine has a very minor profile of side effects and is rather short acting, and is thus controllable. It should be used more frequently whenever the most-important vital function, consciousness, is disturbed or absent for reasons unknown.

References

1. Longo VG (1966) Behavioral and electroencephalographic effects of atropine and related compounds. Pharmacol Rev 18: 965-996
2. Schneck HJ, Rupreht J (1989) Central anticholinergic syndrome (CAS) in anesthesia and intensive care. Acta Anaesthesiol Belg 40: 219-228
3. Rupreht J, Dworacek B (1989) The central anticholinergic syndrome in the postoperative period. In: Nunn JF (ed) General anaesthesia. Butterworth, Oxford, pp 1141-1148
4. Granacher RP, Baldessarini RJ (1975) Physostigmine; its use in acute anticholinergic syndrome with antidepressant and antiparkinson drugs. Arch Gen Psychiatry 32: 375-380
5. Zandstra DF, Kuiper M (1999) Failure to regain consciousness after anesthesia. In: Gullo A (ed) Proceedings of the 14th postgraduate course in critical care medicine. Springer, Milan, pp 225-232
6. Katsanoulas K, Papaioannou A, Fraidakis O, et al (1999) Undiagnosed central anticholinergic syndrome may lead to dangerous complications. Eur J Anaesthesiol 16: 803-809
7. Torline RL (1993) Central anticholinergic syndrome – the forgotten diagnosis? Anesthesiol Rev 20:47-50
8. Link J, Papadopoulos G, Dopjans D et al (1997) Distinct central anticholinergic syndrome following general anaesthesia. Eur J Anaesthesiol 14:15-23
9. Schneck HJ (1988) Besonderheiten der Zentral wirkenden Medikation in Anaesthesiologie und Intensivmedizin. Thesis.Technische Universitat, Munich, pp 47-52
10. Brede S, Dennhardt R (1991) Das zentrale anticholinerge syndrom (ZAS) bei intensivpatienten. Klin Wochenschr 69 [Suppl 26]: 89-94
11. Rathgeber J, Kukowski B, Zenker D (1992) Störungen der Vigilanz bei Intensivpatienten. Anaesthesist 41: 699-701
12. Wise MG, Cassem NH (1992) Behavioral disturbances in the ICU. In: Civetta JM, Taylor RW, Kirby RR (eds) Critical care, 2nd ed. Lippincott, Philadelphia, pp 1523-1533
13. Cook B, Spence AA (1997) Postoperative central anticholinergic syndrome (editorial). Eur J Anaesthesiol 14:1-2
14. De Mas CR (1994) Toxikologischer Notfall: Die Stechapfel-Intoxikation unter dem Bild einer akuten Psychosen. Intensiv Notfallbehandlung 19:143-144
15. Raper RF, Fisher MMD (1992) Poisoning and toxic exposure In: Civetta JM, Taylor RW, Kirby RR (eds) Critical care, 2nd ed. Lippincott, Philadelphia, pp 918-919
16. Giubelli D, Conti L, Bott A, et al (1998) Atropine poisoning. Importance of the clinical diagnosis. Minerva Anesthesiol 64:567-573
17. Beaver KM, Gavin TJ (1998) Treatment of acute anticholinergic poisoning with physostigmine. Am J Emerg Med 16: 505-507
18. De Maar EJW (1956) Side and mode of action in the central nervous system of some drugs used in the treatment of Parkinsonism. Arch Int Pharmacodyn Ther 105:349-365
19. Schmidt W, Lang K (1997) Life-threatening dysrhythmias in severe thioridazine poisoning treated with physostigmine and transient atrial pacing. Crit Care Med 25:1925-1930
20. Daunderer M (1980) Physostigmine salicylate as an antidote. Int J Clin Pharmac Ther Toxicol 18:523-535
21. Riding JE, Robinson JS (1961) The safety of neostigmine. Anaesthesia 16:346-354
22. Rupreht J, Dworacek B, Oosthoek H, et al (1984) Physostigmine versus naloxone in heroin-overdose. J Toxicol Clin Toxicol 21:387-397
23. Torline RL (1992) Extreme hyperpyrexia associated with central anticholinergic syndrome. Anesthesiology 76: 470-471
24. Caroff SN (1980) The neuroleptic malignant syndrome. J Clin Psychiatry 41:79-83
25. Daunderer M (1985) Praktische Erfahrungen bei der Profylaxe des Alkohol – Entzugsdelirs. In: Stoeckel H, Lauven P (eds) Das Zentral – anticholinergische Syndrom: Physostigmin in der Intensivmedizin, Anästhesiologie, Psychiatrie. G Thieme, Stuttgart pp 120-128

26. Woerkom TCAM van, Minderhoud JM, Gottschal T (1982) Neurotransmitters in the treatment of patients with severe head injuries. Eur Neurol 21: 227-234
27. Hartvig P, Wiklund L, Lindström B (1986) Pharmacokinetics of physostigmine after intravenous, intramuscular and subcutaneous administration in surgical patients. Acta Anaesthesiol Scand 38: 177-182
28. Stern Th A (1983) Continuous infusion of physostigmine in anticholinergic delirium: case report. J Clin Psychiatry 44: 463-464
29. Wood M (1990) Cholinergic and parasympathomimetic drugs In: Wood M, Wood AJ (eds) Drugs and anesthesia pharmacology for anesthesiologists, 2nd ed. Williams and Wilkins, Baltimore, pp 83-109
30. Janowsky DS, Risch SC, Huey LY (1985) Central cardiovascular effects of physostigmine in humans. Hypertension 7:140-145
31. Kabatnik M, Heist M, Beiderlinden K et al (1999) Hepatic encephalopathy – a physostigmine--reactive central anticholinergic syndrome? Eur J Anaesthesiol 16:140-142.
32. Nilsson E, Meretoja OA, Neuvonen P (1983) Hemodynamic responses to physostigmine in patients with a drug overdose. Anesth Analg 62:885-888

Blood redistribution during central neural blocks: influence of leg bandaging and other mechanical methods

D. Štifanić, V. Paver-Eržen

Now that the benefits of regional anaesthesia are more widely recognised, both subarachnoid block (SAB) and epidural anaesthesia (EPA) are used with increasing frequency during the perioperative period.

Complete analgesia is necessary for a successful operation. Motor paralysis is often desirable, while sympathetic block is frequently an unwanted but expected effect of SAB and EPA. Preganglionic sympathetic blockade is the main cause of numerous cardiovascular changes, and to a lesser extent, of alterations occurring in the respiratory, gastrointestinal and genitourinary systems. Sympathetic block in the anaesthetized parts of the body may cause severe, potentially fatal complications, but it has many advantages in regional anaesthesia. It is therefore of vital importance for the clinician to be acquainted with the changes caused by SAB and EPA in various organ systems, as well as with the mechanisms triggering these changes.

Blood redistribution during SAB and EPA

The intensity and significance of cardiovascular changes depend on the level and width of the area anaesthetized, as well as on the accompanying cardiovascular diseases and the type and dosage of the local anaesthetic used [1]. In order to get a deeper insight into haemodynamic changes, it is necessary to study blood flow through the anaesthetized and unanaesthetized areas separately. Special attention has to be given to the monitoring of blood flow to the priority areas, i.e., the brain, heart, liver, and kidneys, as circulatory disturbances in these regions can lead to a serious and sometimes irreversible function failure [2].

Haemodynamic changes in the anaesthetized area

A decrease or total loss of sympathetic tone in the anaesthetized area causes dilatation of arteries and veins resulting in changed vascular resistance and volume. Vasodilatation, especially dilatation of subcutaneous veins, results in considerable blood retention in the anaesthetized area [3]. Dilatation of arteries, especially arterioles, reduces vascular resistance and increases blood flow. A considerable increase in vein volume (17%) and blood flow (77%), and a decrease in regional resistance (48%) in the anaesthetized area during SAB and EPA have been demonstrated by occlusive venous plethysmography (sensoric level Th 4-Th 7) [4]. A 3 - 5 fold increase in toe pulse volume depending on the SAB level was determined using the same method [5]. Measurements of the redistribution of radioactive technetium during high thoracic EPA showed that radioactivity increased only in the blocked legs [6]. During SAB, peripheral vein pressure in the lower extremity dropped considerably [7]. Doppler sono-graphy showed a considerable increase in the velocity of blood flow through the femoral vein during lumbar EPA induced with butanilcaine and adrenalin 5 µg/ml. The position of the patient and the level of the block used, which are of importance to the understanding of the results, are not specified in the study [8]. The second group of authors, who studied femoral vein blood flow during SAB and EPA (bupivacaine 0.5%) in patients in the supine position and with the legs elevated did not confirm the results of the previous study [9].

The results of our study showed that both SAB and EPA up to Th 6 (isobaric 0.5% bupivacaine) induced a significant decrease in the velocity of blood flow in the common femoral vein and posterior tibial artery in patients placed in the supine position. At the same time, systolic flow and diastolic reflux velocity through the common femoral artery and posterior tibial artery decreased, indicating considerable vasodilatation in the anaesthetized area [10].

In addition to inducing venous and arterial dilatation, sympathetic vasomo-tor block opens the anatomic arteriovenous anastomosis in the anaesthetized area. The hypothesis advanced some 50 years ago was based on the findings of increased femoral venous oxygen saturation and decreased arteriovenous o-xygen difference during SAB [11-13]. Direct evidence was provided by the analysis of systemic and regional blood flows during SAB using the radioactive micro-sphere technique [14, 15].

Haemodynamic changes in unanaesthetized areas.

An important compensatory mechanism of increased sympathetic activity in unanaesthetized areas is triggered simultaneously with the sympathetic block in the anaesthetized area [16, 17]. Low thoracic SAB reduces blood flow to fingers by more than 50%. Thoracic SAB higher than Th4 that blocks the sympathetic innervation of the arms was found to cause a three-fold increase in blood flow to fingers [2].

High thoracic EPA also enhanced sympathetic activities in the kidney (unanaesthetized area), and blocking the lower thoracic and lumbar segments intensified the sympathetic effect on heart activity. It is generally believed that the barorereflex control of hypotension has the main role in the activation of the above mentioned compensatory mechanisms [18].

A compensatory increase in sympathetic activity in the thoracic area may exert undesired effects in patients with coronary artery disease [19]. In hypovolaemic patients, compensatory increase in the renal sympathetic tone renders the kidney more sensitive to further volume loss [18].

Our study has shown that lumbar SAB and EPA considerably lower the velocity of systolic and diastolic flow through the common carotid artery, which seems to be due to systemic haemodynamic changes rather than to the increased compensatory sympathetic tone [10]. As the autonomic nervous system plays a secondary role in regulating the brain blood flow [20], block of the upper thoracic segments does not cause any significant flow changes [21].

Haemodynamic changes in systemic circulation

The most extensive studies on haemodynamic changes during SAB were conducted some fifty years ago. A significant decrease in arterial pressure, central venous pressure, pulmonary artery pressure, heart rate, stroke volume and cardiac output was noted. Peripheral vascular resistance, venous pressure, hepatic blood flow and total oxygen consumption were decreased. The observed haemodynamic changes were more pronounced in patients receiving high thoracic blocks [2, 22-24]. Later studies showed a very similar course of haemodynamic changes during EPA [3, 25].

Hypotension

Arterial pressure is the basic clinical parameter used to determine the intensity of haemodynamic changes and the effectiveness of compensatory activity during SAB and EPA. The incidence of hypotension may be up to 83% depending on the type and amount of the local anaesthetic used, the level of SAB or EPA and the general physical condition of the patient [26].

A decrease in vascular resistance and venous preload, resulting from marked vasodilatation in the anaesthetized region, is the major contributor to the development of hypotension during these forms of regional anaesthesia. The level of block and the number of blocked segments are the main factors determining the effectiveness of compensatory activities and the size of the area anaesthetized. A block of up to Th 8 prevents release of endogenous catecholamines from the suprarenal glands. In a block as high as Th1, a compensatory increase of sympathetic activity in unanaesthetized parts of the body is completely lost [27].

Treatment of hypotension

There are three basic approaches to the control of hypotension, based on the understanding of basic mechanisms triggering its development during SAB and EPA:

1. administering intravenous infusions (supplement to a decrease in preload);
2. administering sympathomimetic drugs (increase in systemic vascular pressure, heart rate and contractility);
3. various mechanical methods, such as compressing the legs, and changing the patient's position (increase in preload).

Administering intravenous solutions is the most common method of preventing hypotension induced by SAB and EPA. Various crystalloid and colloid solutions are administered to compensate for the decrease in the preload and increase in stroke volume and cardiac output [28].

The basic drawback of administering intravenous solutions is the increase in intra- and extravascular volume in the perioperative period. This can additionally burden the cardiovascular system of the patient with low cardiac reserve, especially during the period when the action of the local anaesthetic diminishes and the vascular tone of the anaesthetized area normalizes. The administration of intravenous solutions causes changes in rheologic characteristics of the blood with a decrease in haematocrit and plasma osmolarity, and lowering of blood temperature [29, 30]. We must not underestimate the risk of allergic reactions and blood clotting disorders as a result of colloid administration [31].

Administering sympathomimetic drugs is a "physiological" approach to treating hypotension in different parts of the body due to sympathetic block. These drugs stimulate alpha and/or beta receptors with the aim of increasing vascular resistance and cardiac output. The main undesired effects of sympathomimetic drugs may include heart arrhythmias and myocardial ischaemia [32-34].

Mechanical methods

Several mechanical methods of compressing the lower limbs are available to increase the preload during SAB and EPA. The basic mechanism is the transfer of outer pressure exerted on legs to all tissues, with the resulting emptying of veins, especially subcutaneous vessels, and an increase in preload.

It has been reported that applying an inflatable cuff exerting pressures of 15 to 20 mmHg afforded a faster flow and better filling of the popliteal and femoral veins, and enhanced venous flow from the legs [35]. The same authors compared the effects of leg compression with elastic bandages and the results obtained with the use of elastic support stockings. On the basis of venous pressure measurements and phlebograms they concluded that pressures of 16 - 20 mmHg proved most effective in decreasing the leg vein area and enhancing venous flow in the legs. Increasing the outer pressure did not improve venous drainage, and the risk of vein occlusion, especially in the popliteal region, was increased. Very good results were obtained in patients with varicose veins [36]. The use of medical antishock trousers exerting a pressure of 40 mmHg after administering EPA produced a rise of systolic arterial pressure and central venous pressure to the pre-anaesthesia levels [37]. Antishock trousers, however, are extremely difficult to use in clinical practice, and the effect of outer pressure of 40 mmHg on microcirculation is questionable. This aspect was not addressed in the study.

Several studies of mechanical methods were carried out in patients receiving SAB for Caesarean section. Wrapping the legs with Esmarch bandages from the ankle to the mid-thigh lowered the incidence of hypotension from 83% to 16% [26] and the use of inflatable full-length leg splints from 83% to 48% [38], but the use of inflatable boots produced no effect [39]. It has to be taken into consideration that various amounts of intravenous solutions were used in these studies: 20 ml/kg BW in the first, 15 ml/kg BW in the second and 10 ml/kg BW in the third.

Leg wrapping during EPA for Caesarean section lowered the incidence of hypotension from 83% to 13% [40], while the use of elastic compression stockings had no effect on the incidence of hypotension [41]. A different volume of intravenous solutions was given in each study : 15 ml/kg BW in the first and only 500 ml in the second.

Pollard [42] analysed the effect of leg wrapping on the incidence of hypotension during SAB for urological procedures. After infusing crystalloid 5-10 ml/kg BW and inducing SAB, the patients had their legs wrapped tightly from mid-ankle to mid-thigh, placed in the racks and raised to approximately 30°. No critical hypotension was noticed during the procedure (mean arterial pressure 65mmHg).

Our study showed that wrapping the legs with elastic bandages from the ankle to the inguinal area prior to anaesthesia in patients with no cardiovascular disease completely prevents any significant changes in the velocity of blood flow through the common carotid artery, common femoral artery and posterior tibial artery, occurring during lumbar SAB and EPA. Full-length leg wrapping also enhances blood flow through the femoral vein, which is very desirable during the perioperative period. The incidence of hypotension was decreased from 20% to 8% during SAB, and from 28% to 12% during EPA. It is important to mention that the patients received only 7 ml/kg BW crystalloids and that all the measurements were performed with the patients placed supine [10].

Conclusion

The mechanical methods of increasing the preload, primarily the application of elastic bandages, can efficiently prevent hypotension during SAB and EPA. Thanks to these methods, a significantly smaller amount of intravenous solutions and vasopressors can be used. Such an approach "aetiologically" prevents the redistribution of blood occurring during SAB and EPA.

Potential side-effects of full-length firm leg compression with elastic bandages can be effectively prevented by testing toe microcirculation using photoelectric plethysmography, the basic component of pulse oximetry, and by reducing the pressure in the popliteal area during bandaging. Elastic leg bandaging is a subjective method, but if we decide to use it, it is more important not to apply ineffective loose bandaging than to wrap the legs too tightly, to which we shall be readily alerted by accurate microcirculation monitoring

The use of the above mentioned mechanical methods should be restricted to the operating room. Patients undergoing a lower limb operation should have elastic bandages applied to their contralateral leg. Since the purpose of leg wrapping is to prevent rather than treat hypotension, it should always precede the induction of anaesthesia.

References

1. Greene NM (1981) Physiology of Spinal Anesthesia. 3rd edn. Williams & Wilkins, Baltimore, London, 26-35
2. Sancetta SM, Lynn B, Simeone FA, et al (1952) Studies of hemodynamic changes in humans following induction of low and high spinal anesthesia. I. General considerations of the problem. Circulation 6:559
3. Bromage PR (1967) Physiology and pharmacology of epidural analgesia. A review. Anesthesiology 28:592
4. Shimosato S, Etsten BE (1969) The role of the venous system in cardiocirculatory dynamics during spinal and epidural anesthesia in man. Anesthesiology 30:619-628
5. Perchoniemi V, Linko K (1987) Effect of spinal versus epidural anaesthesia with 0.5% bupivacaine on lower limb blood flow. Acta Anaesthesiol Scand 31:117-121
6. Arndt J, Hock A, Stanton-Hicks M, Stuhmeier K-D (1985) Peridural anesthesia and the distribution of blood in supine humans. Anesthesiology 63:616-623
7. Adriani J, Rovenstine EA (1940) Effects of spinal anesthesia upon venous pressure in man. Proc Soc Exp Biol Med 45:415
8. Poikolainen E, Hendolin H (1983) Effects of lumbar epidural analgesia and general anaesthesia on flow velocity in the femoral vein and postoperative deep vein thrombosis. Acta Chir Scand 149:361-364
9. Perchoniemi V, Linko K (1987) Effect of spinal versus epidural anaesthesia with 0.5% bupivacaine on lower limb blood flow. Acta Anaesthesiol Scand 31:117-121
10. Štifanic D (2001) Analysis of haemodynamic changes in peripheral and cerebral circulation during subarachnoidal and epidural anaesthesia. Disertation
11. Dorlas JC, Nijboer JA (1985) Photoelectric plethysmography as a monitoring device in anaesthesia. Br J Anaesth 57:524-530
12. Sinha PK, Dubey PK, Gaur A et al (1999) Plethysmographic pulse oximeter waveform variation as an indicator of successful epidural blockade: a prospective study. Anesthesiology 91:899-901
13. Irwin ST, Gilmore J, McGrann S, Hood J, Allen JA (1988) Blood flow in diabetic with foot lesions due to "small vessel disease". Br J Surg 75:1201-1206
14. Sivarajan M, Amory DW, Lindbloom LE, Schwettmann RS (1975) Systemic and regional blood-flow changes during spinal anesthesia in the rhesus monkey. Anesthesiology 43:78-88
15. Sivarajan M, Amory DW, Lindbloom LE, et al (1976) Systemic and regional blood flow during epidural anesthesia without epinephrine in the rhesus monkey. Anesthesiology 45:300
16. Neumann C, Foster AD Jr, Rovenstine FA (1945) The importance of compensatory vasoconstriction in unanesthetized areas in the maintenance of blood pressure during spinal anesthesia. J Clin Invest 24:345
17. Foster AD, Neumann C, Rovenstine EA (1945) Peripheral circulation during anesthesia, shock and hemorrhage. The digital plethysmograph as a clinical guide. Anesthesiology 6:246
18. Taniguchi M, Kasaba T, Takasaki M (1997) Epidural anesthesia enhances sympathetic nerve activity in the unanesthetized segments in cats. Anesth Analg 84:391-397
19. Krantz EM, Viljoen JF, Gilbert MS (1980) Prinzmetal's variant angina during extradural anaesthesia. Br J Anaesth 52:945-949
20. Schmidt CF (1950) The cerebral circulation in health and disease. 1st ed Thomas, Springfield, Illinois, 72-78
21. Cleinerman J, Sancetta SM, Hackel DB (1958) Effects of high spinal anesthesia on cerebral circulation and metabolism in man. J Clin Invest 37:285
22. Rovenstine EA, Papper EM, Brodley SE (1942) Circulatory adjustments during spinal anesthesia in normal man with special reference to the autonomy of arteriolar tone. Anesthesiology 3:421
23. Mueller RP, Lynn B, Sancetta SM (1953) Studies of hemodynamic changes in humans following induction of low i high spinal anesthesia. II. Circulation 6:894
24. Burch JC, Harrison TR (1931) The effect of spinal anesthesia on arterial tone. Arch Surg 22:1040

25. Bonica JJ, Berges PU, Morikawa K (1970) Circulatory Effects of peridural block: I. Effect of level of analgesia and dose of lidocaine. Anesthesiology 33:619

26. Bhagwanjee S, Rocke DA, Rout CC, et al (1990) Prevention of hypotension following spinal anaesthesia for elective Caesarean section by wrapping of the legs. Br J Anaesth 65:819-822

27. McCrae AF, Wildsmith JAW (1993) Prevention and treatment of hypotension during neural block. Br J Anaesth 70:672-680

28. Robson S, Hunter S, Boys R, et al (1989) Changes in cardiac output during epidural anaesthesia for Caesarean section. Anaesthesia 44:475-479

29. Odoom JA, Bovill JG, Haerdeman MR, et al (1992) Effects of epidural and spinal anesthesia on blood rheology. Anesth Analg 74:835-840

30. Goldsmith SR, Cowley AW, Francis GS, Cohn JN (1984) Effect of increased intracardiac and arterial pressures on plasma vasopressin in humans. Am J Physiol 246:647-651

31. Stoelting RK (1983) Allergic reactions during anesthesia. Anesth Analg 62:341-356

32. Weiner N (1985) Norepinephrine, epinephrine and the sympathomimetic amines. In: Gilman AG, Goodman LS, Rall TW, Murad F (eds) Goodman and Gilman's The Pharmacological Basis of Therapeutics. Macmillan, New York, pp 145-80

33. Sharrock NE, Urquhart B (1990) Hemodynamic response to low-dose epinephrine infusion during hypotension epidural anaesthesia for total hip replacement. Reg Anaesth 15:295-299

34. Mueller RA, Lundberg DB (1988) Manual of drug interactions for anesthesiology. 1st ed Churchill Livingstone, New York

35. Husni EA, Ximenes J, Hamilton FG (1968) Pressure bandaging of the lower extremity: use and abuse. JAMA 206:2715-2718

36. Husni EA, Ximenes J, Goyette EM (1970) Elastic support of the lower limbs in hospital patients. JAMA 214:1456-1462

37. Baron JF, Decaux Jacolot A, Edouard A, et al (1986) Influence of venous return on baroreflex control of heart rate during lumbar epidural anesthesia in humans. Anesthesiology 64:188-193

38. Goudie TA, Winter AW, Ferguson DJM (1988) Lower limb compression using inflatable splints to prevent hypotension during spinal anaesthesia for Ceasarean section. Acta Anaesthesiol Scand 32:541-544

39. James FM, Greiss FC (1973) The use of inflatable boots to prevent hypotension during spinal anesthesia for Cesaean section. Anesth Analg 52:246-251

40. Gibbs CP, Werba JV, Banner TE, et al (1983) Epidural anesthesia: leg wraping prevents hypotension. Anesthesiology 59:A405

41. Lee A, McKeown D, Wilson J (1987) Evaluation of the efficacy of elastic compression stockings in prevention of hypotension during epidural anaesthesia for elective Caesarean section. Acta Anaesthesiol Scand 31:193-195

42. Pollard J (1995) Wrapping of the legs reduced the demands in blood pressure following spinal anaesthesia. Reg Anaesth 402-406

Management of the postoperative critically ill patient

J. Besso, E. Rivero, A. Bolivar

A number of developments occurred in the twentieth century that were absolutely essential to the development of the care of the postoperative critically ill patient [1]. Some of the necessary procedures include the following:

1900	Blood typing–Landsteiner
1901	Imaging–Roentgen
1923	Intensive care unit (ICU) (neuro)–First ICU
1940	Dialysis-Kolff
1940	Antibiotics
1952	Ventilation (Denmark)
	Developed originally to manage the polio epidemic
1953	Open heart surgery
1956	Defibrillator-Zoll
1960	(CPR)-Kouiuenhoven
1960	Adult ICU and critical care unit (CCU)
1965	95% Hospital ICU
1970	Triage, resuscitation, fluids, ARDS
1971	Ultrasound
1972	Computed tomographic (CT) scan
1973	Magnetic resonance imaging (MRI)
1980	Trombolytic therapy
1981	Organ transplantation

For a better management of the postoperative critically ill patient emphasis must be placed on determining the limit of physiological reserve, particularly of the cardiorespiratory system. The intention is to identify those patients who will benefit from further research and more-complex perioperative management in the ICU [2, 3].

History should also inquire into the limitation of physiological reserve in other organ systems. Elucidation of the underlying dysfunction must depend upon the time-honoured triad of history, examination, and special research.

Perioperative and recovery from anaesthesia

Management of the postoperative critically ill begins during the perioperative period, where the anaesthesiologist has multiple treatment goals for the patient. Provision of physiological stability during the operative procedure must always serve as the most-important principle. During the perioperative period, there are changes in organ metabolic demand and in nutrient and oxygen availability, which lead to an imbalance between supply and demand, and produce life-threatening organ failure. The aim of circulatory management during this perioperative period is to maintain the balance of nutrient and oxygen supply and demand. Management is based on correction of deranged physiology, with particular reference to optimizing blood volume, oxygen-carrying capacity, cardiac output, and organ perfusion.

The degree of monitoring during transport should be influenced by the stability or instability of the patient. Physicians and other personnel notoriously overventilate patients when they use a manual ventilation system; they also often cause extremely high airway pressures.

We advocate that critically ill patients not be awakened in the operating room, but rather in the ICU. This procedure minimizes the risk involved in the rapid awakening usually required in the operating room. In the ICU, the patient can be awakened at a rate that is most advantageous to the maintenance of homeostasis.

Patient assessment

When the critically ill postoperative patient first arrives in the ICU, several goals need to be accomplished almost simultaneously; these include immediate assessment of vital signs, including heart rate, blood pressure, cardiac rhythm, and neurological status, in order to ensure a degree of stability. Simultaneously, blood samples must be sent to the laboratory for the purpose of developing baseline information. Furthermore, any instability requires rapid correction. All this follows the philosophy that maintenance of homeostasis contributes to the patient's safe and rapid recovery. Treatment is by continued monitoring of the cardiovascular system and organ function, with the judicious use of fluids, blood products, and drugs to improve cardiac function and organ perfusion.

Once basic resuscitation has been performed, management should be directed towards optimizing the intravascular volume and cardiac performance in order to maintain tissue perfusion and tissue oxygen supply.

Therefore, one of the objectives will be to maintain an adequate cardiac output, with the criteria and possible interventions presented in Table 1 [4, 5].

Table 1 Improving myocardial and circulation performance (*CNS* central nervous system)

Objective	Adequate cardiac output
Criteria	Cardiac index > 2.2 l/min per m^2 Urine output > 0.5 ml/kg per hour Functioning CNS Peripheral pulses
Interventions	Increase preload Reduce afterload Increase inotropy

Haemodynamic goals

Optimizing cardiac output

Control of cardiac filling pressure

The principle is to ascend the Frank-Starling curve for each individual by obtaining the optimal filling pressure associated with the best afterload (Fig. 1). It is vital to achieve the optimal filling pressure, thus ensuring an adequate blood volume that will provide complete perfusion for all organs and adequate cardiac filling. The simplest method for assessing the intravascular fluid volume is by using a central venous pressure (CVP) line and fluid challenge. In sicker patients, the pulmonary artery catheter (PAC) allows a more-sophisticated version of the fluid challenge to be performed.

The PAC controversy

A recent report of surprising results from a major observational study evaluating the value of pulmonary artery catheterization in critically ill patients has caused considerable controversy [6]. In this study, two groups of patients, those who did and those who did not undergo placement of a PAC during their first 24 h of ICU care were compared. The researchers concluded that placement of a PAC during the first 24 h of stay in an ICU is associated with a significant increase in the risk of mortality, even when statistical methods are used to

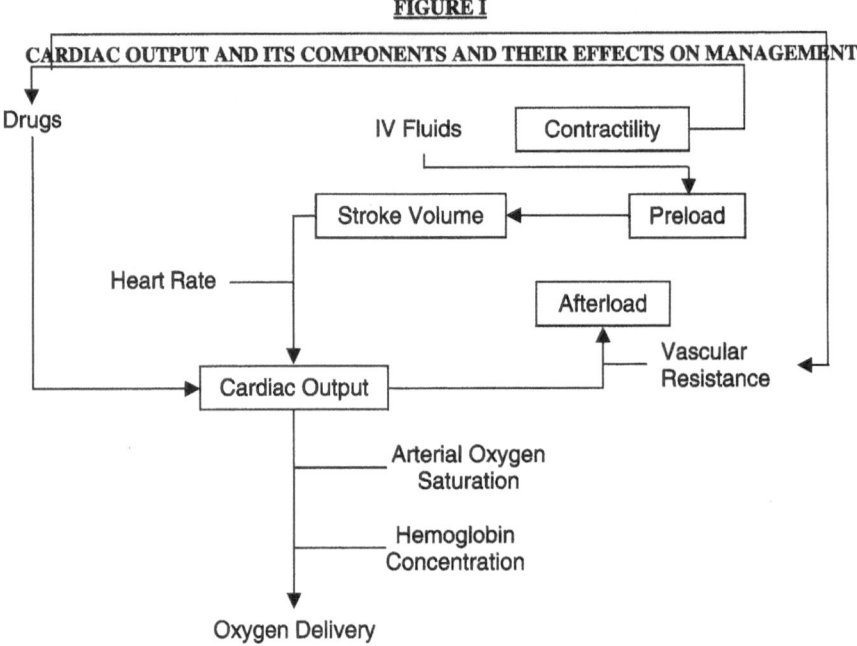

Fig. 1 Cardiac output and its components and their effects on management

account for severity of illness. The value of this analysis was completely dependent on the robustness of their methodology for case-matching, because sicker patients (i.e., those at greater risk of mortality based upon the severity of their illness) were presumably more likely to undergo pulmonary artery catheterization. Accordingly, the authors used sophisticated statistical methods to generate a cohort of study (i.e., PAC) patients, each one having a paired control matched carefully for severity of illness. A critical assessment of their published findings supports the view that the cases and their controls were indeed remarkably well matched with respect to a large number of relevant clinical parameters.

These results actually confirmed those of two prior observational studies. The first of these studies used as a database 3,236 patients with acute myocardial infarction treated as part of the Worcester Heart Attack study [7].

For all patients, hospital mortality was significantly higher for patients treated using a PAC, even when multivariable statistical methods were employed to control key potential confounding factors, such as age, peak circulating creatine kinase concentration, and presence or absence of new Q waves on the electrocardiogram. The second large observational study of patients with acute myocardial infarction also found that hospital mortality was significantly higher for patients managed with the help of a PAC [8]. Even when the presence or absence of "pump failure" was considered in the statistical analysis, in neither of these earlier reports did the authors conclude that placement of a PAC was truly the cause of worsened survival after myocardial infarction. In the case of pulmonary artery catheterization, much of the data available regarding the effect of this intervention on outcomes derive from observational studies such as those cited [6, 8]. The data thereby generated should not be ignored by prudent clinicians. Nevertheless, experts in the field have questioned the value of bedside pulmonary artery catheterization [9, 10], and some have called for a moratorium on the use of the Swan-Ganz catheter [9, 11]. Relatively few prospective, randomized controlled trials of pulmonary artery catheterization have been performed [12, 13].

All the individual single institution studies of vascular surgery patients were relatively underpowered [13-16] and all excluded at least certain categories of patients (e.g., those with a history of recent myocardial infarction). Notwithstanding the weight of current evidence, the limitations of these studies suggest that routine pulmonary artery catheterization is not necessary in patients undergoing cardiac or major peripheral vascular surgical procedures. Based upon the exclusion criteria used in two recent prospective randomized trials, reasonable criteria for perioperative monitoring with the use of a PAC are presented in Table 2.

Table 2 Suggested criteria for perioperative monitoring with the use of a pulmonary artery catheter in patients undergoing cardiac or major vascular surgical procedures

Anticipated need of suprarenal or supraceliac aortic cross-clamping
History of myocardial infarction within 3 months of the operation
History of poorly compensated congestive heart failure
History of coronary artery bypass graft surgery within 6 weeks of the operation
History of ongoing symptomatic mitral or aortic valvular heart disease
History of ongoing unstable angina pectoris

One of the reasons for using a PAC to monitor critically ill patients is to optimize cardiac output and systemic oxygen delivery. Based upon an extensive observational database and comparisons of the haemodynamic and oxygen transport values recorded in survivors and non-survivors, Shoemaker et al. [18] proposed that "goal-directed" haemodynamic resuscitation should achieve a Qt 4.5 L/min per m^2 and DO$_2$ 600 ml/min per m^2. Prompted by these observational findings, a number of researchers have conducted randomized trials designed to evaluate the effect on outcome of goal-directed compared with conventional haemodynamic resuscitation. Some studies provide support for the notion that interventions designed to achieve supraphysiological goals for DO_2, VO_2, and Qt improve outcomes. However, other published studies do not support this view [20, 21] and a recent meta-analysis concluded that interventions designed to achieve supraphysiological goals for oxygen transport do not significantly reduce mortality rates in critically ill patients [22].

Intuitively, invasive monitoring using a PAC should improve outcome, particularly in subgroups of patients at high risk of major derangements in cardiac performance and perfusion of vital organs. Yet, as summarized here, convincing evidence that such monitoring is beneficial is lacking. Indeed, a number of studies suggest quite the opposite. What explanations can be offered for the apparent lack of effectiveness of pulmonary artery catheterization? Although no firm answer to this question can be provided, Connors [23] has offered several suggestions. First, even though bedside pulmonary artery catheterization is quite safe, the procedure is associated with a finite incidence of serious complications, including ventricular arrhythmias, catheter-related sepsis, central venous thrombosis, and pulmonary artery perforation. The adverse effects of these complications on outcome may equal or even outweigh any benefits associated with the use of a PAC to guide therapy. Second, the data generated by the PAC may be inaccurate, leading to inappropriate therapeutic interventions. Third, the measurements, even if accurate, are often misinterpreted in practice. In one famous study, Iberti et al. [24] showed that 47% of 496 clinicians were unable to accurately interpret a straightforward recording of PaO_2 tracing and 44% could not correctly identify the determinants of systemic DO_2 . A more-recent study has confirmed that even well-trained intensivists are capable of misinterpreting the results provided by pulmonary artery catheterization [25].

Intravenous fluid therapy

The aim of intravenous fluid therapy is to increase tissue oxygen delivery by restoring normal intravascular fluid volume with an appropriate haematocrit. This will increase preload and hence cardiac output and oxygen delivery.

In some cases, the choice of intravenous fluid is obvious. If the patient is bleeding and losing blood, fluid replacement will be primarily blood. If the patient has a fistula or large burns, the initial fluid therapy should be matched to replace these losses. However, in many patients the cause of reduced intravascular volume is not immediately obvious. In these cases the intravascular volume should be restored and the haematocrit maintained.

There have been numerous attempts to establish whether intravenous crystalloids or artificial colloidal solutions are most appropriate for resuscitation in these patients and this issue is unresolved.

Some considerations in relation to volume replacement are included in Table 3 and Table 4 [26].

Table 3 Volume replacement

Optimal haematocrit??
< 28% compromises DO_2
Viscosity increases > 40%
Mean haematocrit post open heart surgery is 29.4 ± 4.3

Crystalloids
Less expensive ($ 0.62 per 500 ml)
12% decreases in COP after 1 1

Colloids
More expensive ($ 76.92 per 500 ml)
Remain in intravascular space
11% increases in COP
? Reduced risk of pulmonary oedema
No conclusive studies supporting choice of colloid over crystalloid

Table 4 University Hospital Consortium guidelines for fluid replacement [26]

Haemorrhagic shock	Crystalloid colloid. Blood products prn
Maldistributive shock	Crystalloid unless capillary leak
Hepatic resection	Crystalloid or colloid
Thermal injury	Crystalloids; colloids for burns 50%; 24 h or failure of crystalloid to correct hypovolaemia
Cerebral ischaemia	Crystalloid except special circumstances
Cardiac surgery	Crystalloid as prime and postoperatively; colloid in addition for systemic oedema
Cirrhosis and pancreatitis	Crystalloid; colloid as second line for prevention of complications following ascites removal 4 l
Nephrotic syndrome	Short-term albumin use plus diuretics
Plasmapheresis	Albumin for large exchange (20 ml/kg)

Blood products

When transfusing blood, the improvement in oxygen-carrying capacity must always be balanced against the reduction in flow accompanying the increase in blood viscosity with increasing haemoglobin concentration, the risk of transfusion reaction, and the increasing risk of blood-borne infections.

There is no absolute agreement on the optimal haematocrit; however, the aim should be to maintain the optimum oxygen-carrying capacity while maintaining viscosity as low as possible. Guidelines have been provided [27] (Table 5).

Table 5 Summary of evidence-based guidelines for red blood cell transfusions for acute blood loss. Practice parameter of the College of American Pathologists. If tissue oxygen delivery is not satisfactory when an adequate and appropriate intravascular volume has been ensured, drugs (Table 6) which enhance myocardial performance should be considered.

Evaluate risk of ischaemia

Estimate/anticipate degree of blood loss

< 30% rapid volume loss probably does not require transfusion in a previously healthy person

Measure haemoglobin concentration
< 6 g/dl transfusion usually needed
 6-10 g/dl transfusion dictated by clinical circumstance
> 10 g/dl transfusion rarely needed

Measure vital signs/tissue oxygenation when haemoglobin 6-10 g/dl and extent of blood loss is unknown
– 	Tachycardia, hypotension refractory to volume: transfusion needed
– 	Decrease PVO_2, O_2 extraction ratio 50 %, VO_2 50% of baseline: transfusion usually needed.

Table 6 inotropic support

Beta-adrenergic agents

– 	Dobutamine

– 	Dopamine

– 	Epinephrine

Phosphodiesterase inhibitors

– 	Amrinone

– 	Milrinone

Haemodynamic goals II

Adequate perfusion pressure

Another haemodynamic goal in the management of the critically ill patient is to maintain an adequate perfusion pressure and to minimize stress at the suture lines. This goal is accomplished by maintaining mean arterial pressure 70-100 mmHg with evidence of good systemic perfusion. Interventions will vary in accordance with the clinical situation and may be accomplished through adjustments of preload and afterload, sedation of the agitated or hypertensive patient, or with the use of drugs such as vasodilators or vasopressors according to the clinical situation. In some cases post open heart surgery cardiac assistance devices may be needed.

Hypotension and hypertension

Several causes are responsible for the production of hypotension or hypertension in the postoperative critically ill patient (Table 7).

Table 7 Causes of postoperative hypo- and hypertension

Hypotension	Hypertension
Spurious	Spurious
Hypovolaemia	Preoperative hypertension
Ventricular dysfunction	Enhanced autonomic activity
Myocardial ischaemia	Medications
Cardiac dysrhythmias	
Lowered systemic vascular resistance	

Hypertension can be treated with either continuous or intermittent therapy (Table 8).

Table 8 Postoperative drugs for the treatment of hypertension

Drug	Dosage
Opioids	3-10 mg/h
Labetalol	15-15 mg IV bolus
	10/80 mg/h
Nitroprusside	0.5-5.0 ug/kg per min
Nitroglycerine	0.5-4.0 ug/kg per min
Nicardipine	5.0-25 mg/h

Balance oxygen supply to demand

Another haemodynamic goal will be to balance the oxygen supply to demand. In order to accomplish this goal, several interventions can be used, as seen in Tables 9 and 10.

Table 9 Balanced oxygen supply/demand

Criteria	Absence of ischaemic heart rate < 100
	Low intravascular pressures
	Adequate O_2 content
Interventions	Reduce ventricular rate
	Reduce contractility
	Adjust preload/afterload
	Treat shivering and agitation

Table 10 Myocardial oxygen balance

	O$_2$ supply		O$_2$ demand
1.	Coronary blood flow	1.	Blood pressure afterload
2.	Oxygen delivery	2.	Ventilation volume (preload)
	a. O$_2$ saturation	3.	Heart rate
	b. Haematocrit	4.	Contractility

A study published by Slogoff and Keats [28] showed that anaesthesiologists with the highest rates of ischaemia and tachycardia had the highest rates of postoperative myocardial infarction.

Respiratory management

Postoperative respiratory complications may be due to mechanical, haemodynamic, or pharmacological factors related to surgery and anaesthesia. The preoperative respiratory status and ventilatory reserves of the patient also play an important role in postoperative outcomes. In order to simplify the diagnosis of respiratory problems and direct appropriate therapy, it is useful to categorize respiratory complications as being due to abnormalities in ventilation, arterial oxygenation, or airway patency, and protection problems [29] (Tables 11 and 12).

Table 11 Postoperative respiratory complications inadequate ventilation (*PEEP* positive end expiratory pressure)

Primary factor	Causes
Lowered respiratory drive	Residual effects of anesthetics
	Postoperative opioids/hypnotics
	CO$_2$ retainer, morbid obesity
Increased airway resistance	Obstruction of the upper airways
	Bronchospasm
Lowered compliance	Obesity, atelectasis, restrictive lung disease
Neuromuscular problems	Incomplete reversal of muscle relaxants, thoracic spinal or epidural blockade
Increased dead space	Excessive PEEP or CPAP
	Pulmonary emboli
Increased CO$_2$ production	Shivering, higher work of breathing, sepsis, higher sympathetic tone

Table 12 Postoperative respiratory complications inadequate oxygenation (*BP* blood pressure)

Primary factors	Causes
Altered distribution of ventilation	V/Q mismatch, lower funct. resid. capac., obesity, pulmonary oedema, gastric distention, pulmonary aspiration
Altered distribution of perfusion	Raised pulmonary vascular resistance secondary to pain, hypoxaemia, higher airway pressure, effect of anaesthetics
Inadequate PaO_2	Severe hypoventilation, apnoea, airway obstruction, laryngospasm, diffusion hypoxia
Raised mixed various PaO_2	Lower CO, lower BP, shivering, hypovolaemia

Respiratory management is summarized in Table 13.

Table 13 Respiratory management

Goals	Optimize O_2 saturation
	Normocarbia for patient
	Avoid haemodynamic effects
	Maintain airway protection
	Facilitate early extubation
Criteria	ABG's and CXR haemodynamics
Interventions	• Adjust rate and tidal volume
	• Adjust FiO_2 and PEEP
	• Alternate modes PSV, PCV
	• Short-term sedation

Weaning and extubation

In general, in the surgical patient weaning and extubation require the following.

1. Assessment of the neurological response, haemodynamic stability, urine output and output of any drains.
2. Assessment of TOF and reverse neuromuscular blockade, if not already reversed.
3. It may be able to wean rapidly to CPAP/PSV if the respiratory drive is adequate.
4. Ability to maintain pH 7.35, adequate ABGs, or minimal support (PSV5) suggests readiness.
5. Respiratory mechanics could be considered optimal (Vt, Ve, rate, MIP)

Table 14 lists a number of parameters that can contribute to failed attempts at weaning; efforts to optimize these variables can help shorten the duration of weaning.

Table 14 Parameters that can contribute to failed attempts at weaning

Increased lung water	Muscle weakness
Changes in mental status	Malnutrition
Bronchoconstriction	Overfeeding
Infection	Electrolyte imbalance
Increase lung water	Muscle weakness
Mental status changes	Malnutrition

Several strategies for discontinuation of ventilation have been recently compared [30]. For patients requiring mechanical ventilation for less than 2 weeks' duration, the data indicate that weaning using PSV and/or daily trials of spontaneous breathing is most effective [31-33]. For these patients, it appears that the most-important determinant is healing of the injured lung, because weaning does not appear to improve lung function per se. The most-important part of weaning, therefore, may be simply recognizing when the patient is capable of unassisted breathing. There is insufficient information to determine the best method of weaning for patients who require ventilation for several weeks to months.

Neurological dysfunction

Brain dysfunction presents as an alteration in mental function that spaces the spectrum from delirium to coma. The pathophysiology of brain dysfunction is poorly understood, in part because of the complexities of consciousness and neuronal function. As a result, the etiology is usually listed as multifactorial. (Tables 15 and 16).

Table 15 Etiology of brain dysfunction in the postoperative critically ill

Hepatic encephalopathy
Septic encephalopathy
Neurotoxin accumulation secondary to renal dysfunction
Neuroactive drugs (H_2 blockers, acyclovir)
Catecholamine excess associated with the neurohumoral response to stress
Cerebrovascular event (stroke)
Meningitis·   "Sundowning" (night-time psychomotor agitation)
Electrolyte disturbance
Hypotension, hyper- or hypoglycemia

Table 16 Etiology of delayed recovery from anaesthesiaTreatment of brain dysfunction is supportive

Pre-existing mental dysfunction
Heavy premedication
Residual sedation from anaesthetics
Persistent paralysis
Metabolic
Hypothermia < 33°C
Respiratory: CO_2 narcosis, hypoxemia
SNC: haemorrhage, stroke

Renal dysfunction

Oliguria and anuria are among the most-common problems seen postoperatively. Causes include hypovolemia or low cardiac output despite adequate intravascular volume. Other causes can include an obstructed catheter, acute renal failure (ARF), or damage to the collecting system, such as ureteral obstruction, bladder perforation, and leak.

ARF can follow suprarenal cross-clamping of the aorta. Severe or prolonged intraoperative hypotension can also be the culprit. Acute renal artery thrombosis is rare, but occurs occasionally; a renal scan will demonstrate the absence of blood flow. No specific guidelines exist that routinely and simultaneously produce the least compromise to the kidneys, lungs, and heart. Instead, therapy needs to be individualized, based on the apparent risk to each system. Lacking an easy cookbook approach to prevent the progression from acute prerenal oliguria to ARF, the following generalizations form the basis of a logical approach.
1. Renal hypoperfusion most commonly causes ARF.
2. The duration and magnitude of the initial renal insult determine the severity of ARF.
3. Prevention of ARF reduces mortality more effectively than does dialytic therapy.

Hypothermia

Postoperative hypothermia can cause significant problems in the critically ill patient. The usual causes of hypothermia include a relatively cool operating room and failure to keep the patient warm.

This situation is further aggravated by the use of fluids kept at room temperature. Paralysis prevents heat generation by muscle shivering. Hypothermia can lead to or cause significant complications (Table 17).

Table 17 Complications of hypothermia Postoperatively, hypothermia requires aggressive therapy: rewarming, and, if intravascular volume is adequate, sodium nitroprusside can dramatically aid in the warming process

Bleeding	Despite a normal amount of coagulation factors
Platelet dysfunction	
Cardiovascular dysfunction	– Decreased cardiac output – Hypertension – Bradycardia
Metabolic acidosis with high anion gap	
Neurological dysfunction	
Reduced body immune system	
Depressed liver function	
Pancreatic inhibition	

Nutrition

Enteral versus parenteral versus no specialized nutrition support

Several class I randomized, prospective studies have researched the route of nutrient administration in general surgical patients [34-36]. Most studies show improved outcome with early enteral feeding [37-39]. The benefits of reduced infectious complications with enteral feeding increase as the severity of the injury increases.

In patients in whom gastroparesis does not resolve within 6 - 7 days, parenteral nutrition or transpyloric placement of an enteral tube is clinically indicated, with the transition to intragastric feeding as soon as the gastroparesis resolves.

Postoperative complications

Management of the postoperative critically ill patient implies the knowledge of:
- What are the most-common complications?
- When do they occur?

- Can we identify the high-risk patient?
- How can they be prevented?

Specific concerns in the postoperative heart patient are shown in Table 18.

Table 18 Concerns in the postoperative heart patient

Myocardial ischaemia	Low cardiac output syndrome
Atrial fibrillation and other arrhythmias	Rewarming
Bleeding and need for re-exploration	Early extubation
Diaphragmatic complications	

Specific concerns in the post-craniotomy patient are shown in Table 19.

Table 19 Concerns in the post craniotomy patient

Blood pressure control [CPP = MAP – ICP (intracranial pressure)]

Awakening and neurological status

Seizures

Watch for osmolality and electrolytes

Monitoring ICP: goal is ICP 15 mmHg [20]

Effect of PEEP and other ventilation manoeuvres [40]:
– PEEP raises intrathoracic pressure, decreases venous return, and increases ICP in normal patients
– In injured patients, depends on lung compliance
– Unlikely to affect the ICP at PEEP ≤ 10; if PEEP > 15 better to monitor the ICP.

Therapeutic manoeuvres to decrease the intracranial pressure (ICP) are [41]:
- Head elevation 20-30°
- If ventricular catheter in place, cerebrospinal fluid drainage
- Mannitol load 0.5-1.5 g/kg IV and bolus later 0.25-0.5 g/kg IV every 4-6/h.
  – It increases the osmotic gradient across the blood brain barrier.
  – Onset within 15 min, effect lasts 1 to several hours.
  – Aiming for serum osmolality of 320 mosmol
- Furosemide may decrease the ICP (10-20 mg every 4-6 h prn). We also have to watch for hypovolemia, azotemia, metabolic alkalosis, electrolyte abnormalities, and nephrotoxicity.
- Barbiturates (thiopental 1-4 mg/kg per hour infusion)
  – Titrate to burst suppression, discontinue when:

-ICP remains < 15 mmHg for 48 h
-No response to loading on two consecutive hourly doses
-Escape phenomenon (unable to control with high doses)
- Hyperventilation (typically to $PaCO_2$ of 25-35 mmHg)
  –Useful for very rapid ICP reduction (plateau waves)
  –Ultimately (< 24 h) cerebral blood flow returns to baseline levels
- Corticosteroids

Benefit for oedema-causing tumours

- Mild hypothermia
- Decompressive craniectomy

General concerns following abdominal surgery are:

- Fluid balance, taking into account evaporative and bleeding losses and that "third space" will occur
- Coagulopathy may be a concern
- Bowel ischemia may become manifested with lactic acidosis and development of multisystem failure
- Increased intra-abdominal pressure may have adverse effects on renal perfusion and on ventilation.

Some of the expected management problems following abdominal procedures are listed in Table 20.

Table 20 Expected management problems following abdominal procedures

Splenectomy	Blood loss, risk for GPC
Cholecystectomy	Atelectasis R base
Partial hepatectomy	Blood loss, coagulopathy
Pancreatectomy	Hypocalcaemia
Whipple procedure	Fluid and heat loss
Small bowel resection	Hypotension, hypovolemia

Specific concerns following vascular surgery are shown in Table 21.

Table 21 Concerns following vascular surgery

Myocardial ischaemia
– Arrhythmia control
– Blood pressure control
– Augmentation of poor contractility

Renal and fluid status
– "Third spacing" is common
– Acute tubular necrosis following aortic cross-clamping
– Diuresis following intraoperative mannitol

Anterior spinal artery syndrome

Ischaemic bowel

Specific concerns following thoracotomy are shown in Table 22.

Table 22 Concerns following thoracotomy

Postoperative analgesia is necessary

Dysrhythmias, especially atrial fibrillation

Airway oedema and stridor

Atelectasis, secretions and lobar collapse

Ventilator dependency can be a problem in some patients

In summary, there are issues common to all surgical patients. These include:

- From a cardiovascular standpoint, we watch for haemodynamics and ischaemia
- Respiratory, weaning and extubation, atelectasis
- Fluid management and electrolytes need to be evaluated
- Watch for bleeding and coagulation
- Proper management of sedation and agitation
- Prevention or treatment of infections

The knowledge of the likely complications and course for specific common surgical procedures may affect the outcome.

References

1. Calvin JH, Habert K, Parillo JE (1997) Critical care in the United States: who are we and how we did get there. Crit Care Clin, 13:363-376
2. Boyd O, Grounds RM, Bennett ED (1993) A randomized clinical trial of the effect of deliberate increase of oxygen delivery on mortality in high-risk surgical patients. J Am Med Assoc, 270: 2699-2707
3. Shoemaker WC, Appel PL, Kram HB et al (1988) Prospective trial of supranormal values of survivors as therapeutic goals in high-risk surgical patients. Chest 94:1176-1186
4. Moscucci M, Bates ER (1995) Cardiogenic shock. Cardiol Clin 13:391-406
5. Califf RM, Bengtson JR (1994) Cardiogenic shock. N Engl J Med 330:1724-1730
6. Connors AF Jr, Speroff T, Dawson NV et al (1996) The effectiveness of right-heart catheterization in the initial care of critically ill patients. JAMA 276:889-897
7. Gore JM, Goldberg Rj, Spodick DH et al (1987) A community-wide assessment of the use of pulmonary artery catheters in patients with acute myocardial infarction. Chest 92:721-727
8. Zion MM, Balkin J, Rosenmann D et al (1990) Use of pulmonary artery catheters in patients with acute myocardial infarction: analysis of experience in 5841 patients in the Sprint registry. Chest 98:1331-1335
9. Dalen JE (1990) Does pulmonary artery catheterization benefit patients with acute myocardial infarction? Chest 98:1313-1314
10. Dalen JE, Bone RC (1996) Is it time to pull the pulmonary artery catheter? JAMA 276:916-918
11. Robin ED (1987) Death by pulmonary artery flow-directed catheter. Time for a moratorium? Chest 92:727-730
12. Pearson KS, Gomez MN, Moyers JR et al (1989) A cost/benefit analysis of randomized invasive monitoring for patients undergoing cardiac surgery. Anesth Analg 69:336-341
13. Valentine RJ, Duke ML, Inman MH et al (1998) Effectiveness of pulmonary artery catheters in aortic surgery: a randomized trial. J Vasc Surg 27:203-211
14. Isaacson IJ, Lowdon JD, Berry AJ et al (1990) The value of pulmonary artery and central venous monitoring in patients undergoing abdominal aortic reconstructive surgery, a comparative study of two selected randomized groups. J Vasc Surg 12:754-760
15. Joyce WP, Provan JL, Ameli FM et al (1990) The role of central hemodynamic monitoring in abdominal aortic surgery. A prospective randomized study. Eur J Vasc Surg 4:633-639
16. Bender JS, Smith-Meek MA, Jones CE (1997) Routine pulmonary artery catheterization does not reduce morbidity and mortality of elective vascular surgery: results of a prospective, randomized trial. Ann Surg 226:229-236
17. Bland RD, Shoemaker WC, Abraham E, Cobo JC (1985) Hemodynamic and oxygen transport patterns in surviving and nonsurviving postoperative patients. Crit Care Med 13:85-90
18. Shoemaker WC, Appel PL, Kram HB et al (1988) Prospective trial of supranormal values of survivors as therapeutic goals in high-risk surgical patients. Chest 94:1176-1183
19. Yu M, Burchell S, Hasaniya NWMA et al (1998) Relationship of mortality to increasing oxygen delivery in patients 50 years of age: a prospective, randomized trial. Crit Care Med 26:1011-1019
20. Yu M, Levy MM, Smith P et al (1993) Effect of maximizing oxygen delivery on morbidity and mortality rates in critically ill patients: a prospective, randomized controlled study. Crit Care Med 21:830-838
21. Alía A, Esteban A, Gordo F et al (1999) A randomized and controlled trial of the effect of treatment aimed at maximizing oxygen delivery in patients with sever sepsis or septic shock. Chest 115:453-461
22. Heyland D, Cook DJ, King D et al (1996) Maximizing oxygen delivery in critically ill patients: a methodologic appraisal of the evidence. Crit Care Med 24:577-524
23. Connors AF Jr (1997) Right heart catheterization: is it effective? New Horiz 5:195-200
24. Iberti TJ, Fischer EP, Leibowitz AB et al (1990) A multicenter study of physicians' knowledge of the pulmonary artery catheter. JAMA 264:2928-2932

25. Gnaegi A, Feihl F, Perret C (1997) Intensive care physicians' insufficient knowledge of right-heart catheterization at the bedside: time to act? Crit Care Med 25:213-220
26. Vermeulen LC, Ratko MA, Estad BL (1995) Guidelines for fluid replacement. Arch Intern Med 155-373
27. Simon TL, Alverson DC, AuBuchon J et al (198) Practice parameter for the use of red blood cell transfusions: developed by the Red Blood Cell Administration Practice Guideline Development Task Force of the College of American Pathologists. Arch Pathol Lab Med 122:130-138
28. Slogoff S, Keats JR (1985) Perioperative ischemia and outcome. Anesthesiology 62:107
29. Mecca RS (1992) Postoperative recovery in clinical anesthesia 2nd edn, Lippincott, Philadelphia, pp 1515-1546
30. Kollef MH, Shapiro SD, Silver P et al (1997) A randomized controlled trial of protocol-directed versus physician-directed weaning from mechanical ventilation. Crit Care Med 25:567-574
31. Esteban A, Frutos F, Tobin MJ et al (1995) A comparison of four methods of weaning patients from mechanical ventilation. Spanish Lung Failure Collaborative Group. N Engl J Med 332: 345-350
32. Ely EW, Baker AM, Dunagan DP et al (1996) Effect on the duration of mechanical ventilation of identifying patients capable of breathing spontaneously. N Engl J Med 335:1864-1869
33. Brochard L, Rauss A, Benito S et al (1994) Comparison of three methods of gradual withdrawal from ventilatory support during weaning from mechanical ventilation. Am J Respir 150: 896-903
34. Shirabe K, Matsumata T, Shimada M et al (1997) Comparison of parenteral hyperalimentation and early enteral feeding regarding systemic immunity after major hepatic resection: the result of a randomized prospective study. Hepatogastroenterology 44:205-209
35. Gianotti L, Braga M, Vignali A et al (1997) Effect of route of delivery and formulation of postoperative nutritional support in patients undergoing major operations for malignant neoplasms. Arch Surg 132:1222-1229
36. Windsor AC, Kanwar S, Li AG et al (1998) Compared with parenteral nutrition, enteral feeding attenuates the acute phase response and improves disease severity in acute pancreatitis. Gut 42:431-435
37. Moore EE, Jones TN (1986) Benefits of immediate jejunostomy feeding after major abdominal trauma. J Trauma 26:874-879
38. Kudsk KA, Croce MA, Fabian TC et al (1992) Enteral vs parenteral feeding. Effects on septic morbidity after blunt and penetrating abdominal trauma. Ann Surg 215:503-511
39. Kudsk KA, Minard G, Croce MA et al (1996) A randomized trial of isonitrogenous enteral diets after severe trauma: an immune-enhancing diet reduces septic complications. Ann Surg 224: 531-542
40. Mc Guire, Crossley D, Richards J, Wong D (1997) Effects of varying levels of PEEP on ICP and CPP. Crit Care Med 25:1059-1062
41. Brain Trauma Foundation and American Association of Neurological Surgeons (2000) Guidelines for the management of severe traumatic brain injury

HIV infection in critical care

G. Dominguez-Cherit, D. Borunda, J. Sierra

The human immunodeficiency virus (HIV) pandemic has spread to every country in the world and has infected over 2.5 million persons world wide. While initially limited, infection with the HIV has literally exploded over the past 2 decades to become the worst epidemic of the twentieth century. With more than 20 million fatalities, the AIDS epidemic now ranks alongside the influenza pandemic of the early 1900s and the Bubonic plague of the fourteenth century in terms of fatalities. The impact of this disease on human suffering, cultures, demographics, economics, and even politics has been felt in nearly every society across the globe.

Stages of HIV-1 infection

HIV-1 infection is divided into the following stages:
- Viral transmission
- Primary HIV infection (also called acute HIV infection or acute seroconversion syndrome)
- Seroconversion
- Clinical latent period with or without persistent generalized lymphadenopathy (PGL)
- Early symptomatic HIV infection (previously known as "AIDS-related complex" or ARC and more recently referred to as "B symptoms" according to the 1993 CDC classification)
- AIDS (AIDS indicator condition according to the 1987 CDC criteria and revised 1993 CDC criteria that include a CD4 cell count below 200/mm^3)
- Advanced HIV infection characterized by a CD4 cell count below 50/mm^3

Patients with HIV infection are also divided into three clinical categories.

A   includes primary HIV infection, asymptomatic infection, and PGL.
B   refers to symptomatic patients who do not have conditions specific to A or C.
C   includes patients with AIDS indicator conditions.

The clinical conditions that define a patient as having AIDS will be described below. The diagnosis is infrequently recognized due to the non-specific nature of the complaints and findings [1]. The following symptoms were identified in a review of 209 such cases (in order of frequency, fever, adenopathy, pharyngitis, rash, myalgias or arthralgias, diarrhea and headache, nausea and vomiting, hepatosplenomegaly, thrush, weight loss, and fatigue) [2].

The presence of primary HIV-1 infection should be considered in any patient with a history of potential exposure and the aforementioned clinical features. The diagnosis is best established by the demonstration of p24 antigen, quantitative HIV RNA, or qualitative HIV DNA in association with negative or indeterminate HIV serology. The most-sensitive method is HIV DNA detection, although HIV RNA, levels are readily available and also show good sensitivity, because the acute illness is generally accompanied by a high level of HIV viremia [1, 3].

The presence of symptoms and a prolonged illness (14 days) appear to correlate with more-rapid progression to AIDS [5, 10]. Pedersen et al. [4] described that the risk of progression to an AIDS-defining diagnosis within 3 years following seroconversion was substantially higher in those with acute symptoms lasting more than 14 days than in those who were asymptomatic or had only mild symptoms (78% versus 10%) [4].

Seroconvertion to positive HIV serology within 6 months occurs in over 95% of patients following HIV transmission using standard serological tests [5-8]. Seroconversion generally occurs at 6 - 12 weeks, with a median interval of 63 days [5, 9].

The stage of early symptomatic HIV infection is also called B symptoms and was formerly called AIDS-related complex. Although these diseases occur in association with many disorders, they are more frequent and more severe when associated with HIV infection. The B conditions are not AIDS-indicator conditions.

The definition of AIDS established in 1987 included conditions indicative of severe immunosuppression, especially defective cell-mediated immunity [10]. The more recently revised CDC classification has three ranges of CD4 cell counts and uses a matrix of nine mutually exclusive categories.

The 1993 definition of AIDS includes all of the AIDS-indicator diseases in the 1987 version with three additions: recurrent bacterial pneumonia, invasive cervical cancer, and pulmonary tuberculosis (Table 1). The most-substantive change in the classification was the inclusion of all patients with a CD4 cell count below 200/mm^3.

Table 1 The 1993 definition of AIDS

Candidiasis of esophagus, trachea, bronchi, or lungs

Cervical cancer, invasive [a,b]

Coccidioidomycosis, extrapulmonary [a]

Cryptococcosis, extrapulmonary

Cryptosporidiosis with diarrhea for > 1 month

Cytomegalovirus of any organ other than liver, spleen, or lymph nodes

Herpes simplex with mucocutaneous ulcer for > 1 month or bronchitis, pneumonitis, esophagitis

Histoplasmosis, extrapulmonary

HIV-associated dementia: disabling cognitive and/or motor dysfunction interfering with occupation or activities of daily living [b]

HIV-associated wasting: involuntary weight loss of > 10% of baseline plus chronic diarrhea (>2 loose stools/day for > 30 days) or chronic weakness and documented enigmatic fever for > 30 days [a]

Isosporosis with diarrhea for > 1 month [a]

Kaposi's sarcoma in patient younger than age 60 years (or older than age 60 years [a])

Lymphoma or brain tumor in patient younger than age 60 years (or older than age 60 years [a])

Lymphoma, non-Hodgkin's of B cell or unknown immunological phenotype and histology showing small, non-cleaved lymphoma or immunoblastic sarcoma

Mycobacterium avium or *M. kansasii*, disseminated

Mycobacterium tuberculosis, disseminated

Mycobacterium tuberculosis, pulmonary

Nocardiosis [a]

Pneumocystis carinii pneumonia

Pneumonia, recurrent bacteria [a, b]

Progressive multifocal leukoencephalopathy

Salmonella septicemia (non-typhoid)

Strongyloidosis, extraintestinal

Toxoplasmosis of internal organ

---

[a] Requires positive HIV serology
[b] Added in the revised case definition 1993

The median CD4 count at the time of an AIDS-defining complication is $67/mm^3$ [11]. However, approximately 10% of patients develop an AIDS-defining diagnosis with a CD4 count above $200/mm^3$. The median time from the onset of severe immunosuppression (defined as a CD4 cell count below $200/mm^3$) to an AIDS-defining diagnosis (1987 criteria) is 12 - 18 months in persons not receiving antiretroviral treatment [12].

The CDC reported 71,704 new cases in the 1997 fiscal year. The rank order of first AIDS-defining conditions is given in the CDC Adult/Adolescent Spectrum of HIV Disease Sentinel Surveillance Project [13].

Patients with advanced HIV infection have a CD4 cell count below 50/mm^3. Their median survival is 12 - 18 months in the absence of antiretroviral therapy [14-16]. Virtually all patients who die of HIV-related complications have CD4 cell counts in this range.

Rate of progression

The average life expectancy for a HIV-infected patient in the absence of treatment is approximately 10 years. The rate of progression to AIDS may vary depending upon the mode of transmission. For example, a summary of 20 reports showed that the median time from HIV seroconversion to AIDS (1987 definition) is about 7 years for transfusion recipients, 10 years for hemophiliacs, 10 years for intravenous drug users, and 8 - 12 years for gay men [9]. Rates of progression appear similar by sex, race, and risk category if adjusted for the quality of care [17,18-21]. Patients with symptomatic primary HIV infection progress more rapidly than those with asymptomatic seroconversion.

Age

Age is also an important variable. In one series, for example, the median time from seroconversion to AIDS was 15 years for patients aged 16 - 24 years at seroconversion, compared with 6 years for those 35 years or older at seroconversion [22]. These data are from population-based studies, and the variation between individual patients is extensive.

Characteristics of the virus

Characteristics of the virus itself may also influence the rate of progression. A cohort of patients from Australia (one blood donor and eight recipients), infected with an HIV-1 strain, with a deletion in the region where nef and the long terminal repeat overlap, have been followed for 14 - 18 years [23]. This HIV strain appears to be attenuated since three of the recipients have an undetectable viral load and normal CD4 counts (two recipients died at an advanced age of causes unrelated to HIV). However, three of the four patients with a detectable viral load, including the donor, have shown a decline in CD4 counts.

CD4 count and viral load

Two important laboratory determinants of the rate of progression are the CD4 count and the viral load [24, 25]. The average rate of decline of CD4 cells ("CD4 slope") is about 50/mm^3 per year and the average viral burden (without therapy) is 30,000 - 50,000 copies/ml. The prognosis is worse in patients with a lower CD4 count, a steeper CD4 decline, and a higher viral burden (see Table 2) [25, 26].

Table 2 Opportunistic infections

	Percentage
Pneumocystis carinii pneumonia	42.6
Esophageal candidiasis	15.0
Wasting	10.7
Kaposi's sarcoma	10.7
Disseminated *Mycobacterium avium* infection	4.8
Tuberculosis	4.5
Cytomegalovirus disease	3.7
HIV-associated dementia	3.6
Recurrent bacterial pneumonia	3.0
Toxoplasmosis	2.6
Immunoblastic lymphoma	1.9
Chronic cryptosporidiosis	1.5
Burkitt lymphoma	1.5
Disseminated histoplasmosis	1.0
Invasive cervical cancer	0.9
Chronic herpes simplex	0.5

From reference [13]

ICU management

The admission of patients with HIV to the intensive care unit (ICU) has been decreasing during the last few years, approximately 4%-5% of hospitalized patients with HIV are admitted to the ICU, and the main goal is for closer observation or life-sustaining support.

Among the most-frequent causes for admitting the patients to the ICU are

infections, opportunistic and common bacterial, electrolyte disturbances, neurological alterations, and gastrointestinal disturbances.

Electrolyte disturbances with HIV infection

Fluid loss in these patients most often occurs from the gastrointestinal tract,
due primarily to infectious diarrhoea [27-29]. This disorder can be distinguis-
hed from the SIADH by the low urine sodium concentration (usually below 15
mEq/l) and correction of the hyponatremia with fluid repletion.

Another cause of hyponatremia is adrenal insufficiency, which is less
common than the SIADH or hypovolemia [27, 28]. In general, the fall in the
plasma sodium concentration is due to cortisol deficiency (which appears to
directly enhance hypothalamic ADH release), while the frequently associated
hyperkalemia is due to aldosterone deficiency. The adrenal injury seen in AIDS
or ARC is often due to an adrenalitis, an abnormality that may be infectious in
origin, perhaps being induced by cytomegalovirus, *Mycobacterium avium-in-
tracellulare*, or HIV itself [27, 30, 31]. Adrenal haemorrhage and infiltration
with Kaposi's sarcoma also may be seen [30, 31].

Hyperkalemia is less common than hyponatremia, affecting up to 15 - 20%
of hospitalized patients [32, 33]. This is usually caused by adrenal insufficiency,
the syndrome of hyporeninemic hypoaldosteronism [32], or the administration
of trimethoprim or pentamidine [34-36]. Some other factors, such as coexisting
renal failure due to HIV itself or to the administration of nephrotoxins to treat
infection, can contribute to the tendency for potassium retention. The mechanism responsible for the low renin release in HIV-infected patients is not
known, nor are the relative roles of hyporeninemia and direct adrenal injury in
the decreased aldosterone release. Hyperkalemia induced by hypoaldosteronism can be corrected with replacement (starting with 0.05 - 0.10 mg of
fludrocortisone per day) [32].

Another important cause of hyperkalemia in these patients is trimethoprim,
which is usually given in combination with sulfamethoxazole or dapsone for
Pneumocystis carinii pneumonia. It causes an increase in the plasma potassium
concentration of 0.5 - 1 mEq/l with occasional cases of severe hyperkalemia
[34-36]. Trimethoprim is cationic, like amiloride and triamterene, and appears
to act as a potassium-sparing diuretic, decreasing the number of open sodium
channels in the luminal membrane of the cortical collecting tubule cells [34,
36]. The ensuing reduction in sodium reabsorption then minimizes potassium
secretion. Trimethoprim doses in HIV-infected patients are often 5 to 10 times
higher than that given for conventional infections and this probably explains
the more frequent development of hyperkalemia in the latter setting. However,

conventional doses of trimethoprim can also raise the plasma potassium concentration.

Pentamidine appears to act by the same mechanism as trimethoprim, blocking distal potassium secretion, causing elevation in the plasma potassium concentration.

Lactic acidosis can occur and this is given the increased propensity to serious infection (sepsis) in patients with AIDS [37]. There are some rare cases in which lactic acidosis appears to result from drug-induced mitochondrial dysfunction in the absence of sepsis or hypoperfusion (type B lactic acidosis). The following mechanisms may be involved:

- Drug-induced hepatic steatosis and hepatic failure due, for example, to zidovudine or stavudine [38, 39]. This complication may, in some cases, result from concurrent deficiency of riboflavin, a precursor to a number of cofactors necessary for mitochondrial energy production. In several patients, nucleoside-induced lactic acidosis has been reversed by riboflavin therapy [40, 41].
- Zidovudine-induced myopathy characterized by elevated plasma creatine kinase concentrations and proximal muscle weakness [42].
- A seemingly idiopathic form that can occur in the absence of zidovudine [37]

Neurology disorders

Neurological features of primary HIV-1 infection are uncommon, but include meningoencephalitis, peripheral neuropathy, and, rarely, facial palsy, Guillain--Barré syndrome, brachial neuritis, radiculopathy, cognitive impairment, or psychosis.

Cytomegalovirus

Cytomegalovirus (CMV) neurological disease is an uncommon serious complication of AIDS that can cause paralysis or rapidly fatal encephalitis. Prior to the availability of highly active antiretroviral therapy (HAART), CMV neurological disease occurred in up to 2% of patients with AIDS [43], primarily in those with a CD4 T cell count below $50/mm^3$. However, the incidence of CMV neurological disease has decreased since HAART became available [44,45].

CMV neurological disease can involve the brain, spinal cord, dorsal column nerve roots, or peripheral nerves. CMV inclusions have been identified in astrocytes, neurons, oligodendrocytes, and capillary endothelia of neural tissue.

Clinical manifestations

The symptoms of CMV neurological disease are determined by anatomical location.

Encephalitis

CMV encephalitis is essentially a disease of immunosuppressed subjects. In a review of 676 patients, 85% had AIDS, 12% had other causes of immunosuppression, and only 3% were immunocompetent [46]. CMV ventriculoencephalitis is a distinct entity found almost exclusively in patients with advanced HIV infection [46]. There is a tendency to present dementia that is difficult to distinguish clinically from the dementia caused by HIV itself. However, delirium, confusion, and focal neurological abnormalities are more commonly associated with CMV-related than HIV-related dementia [47].

The presence of CMV encephalitis should be suspected in patients with advanced HIV disease (especially those with prior CMV disease in another site) who have a progressive change in mental status, delirium, rapidly progressive cognitive impairment, or signs and symptoms of brain stem injury. A magnetic resonance imaging (MRI) or contrast computed tomographie (CT) scan must be performed to exclude toxoplasmosis, lymphoma, progressive multifocal leukoencephalopathy, or other intracranial processes. Evidence of periventricular inflammation or meningeal enhancement helps support the diagnosis of CMV encephalitis, but are not specific for the disease. Recent studies suggest that the detection of CMV DNA (e.g., by polymerase chain reaction) or CMV antigen in the cerebrospinal fluid (CSF) is highly sensitive and specific for CMV neurological disease involving the brain or cord [48-50].

Myelitis

The presence of CMV myelitis should be suspected in patients with advanced HIV disease (especially those with prior CMV disease in another site) who have progressive lower extremity weakness and hyperactive reflexes on neurological examination. A MRI or contrast CT scan of the spinal cord (or myelogram) should be performed to exclude mass lesions. Evidence of enhancement of the cord also helps support the presumptive diagnosis of CMV myelitis.

Polyradiculopathy

Patients with CMV polyradiculopathy present with decreased lower extremity strength, decreased or absent reflexes, and, in some cases, urinary retention. The onset of symptoms usually occurs over a period of days to weeks. A myelogram or MRI reveals no mass lesions but may show that lower spinal nerve roots are thickened. CSF abnormalities, in particular a polymorphonuclear pleocytosis, are characteristic of this condition.

In the appropriate clinical setting, a CSF polymorphonuclear pleocytosis with a negative CSF bacterial culture is very strong evidence for CMV radiculomyelopathy in a patient with AIDS who has a CD4 cell count below 50/mm³. A positive test for CMV DNA in the CSF also supports this diagnosis.

Peripheral neuropathy

Patients with CMV peripheral nerve disease usually present with the syndrome of mononeuritis multiplex, consisting of multifocal or asymmetric sensory and motor deficits in the distribution of major peripheral or cranial nerves (especially the laryngeal nerves) [51]. Biopsy of an involved peripheral nerve can confirm the diagnosis.

Natural history

Knowledge of the outcome of CMV neurological disease is limited to data from several small series [47]. Whether treated or not, median survival of patients with CMV neurological disease was less than 3 months in the pre-HAART era. HAART could alter the natural history of CMV neurological disease, even if in such patients HAART is first initiated after being diagnosed with CMV disease. Patients with extraocular CMV disease often have prior or concurrent CMV retinitis. As a result, any patient diagnosed with CMV neurological disease not already known to have retinitis should undergo formal ophthalmological screening for retinitis.

Treatment

The efficacies and toxicities of approved treatments for CMV retinitis have been established by many randomized prospective trials. In contrast, there have been no prospective randomized trials of treatment for CMV neurological disease.

Based upon a few published case reports [52, 53], the consensus of clinical experts is that patients with CMV neurological disease should receive 3-6 weeks of twice daily intravenous (IV) ganciclovir or foscarnet, or both agents in combination [54]. Chronic IV maintenance therapy is indicated for those patients who have a clinical response. For patients who have failed or are intolerant to IV ganciclovir and foscarnet, cidofovir may be an effective alternative treatment [55].

Neutropenia and thrombocytopenia have been the main toxicities of chronic ganciclovir therapy in patients with AIDS, and have been dose-limiting in 16% and 5% of patients, respectively. Ganciclovir-induced severe neutropenia usually can be reversed by the administration of granulocyte-colony stimulating factor [56].

Reversible increases in serum creatinine (due to acute tubular necrosis) and symptoms of hypocalcemia during drug infusions [caused by transient, foscarnet chelation of serum ionized calcium, which can fall by 0.7 - 1.1 mg/dl (0.17 - 0.28 mmol/l)] are the most-serious toxicities of foscarnet, and have been dose limiting in approximately 20% of patients [57, 58]. Foscarnet can also cause transient hypomagnesemia by chelation [59].

Cidofovir has caused serious, irreversible nephrotoxicity via dose-dependent proximal tubular cell injury. The initial manifestations of renal toxicity are proteinuria and increased serum creatinine concentrations; with continued treatment some patients have had a life-threatening Fanconi-like syndrome and renal failure. Saline hydration and high-dose probenecid therapy (which can block cidofovir uptake by proximal renal tubular cells) have been given concomitantly with cidofovir in an attempt to reduce the risk of serious renal injury [60,61]. The oral probenecid regimen is 2 g 3 h before the infusion and 1 g at both 2 and 8 h after the infusion. Because of a possible interaction between probenecid and zidovudine to produce an increased rate of skin reactions, zidovudine should be withheld on the days of cidofovir administration.

Valganciclovir is a valine ester of ganciclovir and is rapidly and completely de-esterified to ganciclovir after oral intake. The ganciclovir component of valganciclovir has approximately 60% oral bioavailability. Valganciclovir has been demonstrated to be effective therapy for CMV retinitis, with no more toxicity than intravenous ganciclovir therapy. The exact incidence of nephrotoxicity is not known.

Pulmonary complications

Among the main pulmonary complications in patients with HIV infection are the infections, mainly due to *P. carinii*, but other bacteria are also present.

Pneumocystis

The AIDS epidemic has been accompanied by an explosion in the number of cases of *P. carinii* pneumonia (PCP). Prior to 1981, there were fewer than 100 cases of PCP reported annually in the United States. These were seen in patients with underlying malignancy and other forms of immunosuppression, especially defects in cell-mediated immunity. The incidence of PCP probably peaked between 1987 and 1988 and has been declining since that time, due to the increased use of PCP prophylaxis. Nevertheless, there are still tens of thousands of anticipated cases of PCP per year. Despite prophylaxis, 15% - 28% of HIV-infected patients can be expected to develop PCP annually.

The organism is believed to be transmitted by the respiratory-aerosol route, and 75% of humans are infected by age 4 years [62]. These primary infections are probably asymptomatic. Although most cases of PCP are believed to represent reactivation of latent disease, there are animal data suggesting that animal-to-animal transmission is possible. Reports of cluster outbreaks in oncology units and among HIV-infected patients suggest that human-to-human transmission is possible, but genotypic analyses indicate that acquisition of infection in such a manner is relatively infrequent and accounts for a minority of cases [63,64]. When cases of PCP among HIV-infected patients are retro-spectively analyzed by geographic location, clustering by zip code has been demonstrated [65, 66]. These data raise, but do not confirm, the possibility of a common environmental exposure.

The incidence of PCP in HIV-infected patients increases as the CD4 count decreases [67-69]. Generally, PCP does not occur until the CD4 count drops below 200 cells/mm^3. In the multicenter AIDS Cohort Study, for example, the incidence of PCP with a CD4 count of 201 - 350 cells/mm^3 was 0.5% [70]. Within 6 months of the CD4 count falling below 200 cells/mm^3, 8% of patients developed PCP.

In a study of over 1,100 individuals with HIV infection, the Pulmonary Complications of HIV Infection Study Group confirmed the relationship be-tween CD4 cell count and PCP [68]; 95% of patients who developed PCP had a CD4 count below 200 cells/mm^3. HIV transmission category, age, smoking history, and use of antiretroviral therapy did not predict development of PCP; black subjects had one-third the risk of PCP compared with white patients.

Clinical manifestations

In HIV-infected patients, PCP is generally gradual in onset and characterized by fever (79 - 100%), cough (95%), and progressive dyspnea (95%) [71]. The cough is generally non-productive, but as many as 30% of patients may have some sputum production. Other symptoms include fatigue, chills, chest pain, and weight loss. Approximately 7% of patients are asymptomatic.

The most-common findings on physical examination are fever (84% of patients have a temperature exceeding 38.1°C) and tachypnea (62%). The most--common adventitial sounds are crackles and rhonchi, but a normal chest examination occurs in 50% of cases. Extrapulmonary manifestations of *P. carinii* infection, such as hepatosplenomegaly, skin lesions, and pleural effusions, are increasing, in part due to localized PCP prophylaxis with aerosolized pentamidine.

Chest radiographs are initially normal in up to 0.25% of patients with PCP. The most-common radiographic abnormalities are diffuse, bilateral interstitial, or alveolar infiltrates [72]. Although upper lobe infiltrates can be seen de novo, a higher incidence of predominantly apical infiltrates is reported in patients using aerosolized pentamidine prophylaxis [73]. Other, less-common presentations include pneumothoraces, lobar or segmental infiltrates, cysts, nodules, and pleural effusions [71, 74].

High-resolution computed tomography (HRCT) has a high sensitivity for PCP among HIV-positive patients [75, 76]. One study, for example, evaluated 51 patients with suspected PCP and normal, equivocal, or non-specific chest X-ray findings; HRCT had a sensitivity of 100% and a specificity of 89% when the presence of patchy or nodular ground-glass attenuation was used to indicate possible PCP [76]. A negative HRCT may allow exclusion of PCP in such patients.

Gallium-67 citrate scanning is a highly sensitive test in patients with PCP, demonstrating intense, diffuse, bilateral uptake [77]. However, its role is limited by lack of specificity, its high cost, and a 2-day delay in obtaining final results. Nevertheless, it may have some usefulness as a screening test when there is a question of active pulmonary infection, especially in patients with normal chest radiographs.

Other screening tests for PCP include measurement of the diffusing capacity for carbon monoxide (DLCO). PCP is highly unlikely if the DLCO is normal, defined by 70% of the predicted value or greater. As an example, one prospective study of 306 HIV-positive patients with 467 episodes of worsening respiratory symptoms found that PCP was present in less than 2% of patients with a normal or unchanged chest X-ray and a single-breath DLCO 75% of the predicted value [78].

Assessment of oxygenation at rest and with exercise is also used to screen for PCP [79]. The presence of PCP is highly unlikely if the response to exercise is normal, i.e., a decrease in the alveolar-arterial oxygen gradient or an increase in the oxygen saturation with exercise.

The two most-common abnormal laboratory values associated with PCP in HIV-infected patients are a CD4 count below 200 cells/mm^3 and an elevated lactate dehydrogenase level (LDH) [70, 80]. The latter is present in 90% of HIV-infected patients with PCP and has some prognostic significance. In one study, for example, the mean LDH of PCP survivors was 340 IU, while the mean level of non-survivors was 447 IU [80]. More importantly, a rising LDH level despite appropriate treatment portends a poor prognosis.

Establishing a definitive diagnosis of PCP is usually recommended for two reasons:

1. PCP has many atypical presentations.
2. Therapy may be toxic or even contraindicated (e.g., the use of steroids in patients presumed to have PCP but actually infected with *Mycobacterium tuberculosis*).

Some clinicians advocate empirical treatment for PCP in high-risk patients. One study investigated the relationship between health-care coverage and diagnostic procedures in HIV-infected patients with PCP, and correlated these factors with patient outcome. Medicaid patients were more likely to be empirically treated for PCP and also were more likely to die in hospital [81]. The higher mortality in this group may have been due to a failure to diagnose pathogens other than *P. carinii*, because procedures that could make a specific diagnosis were less likely to be performed in these patients [82].

Specific diagnosis of PCP requires documentation of the organism in respiratory specimens. Conventional stains such as toluidine blue O, Grocott's methenamine silver, or Giemsa can be used to identify the organism.

The most-rapid and least-invasive method of diagnosing PCP is by analysis of sputum induced by the inhalation of hypertonic saline. While the specificity of this method approaches 100%, the sensitivity ranges from 55% to 92% [83]. This variability is related to the prevalence of PCP in the patient population, the skill of the team inducing the sputum, and the expertise of the laboratory processing and interpreting the specimen.

PCP prophylaxis, especially with aerosolized pentamidine, seems to lower the diagnostic sensitivity of sputum induction. In one study, for example, the yield of sputum induction in patients not receiving prophylaxis was 92%, compared with 64% in patients receiving aerosolized pentamidine prophylaxis [84]. The specificity of a positive induced sputum is reduced following an acute episode of PCP, because visible organisms may persist in the sputa of successfully treated patients. One series of 24 patients found residual cysts in 16 patients (76%) after the completion of 3 weeks of appropriate antimicrobial therapy, but this finding was not associated with an increased risk of relapse [85]. Three weeks later, 24% of all patients still had positive induced sputa.

Immunofluorescent staining, using monoclonal antibodies against glycoproteins in the cell walls of the cysts and trophozoites of *P. carinii*, may increase the yield of sputum induction. One report showed that when antibody staining techniques were applied to induced sputum, the sensitivity for PCP was 95% and the specificity was 100% [86].

If sputum induction is non-diagnostic or cannot be performed (e.g., the patient cannot cooperate, is too dyspneic, or has an altered mental status), then fiberoptic bronchoscopy with bronchoalveolar lavage (BAL) is recommended, with or without transbronchial biopsy. BAL alone has a diagnostic yield of 97% - 100% in HIV-infected patients. However, it has been suggested that the diagnostic sensitivity of BAL in patients using aerosolized pentamidine prophylaxis may be as low as 62% [73]. In these patients, transbronchial biopsy, which has a diagnostic yield of up to 100%, can be added.

Site-directed lavage, which involves sampling the most heavily involved lobes on chest radiograph, can also increase the yield in patients with focal infiltrates. One group has shown that the combination of site-directed lavage and immunofluorescent antibody staining increased the sensitivity of BAL from 80% to 98% [87].

The major complications of BAL include respiratory failure (rare) and fever (common). Transbronchial biopsy can be complicated by hemoptysis and pneumothorax (the latter occurring in less than 2%). Of note, BAL can be performed without a bronchoscope by introducing a BAL catheter blindly into the lung [88]. The diagnostic yield is similar to that of BAL, but it is rarely used since most physicians are unfamiliar with the technique.

Endotracheal aspirates from intubated and mechanically ventilated patients appear to have a high sensitivity for the detection of PCP. As an example, one study of 31 intubated patients found that endotracheal aspirates examined with immunostaining techniques had a sensitivity of 92% for PCP, with immuno-stained BAL specimens serving as the reference standard [89]. Thus, examination of endotracheal aspirates in intubated patients may obviate the need for bronchoscopy in many cases.

Transthoracic needle biopsy, which has a high diagnostic yield, is rarely used because of the 30% incidence of pneumothorax. Although lung biopsy, either by thoracotomy or by video-assisted thoracoscopic surgery, can be performed with an assurance of 100% sensitivity and specificity for the diagnosis of PCP, it is used very infrequently because of its cost and invasiveness.

The diagnosis of breakthrough PCP (i.e., PCP occurring despite adequate prophylaxis) may be more complicated than that of PCP occurring without prophylaxis. The problems associated with breakthrough PCP have been closely examined in patients receiving aerosolized pentamidine prophylaxis, but no good data exist for patients receiving systemic prophylaxis. In breakthrough PCP, the clinical course may be less severe, the radiographic findings may be atypical, and the diagnostic yield of traditional BAL (i.e., from the lingula and right middle lobe) may be lower [73].

There is also evidence that higher rates of pneumothorax may be seen in patients on aerosolized pentamidine prophylaxis [74]. One study found that cigarette smoking, active PCP, the presence of pneumatocoeles on chest radiographs, and aerosolized pentamidine prophylaxis were risk factors for the development of pneumothorax [90]. Because the presence of PCP correlates so closely with the development of pneumothorax, all HIV-infected patients who develop a pneumothorax should be investigated for the presence of *P. carinii*.

The application of polymerase chain reaction (PCR) technology to the diagnosis of PCP is under investigation. One small study showed that circulating *Pneumocystis* DNA was present in the blood of 86% of patients with active PCP but none of the HIV-infected patients without pneumonia [91]. Studies looking at the diagnostic utility of PCR in diagnosing *Pneumocystis* from sputum and BAL specimens have yielded sensitivities ranging from 81% to 100% and specificities of 86% -100% [92-94]. Another group evaluated PCR on nasopharyngeal samples (nasal or throat swabs or saliva) in AIDS patients with pulmonary infections and controls [95]. Eleven AIDS patients had PCP diagnosed by BAL and PCR was positive in all of these; none of 31 patients with AIDS or cancer who had negative BALs were positive by PCR. In addition, 258 samples from 86 control patients without pneumonia and with AIDS, cancer, or no underlying disease were all negative for PCP by PCR.

Although these data look promising, the clinical impact may be small, because other methods of diagnosis have such high yields. Additionally, PCR is not readily available and its cost is high. One approach to diagnosing PCP may be to use conventional staining first and apply PCR or immunofluorescent staining only to the negative samples.

Management

Although both trimethoprim- sulfamethoxazole (TMP-SMX) and pentamidine are effective treatment for PCP, TMP-SMX remains the initial drug of choice, independent of the severity of the pneumonia.

TMP-SMX is inexpensive, readily available, and also has activity against other pathogens. Mild PCP can be treated with oral TMP-SMX, but patients with severe pneumonia or those who cannot tolerate the drug orally should receive IV therapy [96]. High-dose therapy often causes hyperkalemia, since trimethoprim acts as a potassium-sparing diuretic.

Adverse reactions occur in 50% - 100% of HIV-infected patients [97, 98]. If an adverse allergic reaction is mild or the patient cannot tolerate other effective medications for PCP, desensitization to TMP-SMX is recommended.

Pentamidine is the drug of choice for severe cases of PCP in patients with intolerance to TMP-SMX. However, adverse reactions occur in up to 70% of patients, including hyperkalemia by a mechanism similar to that with trimethoprim. Despite the appeal of aerosolized pentamidine, high relapse rates make it unacceptable as a treatment option [99].

There are few prospective studies directly comparing TMP-SMX and pentamidine. One report compared these drugs in patients with their first episode of PCP. The survival rate of patients receiving TMP-SMX was 75%, with 41% of patients experiencing major adverse reactions. In comparison, the survival rate for the pentamidine group was 95%, with a major adverse reaction rate of 44% [100]. These differences were not statistically significant.

In another report, Sattler et al. [101] found that the survival rate for patients treated with TMP-SMX was significantly higher than that in patients treated with pentamidine (86% versus 61%).

Meanwhile, another prospective trial (with crossover to the other agent if primary therapy failed) revealed a survival rate of 67% for the TMP-SMX group and 74% for the pentamidine group, a difference that was not statistically significant [102]. Conclusions from these prospective studies, as well as wide clinical experience indicate that both drugs have efficacy, but both have high rates of toxic side effects.

Some other alternative drugs have been evaluated since both TMP-SMX and pentamidine have significant toxicity. The combination of clindamycin and primaquine is an alternative for mild to moderate PCP. One study reported an 86% survival with this regimen in patients who failed or were intolerant to conventional regimens [103]. Clindamycin-primaquine can be given as an oral regimen, which makes it an attractive option for outpatient treatment.

Dapsone alone is not recommended for treatment of PCP, but the combination of dapsone and trimethoprim can be effective for mild-to-moderate PCP [104]. When compared with oral TMP-SMX, one study found dapsone-TMP equally effective for mild-to-moderate PCP, but with half the frequency of adverse reactions [96].

Although atovaquone exhibits variable absorption rates and unpredictable bioavailability, it has been approved for mild-to-moderate PCP in patients who cannot tolerate TMP-SMX. One study comparing oral TMP-SMX and atovaquone found 10% non-responders in the TMP-SMX group versus 20% with atovaquone. There were adverse reactions in 25 % with TMP-SMX versus 9% with atovaquone [105]. Another study found that atovaquone was as effective as IV pentamidine [106].

However, less-promising results have also been observed. One report found that 7 of 34 patients (21%) failed therapy with atovaquone, and 7 of the 27 initial responders (26%) had early relapses [107].

Trimetrexate has been approved for PCP in patients who are unable to tolerate TMP-SMX or pentamidine and require IV therapy. In one study, trimetrexate had a 38% failure rate versus 20% with TMP-SMX [108]. Only 9% of patients in the trimetrexate group had adverse reactions. Leucovorin is given with trimetrexate to minimize haematological side effects.

Difluoromethylornithine (DFMO) can be used as a last resort for patients who have failed other forms of therapy. Although the drug has activity against *P. carinii*, one study showed a failure rate of 58% compared with a 20% failure rate for TMP-SMX [109].

Because corticosteroids given in conjunction with anti-*Pneumocystis* therapy have significantly decreased the mortality associated with PCP, their use is recommended in moderate-to-severe cases of PCP (defined by an arterial O_2 tension of 70 mmHg or less and/or an alveolar-arterial oxygen gradient of 35 mmHg or more while breathing room air). One study, for example, found that early deterioration (which occurs in the first 5 - 10 days after institution of PCP treatment) occurred in only 6% of steroid-treated patients, compared with 42% of those not taking steroids [110]. Although there are no studies that show the optimal dose or duration of therapy.

Other prospective studies have shown statistically significant decreases in both mortality and the rate of respiratory failure in patients receiving steroids early in the course of treatment for PCP, with no major adverse side effects [111, 112]. Several case reports have raised concerns that corticosteroid-related immunosuppression increases the risk of subsequent opportunistic infections [113, 114], but this belief is not well supported in larger series. As an example, one series of 174 patients found that after adjustment for CD4 count, adjunctive corticosteroids increased the likelihood of subsequent esophageal candidiasis, but not CMV disease, *Mycobacterium avium* complex disease, cryptococcal meningitis, toxoplasmosis, Kaposi's sarcoma, herpes simplex, or herpes zoster [115].

Three patients from France have been described who received early initiation of highly active antiretroviral therapy (HAART) following a diagnosis of PCP and developed late respiratory failure after an initial favorable response to PCP therapy, which had included corticosteroids [116]. The authors suggest that this may have reflected increased inflammation due to an immune reconstitution phenomenon, which might respond to a further short course of corticosteroids.

Prognosis

Despite adequate treatment, some patients with PCP develop respiratory failure. Early in the HIV epidemic, mortality in HIV-infected patients with PCP requiring mechanical ventilation approached 100%. However, in the early 1990s, mortality in this group dropped to 60% - 80%, probably due in part to the widespread use of corticosteroids [117]. Data suggest that mortality among patients with PCP and respiratory failure have stabilized around 60%, despite the fact that patients with PCP and respiratory failure currently may have more--advanced disease than was the case a decade ago. As an example, one analysis of 1,660 patients treated for PCP at 71 hospitals between 1995 and 1997 found that mortality among mechanically ventilated patients with PCP was 62% [118].

The effect of PCP on survival was studied over a 7-year period in 4,412 patients with 5,222 episodes of the infection [119]. Survival at more than 1 month was 82% in the whole cohort and 47% at [3]12 months. Antiretroviral therapy was associated with early survival, and survival at 1 year improved from 40% in 1992 to 1993 to 63% in 1996 through 1998. Risk factors for early death by multiple logistic regression were previous history of PCP, older age, and CD4 cell count <50/µl. This study countered a small report from Denmark of reduced survival in PCP patients with mutations in the *P. carinii* dihydropteroate synthase gene, which has been associated with sulfonamide resistance [120].

Bacterial pneumonia

Bacterial pneumonia occurs more frequently in HIV-seropositive patients, with an annual incidence ranging from 5.5 to 29 per 100 compared with 0.9 to 10 per 100 in HIV-seronegative patients [121, 122]. Bacteria have been reported to account for 3 - 45% of all respiratory infections in HIV-infected hosts [123-126].

Although bacterial pneumonias can occur throughout the course of HIV infection, they tend to develop more frequently in individuals with advanced immunosuppression [122, 127]. A direct relationship between the CD4 count and the incidence of bacterial pneumonia was noted in a 1995 report: 2.3, 6.8, and 10.8 episodes per 100 patient years with respective CD4 counts of >500, 200 - 500, and < 200 cells/mm³ [122].

Based on the latter, the CDC added recurrent bacterial pneumonia as an AIDS-defining condition in 1992 [128]. Among HIV-infected patients, injection drug users, inner city inhabitants, smokers, and persons from developing countries are at highest risk for bacterial pneumonias [121, 122, 124, 125].

Regimens containing protease inhibitors significantly decreased the risk of developing bacterial pneumonia in a multivariate analysis. Depressed CD4 count, prior episode of PCP, and injection drug use remained as significant risk factors for pneumonia regardless of the specific antiretroviral therapy.

The most-common bacterial pathogens reported to cause community acquired pneumonia in HIV-infected patients are *Streptococcus pneumoniae*, *Haemophilus influenzae*, and *Staphylococcus aureus* [122, 124, 125]. In addition, *Pseudomonas aeruginosa* has been reported with increased frequency as a cause of recurrent community acquired pneumonia in patients with advanced HIV infection [138-140].

Several pathophysiological mechanisms, such as deficiencies in humoral immunity, defective neutrophil function, and alveolar macrophage dysfunction, underlie the susceptibility to infection with encapsulated, pyogenic organisms [141-145].

Smoking HIV-infected patients experience decreases in the percentage and absolute numbers of pulmonary CD4+ lymphocytes and suppression of the production of IL-1 β and TNF-α within the lung.

Bacterial tracheitis and recurrent bacterial bronchitis, often associated with bronchiectasis, have also been reported in HIV-infected individuals. The isolated bacterial pathogens are similar to those causing pneumonia [142-144].

Nosocomial pneumonia in HIV-infected patients is most commonly caused by *S. aureus* and Gram-negative organisms, including *P. aeruginosa, Klebsiella pneumoniae,* and *Enterobacter* species [123, 125].

The clinical presentation of bacterial pneumonia in the HIV-seropositive patient is similar to that in patients not infected with HIV. Most patients have an abrupt onset of fever, chills, cough with sputum production, dyspnea, and pleuritic chest pain [146,147]. The leukocyte count is generally elevated. Bacteremia is frequently associated with pneumonia, with rates as high as 75% reported with *S. pneumoniae* infection [146, 148, 149].

Bronchitis with bronchiectasis often presents in a similar fashion with fever and copious purulent sputum production. In comparison, bacterial tracheitis may present with signs and symptoms of upper airway obstruction.

The chest X-ray of bacterial pneumonia in the HIV-infected patient is segmental or lobar consolidation, although diffuse reticulonodular infiltrates and patchy lobar infiltrates may also be seen [124,126]. Certain patterns have been associated with specific infections.

The infection caused by *S. pneumoniae* was isolated in all cases with lobar consolidation, and *H. influenzae* in two-thirds of those with diffuse infiltrates [124].

Rhodococcus equi pneumonia, an unusual infection, has been reported with increasing frequency in HIV- infected patients with reduced CD4 counts. The chest radiograph commonly reveals upper lobe nodules and/or cavitation, mimicking tuberculosis [16].This pattern has also been observeded in pulmonary nocardiosis. Other radiographic findings described in association with *Nocardia* infection include diffuse interstitial infiltrates, pleural effusions, and solitary masses [134].

The chest radiographs in patients with bronchitis and bronchiectasis may be normal or show only increased bronchovascular markings. The presence of bronchiectasis can be confirmed by CT scan.

Diagnostic evaluation and treatment

The initial evaluation of a patient suspected of having a bacterial pneumonia should consist of Gram stain and culture of an expectorated or induced sputum specimen and blood cultures. *S. pneumonie* can be isolated in blood cultures in up to 60% of HIV-infected patients with pneumococcal pneumonia [146]. Some authors have advocated the use of protected bronchoalveolar lavage with quantitative cultures as part of the initial management [125], but the utility of this or the protected brush catheter in this setting is unknown.

Management before the results of the culture is known will depend upon the clinical presentation. In a patient presenting with typical symptoms of a bacterial pneumonia plus focal consolidation on chest radiograph, initial antibiotic therapy should be directed at the most-common pathogens, using agents such as amoxicillin-clavulanate or a second-generation cephalosporin while awaiting culture results. Rates of penicillin-resistance by *S. pneumoniae* are 20% - 30%. Seriously ill patients should receive a third- or fourth-generation cephalosporin or a fluoroquinone. *Legionella* infection, which is uncommon in general, is 40 times more frequent in patients with AIDS than in the general population. If this is suspected, initial therapy should consist of a macrolide or a fluoroquinone. HIV-infected patients generally defervesce within 5 days of starting therapy [146]. Proceeding to bronchoscopy may be necessary in those patients who fail to respond.

When culture results are available, specific therapy should be provided. Some considerations regarding the pathogen are described. *P. aeruginosa* pneumonia should be treated with two synergistic intravenous antibiotics for 2 weeks . Maintenance therapy with an aerosolized aminoglycoside may be a consideration in patients with advanced HIV disease and documented relapse is associated with high relapse and recurrence rates [138].

R. equi infection therapy includes erythromycin, clarithromycin, vancomycin, tetracycline, rifampin, clindamycin, ciprofloxacin, and aminoglycosides. Some authors recommend IV therapy with at least two antibiotics for 3-6 weeks, followed by treatment with two oral agents [136]. The optimal duration of therapy is unknown, but prolonged treatment is recommended because of a high frequency of relapse.

Nocardia respond successfully to sulfonamides; alternative antibiotics include imipenem, amikacin, and third-generation cephalosporins when adverse reactions to the sulfonamides prohibit their use. Prolonged treatment (6-12 months) is recommended for this infection, followed possibly by low-dose, life-long maintenance therapy. Bacterial tracheitis and bronchitis respond well to antibiotics. Therapy should be guided by the results of sputum Gram stain and culture.

Strategies for prophylaxis in AIDS patients continue to be investigated due to the increased incidence of bacterial pneumonia, recurrence rates ranging from 8% to 50%, and mortality rates of greater than 50% associated with bacteremic pneumococcal pneumonia [123, 124, 146, 148, 149]. Pneumococcal and *H. influenzae* vaccine are recommended.

Gastrointestinal complications

Gastrointestinal (GI) and hepatobiliary symptoms are among the most-frequent complaints in patients HIV infection and AIDS. Indeed, recent studies suggest the prevalence of these GI complications is falling [150]

The most-common GI symptoms are intolerance to medications, thrush, and diarrhea; the diarrhea is often chronic and associated with weight loss and malnutrition. Odynophagia and dysphagia, abdominal pain, jaundice, and ano-rectal disease are less frequent but are equally difficult diagnostic and management challenges for the clinician caring for patients with AIDS. In contrast to these other symptoms, GI bleeding is unusual; when it occurs, non-AIDS-related disorders are more probable than specific opportunistic infections or neoplasms. The high prevalence of GI disorders in patients with HIV infection was illustrated in a study involving 671 HIV-infected men and women in whom 88% had a least one abnormality of GI function, including low D-xylose absorption (48%), a history of liver disease (40%), chronic diarrhea (28%), and borderline low serum vitamin B_{12} levels (23 %) [151].

When evaluating a patient with AIDS and GI symptoms the following general considerations should be applied:

- Clinical signs and symptoms alone rarely will be diagnostic.
- Less-invasive diagnostic maneuvers such as stool collection should precede more invasive ones, and which be dictated by the severity and acuity of symptoms.
- Multiple infections are common.
- The main goal is to identify treatable disorders. The absence of a specific diagnosis after adequate evaluation is not unusual; further work-up can await the development of more symptoms.
- Likely diagnoses can be predicted based upon the degree of immunocompromise in the host (as example *Cryptosporidia* are usually found in patients with CD4 less than 100 /mm3).
- In late-stage AIDS, GI manifestations are usually part of a systemic infection such as CMV or MAC.
- Lymphomas, Kaposi's sarcoma, and anal carcinoma are the most-common neoplasms associated with GI symptoms

Stool examinations should be the first diagnostic tests ordered; this includes culture for enteric bacterial pathogens, *Clostridium difficile* toxin assay and two to three stools for ova and parasites. An acid-fast smear should also be requested to look for *Cryptosporidium, Isospora*, and *Cyclospora. Microsporidium* can be diagnosed by trichrome staining of a stool specimen [152]. *Salmonella* is the most-frequent enteric bacterial pathogen associated with immunodeficiency complicating HIV infection, and *C. difficile*-associated diarrhea is common in patients receiving antibiotics, especially ampicillin, clindamycin, or cephalosporins.

If a diagnosis is not made with careful stool analysis, we recommend proceeding with more-invasive testing in the majority of patients. We recommend sigmoidoscopy with biopsy as the first procedure. Biopsies should be taken of any abnormal-appearing mucosa or otherwise randomly from rectal mucosa. While colonoscopy, rather than sigmoidoscopy, has been advocated for enhanced diagnosis of CMV confined to the right colon [153,154] we recommend reserving this procedure for patients in whom the sigmoidoscopy is negative as a more cost-effective approach.

If stool evaluations and flexible sigmoidoscopy are non-diagnostic, another alternative approach to proceeding with colonoscopy and upper endoscopy is a limited trial of empirical antibiotics. Empirical therapy may include a quinolone and metronidazole to treat possible small bowel overgrowth, culture-negative *Campylobacter*, or *Giardia*. There have been no studies to document the utility of a trial of empirical therapy, although this tactic has established merit in immunocompetent patients given quinolones for severe enigmatic diarrhea.

Abdominal pain

Acute abdominal pain is often a serious finding in patients with AIDS. In the majority of patients with AIDS, abdominal pain is directly related to HIV and its consequences [155], but the more-common causes of abdominal pain in the general population also need to be considered. Many studies of abdominal pain in AIDS stress the broad spectrum of potential causes for this symptom [155, 156].

The history is important in localizing the origin of the abdominal pain; associated symptoms and signs should suggest the particular organ involved. Perforation with peritonitis and obstruction are the most-serious causes of abdominal pain and need to be excluded quickly; perforation of the distal small bowel or colon is most commonly caused by CMV and obstruction by tumors. Intussusception may be an unusual form of lymphomatous obstruction, but may also be caused by an infection [157].

Infectious enteritis can produce dull, intermittent abdominal pain or acute pain in the absence of obstruction or perforation; diarrhea usually accompanies the pain. The portion of the bowel involved (large versus small bowel) will dictate the specific symptoms and signs.

Pancreatitis is also a common complication in patients with AIDS [158]. It can be part of primary HIV infection [159], but more frequently occurs as a complication of medications taken to combat the virus or treat opportunistic infections (usually didanosine or pentamidine) [160-162]. The presentation of this entity in HIV patients is similar to non-HIV patients, and the prognosis correlates with APACHE II score [163].

The work-up undertaken for abdominal pain in an AIDS patient is the same as for a patient without AIDS. The duration and severity of symptoms will dictate the urgency of evaluation. As an example, patients with dull, insidious abdominal pain can be evaluated with less urgency than the patient who develops acute, severe abdominal pain with evidence of peritonitis.

Abdominal sonography and CT scanning are useful early in the assessment of abdominal pain, and may detect disease not suspected clinically [164]. Examples of frequent unsuspected findings include:
- Gallbladder or colonic wall thickening
- Focal hepatic lesions
- Biliary ductal dilatation
- Pancreatic infiltration
- Abdominal adenopathy
- Peritoneal thickening

Paracentesis is a safe procedure in AIDS patients with ascites. In one study of 24 such patients, paracentesis led to a major diagnosis in 33% of patients 165]. These diagnoses included spontaneous bacterial peritonitis, tuberculous or fungal peritonitis, and lymphoma. High-protein ascites of uncertain etiology has also been reported; laparoscopy may be necessary to attempt to define a cause [166].

AIDS patients with pancreatitis usually have elevations of serum amylase and lipase except those with preexisting chronic pancreatitis. Infectious pancreatitis (CMV and, less often, mycobacteria, *Cryptococcus*, and herpes simplex) may not always be clinically obvious, but should be considered in any patient with abdominal pain and elevated serum amylase [160,167]. In CMV--induced pancreatitis, inclusions can be demonstrated either in ductal epithelium or acinar cells by fine-needle aspiration [167]. ERCP findings are non--specific.

Hepatomegaly and jaundice

Hepatomegaly, with or without jaundice, is a frequent finding in patients with

AIDS. It is present clinically in up to 50% of patients [168] and at autopsy in up to 84%. Hepatomegaly is usually associated with one or more liver function test abnormalities, although significant jaundice due to parenchymal disease is uncommon. The spectrum of hepatic infections in patients with HIV changes with the degree of immunocompromise. Chronic hepatitis due to HBV or HCV is especially common and easily detected by serology for HBVsAg and anti-HCV. The frequency of chronic hepatitis due to HCV in patients with hemophilia or injection drug use is 70% - 90%; this currently represents the most--common cause of hepatic failure in HIV care programs serving urban populations. Clinical manifestations in patients with HIV and hepatobiliary disease, including hepatitis, can range from the asymptomatic to overt liver failure.

The early use of abdominal CT scan and ultrasonography are specially useful in identifying ductal dilatation, gallbladder pathology, and focal hepatic lesions. An extrahepatic cause for jaundice is suggested on CT or ultrasound scan by the presence of dilated ducts or other biliary abnormalities.

If extrahepatic obstruction is documented, possible papillary stenosis associated with AIDS cholangiopathy must be considered promptly. If CT or ultrasound scan demonstrates extension of dilated ducts to the duodenum, an ERCP may be indicated. ERCP is useful for collecting ampullary and duodenal biopsy specimens or bile and/or biliary cytology. Bile can be examined for neoplastic cells or specifically stained for viruses or protozoa.

References

1. Schacker, T, Collier AC, Hughes J et al (1996) Clinical and epidemiologic features of primary HIV infection. Ann Intern Med 125:257
2. Niu MT, Stein DS, Schnittman SM (1993) Primary human immunodeficiency virus type 1 infection: review of pathogenesis and early treatment intervention in humans and animal retrovirus infections. J Infect Dis 168:1490
3. Henrard DR, Phillips J, Windsor I et al (1994) Detection of human immunodeficiency virus type 1 p24 antigen and plasma RNA: relevance to indeterminate serologic tests. Transfusion 34:376
4. Pedersen C, Lindhardt BO, Jensen BL et al (1989) Clinical course of primary HIV infection: consequences for subsequent course of infection. BMJ 299:154
5. Horsburgh CR Jr, Ou CY, Jason J et al (1989) Duration of human immunodeficiency virus infection before detection of antibody. Lancet II:637
6. Coutlee F, Olivier C, Cassol S et al (1994) Absence of prolonged immunosilent infection with human immunodeficiency virus in individuals with high-risk behaviors. Am J Med 96:42
7. Simmonds P, Lainson FA, Cuthbert R et al (1988) HIV antigen and antibody detection: variable responses to infection in the Edinburgh haemophiliac unit. B M J 296:593
8. Sheppard HW, Busch MP, Louie PH et al (1993) HIV-1 PCR and isolation in seroconverting and seronegative homosexual men: absence of long-term immunosilent infection. J Acquir Immune Defic Syndr 6:1339
9. Alcabes P, Munoz A, Vlahav D, Friedland GH (1993) Incubation period of human immunodeficiency virus. Epidemiol Rev 15:303

10. Revision of the CDC surveillance case definition for acquired immunodeficiency syndrome (1987) MMWR Morb Mortal Wkly Rep 36:15

11. Taylor JM, Sy JP, Visscher B, Giorgi JV (1995) CD4+ T-cell number at the time of acquired immunodeficiency syndrome. Am J Epidemiol 141:645

12. Karon JM, Buehler JW, Byers RH et al (1992) Projections of the number of persons diagnosed with AIDS and the number of immunosuppressed HIV-infected persons - United States, 1992-1994. MMWR Morb Mortal Wkly Rep 41:1

13. CDC Surveillance for AIDS: defining opportunistic illnesses 1992-1997 (1999) MMWR Morb Mortal Wkly Rep 48:1

14. Yarchoan R, Venzon DJ, Pluda JM et al (1991) CD4 count and the risk for death in patients infected with HIV receiving antiretroviral therapy. Ann Intern Med 115:184

15. Phillips AN, Elford J, Sabin C et al (1992) Immunodeficiency and the risk of death in HIV infection. JAMA 268:2662

16. Easterbrook PJ, Emami J, Moyle G, Gazzard BG (1993) Progressive CD4 cell depletion and death in zidovudine-treated patients. J Acquir Immune Defic Syndr 6:927

17. Galai N, Vlahov D, Margolick JB et al (1995) Changes in markers of disease progression in HIV-1 seroconverters: a comparison between cohorts of injecting drug users and homosexual men. J Acquir Immune Defic Syndr Hum Retrovirol 8:66

18. Margolick JB, Munoz A, Vlahov D et al (1994) Direct comparison of the relationship between clinical outcome and change in CD4+ lymphocytes in human immunodeficiency virus-positive homosexual men and injecting drug users. Arch Intern Med 154:869

19. Melnick SL, Sherer R, Louis TA et al (1994) Survival and disease progression according to gender of patients with HIV infection. The Terry Beirn Community Programs for clinical research on AIDS. JAMA 272:1915

20. Vella S, Giuliano M, Floridia M et al (1995) Effect of sex, age and transmission category on the progression to AIDS and survival of zidovudine-treated symptomatic patients. AIDS 9:51

21. Chaisson RE, Keruly JC, Moore RD (1995) Race, sex, drug use, and progression of human immunodeficiency virus disease. N Engl J Med 333:751

22. Mariotto AB, Mariotti S, Pezzotti P et al (1992) Estimation of the acquired immunodeficiency syndrome incubation period in intravenous drug users. Am J Epidemiol 135:428

23. Learmont JC, Geczy AF, Mills J et al (1999) Immunologic and virologic status after 14 to 18 years of infection with an attenuated strain of HIV-1. A report from the Sydney Blood Bank Cohort. N Engl J Med 340:1715

24. Mellors JW, Rinaldo CR Jr, Gupta P et al (1996) Prognosis in HIV-1 infection predicted by the quantity of virus in plasma. Science 272:1167

25. Mellors JW, Munoz A, Giofgi JV et al (1997) Plasma viral load and CD4+ lymphocytes as prognostic markers of HIV-1 infection. Ann Intern Med 126:946

26. Vlahov D, Graham N, Hoover D et al (1998) Prognostic indicators for AIDS and infectious disease death in HIV-infected injection drug users. Plasma viral load and CD4+ cell count. JAMA 279:35

27. Glassock RJ, Cohen AH, Danovitch G, Parsa KP (1990) Human immunodeficiency virus (HIV) infection and the kidney. Ann Intern Med 112:35

28. Vitting KE, Gardenswartz MH, Zabetakis PM et al (1990) Frequency of hyponatremia and nonosmolar vasopressin release in the acquired immune deficiency syndrome. JAMA 263:973

29. Tang WW, Kaptein EM, Feinstein EI, Massry SG (1993) Hyponatremia in hospitalized patients with the acquired immunodeficiency syndrome (AIDS) and the AIDS-related complex. Am J Med 94:169

30. Freda PU, Wardlaw SL, Brudney K, Goland RS (1994) Clinical case seminar. Primary adrenal insufficiency in patients with the acquired immunodeficiency syndrome. A report of five cases. J Clin Endocrinol Metab 79:1540

31. Glasgow BJ, Steinsapir KD, Anders K, Layfield LJ (1985) Adrenal pathology in the acquired immune deficiency syndrome. Am J Clin Pathol 84:594

32. Kalin MF, Poretsky L, Seres DS, Zumoff B (1987) Hyporeninemic hypoaldosteronism associated with AIDS. Am J Med 82:1035
33. Guy RJ, Turberg Y, Davidson RN et al (1989) Mineralocorticoid deficiency in HIV infection. BMJ 298:496
34. Choi MJ, Fernandez PC, Patnaik A et al (1993) Trimethoprim-induced hyperkalemia in a patient with AIDS. N Engl J Med 328:703
35. Greenberg S, Reiser IW, Chou SY, Porush JG (1993) Trimethoprim-sulfamethoxazole induces reversible hyperkalemia. Ann Intern Med 119:291
36. Velazquez H, Perazella M, Wright FS, Ellison DH (1993) Renal mechanism of trimethoprim-induced hyperkalemia. Ann Intern Med 119:296
37. Chattha G, Arieff AI, Cummings C, Tierney LM Jr (1993) Lactic acidosis complicating the acquired immunodeficiency syndrome. Ann Intern Med 118:37
38. Sundar K, Suarez M, Banogon PE, Shapiro JM (1997) Zidovudine-induced fatal lactic acidosis and hepatic failure in patients with acquired immunodeficiency syndrome: report of two patients and review of the literature. Crit Care Med 25:1425
39. Lenzo NP, Garas BA, French MA (1997) Hepatic steatosis and lactic acidosis associated with stavudine treatment in an HIV patient: a case report. AIDS 11:1294
40. Fouty B, Frerman F, Reves R (1998) Riboflavin to treat nucleoside analogue-induced lactic acidosis. Lancet 32:291
41. Luzzati R, Del Bravo P, Di Perri G et al (1999) Riboflavine and severe lactic acidosis. Lancet 353:901
42. Gopinath R, Hutcheon M, Cheema-Dhadli S, Halperin M (1992) Chronic lactic acidosis in a patient with acquired immunodeficiency syndrome and mitochondrial myopathy: biochemical studies. J Am Soc Nephrol 3:1212
43. Gallant J, Moore R, Richman D et al (1992) Incidence and natural history of cytomegalovirus disease in patients with advanced human immunodeficiency virus disease treated with zidovudine. J Infect Dis 166:1223
44. Baril L, Jouan M, Caumes E et al (1997) The impact of highly active antiretroviral therapy on the incidence of CMV disease in AIDS patients (abstract). 37th Interscience Conference on Antimicrobial Agents and Chemotherapy, Toronto, Canada
45. Hammer SM, Squires KE, Hughes MD et al (1997) A controlled trial of two nucleoside analogues plus indinavir in persons with human immunodeficiency virus infection and CD4 cell counts of 200 per cubic millimeter or less. N Engl J Med 337:725
46. Arribas JR, Storch GA, Clifford DB, Tselis AC (1996) Cytomegalovirus encephalitis. Ann Intern Med 125:577
47. McCutchan JA (1995) Cytomegalovirus infections of the nervous system in patients with AIDS. Clin Infect Dis 20:747
48. Revello MG, Percivalle E, Sarasini et al (1994) Diagnosis of human cytomegalovirus infection of the nervous system by pp65 detection in polymorphonuclear leukocytes of cerebrospinal fluid from AIDS patients. J Infect Dis 170:1275
49. Arribas JR, Clifford DB, Fichtenbaum CJ et al (1995) Level of cytomegalovirus (CMV) DNA in cerebrospinal fluid of subjects with AIDS and CMV infection of the central nervous system. J Infect Dis 172:527
50. Flood J, Drew WL, Miner R et al (1997) Diagnosis of cytomegalovirus (CMV) polyradiculopathy and documentation of in vivo anti-CMV activity in cerebrospinal fluid by using branched DNA signal amplification and antigen assays. J Infect Dis 176:348-354
51. Small PM, McPhaul LW, Sooy CD et al (1989) Cytomegalovirus infection of the laryngeal nerve presenting as hoarseness in patients with acquired immunodeficiency syndrome. Am J Med 86:108
52. Kim YS, Hollander H (1993) Polyradiculopathy due to cytomegalovirus: report of two cases in which improvement occurred after prolonged therapy and review of he literature. Clin Infect Dis 17:32

53. Decker CF, Tarver JH, Murray DF, Martin GJ (1994) Prolonged concurrent use of ganciclovir and foscarnet in the treatment of polyradiculopathy due to cytomegalovirus in a patient with AIDS (letter). Clin Infect Dis 19:548

54. Whitley RJ, Jacobson MA, Friedberg DN et al (1998) Guidelines for the treatment of cytomegalovirus diseases in patients with AIDS in the era of potent antiretroviral therapy: recommendations of an international panel. Arch Intern Med 158:957

55. Sadler M, Morris-Jones S, Nelson M, Gazzard BG (1997) Successful treatment of cytomegalovirus encephalitis in an AIDS patients using cidofovir (letter). AIDS 10:1293

56. Jacobson MA, Stanley HD, Heard SE (1992) Ganciclovir with recombinant methionyl human granulocyte colony-stimulating factor for treatment of cytomegalovirus disease in AIDS patients (letter). AIDS 6:515

57. Jacobson MA, Gambertoglio JG, Aweeka FT et al (1991) Foscarnet-induced hypocalcemia and effects of foscarnet on calcium metabolism. J Clin Endocrinol Metab 72:1130

58. Studies of Ocular Complications of AIDS Research Group (1992) Mortality in patients with the acquired immunodeficiency syndrome treated with either foscarnet or ganciclovir for cytomegalovirus retinitis. N Engl J Med 326:213

59. Palestine AG, Polis MA, De Smet MD et al (1991) A randomized, controlled trial of foscarnet in the treatment of cytomegalovirus retinitis in patients with AIDS. Ann Intern Med 115:665.5

60. Studies of Ocular Complications of AIDS Research Group in collaboration with the AIDS Clinical Trials Group (1997) Parenteral cidofovir for cytomegalovirus retinitis in patients with AIDS: The HPMPC peripheral cytomegalovirus retinitis trial. Ann Intern Med 126:264

61. Lalezari JP, Stagg RJ, Kuppermann BD et al (1997) Intravenous cidofovir for peripheral CMV retinitis in patients with AIDS. Ann Intern Med 126:257

62. Pifer LL, Hughes WT, Stango S, Woods D (1978) Pneumocystis carinii infection: evidence of high prevalence in normal and immunosuppressed children. Pediatrics 61:35

63. Singer C, Armstrong D, Rosen PP, Schottenfeld D (1975) Pneumocystis carinii pneumonia: a cluster of eleven cases. Ann Intern Med 82:772

64. Helweg-Larsen J, Tsolaki AG, Miller RF et al (1998) Clusters of Pneumocystis carinii pneumonia: analysis of person-to-person transmission by genotyping. QJM 91:813

65. Dohn MN, White ML, Vigdorth EM et al (2000) Geographic clustering of pneumocystis carinii pneumonia in patients with HIV infection. Am J Respir Crit Care Med 162:1617

66. Morris AM, Swanson M, Ha H, Huang L (2000) Geographic distribution of human immunodefieicny virus-associated Pneumocystis carinii pneumonia in San Francisco. Am J Respir Crit Care Med 162:1622

67. Hoover DR, Saah AJ, Bacellar H et al (1993) Clinical manifestations of AIDS in the era of Pneumocystis prophylaxis. N Engl J Med 329:1922

68. Stansell JD, Osmond DH, Charlebois E et al (1997) Predictors of Pneumocystis carinii pneumonia in HIV-infected persons. Am J Respir Crit Care Med 155:60

69. Bozzette SA, Finkelstein DM, Spector DA et al (1995) A randomized trial of three antipneumocystis agents in patients with advanced human immunodeficiency virus infection. N Engl J Med 332:693

70. Phair J, Muñoz A, Detels R et al (1990) The risk of Pneumocystis carinii pneumonia among men infected with the human immunodeficiency virus type I. Multicenter AIDS cohort study group. N Engl J Med 322:161

71. Kales CP, Murren JR, Torres RA, Crocco JA (1987) Early predictors of in-hospital mortality for Pneumocystis carinii pneumonia in acquired immunodeficiency syndrome. Arch Intern Med 147:1413

72. De Lorenzo LJ, Huang CT, Maguire GP, Stover DE (1987) Roentgenographic patterns of Pneumocystis carinii pneumonia in 104 patients with AIDS. Chest 91:323

73. Jules-Elysee K, Stover DE, Zaman MB et al (1990) Aerosolized pentamidine: effect on diagnosis and presentation of Pneumocystis carinii pneumonia. Ann Intern Med 112:750

74. Sepkowitz KA, Telzak EE, Gold JWM et al (1991) Pneumothorax in AIDS. Ann Intern Med 114:455

75. Gruden JF, Huang L, Turner J et al (1997) High-resolution CT in the evaluation of clinically suspected *Pneumocystis carinii* pneumonia in AIDS patients with normal, equivocal, or nonspecific radiographic findings. AJR Am J Roentgenol 169:967

76. Hartman TE, Primack SL, Muller NL, Staples CA (1994) Diagnosis of thoracic complications in AIDS: accuracy of CT. AJR Am J Roentgenol 162:547

77. Tuazon CN, Delaney MD, Simm GL et al (1985) Utility of gallium-67 scintigraphy and bronchial washings in the diagnosis of *Pneumocystis carinii* pneumonia in patients with the acquired immune deficiency syndrome. Am Rev Respir Dis 132:1087

78. Huang L, Stansell J, Osmond D et al (1999) Performance of an algorithm to detect *Pneumocystis carinii* pneumonia in symptomatic HIV-infected persons. Chest 115:1025

79. Stover DE, Meduri GU (1988) Pulmonary function tests. Clin Chest Med 9:473

80. Zaman MK, White DA (1988) Serum lactate dehydrogenase levels and *Pneumocystis carinii* pneumonia: diagnostic and prognostic significance. Am Rev Respir Dis 137:796

81. Horner RD, Bennett CL, Rodriguez D et al (1995) Relationship between procedures and health insurance for critically ill patients with *Pneumocystis carinii* pneumonia. Am J Respir Crit Care Med 152:1435

82. Glenny RW, Pierson DJ (1992) Cost reduction in diagnosing *Pneumocystis carinii* pneumonia. Sputum induction versus bronchoalveolar lavage as the initial diagnostic procedure. Am Rev Respir Dis 145:1425

83. Zaman MK, Wooten OJ, Suprahmanya B et al (1988) Rapid non-invasive diagnosis of *Pneumocystis carinii* from induced liquified sputum. Ann Intern Med 109:7

84. Levine SJ, Masur H, Gill VJ et al (1991) Effect of aerosolized pentamidine prophylaxis on the diagnosis of *Pneumocystis carinii* pneumonia by induced sputum examination in patients infected wit the human immunodeficiency virus. Am Rev Respir Dis 144:760

85. O'Donnell WJ, Pieciak W, Chertow GM et al (1998) Clearance of *Pneumocystis carinii* cysts in acute *P. carinii* pneumonia. Assessment by serial sputum induction. Chest 114:1264

86. Willocks L, Burns S, Cossar R, Brettle R (1993) Diagnosis of *Pneumocystis carinii* pneumonia in a population of HIV-positive drug users, with particular reference to sputum induction and fluorescent antibody techniques. J Infect 26:257

87. Levine SJ, Kennedy D, Shelhamer JH et al (1992) Diagnosis of *Pneumocystis carinii* pneumonia by multiple site-directed bronchoalveolar lavage with immunofluorescent monoclonal antibody staining in human immunodeficiency virus-infected patients receiving aerosolized pentamidine chemoprophylaxis. Am Rev Respir Dis 146:838

88. Bustamante EA, Levy H (1994) Sputum induction compared with bronchoalveolar lavage by Ballard catheter to diagnose *Pneumocystis carinii* pneumonia. Chest 105:816

89. Alvarez F, Bandi V, Stager C, Guntupalli KK (1997) Detection of *Pneumocystis carinii* in tracheal aspirates of intubated patients using calcofluor-white (Fungi-Fluor) and immunofluorescence antibody (Genetic Systems) stains. Crit Care Med 25:948

90. Metersky ML, Colt H, Olson LK, Shanks TG (1995) AIDS-related spontaneous pneumothorax. Chest 108:946

91. Schluger N, Godwin T, Sepkowitz K et al (1992) Application of polymerase chain reaction to pneumocystis and frequent detection of *Pneumocystis carinii* in serum of patients with *Pneumocystis* pneumonia. J Exp Med 176:1327

92. Lipschik GY, Gill VJ, Lundgren JD et al (1992) Improved diagnosis of *Pneumocystis carinii* infection by polymerase chain reaction on induced sputum and blood. Lancet 340:203

93. Olsson M, Elvin K, Löfdahl S, Lindner E (1993) Detection of *Pneumocystis carinii* DNA in sputum and bronchoalveolar samples by polymerase chain reaction. J Clin Microbiol 31:221

94. Torres J, Goldman M, Wheat LJ et al (2000) Diagnosis of *Pneumocystis carinii* pneumonia in human immunodeficiency virus-infected patients with polymerase chain reaction: a blinded comparison to standard methods. Clin Infect Dis 30:141

95. Oz HS, Hughes WT (2000) Search for *Pneumocystis carinii* DNA in upper and lower respiratory tract of humans. Diagn Microbiol Infect Dis 37:161

96.Medina I, Mills J, Leong G et al (1990) Oral therapy for *Pneumocystis carinii* pneumonia in the acquired immunodeficiency syndrome. N Engl J Med 323:776

97.Fischl MA, Dickinson GM, La Voie L (1988) Safety and efficacy of sulfamethoxazole and trimethoprim chemoprophylaxis of *Pneumocystis carinii* pneumonia in AIDS. JAMA 259:1185

98.Gordon FM, Simon GL, Wofsy CB, Mill J (1984) Adverse reactions to trimethoprim-sulfamethoxazole in patients with the acquired immunodeficiency syndrome. Ann Intern Med 100:495

99. Conte JE, Chernoff D, Feigel DW et al (1990) Intravenous or inhaled pentamidine for treating *Pneumocystis carinii* pneumonia in AIDS. Ann Intern Med 113:203

100. Wharton JM, Coleman DL, Wofsky CB et al (1986) Trimethoprim-sulfamethoxazole or pentamidine for *Pneumocystis carinii* pneumonia on the acquired immunodeficiency syndrome. Ann Intern Med 105:37

101. Sattler FR, Cowan R, Nielsen DM, Ruskin J (1988) Trimethoprim-sulfamethoxazole compared with pentamidine for treatment of *Pneumocystis carinii* pneumonia in the acquired immunodeficiency syndrome. Ann Intern Med 109:280

102. Klein NC, Duncanson FP, Lenoa TH et al (1992) Trimethoprim-sulfamethoxazole versus pentamidine for *Pneumocystis carinii* pneumonia in AIDS patients: results of a large prospective randomized treatment trial. AIDS 6:301

103. Noskin GA, Murphy RL, Black JR, Phair FP (1992) Salvage therapy with clindamycin/primaquine for *Pneumocystis carinii* pneumonia. Clin Infect Dis 14:183

104. Leoung GS, Mills J, Hopewell VC et al (1994) Dapsone-trimethoprim for *Pneumocystis carinii* pneumonia in the acquired immunodeficiency syndrome. Ann Intern Med 121:174

105. Hughes WT, Leoung G, Kramer F et al (1993) Comparison of atovaquone (566C80) with trimethoprim-sulfamethoxazole to treat *Pneumocystis carinii* pneumonia in patients with AIDS. N Engl J Med 328:1521

106. Dohn MN, Weinberg WG, Torres RA et al (1994) Oral atovaquone compared with intravenous pentamidine for *Pneumocystis carinii* pneumonia in patients with AIDS. Ann Intern Med 121:174

107. Falloon J, Kovacs J, Hughes W et al (1991) A preliminary evaluation of 566C80 for the treatment of *Pneumocystis carinii* pneumonia in patients with the acquired immunodeficiency syndrome. N Engl J Med 325:1534

108. Sattler FR, France D, Davis R et al (1994) Trimetrexate with leucovorin versus trimethoprim--sulfamethoxazole for moderate to severe episodes of *Pneumocystis carinii* pneumonia in patients with AIDS: a prospective, controlled, multicenter investigation of the AIDS Clinical Trials Group Protocol 029/031. J Infect Dis 170:165

109. Smith D, Davies S, Smithson J et al (1992) Elfornithine versus cotrimoxazole in the treatment of *Pneumocystis carinii* pneumonia in AIDS patients. AIDS 6:1489

110. Montaner JSG, Lawson LM, Levitt N et al (1990) Corticosteroids prevent early deterioration in patients with moderately severe *Pneumocystis carinii* pneumonia and the acquired immunodeficiency syndrome (AIDS). Ann Intern Med 113:14

111. Gagnon S, Boota AM, Fischl MA et al (1990) Corticosteroids as adjunctive therapy for severe *Pneumocystis carinii* pneumonia in the acquired immunodeficiency syndrome. N Engl J Med 323:1444

112. Bozzette SA, Sattler Fr, Chin J et al (1990) A controlled trial of early adjunctive treatment with corticosteroids for *Pneumocystis carinii* pneumonia in the acquired immunodeficiency syndrome. N Engl J Med 323:1451

113. Nelson MR, Erskine D, Hawkins DA, Gazzard BG (1993) Treatment with corticosteroids-a risk factor for the development of clinical cytomegalovirus disease in AIDS. AIDS 7:375

114. Horsburgh CR (1991) *Mycobacterium avium* complex in the acquired immune deficiency syndrome. N Engl J Med 324:1332

115. Gallant JE, Chaisson RE, Moore RD (1998) The effect of adjunctive corticosteroids for the treatment of *Pneumocytis carinii* pneumonia on mortality and subsequent complications. Chest 114:1258

116. Wislez, M, Bergot, E, Antoine, M et al (2001) Acute respiratory failure following HAART introduction in patients treated for *Pneumocystis carinii* pneumonia. Am J Respir Crit Care Med 164:847
117. Wachter RM, Russi MB, Bloch DA et al (1991) *Pneumocystis carinii* pneumonia and refractory respiratory failure in AIDS. Am Rev Respir Dis 143:251
118. Curtis JR, Yarnold PR, Schwartz DN et al (2000) Improvements in outcomes of acute respiratory failure for patients with human immunodeficiency virus-related *Pneumocystis carinii* pneumonia. Am J Respir Crit Care Med 162:393
119. Dworkin MS, Hanson DL, Navin TR (2001) Survival of patients with AIDS, after diagnosis of *Pneumocystis carinii* pneumonia, in the United States. J Infect Dis 183:1409
120. Helweg-Larsen J, Benfield TL, Eugen-Olsen J et al (1999) Effects of mutations in *Pneumocystis carinii* dihydropteroate synthase gene on outcome of AIDS-associated *P. carinii* pneumonia. Lancet 354:1347
121 Caiaffa WT, Graham NM, Vlahov D (1993) Bacterial pneumonia in adult populations with human immunodeficiency virus (HIV) infection. Am J Epidemiol 138:909
122. Hirschtick R, Glassroth J, Jordan M et al (1995) Bacterial pneumonia in persons infected with the human immunodeficiency virus. N Engl J Med 333:845
123. Murray JF, Felton CP, Garay SM et al (1984) Pulmonary complications of the acquired immunodeficiency syndrome. Report of a National Heart, Lung, and Blood Institute workshop. N Engl J Med 310:1682
124. Polsky B, Gold JWM, Whimbey E et al (1986) Bacterial pneumonia in patients with the acquired immunodeficiency syndrome. Ann Intern Med 104:38
125. Witt DJ, Craven DE, McCabe WR (1987) Bacterial infections in adult patients with the acquired immunodeficiency syndrome (AIDS) and AIDS-related complex. Am J Med 82:900
126. Jean-Luc M, Nicod LP, Auckenthaler R, Junod AF (1991) Mode of presentation and diagnosis of bacterial pneumonia in human immunodeficiency virus-infected patients. Am Rev Respir Dis 144:917
127. Farizo KM, Buehler JW, Chamberland ME et al (1992) Spectrum of disease in persons with human immunodeficiency virus infection in the United States. JAMA 267:1798
128. Centers for Disease Control (1992) 1993 revised classification system for HIV infection and expanded surveillance case definition for AIDS among adolescents and adults. MMWR Morb Mortal Wkly Rep 41:1
129. Sullivan JH, Moore RD, Keruly JC, Chaisson RE (2000) Effect of antiretroviral therapy on the incidence of bacterial pneumonia in patients with advanced HIV infection. Am J Respir Crit Care Med 162:64
130. Steinhart R, Reingold AL, Taylor F et al (1992) Invasive *Haemophilus influenzae* infections in men with HIV infection. JAMA 268:3350
131. Casadevall A, Dobroszycki J, Small C, Pirofski L (1992) *Haemophilus influenzae* type B bacteremia in adults with AIDS and at risk for AIDS. Am J Med 92:587
132. Schlamm HT, Yancovitz SR (1989) Haemophilus influenzae pneumonia in young adults with AIDS, ARC, or risk of AIDS. Am J Med 86:11
133. Levine SJ, White DA, Fels AOS (1990) The incidence and significance of *Staphylococcus aureus* in respiratory cultures from patients infected with the human immunodeficiency virus. Am Rev Respir Dis 141:89
134. Javaly K, Horowitz HW, Wormser GP (1992) Nocardiosis in patients with human immunodeficiency virus infection: report of 2 cases and review of the literature. Medicine (Baltimore) 71:128
135. Doebbeling BN, Feilmeier ML, Hersaldt LA (1990) Pertussis in an adult man infected with human immunodeficiency virus. J Infect Dis 161:1276
136. Cury JD, Harrington PT, Hosein IK (1992) Successful medical therapy of *Rhodococcus equi* pneumonia in a patient with HIV infection. Chest 102:1619
137. Drabick JJ, Gasser RA, Saunders NB et al (1993) *Pasteurella multocida* pneumonia in a man with AIDS and nontraumatic feline exposure. Chest 103:7

138. Baron AD, Hollander H (1993) *Pseudomonas aeruginosa* bronchopulmonary infection in late human immunodeficiency virus disease. Am Rev Respir Dis 148:992
139. Fichtenbaum CJ, Woeltje KF, Powderly WG (1994) Serious *Pseudomonas aeruginosa* infections in patients infected with human immunodeficiency virus: a case-control study. Clin Infect Dis 19:417
140 Afessa B, Green W, Chiao et al (1998) Pulmonary complications of HIV infection. Autopsy findings. Chest 113:1225
141. Lane HC, Masur H, Edgar LC et al (1983) Abnormalities of B-cell activation and immunoregulation in patients with the acquired immunodeficiency syndrome. N Engl J Med 309:453
142. Ellis M, Gupta S, Galant S et al (1988) Impaired neutrophil function in patients with AIDS or AIDS-related complex: a comprehensive evaluation. J Infect Dis 158:1268
143. Parkin JM, Helbert M, Hughes CL et al (1989) Immunoglobulin G subclass deficiency and susceptibility to pyogenic infections in patients with AIDS-related complex and AIDS. AIDS 3:37
144. Moja P, Jalil A, Quesnel A et al (1997) Humoral immune response within the lung in HIV-1 infection. Clin Exp Immunol 110:341
145. Wewers MD, Diaz PT, Wewers ME et al (1998) Cigarette smoking in HIV infection induces a suppressive inflammatory environment in the lung. Am J Respir Crit Care Med 158:1543
146. Janoff EN, Breiman RF, Daley CL, Hopewell PC (1992) Pneumococcal disease during HIV infection: epidemiologic, clinical. and immunologic perspectives. Ann Intern Med 117:314
147 Chaisson RE (1989) Bacterial pneumonia in patients with human immunodeficiency virus infection. Semin Respir Infect 4:133
148 Gerberding JL, Drieger J, Sand MA (1986) Recurrent bacteremic infection with *S. pneumoniae* in patients with AIDS virus (AV) infection. Program and abstracts of the Twenty-sixth Interscience Conference on Antimicrobial Agents and Chemotherapy, New Orleans. American Society of Microbiology, p 177
149. Pesola GR, Charles A (1992) Pneumococcal bacteremia with pneumonia: mortality in acquired immunodeficiency syndrome. Chest 101:150
150. Monkemuller KE, Call SA, Lazenby AJ, Wilcox CM (2000) Declining prevalence of opportunistic gastrointestinal disease in the era of combination antiretroviral therapy. Am J Gastroenterol 95:457
151. Knox TA, Spiegelman D, Skinner SC, Gorbach S (2000) Diarrhea and abnormalities of gastrointestinal function in a cohort of men and women with HIV infection. Am J Gastroenterol 95:3482
152. Chioralia G, Trammer T, Kampen H, Seitz HM (1998) Relevant criteria for detecting microsporidia in stool specimens. J Clin Microbiol 36:2279
153. Wilcox CM, Schwartz DA, Cotsonis G, Thompson SE 3rd (1996) Chronic unexplained diarrhea in human immunodeficiency virus infection: determination of the best diagnostic approach. Gastroenterology 110:30
154. Dieterich DT, Rahmin M (1991) Cytomegalovirus colitis in AIDS: presentation in 44 patients and a review of the literature. J Acquir Immune Defic Syndr 4:S29
155. Parente F, Cernuschi M, Antinori S et al (1994) Severe abdominal pain in patients with AIDS: frequency, clinical aspects, causes and outcome. Scand J Gastroenterol 29:511
156. Ferguson CM (1988) Surgical complications of human immunodeficiency virus infection. Am Surg 54:4
157. Wood BJ, Kumar PN, Cooper C et al (1995) AIDS-associated intussusception in young adults. J Clin Gastroenterol 21:158
158. Dassopoulos T, Ehrenpreis ED (1999) Acute pancreatitis in human immunodeficiency virus-infected patients: a review. Am J Med 107:78
159. Rizzardi GP, Tambussi G, Lazzariin A (1997) Acute pancreatitis during primary HIV-1 infection. N Engl J Med 336:1836
160. Bonacini M (1991) Pancreatic involvement in human immunodeficiency virus infection. J Clin Gastroenterol 13:58

161. Floridia M, Vella S, Seeber AC et al (1997) A randomized trial (ISS 902) of didanosine versus zidovudine in previously untreated patients with mildly symptomatic human immunodeficiency virus infection. J Infect Dis 175:255

162 Pauwels A, Eliaszewicz M, Larrey D (1990) Pentamidine-induced acute pancreatitis in a patient with AIDS. J Clin Gastroenterol 12:457

163. Cappell MS, Marks M (1995) Acute pancreatitis in HIV-seropositive patients: a case control study of 44 patients. Am J Med 3:243

164. Jeffrey RB (1988) Gastrointestinal imaging in AIDS - abdominal computed tomography and ultrasound. Gastroenterol Clin North Am 17:507

165. Cappell MS, Shetty V (1994) A multicenter, case-controlled study of the clinical presentation and etiology of ascites and of the safety and clinical efficacy of diagnostic abdominal paracentesis in HIV seropositive patients. Am J Gastroenterol 89:2172

166. Wilcox CM, Forsmark CE, Darragh J et al (1991) High-protein ascites in patients with acquired immunodeficiency syndrome. Gastroenterology 100:745

167. Wilcox CM, Forsmark CE, Grendell JH et al (1990) Cytomegalovirus-associated acute pancreatic disease in patients with acquired immunodeficiency syndrome. Gastroenterology 99:263

168. Glasgow BJ, Anders K, Layfield LJ (1985) Clinical and pathologic findings of the liver in the acquired immune deficiency syndrome (AIDS). Am J Clin Pathol 83:582

Anaesthesia for transurethral prostatoctomy

C. MELLONI, F. SFOGLIAFERRI, S. PISTOCCHI

Anaesthesia for transurethral prostatectomy (TURP) is not always routine; even though it can be considered a simple and safe procedure, between 2.5% and 20% of patients suffer major complications, and perioperative mortality rate varies between 0.5% and 6% [1-4], so that there is no difference in mortality rate in comparison with retropubic or suprapubic prostatectomies (open procedures). Moreover, in recent years even TURP has undergone important technical changes, one of which involves laser vaporization of the prostatic tissue (Vapo TURP); advantages claimed for vapo TURP are described below.

Complications during TURP derive basically from:
- Patients, their intrinsic risk factors and anaesthesia-related risks;
- Surgical procedure; its complications, some peculiar to the technique used;
- Utilization of irrigating fluids.

Patients

Prostatic benign hypertrophy (and carcinoma) represent a typical pathology of old age; therefore patients are generally affected by all the diseases common in this age group. This group constitutes a risk group for cardiovascular complications, but the extraperitoneal nature of the procedure and the absence of wounds interfering with the physiology of respiration pose no special risk toward the development of respiratory insufficiency. The TUR approach has been recommended to protect the respiratory system of patients against the development of complications. Meyhoff et al. [5] found that the TUR approach allowed earlier discharge of the patients with less in-hospital morbidity, a shorter period of sick leave, and therefore calculated substantial savings for the institutions and the health system as a whole. The major complications of the TUR approach are restricted to the cardiovascular system, with some hints that myocardial damage is particularly frequent in the perioperative period (6% -10%).If this is the case, it may result from the volume of fluid absorbed and be secondary to volume shifts or attributed to the solute, with suggestions that glycine might be more toxic to the myocardium than other solutions [6-8]. Recently [9] no difference was found with either glycine or sorbitol-mannitol in the frequency of troponin I increases, while the overall incidence of cardiac damage varied between 8.4% and 6.5%, quite an alarming incidence.

Surgical procedure

Despite the advantages claimed for the endoscopic procedures, it soon became clear that TURP possessed intrinsic problems related to the nature of the irrigating fluid used, which were collected under the pseudonym of "TURP syndrome".

Theoretically a laser procedure could be safer because with the sealing of blood vessels by laser beam there is minimal blood loss and less systemic absorption of irrigating fluid, together with excellent control of any bleeding during the procedure; however even in the field of traditional TURP, technical improvements like video monitoring and attention to the earlier signs of the so--called TURP syndrome have markedly decreased the occurrence of complications, so that today many surgeons are uncertain about which is the technique of choice for uncomplicated prostatic resection.

The TURP syndrome

Under this name many complications have been reported and all of them (hopefully) will be discussed in the following sections; diagnosis may be difficult because the syndrome does not have a consistent appearance and there are many confounding effects, like hypotension associated with regional anaesthesia.

Signs and symptoms

TURP syndrome can occur at any time perioperatively, sometimes as early as 10 min following the beginning of the procedure and sometimes a few hours following the completion of the operation.

Signs and symptoms have varied and can be divided according to the systems involved:

- Cardiovascular; hypotension, hypertension, dysrhythmias, shock, pulmonary oedema, cardiac arrest;
- Respiratory; tight feeling in the chest or throat, shortness of breath, hyperventilation, dyspnea, pulmonary oedema;
- Cerebral; dizziness, mental confusion, and lethargy lapsing into coma, headaches, nausea, restlessness, retching, blindness, twitches, and seizures.

The full clinical manifestation of symptoms appear under regional anaesthesia, while under general anaesthesia all the symptoms are absent except the rise and fall in blood pressure, respiratory arrest, and severe bradycardia, with a variety of electrocardiogram (ECG) modifications; recovery from general anaesthesia and muscle relaxation may take a long time, if occurring at all.

In view of the possibility of early detection of TUR syndrome due to the signs and symptoms described above, regional anaesthesia may be the first choice for TURP, since the patients may exhibit symptoms and signs that are clouded by general anaesthesia.

Problems ascribed to the irrigating solutions

The ideal irrigating solution should be isotonic, electrically inert, non-toxic, clear transparent, easy to sterilize and handle, and not too expensive, nor toxic to the body. The main problem of the solutions used for irrigation depends on the fact that during the continuous infusion of the solution some passes into the general circulation, being absorbed through the venous and capillary bed of the prostate because of the hydrostatic pressure present, higher than the venous and capillary pressures. Moreover, fluids can be absorbed through the retroperitoneal and paravesical spaces, even in the absence of surgical perforation. The entrainment of the solution causes circulatory overload, haemodilution, hypotonia and hypo-osmolality, and may progress to haemolysis, shock, and renal failure.

Because there is no time to discuss all the solutions used in the past, the present article will discuss the solutions more widely used today, i.e., glycine 1.2%-1.5%, mannitol 3%, mannitol/sorbitol (2.7%-0.54% respectively) mixtures.

When a significant amount of any solution is absorbed it may cause circulatory overload and hyponatremia, which are the main causes of pulmonary oedema, cardiac insufficiency, and all the signs and symptoms quoted above. Beside these problems common to all solutes, glycine possess significant cardiac and retinal toxicity and may cause hyperammonemia, because its metabolites overload the urea synthesis cycle; glucose may cause severe hyperglycemia, and mannitol and sorbitol may cause lactic acidosis and hyerglycemia due to shift in the glycolysis pathways. Moreover, acidosis may be exacerbated by the concurrent hypoperfusion of shock and circulatory failure and hypoxemia, initiating a vicious circle where etiology and hence therapy become difficult.

Circulatory overloading. Intravascular volume expansion

Both hypertension and hypotension occur during TURP syndrome; the rapid volume expansion from absorbed irrigant during TURP can explain hypertension with reflex bradycardia [10]. Absorption rates can reach 200 ml/min [11] and numerous measurements of the volume absorbed have reported volume gains up to 8 l; with average weight gain about 2 kg. Patients with poor left ventricular function may develop pulmonary oedema from acute circulatory volume overload. A report of five patients [12] with severe TURP syndrome (two deaths, two seizures, and one ventricular arrhythmia) found "no significant variations" in serum osmolalities before and after TURP, which suggests that intravascular volume changes independent of osmolality may play an important role in the morbidity and mortality associated with TURP syndrome. Several factors contribute to the volume gained, prominent among which are:

- the intravesical pressure (governed by the height of the irrigation bag above the prostatic sinuses)
- the number of prostatic sinuses opened

Therefore the length of the procedure, experience of the surgeon (or inexperience), and difficulty of resections also play a role in the genesis of the complications. Many authors suggest an elevation of the irrigating fluid at no more that 60 cm from the table and a reduction in the resection time, even if no correlation has been consistently found with duration of surgery. Evans et al. [13] found that stroke volume and cardiac index were depressed over time, but these changes were reversed by infusing the irrigating fluids at body temperature, so that iatrogenic hypothermia plays a role in the genesis of the depression of cardiac function and should be avoided. A drop in body temperature of as little as 1°C produces significant haemodynamic alterations and patient discomfort, frequently reported as feeling cold, resulting in shivering that increases oxygen consumption. Inadvertent intraoperative hypothermia has his own list of complications [14], so that the use of a continuous warm irrigating fluid is recommended in order to maintain temperature homeostasis and increase patient satisfaction [15, 16].

Therapeutic suggestions include continuous infusion of warm irrigating medium or prewarmed irrigating fluids; warm the patients, administer oxygen by mask and monitor the body temperature.

Antidiuretic hormone produced by the stress of surgery, increased renin, and aldosterone secretion may also contribute to volume expansion by promoting water retention.

Intravascular volume loss

Perioperative hypotension during TURP is sometimes preceded by hypertension. Profound hyponatremia by itself does not explain the hypotension; however, hyponatremia with hypertension may lead to net water flux along osmotic and hydrostatic pressure gradients out of the intravascular space and into the lungs, which triggers pulmonary oedema and hypovolemic shock. This concept is consistent with the findings of Hahn [17] who hypothesized that the absorption of fluids derives from two sources, one from direct absorption into the circulation (early phase) and the second from interstitial accumulation, both from periprostatic and retoperitoneal spaces and from fluid shifts along physiological gradients, according to the Starling equation. The excretion of urine is rapidly increased by all irrigating fluids, especially mannitol [18], resulting in an osmotic diuresis and hence a net loss of circulating volume, but the situation changes according to the volume administered, since excretion of glycine is less than that of mannitol or sorbitol, with a greater intracellular accumulation of glycine [19, 20].

Sympathetic blockade induced by regional anaesthesia may compound TURP syndrome. Absorption of distilled water during TURP can cause acute hypo-osmolality with massive haemolysis. Bleeding and red blood cell destruction are additional sources of volume and oxygen-carrying capacity losses. The haemoglobinemia that follows such haemolysis, coupled with hypotension, can cause acute renal failure and death.

Blood loss during TURP is usually modest, but sometimes large loss can occur; the blood loss correlates with the size of the gland, the duration of surgery, and the surgical skills. Total blood loss after TURP is significantly correlated with the prostatic tissue weight; but when the tissue weight resected exceeds 35 g, blood loss was in excess of the linear correlation [21]. There was no significant difference in measured coagulation variables [fibrinogen, factor V, plasminogen, antithrombin III, and fibrin degradation products (FDP)] between the spinal and general anaesthesia groups, but there were significant decreases in postoperative fibrinogen and factor V levels compared with preoperative values in both spinal and general anaesthesia groups. Three patients (6%) had increased FDP levels 1 h postoperatively. The prostatic tissue weight and the surgical duration was significantly higher in these patients. The authors concluded that perioperative blood loss in TURP patients is not affected by the anaesthetic technique, but 6% of TURP patients developed subclinical intravascular coagulopathies that correlated with mass of resected prostate tissue. Coagulopathies may be caused by dilutional thrombocytopenia or the appearance of a systemic coagulopathy with the characteristics of disseminated intravascular coagulation. Particles of prostatic tissue, rich in thromboplastin, enter the blood and start bleeding, with very low levels of platelets and fibrinogen and a rise in FDP, probably due to secondary fibrinolysis. In suspected cases, a full coagulation profile should be obtained and deficitary components corrected.

Of course blood loss contributes to hypovolemia and worsens the vicious circle initiated by the mechanisms above. It should be noted that, from a purely theoretical point of view, low venous pressure would promote not only absorption of irrigating fluid into the circulation but also uptake of resected prostatic tissue into the open venous sinuses, providing the stimulus for fibrinolysis. However, that was not evidenced in the study of Smyth et al. [21].

Bacteremia, septicemia

The prostatic gland harbours a variety of bacteria and it is a common source of postoperative bacteremia despite the use of prophylactic antibiotics. Indwelling preoperative bladder catheters promote the growth of bacteria and their entry into the bloodstream is facilitated by high irrigation pressures, so that 5%-6% of all patients develop septicemia.

Osmotically active solutes

Glycine, sorbitol, and mannitol are electrically non-conducting, but osmotically active solutes that are added to irrigation fluids to decrease the risk of massive intravascular haemolysis. Their use in irrigation solutions has reduced the occurrence of significant haemolysis and death by more than 50%.

Although distilled water may still be used by some clinicians, the irrigation solutions most often used now range in calculated osmolality from 178 mosmol/kg water for 3% sorbitol to 200 mosmol/kg for 1.5% glycine solutions or to isotonic sorbitol or glycine solutions. Osmolality calculations for irrigation solutions assume that there is no interaction between solute particles. Since these interactions do occur, calculated osmolality values are slightly greater (10–20 mosmol/kg) than the solution's measured osmolality.

Treatment of intravascular fluid volume shift

Massive absorption is more likely if intravesicular pressure increases above 30 mmHg. Limiting the height of the irrigation bag to 40 cm above the prostate [22] or using continuous irrigating resectoscopes or suprapubic trocar drainage can minimize absorption [23]. If intravesical pressure is kept below 15 cm H_2O, absorption virtually ceases.

Resection time under 1 h and leaving a rim of tissue on the capsule until near the end of the procedure, where it can either be left (if signs of TURP syndrome are evident) or removed all at once, may reduce the time that a large number of prostatic sinuses are open and thus capable of absorbing fluid.

The most widely used indicator of volume gain is serum sodium dilution [24] or breath alcohol level, when ethanol is used as a tracer in the irrigation solution [25]. Other methods follow volumetric fluid balance, central venous pressure trend, plasma electrolyte concentrations (e.g., magnesium and calcium), serial concentrations of irrigation solutes (glycine, sorbitol), transthoracic impedance change, and the patient's weight gain.

No method guarantees that TURP syndrome will be avoided. Symptomatic cardiovascular or pulmonary compromise requires aggressive intervention. After adequate pulmonary gas exchange and haemostasis are established, administration of blood, positive inotropic agents, calcium and magnesium, or diuretics, or augmentation of intravascular volume may be needed; hypertonic saline should be used judiciously.

TURP syndrome: plasma solute effects

Neurological function is largely independent of volume-related effects, but acute hyponatremia (water intoxoxation) caused by the rapid absorption of a large volume of sodium-free irrigation fluid can trigger the central nervous system (CNS) complications, where other factors also play a role, including derangements of osmolality, production of ammonia, hyperglycaemia, administration of benzodiazepines, and opiates, and spinal anaesthesia (nausea and vomiting following hypotension).

Hyponatremia

Profound hyponatremia has been implicated as the cause of visual aberrations, encephalopathy, pulmonary oedema, cardiovascular collapse, seizure, and death. The incidence of serum sodium concentration less than 125 mmol/l after

TURP may reach 15% with a mortality of 40% [26] when hyponatremia is symptomatic (headache, nausea, vomiting). Dilutional hyponatremia may be aggravated by electrolyte losses into accumulations of infused extravasated non-electrolyte fluid.

Hyponatremia is common, and serum sodium concentration decreases of 6 - 54 mmol/l have an incidence ranging from 7% to 26%; however, even markedly hyponatremic patients may show no signs of water intoxication. There could be a difference in measured against calculated osmolality when mannitol is infused because the osmotic effect of mannitol could not be accounted for by the calculation. Although severe hyponatremia has been associated with haemolysis and renal failure, cardiovascular and electrocardio-gram changes, respiratory and neurological compromise, many hyponatremic patients do well, suggesting that hyponatremia may not be the sole or even the primary cause of the neurological manifestations of TURP syndrome. Dilution alone could not be the determinant of all the symptoms, otherwise it could be found in all patients, and diuretic therapy should not be considered the main therapy [27, 28] because there is loss of sodium during the osmotic diuresis associated with irrigating fluids; moreover large amounts of glycine stimulate the release of atrial natriuretic peptide in excess of that expected by the volume load, further promoting diuresis [29]. The urinary excretion of sodium repre-sents an absolute loss as the irrigant fluid contains no electrolytes and this loss increases linearly with the volume of fluid absorbed, amounting to 100 mmol when 4 l of fluid has been taken up [17]; therefore there is a summation between hyponatremia by fluid absorption (dilution) and natriuresis. Further loss of sodium may occur along with blood loss, electrolytes entering into the circu-lation from the interstitial fluid when irrigating fluids are absorbed, while water travels in the opposite direction, therefore contributing to net electrolyte losses from bleeding vessels and by urine excretion derived from interstitial fluid;the magnitude of this sodium entrapment is further aggravated by blood loss. Actually, hypo-osmolality is known as the most-important determinant because it is the cause of widespread cellular and particularly cerebral oedema. It is difficult for the kidney to maintain a high level of water excretion without losing large amounts of osmotically active solutes; therefore the osmotic diuresis induced by all irrigating fluids is associated with a progressive loss of extracel-lular ions, such as sodium, while the solutes present in the irrigating fluid diffuse intracellulary, with the exception of mannitol. Therefore a situation develops where a persistent slightly reduced serum osmolality coexists with a gradually increasing cellular oedema and this is particularly true for glycine and without any evidence of self correction at least for some hours after overhydration [17].

A quick estimation of the volume of irrigating solution absorbed into the circulation based on the quotient between preoperative and postoperative is still useful.

Sodium levels:

Volume absorbed = [(preoperative serum Na/postoperative serum NA)*ECF in KG)]-ECF in kg

e.g., if the preoperative sodium was 140 and postoperative 110, the calculation yields for an estimate of EC as 30% of body weight for a 70 kg man=21 kg:

1)   140/110=1.2
2)   1.2*21=26.6
3)   26.6-21=5.6,volume gain in kg (or l).

Hypoosmolality

Having defined the crucial physiological derangement of CNS function as due not to hyponatremia per se, but to acute hypo-osmolality, we will explore further these concepts that were expected because the blood-brain barrier is essentially impermeable to sodium but freely permeable to water. Human and experimental research has pointed out that correction of osmolality is more important than hyponatremia [30]; calculating the electrical alterations according to the Nernst equation the decrease in extracellular sodium concentration that accompanies the hypo-osmolality seen with TURP only minimally alters neuronal excitability. Replacing a Na^+ value of 140 mmol/l with 100 mmol/l in the Nernst equation increases the calculated transmembrane resting potential of -60 mV by 9 mV. Thus, theoretically, serum sodium concentration should not substantially contribute to neuronal excitability independent of serum osmolality, even when these changes are of the magnitude typically associated with severe TURP syndrome.

The brain reacts to a sustained hypo-osmotic stress within seconds to minutes, with intracellular decreases in Na^+, K^+, Cl^-, and in so-called idiogenic osmoles, which act to decrease intracellular osmolality and prevent swelling. However, with acute osmotic change (within hours or even minutes), such compensatory mechanisms may not work fast enough. Cerebral oedema caused by acute hypo-osmolality can increase intracranial pressure, which results in bradycardia and hypertension by the Cushing reflex. Furthermore, cerebral oedema is not caused by decreased serum colloid oncotic pressure, but by decreased osmolality.

Only a few studies correlate a patient's fate after TURP with both serum sodium concentration and osmolality. In a series of 72 patients [31] undergoing TURP, serum sodium concentration decreased by 10 to 54 mmol/l in 19 (26%), while osmolality changed in only 2 (3%). The 2 patients who had both hyponatremia (serum sodium concentration decreases of 27 and 30 mmol/l) and hypo-osmolality (serum osmolality of 260 and 256 mmol/l) developed pulmonary oedema and encephalopathy. The 5 patients in this series with the largest decreases in serum sodium concentration (by 34 - 54 mmol/l) had no changes in serum osmolality and no signs of TURP syndrome.

A review of a series of 2,000 consecutive patients [32] revealed 14 coma cases postoperatively, with sodium levels 15-20 mEq/l below the normal level. The coma was, at that time, correctly, ascribed to water intoxication and associated surgical risk factors were identified, because in 9 of these cases the prostatic capsule was surgically violated or large venous sinuses were opened; all 14 patients eventually awoke without sequelae.

Treatment of hyponatremia and hypo-osmolality

Diuretics may not be indicated in the treatment of the TURP syndrome, since when used routinely or to treat hypervolemia after TURP, they may worsen hyponatremia and hypo-osmolality and, thus, lead to TURP syndrome [34]. Furosemide acts within minutes on the ascending loop of Henle, inhibiting chloride uptake and causing urinary sodium loss and promoting salt wasting after TURP. Mannitol also causes sodium losses during the first 12 h after TURP, but does not lower the serum level during the first 3-5 postoperative hours, contributing a partial correction of hypo-osmolality [35]. A patient's serum sodium concentration and osmolality may continue to decrease for some time after the procedure, because much irrigant is slowly absorbed from the perivesicular and retroperitoneal spaces. The TURP syndrome can start 4 - 24 h later with coma, blindness, grand mal seizures, and hemiplegia [36, 37]. Some of these cases could be ascribed to instrumental perforation of the prostatic capsule (and more rarely of the bladder) with fluid deposited in a pool in the retroperitoneal space; the fluid may compress the caval veins and diffuse through the peritoneal membrane, again creating flows according the Starling laws; electrolytes entering the pool of fluid and solutes contributing to plasma volume decrease as the solutes travel in the opposite direction, i.e., toward the cell, where they are metabolized or accumulate. In these cases moderate hyponatremia and hypo-osmolality develop with a time delay, some hours following the operation. Clinically there is a tendency toward an increased incidence of abdominal pain, bradycardia, and hypotension [38].

From the aforementioned considerations a more-appropriate therapy could be the concomitant administration of diuretics with saline, even in the presence of a near-normal serum sodium concentration; there is actually a debate on the timing of administration of the hypertonic saline, as a pretreatment or as therapy; this approach may decrease the incidence of TURP syndrome caused by hypo-osmolality, but likely will exacerbate the incidence and severity of the syndrome's hypervolemia manifestations. Because the serum sodium concentration need not reflect serum osmolality, serum sodium concentration should be reported together with osmolality when the irrigant solution contains osmotically active solutes (such as glycine, mannitol, or sorbitol). If osmolality is near normal, no intervention to correct sodium is recommended for asymptomatic patients, even in the face of reduced serum sodium concentration. Hypertonic saline restores for two-thirds serum sodium and osmolality while for one-third redistributes water from the cells to the extracellular space where it is available to diuretic treatment; in the absence of saline infusion the use of furosemide is contraindicated because it acts by promoting sodium excretion and its effect may be poor in hyponatremia. In the absence of pulmonary oedema diuretic therapy should not be instituted until the cardiovascular stability has been attained.

The most-feared complication of correcting hyponatremia is central pontine myelinolysis (CPM). Because demyelination can occur in extrapontine areas, the disease is also referred to as "osmotic demyelination syndrome" [39]. CPM has been reported after rapid as well as slow correction of serum sodium concentration in TURP patients; we suggest a prompt treatment with increases in the serum sodium concentration not greater than 2 mmol/l per hour [40]; in general the correction dose not require doses > 100 ml/h.

When treatment is instituted too slowly for symptomatic hyponatremia ($\leq$ 0.7 mmol/l per hour), it has been associated with a higher morbidity and mortality than has rapid correction ($\geq$1.0 mmol/l per hour) [41]. Many reports suggesting that a 1.5- to 2.0-mmol/l per hour correction rate is safe have failed to consider changes in osmolality. Several investigators have suggested that osmotic stress is probably greater when correcting chronic compared with acute hyponatremia.

The presence of symptoms has been described as the single most-important factor determining morbidity and mortality from hyponatremia. The safest treatment of hyponatremia and hypo-osmolality may be symptomatic [42]. Instituting therapy in the absence of symptoms risks too rapid a correction because the correction rate is difficult to control. Therefore, osmolality should be monitored and corrected aggressively only until symptoms substantially resolve; then correction should be continued slowly (Na+ correction around 1.5 mmol/l per hour) [43].

Hypocalcemia

Chassard et al. [44] found a close correlation between serum sodium and free (ionized) calcium concentrations during the first 20 min of their study. Thereafter, serum calcium remained essentially unchanged, although the glycine infusion continued for another 40 min. These findings suggest that the mechanisms compensating for a diluted serum calcium concentration have the same strength as for serum sodium during 20–30 min of a glycine infusion, after which they become stronger for calcium.

During infusion of the irrigating fluid, there was a close correlation between changes in serum sodium and albumin-corrected serum calcium concentrations; after infusion, however, serum calcium concentration was restored more rapidly than serum sodium concentration.

Dilution of serum sodium during glycine infusions is governed mainly by the volume of irrigant absorbed. Correction occurs by diffusion of glycine and irrigant water from the extracellular to the intracellular fluid compartment, and marked, but delayed, cellular oedema develops. Urine excretion also plays a part, but the urine contains large amounts of sodium, particularly when a large volume of glycine solution is given. The principal difference between the correction of diluted concentrations of sodium and calcium is that the latter ion can be mobilized easily from loosely bound bone stores, and equilibration has been claimed to occur with a half-time of 70 min. The relatively poor perfusion of bone certainly explains some of this delay. This indicates that hypocalcaemia probably does not get worse after 20–40 min of glycine absorption in the clinic either. When irrigating fluid is absorbed very rapidly, however, severe hypocalcaemia may develop within this time and then contribute to the hypokinetic circulation seen in the TURP syndrome. A role for calcium in the treatment of this syndrome has also been suggested by two reports of patients in whom cardiac arrest and hyponatraemia developed during prostatectomy [45]. Some degree of "self-treatment" of the hypocalcaemia can be expected as the TURP syndrome is associated with metabolic acidosis, although this is usually fully compensated until circulatory disturbances occur.

Further clinical studies, including monitoring calcium concentrations during acute TURP, should be encouraged. This could help in the decision to introduce calcium therapy in the resuscitation of cardiovascular disturbances in this syndrome.

Hyperglycinemia

Glycine in large amounts exerts toxic effects, especially on the heart and retina and the syndrome of hyperglycinemia resembles a disease characterized by a defect in the glycine cleavage enzyme system, disturbed electrophysiological function, intractable seizures, lethargy, spasticity, mental retardation, and death within the first few months of life. These infants have a plasma glycine level up to 10 times greater than that of normal infants (mean range 266–2,027 mmol/l; normal infant level 209 mmol/l) [46, 47].

Incidence and severity of circulatory and nervous symptoms are proportional to the amount of glycine absorbed; with < 300 ml, there was a mean of 1.3 symptoms, increasing to 2.3 at 2 l of fluid absorption and 5.8 symptoms at absorption of 3 l [48].

Glycine potentiates the N-methyl-D-aspartate (NMDA) response, an excitatory neurotransmitter, and so may facilitate excitatory transmission in the brain and contribute to seizures [49]. A large concentration of glycine may be harmless in plasma but can be fatal in the brain. Signs of glycine toxicity include nausea, vomiting, headache, malaise, and weakness. They manifest at an infusion rate of 3.5 mg/kg per min, which, in a 70-kg man represents an intravascular absorption of 1.5% glycine solution at the rate of 54 ml/min. Serum glycine after TURP has been reported at a level greater than 14,300 mmol/l. This concentration is 17 times greater than that in children dying from glycine encephalopathy and over 65 times that in adults (normal adult level 219 mmol/l) [50, 51].

Visual disturbances in TURP syndrome vary in severity from blurred vision to complete blindness; some patients present with sluggish or fixed and dilated pupils and total loss of light/dark discrimination [52, 32].

Atropine [53] or hyponatremia and cerebral oedema from overhydration may contribute to these visual disturbances. Patients with cortical blindness, on the other hand, lose all visual sensation (light perception and the blink reflex) but retain the pupillary responses to light and accommodation. Although it is difficult to separate the effects of serum sodium concentration from those of other retinal transmitters, sodium appears to play only a minor role in the visual disturbances.

Glycine is now gaining acceptance as the most likely cause of visual aberrations during the TURP syndrome. A wide range of serum glycine levels have been documented in patients with visual changes. These have led to speculation of a serum glycine concentration threshold for symptomatic visual impairment (>4,000 mmol/l) [54] and blindness (>13,734 mmol/l) [55]. Glycine is probably a major inhibitory neurotransmitter in the retina. The sensitivity of oscillatory potentials of the electroretinogram and visual evoked potentials to glycine in the absence of large osmolality changes has been demonstrated. Therefore, glycine appears to affect the retinal physiological condition independent of cerebral oedema caused by hypo-osmolality.

Glycine may also exert toxic effects on the kidney [56]. A study in rats found histological evidence of glycine toxicity in their kidneys 6 h after either intravenous or intraperitoneal administration of large doses of 1.5% glycine solution. No toxicity was found after injecting similar volumes of retroperitoneal water or lactated Ringer's solution. This study did not investigate whether the kidney would eventually recover from the apparent toxic insult. Hyperoxaluria from metabolism into oxalate and glycolate has also been proposed as a route whereby glycine could cause renal failure in susceptible patients [57].

In considering the treatment of hyperglycinemia, glycine may be involved with TURP encephalopathy and seizure through its positive action on the NMDA receptor channel system, as it is in glycine encephalopathy. Seizures after TURP associated with hyponatremia and hypo-osmolality are likely to be resistant to benzodiazepine and anticonvulsant therapy; in fact, such treatment may provoke apnoea. Theoretically, a NMDA receptor antagonist or glycine antagonist are better choices. Arginine is capable of preventing the toxic effects of glycine infused before or simultaneously [58, 59].

Magnesium exerts a negative control on the NMDA receptor. A serum magnesium level lowered by dilution may increase susceptibility to seizures. Magnesium may be dramatically lowered after TURP in patients who have been treated with a loop diuretic. Therefore, a trial of magnesium therapy for seizures in patients in whom a glycine irrigant was used during TURP deserves consideration, especially if measured osmolality is near normal.

Vision returns to normal within 24 h as glycine approaches normal. This is predictable because the half-life of glycine is approximately 85 min. Reassurance that unimpaired vision is expected to return may be the best treatment.

Furthermore, there are animal and human proofs that glycine is toxic for isolated cardiomyocytes [60], causes myocardial ischaemic damage in rabbit hearts [61], and subacute effects on the myocardium (t wave inversion) [62]. In an epidemiological study absorption > 500 ml doubled the risk of acute myocardial infarction [63].

Hyperammonemia

Ammonia is the principal byproduct of glycine metabolism and hyperammoniemia has followed glycine irrigation. Symptoms are characteristic, starting with nausea and vomiting and rapidly progressing to coma; blood levels of ammonia rise above 500 mmol/l (normal 11-35): coma persists in general for 10-12 h with progressive awakening when blood ammonia levels start to fall below 150 µg/l. It is not clear why only some patients develop the hyperammoniemic syndrome; it could be that these patients have a relative or absolute deficit of arginine, one of the intermediary products of the cycle with whom ammonia is converted in the liver to urea via the ornithine cycle.

In the treatment of hyperammonemia, L-arginine has been used; it acts in the liver by preventing hepatic release of ammonia and accelerating ammonia conversion to urea. The time necessary to deplete endogenous arginine stores may be as little as 12 h, which approximates preoperative fast time; prophylactic administration of intravenous L-arginine markedly moderated the increase in blood ammonia concentration in fasting patients receiving intravenous glycine. Infusion of L-arginine with or at the conclusion of glycine administration prevented further increases in blood ammonia concentration and accelerated its return to normal. Doses between 4 g (20 mmol) infused over 3 min and 38 g (180 mmol) infused over 120 min have been recommended. No toxicity was noted with either of these regimens [64].

Hyperglycaemia and lactic acidosis

Sorbitol is a natural C6 sugar alcohol found in many fruits and metabolized to fructose by sorbitol dehydrogenase in the liver and to a lesser extent in the kidney. A high dose of sorbitol can induce toxic effects similar to fructose toxicity, such as lactic acidosis, hyperuricaemia, and hyperglycaemia. Diffe-rential diagnosis should exclude other causes of lactic acidosis, like those caused by hypoxemia and tissue hypoperfusion.

A few case reports have described the syndrome of hyperglycemia and lactic acidosis associated with the irrigation of sorbitol; one was a case of massive absorption [65] and the other a less-serious case [66]. These cases demonstrate that acid base changes could occur and became serious during TURP, sugge-sting the usefulness of EGA, blood glucose, and arterial lactate concentration monitoring whenever a significant sorbitol uptake is suspected.

TURP syndrome: other considerations

Benzodiazepines are known to act at the GABA receptor, and thereby may mediate some compromise of vision through the activation of the retinal GABA receptor. Diazepam increases the latency of visual evoked potentials and decreases their amplitude in both rats and rabbits. Narcotics can contribute to sedation and nausea. When these drugs are used their effects must be considered in the differential diagnosis of the TURP syndrome.

Choice of anaesthetic technique and outcome

Most anaesthetists routinely provide spinal anaesthesia for patients undergoing TURP unless there are contraindications, in the belief that spinal is safer; yet this popularity of regional over general is intriguing as there are only a few studies showing convincing differences in variety of endpoints [67]. Comparative studies have investigated blood loss; some studies [68-70] showed that regional was better than general, even if Smyth et al. [71] disputed these results recently, negating differences in incidence of coagulopathies, mortality, and major morbidity [27, 73, 74], heat balance [75], evidence of myocardial ischaemia [76, 77], haemodynamic disturbances [78], mental functioning [79], and length of postoperative hospital stay [80]. Epidural anaesthesia has been demonstrated to reduce the incidence of catheter-related pain after TURP, although being of similar efficacy to oral diazepam [81].This popularity suggests that anaesthesiologists who consider spinal anaesthesia to be superior are basing their convictions on personal experience, a belief that the few studies performed lack the power to detect a true difference or an impression that outcome is improved in a way not easily measured. The most-recent study of Reeves and Myles [82] showed that the likelihood of any adverse event or complication occurring during or after TURP was increased in patients undergoing general anaesthesia; however most of these complications were minor and true differences were limited to length of stay in the recovery room. Some complaints typical of spinal anaesthesia, such as backache, were more frequent in the regional group, while other complaints like sore throat were more frequent in the general anaesthesia group. Postoperative nausea and vomiting was a significant complaint following general anaesthesia.

It is true, however, that even if very often secondary end points fail to demonstrate differences in outcome, almost all the indirect conclusions favour regional anaesthesia; consider the possibility of infection for instance, where the study of Le Cras et al. [83] emphasize that spinal anaesthesia is less immunosuppressive than general anaesthesia based on the measurement of Th1/Th 2 ratios; Th1 cells increased in patients who had undergone TURP under spinal anaesthesia and the percentage of Th2 decreased, with a resultant increase in the Th1/Th2 ratio. Since Th1 cells produce predominantly interferon-gamma and favour cell-mediated immune responses, while Th2 cells secrete predominantly interleukin-4 and favour humoral immunity, these findings tend toward less immunosuppression and better prevention of infection with regional as compared with general anaesthesia. These findings have been anticipated by Whelan and Morris [84], who found a significant reduction in lymphocyte numbers and in the response of lymphocytes to various mitogens and to histocompatibility antigens in mixed lymphocyte cultures in patients after TURP under general anaesthesia, while minimal changes were associated with spinal anaesthesia.

In conclusion, many studies point to a higher safety of regional anaesthesia for TURP, but many of these differences are limited to secondary end points. Because of the low rate of serious complications after TURP, a randomized controlled trial would require many thousands of patients to be assessed and would take many years to complete; a definitive answer may not be applicable given the probable concurrent improvements in surgical and anaesthetic practice. At present regional anaesthesia may be preferred, but even general anaesthesia is safe. Edwards et al. [76] studied the incidence and duration of perioperative myocardial ischaemia using ambulatory electrocardiographic monitoring in 100 patients undergoing transurethral surgery, who were allocated randomly to receive either general or spinal anaesthesia. The overall incidence of myocardial ischaemia increased from 18% to 26% between the preoperative and postoperative periods. Patients with ischaemic heart disease had a significantly greater incidence of myocardial ischaemia after operation than patients without known ischaemic heart disease ($P<0.05$). There was an increase in both the incidence and duration of myocardial ischaemia after operation with both anaesthetic techniques, but no significant difference between the two.

There appears to be no difference in the effects of general, epidural, or spinal anaesthesia on the incidence of postoperative delirium following total knee arthroplasty or TURP procedures. However, cognitive function appears to be better preserved in elderly patients who undergo TURP with regional anaesthesia without intraoperative sedation [85-87]; there are also reports that postoperative patient-controlled epidural analgesia can improve mental status in elderly patients [88]. An interesting point has recently been raised by Gehring et al. [89], measuring absorption with blood and exhaled ethanol measurements they were able to show that absorption of irrigating fluids during TURP is significantly more marked amongst spontaneously breathing patients with regional anaesthesia in comparison with patients undergoing general anaesthesia with IPPV. The markedly lower central venous pressure before the start of irrigation should be considered as a possible cause of this effect absorption rate, and blood ethanol concentration are variables to which the anaesthesiologist can refer directly for assessing the extent of irrigating fluid absorption during anaesthesia; breath monitoring of alcohol facilitates these measurements [90], but determination of the area under the curve and calculation of the absorbed volume from a nomogram are procedures that cannot be implemented immediately whilst surgery is in progress [91].

Ethanol monitoring started routinely in the mid 1980s and one of the earlier instruments (Breathalyzer, Alcolmeter S-D2, Lions, Wales, UK) has proved to be very reliable; recalibration is rarely necessary provided that the battery is fresh and the Breathalyzer is serviced every year. However, staff education is necessary. Data may be wrong if the sampling button is not pressed long enough or the Alcolmeter is placed adjacent to equipment that has just been cleaned with alcohol. When general anaesthesia is used, the Alcolmeter must be positioned close to the tracheal tube because moisture exchangers and soda lime absorb ethanol.

A difficult part of the education is to teach the user to identify large-scale extravascular absorption, which can occur after instrumental perforations and gives rise to a typical pattern of ethanol changes with very low readings and delayed symptomatology of fluid overload. This possibility should be considered in cases similar to that reported by Letheren [92].

TURP can be done under profound sedoanalgesia and local infiltration and this technique deserves attention because its simplicity and low cost [93], allowing early feeding and discharge within 48 h of surgery.

Conclusions

Our understanding of the pathophysiology leading to the TURP syndrome has improved in recent years. Complex changes in intravascular volume, solute, and neurophysiological function mark the TURP syndrome. The prevention, diagnosis, and treatment of TURP syndrome is challenging, because aberrations of solute and volume can occur simultaneously and may suggest opposing diagnoses and treatments.

Therapeutic suggestions:

- Be always vigilant for TURP whenever irrigating fluids are used; refer to ICU in every case where absorption exceeds 3 l
- Maintain temperature homeostasis
- Cardiovascular monitoring; at least NIBP, ECG, SaO2; PVC helpful; hypotension treated with judicious infusion of colloids and adrenergic drugs. Hypertonic (3%-5% saline) should be administered as a slow infusion
- Pulmonary monitoring; auscultation, EGA
- Metabolic monitoring; Na levels and osmolality the most important; Hct; Hb, Ca, MG; in case of use of glycine, glycinemia and ammoniemia; in case of use of sorbitol-mannitol, glycemia and lactic acid. Metabolic acidosis should be judiciously treated with a buffer.
- Monitoring of consciousness and looking for early subtle neurological signs

of TURP syndrome. In case of depression of consciousness, maintenance of a secure airway and positive pressure ventilation recommended.

- Limit the height of the irrigation bag to 40 cm above the prostate; the lower, the better;
- Use a continuous irrigating resectoscopes or suprapubic trocar drainage (minimize absorption)
- Supportive care remains the mainstay of management for renal, pulmonary, and cardiovascular complications of TURP syndrome. Several therapies warrant consideration in formulating a management plan for hyperammonemia, hyperglycinemia, hyponatremia, hypo-osmolality, encephalopathy, and seizures after TURP.
- The introduction of new therapies for the medical and surgical management of prostatic hypertrophy may minimize risks of TURP syndrome in the future.

Early detection of the TURP syndrome could be obtained marking the irrigation fluid with ethanol [94]; plasma and exhaled ethanol concentrations could be measured and absorption calculated assuming that significant fluid absorption has taken place when ethanol concentration in plasma exceeds 0.1/1000. Plasma and exhaled ethanol demonstrated a linear correlation, while plasma ethanol correlated inversely with plasma sodium. The measurements were consistent both in patients under spinal and general anaesthesia, undergoing mechanical ventilation; but ethanol levels were not predictive of sodium concentrations so that the authors recommended additional separate electrolytes determinations whenever exhaled ethanol exceeds 0.2/1,000.

References

1. Holtgrewe HL, Valk VVL (1962) Factors influencing the mortality and morbidity of transurethral prostatectomy: a study of 2,015 cases. J Urol 87:450-459
2. Roos NP, Wennberg JE, Malenka DJ et al (1989) Mortality and re-operation after open and transurethral resection of the prostate for benign prostatic hyperplasia. N Engl J Med 320:1120
3. Malenka DJ, Roos N, Fisher ES et al (1990) Further study of the increased mortality following transurethral prostatectomy: a chart-based analysis. J Urol 144:224
4. Seagroatt V (1995) Mortality after prostatectomy: selection and surgical approach. Lancet 346:1521
5. Meyhoff HH, Nordling J, Hald T (1985) Economy in transurethral prostatectomy. Scand J Urol Nephrol 19:17-20
6. Olsson J, Hahn RG (1996) Survival after high-dose intravenous infusion of irrigating fluids in the mouse. Urology 47:689-692
7. Zhang W, Andersson B, Hahn RG (1995) Effect of irrigating fluids and prostatic tissue extracts on isolated cardiomyocytes. Urology 46:821-824
8. Yeung ST, Yoong C, Spink J et al (1991) Functional myocardial impairment in children treated with anthracyclines for cancer. Lancet 337:816-818

9. Inman RD, Hussain Z, Elves AWS et al (2001) A comparison of 1.5% glycine and 2.7% sorbitol-0.5% mannitol irrigants during transurethral prostate resection. J Urol 166:2216-2220
10. Hahn RG (1990) Fluid and electrolyte dynamics during development of TURP syndrome. Br J Urol 66:79-84
11. Creevy CD, Reiser MP (1963) The importance of hemolysis in transurethral prostatic resection: severe and fatal reactions associated with the use of distilled water. J Urol 89:900-905
12. Norris HT, Aasheim GM, Sherrard DJ, Tremann JA (1978) Symptomatology, pathophysiology and treatment of the transurethral resection of the prostate syndrome. Br J Urol 45:420-427
13. Evans JTA III, Singer M, Coppinger SWV et al (1994) Cardiovascular performance and core temperature during transurethral prostatectomy. J Urol 152:2025-2029
14. Sessler, Daniel I (2001) Complications and treatment of mild hypothermia. Anesthesiology 95:531-543
15. Monga M, Comeaux B, Roberts JA (1996) Effect of irrigating fluid on perioperative temperature regulation during transurethral prostatectomy. Eur Urol 29:26-28
16. Pit MJ, Tegelaar RJH, Venema PL (1996) Isothermic irrigation during transurethral resection of the prostate: effects on perioperative hypothermia, blood loss, resection time and patient satisfaction. Br J Urol 78: 99-103
17. Hahn RG (1997) Irrigating fluids in endoscopic surgery. Br J Urol 79:669-680
18. Nilsson A, Randmaa 1, Hahn RG (1996) Haemodynamic effects of irrigating fluids studied by Doppler ultrasonography in volunteers. Br J Urol 77: 541-546
19. Hahn R, Ess6n P, Wernerman J (1992) Amino acid concentrations in plasma and skeletal muscle after transurethral resection syndrome. Scand Urol Nephrol 26:235-239
20. Madsen PO, Naber KB (1974) Absorption and excretion of sorbitol and mannitol in transurethral resection of the prostate. Invest Urol 11:331-335
21. Smyth R, Cheng D, Asokumar B et al (1995) Coagulopathies in patients after transurethral resection of the prostate: spinal versus general anaesthesia. Anesth Analg 81:680-685
22. Madsen PO, Naber KG (1973) The importance of the pressure in the prostatic fossa and absorption of irrigating fluid during the transurethral resection of the prostate. J Urol 109:446-452
23. Briggs TP, Parker C, Connolly AA, Miller R (1991) Fluid delivery systems: high flow, low pressure, the key to safe resection. Eur Urol 19:150-154
24. Ghanem AN, Ward JP (1990) Osmotic and metabolic sequelae of volumetric overload in relation to the TURP syndrome. Br J Urol 66:71-78
25. Norlén H, Allgén LG, Vinnars E, Bedrelidou-Classon G (1986) Glycine solution as an irrigating agent during transurethral prostatic resection. Scand J Urol Nephrol 20:19-26
26. Dixon B, Ernest D (1996) Hyponatraemia in the transurethral resection of prostate syndrome. Anaesth Intensive Care 24:102-103
27. Mebust WK, Holtgrewe HL, Cockett ATK et al (1989) Transurethral prostatectomy: immediate and postoperative complications. A cooperative study of 13 participating institutions evaluating 3,885 patients. J Urol 141: 243-247
28. Bernstein GT, Loughlin KR, Gittes RF (1989) The physiologic basis of the TUR syndrome. I. Surg Res 46:135-141
29. Flahn RG, Stalberg H, Carlström K et al (1994) Plasma atrial natriuretic peptide concentration and renin activity during overhydration with 1.5% glycine solution in conscious sheep. Prostate 24:55-61
30. Andrew RD (1991) Seizure and acute osmotic change: clinical and neurophysiological aspects. J Neurol Sci 101:7-18
31. Desmond J (1970) Serum osmolality and plasma electrolytes in patients who develop dilutional hyponatremia during transurethral resection. Can J Surg; 13:116-121
32. Henderson DJ, Middleton RG (1980) Coma from hyponatremia following transurethral resection of prostate. Urology 15:267-71
33. Donatucci CF, Deshon GE Jr, Wade CE, Hunt M (1990) Furosemide-induced disturbances of renal function in patients undergoing TURP. Urology 35:295-300

34. Malone PR, Davies JH, Stanfield NJ et al (1986) Metabolic consequences of forced diuresis following prostatectomy. Br J Urol 58:406-411
35. Madsen PO, Knuth OE, Wagenknecht LV, Genster HG (1970) Induction of diuresis following resection of the prostate. J Urol 104:735-738
36. Swaminathan R, Tormey WP (1981) Fluid absorption during transurethral prostatectomy (letter). Br J Urol 282:317
37. Ghanem AN, Ward JP (1990) Osmotic and metabolic sequelae of volumetric overload in relation to the TURP syndrome. Br J Urol 66:71-78
38. Oilsson J, Nilsson A, Hahn RG (1995) Symptoms of the transurethral resection syndrome using glycine as the irrigant. J Urol 154:123-128
39. Sterns RH, Riggs JE, Schochet SS Jr (1986) Osmotic demyelination syndrome following correction of hyponatremia. N Engl J Med 314:1535-1542
40. Ayus JC, Krothapalli RK, Arieff AL (1987) Treatment of symptomatic hyponatraemia and its relation to brain damage. N Engl J Med 317: 1190-1195
41. Ashraf N, Locksley R, Arieff AI (1981) Thiazide-induced hyponatremia associated with death or neurological damage in outpatients. Am J Med 70:1163-1168
42. Sarnaik AP, Meert K, Hackbarth R, Fleischmann L (1991) Management of hyponatremic seizures in children with hypertonic saline: a safe and effective strategy. Crit Care Med 19:758-762
43. Gravenstein D (1997) Transurethral resection of the prostate (TURP) syndrome: a review of the pathophysiology and management. Anesth Analg 84:438-446
44. Chassard D, Berrada K, Tournadre JP, Boulétreau P (1996) Calcium homeostasis during i.v. infusion of 1.5% glycine in anaesthetized pigs. Br J Anaesth 77:271-273
45. Charlton AJ (1980) Cardiac arrest during transurethral prostatectomy after absorption of 1.5% glycine. Anaesthesia 35:804-806
46. Perry TL, Urquhart N, MacLean J et al (1975) Nonketotic hyperglycinemia: glycine accumulation due to absence of glycine cleavage in brain. N Engl J Med 292:1269-1273
47. Perry TL, Urquhart N, Hansen S, Mamer OA (1977) Studies of the glycine cleavage enzyme system in brain from patients with glycine encephalopathy. Pediatr Res 12:1192-1197
48. Hahn RG, Shemais H, Ess6n P (1997) Glycine 1.0% versus glycine 1.5% as irrigating fluid during transurethral resection of the prostate. Br J Urol 79: 394-400
49. Johnson W, Ascher P (1987) Glycine potentiates the NMDA response in cultured mouse brain neurons. Nature 325:529-531
50. Norlén H, Allgén LG, Vinnars E, Bedrelidou-Classon G (1986) Glycine solution as an irrigating agent during transurethral prostatic resection. Scand J Urol Nephrol 20:19-26
51. Hamilton Stewart PA, Barlow IM (1989) Metabolic effects of prostatectomy. J R Soc Med 82:725-728
52. Kaiser R, Adragna MG, Weis FR Jr, Williams D (1985) Transient blindness following transurethral resection of the prostate in an achondroplastic dwarf. J Urol 133:685-686
53. Gooding JM, Holcomb MC (1977) Transient blindness following intravenous administration of atropine. Anesth Analg 56:872-873
54. Wang JM, Creel DJ, Wong KC (1989) Transurethral resection of the prostate, serum glycine levels, and ocular evoked potentials. Anesthesiology 70:36-41
55. Kaiser R, Adragna MG, Weis FR Jr, Williams D (1985) Transient blindness following transurethral resection of the prostate in an achondroplastic dwarf. J Urol 133:685-686
56. Maatman TJ, Musselman P, Kwak YS, Resnick MI (1991) Effect of glycine on retroperitoneal and intraperitoneal organs in the rat model. Prostate 19:323-328
57. Fitzpatrick JM, Kasidas GP, Rose GA (1981) Hyperoxaluria following irrigation for transurethral prostatectomy. Br J Urol 53:250-252
58. Johnson W, Ascher P (1987) Glycine potentiates the NMDA response in cultured mouse brain neurons. Nature 325:529-531
59. Schwarcz R, Meldrum B (1985) Excitatory amino acid antagonists provide a therapeutic approach to neurological disorders. Lancet II:140-143

60. Zhang W, Andersson B, Hahn RG (1995) Effect of irrigating fluids and prostatic tissue extracts on isolated cardiomyocytes. Urology 46: 821-824
61. Hahn RG, Nennesmo 1, Rajs J et al (1996) Morphological and X-ray microanalytical changes in mammalian tissue after overhydration with irrigating fluids. Eur Urol 29: 355-361
62. Hahn R, Ess6n P (1994) ECG and cardiac enzymes after glycine absorption in transurethral prostatic resection. Acta Anaesthesiol Scand 38: 550-556
63. Hahn RG, Nilsson A, Farahmand B et al (1996) Operative factors and the long-term risk of acute myocardial infarction after transurethral resection of the prostate. Epidemiology 6: 93-95
64. Fahey JL (1957) Toxicity and blood ammonia rise resulting from intravenous amino-acid administration in man: the protective effect of L-arginine. J Clin Invest 36:1647-1655
65. Trepanier CA, Lessard MR, Brochu J, Turcotte G (2001) Another feature of TURP syndrome: hyperglycemia and lactic acidosis caused by massive absorption of sorbitol. Br J Anaesth 87:316-319
66. Scheingraber S, Heitmann L, Weber W, Finsterere U (2000) Are there acid base changes during transurethral resection of the prostate (TURP)? Anesth Analg 90:946-950
67. Agin C (1993) Anesthesia for transurethral prostate surgery. Int Anesth Clin 31:25-46
68. Abrams PH, Shah PJR, Bryning K et al (1982) Blood loss during transurethral resection of the prostate. Anaesthesia 37:71-73
69. McGowan SW, Smith GPN (1980) Anaesthesia for transurethral prostatectomy. Anaesthesia 35: 847-853
70. Dobson PMS, Caldicott LD, Gerrish SP et al (1994) Changes in haemodynamic variables during transurethral resection of the prostate: comparison of general and spinal anaesthesia. Br J Anaesth 72:267-271
71. Smyth R, Cheng D, Asokumar B et al (1995) Coagulopathies in patients after transurethral resection of the prostate: spinal versus general anaesthesia. Anesth Analg 81: 680-685
72. Hosking MP, Lobdell CM (1989) Anaesthesia for patients over 90 years of age. Outcomes after regional and general anaesthetic techniques for two common surgical procedures. Anaesthesia 44:142-147
73. Thorpe AC, Cleary R, Coles J et al (1994) Deaths and complications following prostatectomy in 1400 men in the Northern Region of England. Br J Urol 74: 559-565
74. Stjernström R, Hermeberg S, Eklund A et al (1985) Thermal balance during transurethral resection of the prostate. Acta Anaesthesiol Scand 29: 743-749
75. Edwards ND, Callaghan LC, White T et al (1995) Perioperative myocardial ischaemia in patients undergoing transurethral surgery: a pilot study comparing general with spinal anaesthesia. Br J Anaesth 74:68-72
76. Windsor A, French GWG, Sear JW et al (1996) Silent myocardial ischaemia in patients undergoing transurethral prostatectomy. Anaesthesia 51:728-732
77. Dobson PMS, Caldicott LD, Gerrish SP et al (1994) Changes in haemodynamic variables during transurethral resection of the prostate: comparison of general and spinal anaesthesia. Br J Anaesth 72:267-271
78. Asbjorn 1, Jakobsen BW, Pilegaard HK et al (1989) Mental function in elderly men after surgery during epidural analgesia. Acta Anaesthesiol Scand 33: 369-373
79. Kirollos M (1997) Length of postoperative hospital stay after transurethral resection of the prostate. Ann Roy Coll Surg Eng 79: 284-288
80. Nott MR, Jameson PM, Julious SA (1997) Diazepam for relief of irrigation pain after transurethral resection of the prostate. Eur J Anaesthesiol 14: 197-200
81. Reeves MDS, Myles PS (1999) Does anesthetic technique affect the outcome after transurethral resection of the prostate? Brit J Urol 84:982-986
82. LeCras A, Galley HF, Webster NR (1998) Spinal but not general anesthesia increases the ratio of T helper 1 to T helper 2 cell subsets in patients undergoing transurethral resection of the prostate. Anesth Analg 87:1421-1425
83. Whelan P, Morris PJ (1982) Immunological responses after transurethral resection of prostate: general versus spinal anesthetic. Clin Exp Immunol 48:611-618

84. Moller JT, Cluitmans P, Rasmussen LS et al (1998) Long-term postoperative cognitive dysfunction in the elderly ISPOCDI study. ISPOCD investigators. International Study of Post-Operative Cognitive Dysfunction. Lancet 351:857-861
85. Ritchie K, Polge C, Roquefeuil G de et al (1997) Risk factors for dementia. Impact of anaesthesia on the cognitive functioning of the elderly. Int Psychogeriatr 9:309-326
86. Williams-Russo P, Sharrock NE, Mattis S et al (1995) Cognitive effects after epidural vs. general anesthesia in older adults. A randomized trial. JAMA 274:44-50
87. Mann C, Pouzeratte Y, Boccara G et al (2000) Comparison of intravenous or epidural patient-controlled analgesia in the elderly after major abdominal surgery. Anesthesiology 92:433-441
88. Gehring H, Nahm W, Baerwald J et al (1999) Irrigation fluid absorption during transurethral resection of the prostate: spinal versus general anesthesia. Acta Anesthesiol Scand 43:458-463
89. Gehring H, Schmitz A, Nahm W et al (1997) Measurement of breath ethanol concentration in patients with general anesthesia. Anesthesiology 87:A406
90. Hahn RG (1997) Estimation of fluid absorption by using the area under the curve for ethanol in expired air. Urol Int 58:25-29
91. Letheren MJR (1995) A case of hyponatremia while using ethanol labeling for endometrial resection (letter) Anesth Analg 80:212
92. Chander J, Gupta U, Mehra R, Ramteke VK (2000) Safety and efficacy of transurethral resection of the prostate under sedoanalgesia. Brit J Urol Int 86:220-222
93. Heide C, Weninger EW, Ney L et al (1997) Early detection of TUR (transurethral resection) syndrome; ethanol measurement in ventilated patients. Anaesthesiol Intensivmed Notfall Med Schmerzther 32:610-615

BRAIN

GLOBAL AND FOCAL MONITORING IN ACUTE
CEREBRAL DAMAGE

Clinical cerebral monitoring: the role of the jugular O_2 difference

A. BACHER

Jugular bulb oxyhaemoglobin saturation (SjO_2) is a measure of global cerebral oxygen balance, because SjO_2 is closely related to the oxygen content in the venous blood of the jugular bulb (cjO_2). The latter is determined by SjO_2, the hemoglobin concentration (Hb), and the oxygen tension in the venous blood of the jugular bulb (PjO_2). We may therefore conclude that for a given Hb concentration, changes in SjO_2 always indicate changes in cjO_2.

The cerebral metabolic rate of oxygen or cerebral oxygen consumption ($CMRO_2$) is the difference between cerebral oxygen transport (DO_2) and the amount of O_2 leaving the brain with venous blood. Cerebral DO2 is the product of cerebral blood flow (CBF) and arterial oxygen content. Consequently, cjO_2 depends on the relationship between DO_2–$CMRO_2$ to CBF.

Cerebral oxygen consumption underlies changes depending on cerebral activity, which may be modified by anaesthetics, trauma, temperature, or the presence of seizures [1-5]. CBF and, consequently, cerebral DO_2 are continuously being modified by autoregulatory mechanisms in the healthy brain according to changes in $CMRO_2$. However, under the influence of certain diseases (e.g., severe liver disease) or anaesthetics, the coupling between CBF, DO_2, and $CMRO_2$ may be abolished [6, 7].

Venous blood in the jugular bulb is a mixture of the venous drainage of the entire brain. The contribution of a certain brain region to the global cerebral oxygen balance depends on its size, on the amount of venous drainage from this particular region, and on regional $CMRO_2$. For example, if a small brain area with a very high $CMRO_2$ is supplied with an insufficient fraction of global cerebral DO_2, the decrease in SjO_2 from the baseline will eventually be the same, as if a larger brain area with a low $CMRO_2$ is inadequately supplied with oxygen. These considerations are of great importance if we interpret changes in SjO_2 and try to associate these changes with clinical events. Clinical events that are typically related to a decrease in SjO_2 are either caused by a decrease in cerebral DO_2 (cerebral ischaemia, hypotension, occlusion of an intracranial artery, intracranial hypertension, cerebral vasospasm, hyperventilation, decreased arterial oxygen content, hypoxia, anaemia, carbon monoxide intoxication, haemoglobin disorders) or by a pathologically increased $CMRO_2$ (seizures, forced rewarming during cardiopulmonary bypass, hyperthermia).

An additional way to assess the oxygenation status of the brain with a jugular venous bulb catheter is to measure lactate and glucose concentrations in the jugular bulb and to compare these with arterial lactate and glucose concentrations [difference between the lactate concentration in the jugular bulb and the arterial lactate concentration (VADL), difference between the arterial glucose concentration and the glucose concentration in the jugular bulb (AVDG)]. If cerebral DO_2 decreases below a threshold upon which aerobic metabolism cannot be maintained, VADL and AVDG increase due to an increased rate of anaerobic glycolysis and lactate production by astrocytes and neurons. The lactate-glucose index ($LGI = VADL \cdot 100 \cdot 2^{-1} \cdot AVDG^{-1}$) is the proportion of glucose consumption appearing as lactate in the jugular bulb [8]. Normal values in healthy awake volunteers are 0.19 ± 0.10 µmol/ml for VADL, 0.53 ± 0.09 µmol/ml for AVDG, and $3.2 \pm 1.7\%$ for LGI (means±standard deviations) [9]. A cerebral microdialysis study revealed that the cerebral extracellular lactate concentration significantly increases, cerebral extracellular glucose concentration decreases, and LGI increases during ischaemic events [10]. It is therefore likely that changes in VADL and AVDG that can be measured with a jugular bulb catheter correctly reflect the onset of anaerobic metabolism. Another variable that is frequently determined with a jugular bulb catheter is the lactate-oxygen index ($LOI = VADL/AVDO_2$). The LOI may be used to differentiate between compensated or uncompensated states of a low cerebral DO_2 [12]. During states of compensated low cerebral DO_2, VADL remains normal or increases slightly, and AVDO2 increases if $CMRO_2$ remains constant, which will result in an unchanged or slightly decreased LOI [11]. If cerebral DO_2 decreases below the anaerobic threshold, $CMRO_2$ decreases due to the lack of oxygen. Therefore, $AVDO_2$ does not further decrease, but lactate production increases due to the onset of anaerobic metabolism. In this situation of uncompensated oxygen depletion, the LOI increases. It has been found that an increased lactate production indicating cerebral maloxygenation is present if LOI increases to more than 0.08 [11]. In contrast, if $AVDO_2$ is low without a pathological increase in LOI, absolute or relative hyperemia is present [11].

An important question for the interpretation of SjO2 is whether certain thresholds for SjO_2 or cjO_2 exist upon which global cerebral metabolism is predominantly anaerobic. This issue has been studied in patients after rewarming on hypothermic cardiopulmonary bypass [12]. The authors found that VADL, AVDG, and LGI significantly increase if cjO_2 decreases below 6.72 ml

O_2/100 ml blood [12]. The relationship between VADL, AVDG, and LGI and cjO_2 is shown in Fig. 1. This threshold of cjO2 would correspond to an estimated SjO_2 of 51%, if we assume a Hb concentration of 10 g/100 ml blood. The onset of global cerebral anaerobic metabolism or ischemia has therefore been defined as a decrease in SjO_2 to less than 50% lasting for at least 10 min [13, 14]. However, it has to be noted that if the Hb concentration is lower than 10 g/100 ml blood a cjO_2 of 6-7 ml O_2/ 100 ml blood corresponds to a higher SjO_2 (e.g., if Hb concentration is 8 g/100 ml blood a cjO_2 of 7 ml O_2/100 ml blood corresponds to a SjO_2 of approximately 66%). Consequently, the anaerobic threshold of SjO_2 may depend on the actual Hb concentration, and it is more reasonable to measure cjO2 than SjO2, at least if the Hb concentration is not constant over the entire monitoring period.

Technology

Cerebral venous blood samples are usually obtained by inserting catheters into the jugular bulb via a single retrograde puncture of the internal jugular vein. The catheter is introduced by a modified Seldinger technique over a guidewire. The blood sample must be analyzed with a co-oximeter for the determination of SjO_2 and cjO_2 [15]. A pressure flush system (isotonic saline at a flow of 3 ml/h) connected to the catheter inhibits catheter obstruction by clotted blood.

The most-recent technology of SjO_2 monitoring is based on reflection spectrophotometry and allows continuous recording of SjO_2[16]. Modern catheters are 4 F in diameter and consist of fiberoptic elements that transmit light of three different wavelengths (670, 700, and 800 nm) to the tip of the catheter at 1-ms intervals. These three wavelengths of light are absorbed, reflected, and refracted to a distinct degree by oxygenated or reduced Hb molecules. The accuracy of catheter reflection spectrophotometry has been studied by comparing catheter measuring results in vivo with laboratory transmission spectrophotometry [17]. An excellent correlation between the two techniques could be demonstrated [17]. Clinical studies on the reliability of jugular bulb reflection spectrophotometry catheters (three-wavelength systems) for monitoring of SjO_2 have been performed during long-term use (mean duration of monitoring 4.5 days) in patients suffering from severe head injury, as well as during the intraoperative period in patients undergoing cardiac surgery under cardiopulmonary bypass [16, 18]. An excellent agreement (limits of agreement –4.6% to 5.8%, confidence interval of bias 0.38%-1.8%) and a highly significant correlation ($r=0.91$, $P< 0.001$) between SjO_2 measurements with a co-oximeter and with reflection spectrophotometry catheters have been found [16]. However, after 12 h of monitoring, the limits of agreement increased approximately twofold [16]. It has therefore been recommended that this catheter should be recalibrated twice per day [16].

Modern reflection spectrophotometry oximeters are equipped with a signal quality indicator consisting of a digital signal filter that permits the detection of wall artefacts. It is most obvious that the signal quality has to be checked regularly during SjO_2 recording. It is the opinion of some clinicians that one of the greatest problems with SjO_2 monitoring is the high rate of drop out time because of a bad signal quality. However, if a sheath introducer is used, the catheter may be repositioned if a bad signal quality is detected [13]. A moderate-to-good signal quality may then be obtained in up to 80% of the total monitoring period [18]. Sheath introducers are coated with an antimicrobial and heparin-containing layer and are 4.5 F in diameter. In critically ill patients, the maximum time periods of successful SjO_2 monitoring were in the range of 5-10 days [13, 19].

Like any other invasive instrument, the SjO_2 monitoring catheter must be inserted using an aseptic technique. The patient is either in a flat position, or the head and upper body are elevated up to 30°, depending on intracranial pressure. In order to identify the internal jugular vein, the carotid artery is palpated at the level of the inferior edge of the thyroid cartilage, or slightly more caudal [15]. Lateral to the carotid artery, a 21-guage needle with a syringe filled with isotonic saline is advanced in a 30-45° angle towards the ipsilateral external auditory canal. The aspiration of jugular venous blood should be possible within 4 cm from the skin. The sheath introducer is then introduced using a Seldinger technique. After suturing the introducer to the skin, the SjO_2 monitoring catheter is inserted through the introducer with or without preceding in vitro calibration. At a distance of approximately 14-15 cm in adults a resistance may be felt, indicating that the tip of the catheter has reached the base of the skull. Finally, the exact position of the catheter has to be confirmed by a lateral skull and neck X-ray. On the X-ray, the tip of the catheter must be projected at the lower edge of C1. If the catheter is in correct position, no danger arises from venous obstruction by the catheter with regard to increases in intracranial pressure, either in adults or in children [20]. An important question regarding the insertion technique of SjO_2 catheters is the choice of the left or right side for monitoring. Probably, the most-logical approach to solve this problem is to use the following algorithm [16]. The side of predominant cerebral venous drainage is determined by elevating the patient's upper body to 10-15° with the head in mid-position, if it has not been elevated before as part of the intracranial hypertension treatment regimen. Then the internal jugular veins are manually compressed on each side and the maximum increase in intracranial pressure is noted. The side of the greater increase in intracranial pressure is chosen for SjO_2 monitoring. If the increase in intracranial pressure due to manual compression of the internal jugular vein is equal on both sides, the side showing the predominant pathology on the computer tomography scan is chosen. In case of a diffuse injury, the right side is chosen. This procedure might be superior to others, such as simply choosing the right side, or always choosing the side of the predominant lesion [15].

Clinical applications

Continuous monitoring of SjO_2 has been studied in patients suffering from head trauma in order to test its ability for early detection of maloxygenation during intensive care [13]. Further, the effects of various standard treatment regimens in head-injured patients on SjO_2 have been investigated [14, 21]. Different clinical studies on head-injured patients have revealed very similar causes and frequencies of jugular bulb desaturation episodes during intensive care [13, 14, 19]. In a large series of patients (n=189), it has been found that a decrease in SjO_2 below 50% (i.e., a desaturation episode) occurs in approximately 30%-50% of patients presenting with a Glasgow Coma Scale of 3-5 after severe open or closed head injury [14]. Arterial hypotension was associated with a desaturation episode in 31.2%, hypocapnia in 29.5%, intracranial hypertension in 27.7%, hypoxia in 8.0%, anaemia in 1.8%, and seizures in 1.8% [14]. In another study in 25 head-injured patients with a Glasgow Coma Scale ≤8, desaturation episodes were associated with hypocapnia (arterial carbon dioxide tension of 22-34 mmHg) in 45%, low cerebral perfusion pressure (CPP=mean arterial pressure-intracranial pressure) without an increase in intracranial pressure in 22%, intracranial hypertension without a decrease in mean arterial pressure in 9%, arterial hypotension and intracranial hypertension in 5%, and a combination of low CPP, hypocapnia, intracranial hypertension, or arterial hypotension in 24% [22]. The treatment protocol was not different among these patients, and desaturation episodes were observed in 72% of all patients [22]. However, in this study, desaturation episodes were more strictly defined as a decrease in SjO_2 below 55% instead of a decrease below 50% [22]. A further study in ten adults with severe closed head injury revealed almost identical reasons and frequencies of jugular bulb desaturation, which was defined as a decrease in SjO_2 below 55% [19]. Hypocapnia (arterial carbon dioxide tension below 30 mmHg) was related to 50%, low CPP to 21%, intracranial hypertension to 7%, and a combination of these events to 22% of all observed desaturation episodes [19]. It is remarkable that jugular bulb desaturation episodes occurred in all of these studies, although the treatment protocols were actually aimed at avoiding hyperventilation, a decrease in CPP, and intracranial hypertension [14, 19, 22]. The conclusion that may be derived is that the intensivist must be even more alert to maintain these variables within the desired range during clinical routine.

Monitoring of SjO_2 has also been performed in patients after non-traumatic intracerebral or subarachnoid haemorrhage [13]. It has been found that patients suffering from intracerebral haemorrhage are most likely to experience a jugular bulb desaturation episode during intensive care, i.e., 93% of such patients will suffer at least one desaturation episode [13]. A very high rate of jugular bulb desaturation episodes (91%) has also been observed in patients after subarachnoid haemorrhage compared to head-injured patients in whom such events occurred in only 50% [13].

In critically ill patients, abnormally high values of SjO_2 may sometimes be observed. This has commonly been interpreted as absolute or relative hyperaemia due to a pathological reaction of CBF regulatory mechanisms. However, high values of SjO_2 may sometimes be related to pathological increases in cerebral lactate production, as indicated by an increase in the LOI [11, 4]. In a large study in 450 severely head-injured patients, SjO_2 was ≥75% in 19.1% of all patients [4]. CBF was significantly increased, and $CMRO_2$ was significantly decreased compared with patients who showed an average SjO_2 of 74%-56%, or ≤55% [4]. Despite this state of apparent luxury perfusion neurological outcome was significantly worse in patients with a SjO_2 ≥75%, and a considerable proportion of these patients also showed an increased cerebral lactate production [4]. The explanation for this rather surprising result could be that head trauma may sometimes induce an uncoupling of CBF and $CMRO_2$ that may further contribute to intracranial hypertension on the basis of cerebral oedema. Increased cerebral lactate production could be the result of a failure of cerebral oxygen utilization, similar to a systemic oxygenation deficit that is seen in septic patients.

The question remains whether certain treatment protocols are able to reduce the incidence of desaturation episodes in critically ill patients suffering from severe head trauma. Indeed, it has been found that treatment protocols that are CBF targeted instead of intracranial pressure targeted may reduce the risk of jugular bulb desaturation by the factor 2.4 [14]. The CBF-targeted protocol included the maintenance of cerebral perfusion pressure >70 mmHg, arterial carbon dioxide tension at 35 mmHg, and mean arterial pressure >90 mmHg [14]. In contrast, the intracranial pressure-targeted protocol allowed the use of hyperventilation to an arterial carbon dioxide tension of 25-30 mmHg, and cerebral perfusion pressure was only increased if it decreased below 50 mmHg [14]. The incidence of jugular bulb desaturation episodes (defined as a decrease in SjO$_2$ <50%) was 30% in the group with the CBF-targeted protocol and 50.6% in the group with the intracranial pressure-targeted protocol [14]. However, in this study, neurological outcome was not improved by the CBF-targeted protocol [14]. The authors argue that the fact that jugular bulb desaturation was aggressively counteracted in both treatment protocols has probably offset any beneficial effect of the CBF-targeted protocol [14]. Nevertheless, the main conclusion of this study is that the maintenance of a higher CPP and the avoidance of hypocapnia have a positive effect on global cerebral oxygenation [14]. The deleterious effect of hyperventilation on SjO$_2$ has been confirmed in numerous other studies in head-injured patients, as well as in patients suffering from acute cerebrovascular disease or meningitis [21, 23, 24]. The reason for the observation that SjO$_2$ decreases with a decrease in arterial carbon dioxide tension has clearly been identified as a decrease in CBF [24]. Hyperventilation to an arterial carbon dioxide tension of less than 25 mmHg increases the risk of regional cerebral ischaemia after severe head injury by the factor 2.5 [24].

Monitoring of SjO$_2$ has further been applied to assess the effects of cardio-pulmonary bypass (CPB) on global cerebral oxygenation. Cerebral oxygen supply may be endangered by a number of factors associated with CPB, such as hypothermia and rewarming, hypotension, haemodilution, non-pulsatile flow pattern, acid base management, and microembolization. Mental disorders determined by neuropsychiatric testing occur in approximately 38%-40% of patients undergoing CPB procedures [25]. The incidence of cognitive dysfunction after CPB significantly correlated with SjO$_2$ (inversely), with the highest value of intraoperative AVDO$_2$, with preoperative psychometric scores, and with years of education [25]. We may therefore conclude that monitoring of SjO$_2$ during operations under CPB is useful, if it is possible to identify and avoid causes of jugular bulb desaturation. Several clinical studies have been performed to elucidate this important issue [26-30]. In order to avoid episodes of jugular bulb desaturation, it is of great interest during which phases of CPB surgery these episodes are most likely to happen. It has been demonstrated that almost all episodes of jugular bulb desaturation occur during the rewarming phase after deep, mild, or moderate hypothermia [26-30]. Obviously, the shift from a reduced CMRO$_2$ during hypothermia to normal normothermic values is a very vulnerable phase, during which the brain is most susceptible to the acquisition of an oxygen debt. The presence of an oxygen debt during rewarming on CPB has been confirmed by increases in cerebral lactate production, as expressed by pathological increases in LOI, VADL, AVDG, and LGI [26, 29]. A clear and significant relationship between the rewarming speed and the incidence of jugular bulb desaturation has been identified [26, 30]. It has to be pointed out that a rewarming speed of more than 0.3°C/min will result in a 30%

decrease in SjO_2 from the values obtained during hypothermia [30]. Since these values are usually in the range of 70%-80%, a rewarming speed >0.3°C/min is very likely to cause a decrease in SjO_2 below the anaerobic threshold of 50% [30]. A recent publication showed that in diabetic patients, $SjO2$ will decrease below 50% despite a rewarming speed <0.3±0.07°C/min (mean±standard deviation) and that disturbances in cognitive function cannot be avoided by reducing rewarming speed to 0.46±0.09°C/min (mean±standard deviation) [31]. However, in the latter study, the low rewarming speed group also had a rewarming speed that was very close to the threshold of 0.3°C/min [31]. We may therefore hypothesize that an even lower rewarming speed in diabetic patients would possibly prevent jugular bulb Hb desaturation. Apart from a high rewarming speed, arterial hypotension could be responsible for jugular bulb desaturation episodes during CPB. A significant relationship between decreases in mean arterial pressure during CPB and the incidence of jugular bulb desaturation has been demonstrated in several clinical studies [25, 26, 29]. A decrease in mean arterial pressure below 60 mmHg during rewarming on CPB, as well as during the initial normothermic phase of CPB, strongly correlates with a decrease in SjO_2 below 50% [25, 26]. In contrast, arterial hypotension is very well tolerated during the hypothermic phase of CPB, because CBF mainly depends on pump flow rate instead of mean arterial pressure [32, 33]. A low haematocrit is another characteristic of CPB that might contribute to jugular bulb desaturation. A decrease in haematocrit during CPB is usually caused by profound haemodilution due to the priming volume of heart-lung machines. Haemodilution has two well-known effects on tissue oxygen supply. Firstly, whole-blood viscosity decreases exponentially with decreasing haematocrit. This effect perhaps improves microcirculation, which could lead to an amelioration of tissue oxygenation by increasing the number of perfused capillaries and reducing the diffusion distances. Secondly, haemodilution causes a proportional decrease in caO_2. At a given CBF, a lower caO_2 will result in a decrease in cerebral DO_2. During CPB, CBF depends to a certain degree on the pump flow rate [33]. Therefore, a decrease in caO_2 during CPB may easily result in cerebral maloxygenation and a decrease in SjO_2. Indeed, an inverse relationship between haematocrit during CPB and SjO_2 has been observed [26]. Another important issue is the choice of acid-base management during hypothermic CPB. Alpha-stat acid-base management means that the arterial carbon dioxide tension is adjusted to normal values (35-45 mmHg) if it is determined at a temperature of 37°C, regardless of the patient's temperature. pH-stat acid-base management means that the arterial carbon dioxide tension is adjusted to normal values if it is determined at the actual body temperature of the patient. Since gas tensions decrease during hypothermia due to an increase in gas solubility, the alpha-stat management will result in lower arterial carbon dioxide tensions during hypothermia than the pH-stat management. We would therefore expect higher CBF and SjO$_2$ during hypothermia with the pH-stat management than with the alpha-stat management. This assumption has been verified in a clinical study on the relationship between arterial carbon dioxide tension and SjO$_2$ during CPB [26]. Hypercapnia might be effective to inhibit a pathological decrease in SjO2 during the rewarming period after hypothermic CPB, but it has not been beneficial during stable hypothermic CPB [26, 28]. In contrast, the use of an alpha-stat acid-base management during hypothermic CPB is associated with hyperemia and a significantly worse neurological outcome after CPB procedures [28]. Cerebral oxygen balance may not only be improved by increasing CBF and cerebral DO$_2$, but also by reducing CMRO$_2$. This hypothesis has been tested by reducing CMRO$_2$ by the administration of electroencephalographic burst suppression doses of propofol [29]. However, no differences in the incidence and severity of jugular bulb desaturation episodes were observed between the control group and the propofol group [29]. The authors of this study suggested that arterial hypotension, which was more frequently observed in the propofol group, was responsible for the lack of any beneficial effect of propofol on SjO$_2$ [29]. Neurological deficits after CPB may not only be caused by mismatches between CMRO$_2$ and global cerebral DO$_2$, but also by microemboli, either consisting of air bubbles or blood microclots. Microemboli may occlude small cerebral arteries or capillaries, thereby leading to focal cerebral ischaemia and infarction. However, it has been demonstrated that cerebral microembolization and microscopic focal ischaemia cannot be detected by monitoring of SjO$_2$, because such small ischaemic areas do not contribute enough to the total cerebral venous drainage [34].

Monitoring of SjO$_2$ has been used to study changes in global cerebral oxygenation after cardiopulmonary resuscitation (CPR). Since the brain is the most-vulnerable organ with regard to the development of anoxic necrosis, permanent neurological deficits are major determinants of outcome after successful CPR. In order to predict outcome, the brain's condition in survivors of circulatory arrest is the focus of the clinicians' interest. It could be shown that the difference between mixed venous oxygen content and cjO$_2$ may be used as a prognostic indicator of recovery from consciousness after CPR with a sensitivity of 95% and a specificity of 100% [35]. If mixed venous oxygen content is greater than cjO$_2$, patients will most likely recover from unconsciousness, whereas cjO$_2$ is smaller than mixed venous oxygen content in patients who are brain dead or in a vegetative state after CPR [35]. The pathophysiological explanation for this finding is that in patients with severe neurological deficits, large necrotic brain areas do not take up oxygen at all.

High values of SjO_2 and cjO_2 are observed because in such states, the majority of jugular venous blood consists of extracerebral admixture, or because the $CMRO_2$ of the remaining brain areas (i.e., the brain stem in case of a vegetative state) is lower than normal global $CMRO_2$. The latter may be interpreted as a pathological uncoupling of CBF and $CMRO_2$ after the anoxic insult. Another interesting phenomenon has been elucidated with jugular bulb catheterization in patients during CPR [36]. Despite the fact that cerebral lactate production is increased during CPR due to anaerobic metabolism, the brain extracts even more lactate from the systemic circulation, which might be explained by cerebral lactate utilization under conditions of cerebral ischaemia, hypoxia, or lactic acidosis, or by diffusion of unionized lactate into the brain [36].

Limitations and frequent problems

The major limitation of SjO_2 monitoring is the fact that regional disorders of cerebral oxygenation may not be detected. This has been demonstrated for very small, but multiple areas of ischaemia arising from microembolization during transmyocardial laser revascularization [34]. It could further be shown that computer tomography confirmed cerebral infarction occurring during the course of severe head injury is not reflected by decreases in SjO_2, but may be detected by monitoring of $PtiO_2$ [37]. However, it has to be noted that the exclusive use of $PtiO_2$ monitoring may show a similar poor sensitivity for detecting focal cerebral anoxia, particularly if it is placed in an area outside the ischaemic insult [37].

The possibility of side differences in SjO_2 between the right and the left jugular bulb is frequently the subject of debate among clinicians using this monitoring technique. The correct choice of the left or right side for monitoring is probably of great importance, because clinically relevant differences in SjO_2 between the two sides have been demonstrated [38]. In more than 55% of head-injured patients, the difference in SjO_2 between the right and the left jugular bulb was greater than 10%, and in only 25% was it less than 5% [38]. In order to eliminate a bias of the true value of SjO_2, a special algorithm has been suggested to identify the side of predominant cerebral venous drainage [16].

A further problem of SjO_2 monitoring is the unknown amount of admixture of extracerebral venous blood to the cerebral venous drainage in the jugular bulb. Although the fraction of extracerebral venous admixture is probably insignificant under normal conditions, it is possible that strong deviations from this assumption are present during various pathophysiological states. The amount of extracerebral admixture may be considerably increased in cases of a decreased CBF. During cerebral herniation, very high values of SjO$_2$ may sometimes be observed, which is often interpreted as a result of a decrease in CMRO$_2$ due to severe anoxia. However, abnormally high values that are observed during cerebral infarction are probably caused by a significant increase in the proportion of extracerebral admixture to the decreasing cerebral venous drainage. Venous blood of bones, muscles, or skin that may contaminate cerebral venous blood has a high oxygen content, because of a low oxygen consumption of these tissues compared with the brain. It has further been demonstrated that the rate of blood withdrawal affects SjO$_2$ [39]. Withdrawal rates greater than 2 ml/min revealed significantly higher values of SjO$_2$, which is possibly the result of an increased proportion of extracerebral admixture [39]. Particular attention should be paid to the correct aspiration of blood from the jugular bulb for calibrating the oximetry catheter.

Complications related to puncturing of the internal jugular vein and to long-time catheter placement are rare and similar to complications arising from central venous catheterization [15]. Typical complications associated with puncturing are inadvertent carotid artery puncture occurring in approximately 3%, haematoma occurring in 2%, or infection of the catheter occurring in up to 10% [15, 40].

References

1. Hoffman WE, Charbel FT, Ausman JI (1997) Cerebral blood flow and metabolic response to etomidate and ischemia. Neurol Res 19:41-44
2. Cold GE (1978) Cerebral metabolic rate of oxygen (CMRO2) in the acute phase of brain injury. Acta Anaesthesiol Scand 22:249-256
3. Michenfelder JD, Milde JH (1992) The effect of profound levels of hypothermia (below 14 degrees C) on canine cerebral metabolism. J Cereb Blood Flow Metab 12:877-880
4. Cormio M, Valadka AB, Robertson CS (1999) Elevated jugular venous oxygen saturation after severe head injury. J Neurosurg 90:9-15
5. Katsura K, Folbergrova J, Gido G, Siesjo BK (1994) Functional, metabolic, and circulatory changes associated with seizure activity in the postischemic brain. J Neurochem 62:1511-1515
6. Larsen FS, Ejlersen E, Strauss G, et al (1999) Cerebrovascular metabolic autoregulation is impaired during liver transplantation. Transplantation 68:1472-1476
7. Olsen KS, Henriksen L, Owen-Falkenberg A, et al (1994) Effect of 1 or 2 MAC isoflurane with or without ketanserin on cerebral blood flow autoregulation in man. Br J Anaesth 72:66-71
8. Cohen JP, Wollman H, Alexander SC, et al (1964) Cerebral carbohydrate metabolism in man during halothane anesthesia. Anesthesiology 25:185-191
9. Gibbs EL, Lennox WG, Nims LF, Gibbs FA (1942) Arterial and cerebral venous blood. Arterial-venous differences in man. J Biol Chem 144:325-332
10. Goodman JC, Valadka AB, Gopinath SP (1999) Extracellular lactate and glucose alterations in the brain after head injury measured by microdialysis. Crit Care Med 27:1965-1973
11. Robertson CS, Narayan RK, Gokaslan ZL, et al (1989) Cerebral arteriovenous oxygen difference as an estimate of cerebral blood flow in comatose patients. J Neurosurg 70:222-230

12. Sapire KJ, Gopinath SP, Farhat G, et al (1997) Cerebral oxygenation during warming after cardiopulmonary bypass. Crit Care Med 25:1655-1662

13. Schneider GH, v. Helden A, Lanksch WR, Unterberg A (1995) Continuous monitoring of jugular bulb oxygen saturation in comatose patients – therapeutic implications. Acta Neurochir (Wien) 134:71-75

14. Robertson CS, Valadka AB, Hannay HJ, et al (1999) Prevention of secondary ischemic insults after severe head injury. Crit Care Med 27:2086-2095

15. Goetting MG, Preston G (1990) Jugular bulb catheterization: experience with 123 patients. Crit Care Med 18:1220-1223

16. Andrews PJD, Dearden NM, Miller JD (1991) Jugular bulb cannulation: description of a cannulation technique and validation of a new continuous monitor. Br J Anaesth 67:553-558

17. Reinhart K, Moser N, Rudolph T, et al (1988) Accuracy of two mixed venous saturation catheters during long-term use in critically ill patients. Anesthesiology 69:769-773

18. Nakajima T, Ohsumi H, Kuro M (1993) Accuracy of continuous jugular bulb venous oximetry during cardiopulmonary bypass. Anesth Analg 77:1111-1115

19. Lewis SB, Myburgh JA, Thornton EL, Reilly PL (1996) Cerebral oxygenation monitoring by near-infrared spectroscopy is not clinically useful in patients with jugular venous bulb oximetry. Crit Care Med 24:1334-1338

20. Goetting MG, Preston G (1991) Jugular bulb catheterization does not increase intracranial pressure. Intensive Care Med 17:195-198

21. Thiagarajan A, Goverdhan PD, Chari P, Somasunderam K (1998) The effect of hyperventilation and hyperoxia on cerebral venous oxygen saturation in patients with traumatic brain injury. Anesth Analg 87:850-853

22. Lewis SB, Myburgh JA, Reilly PL (1995) Detection of cerebral venous desaturation by continuous jugular bulb oximetry following acute neurotrauma. Anaesth Intensive Care 23:307-314

23. Tateishi A, Maekawa T, Soejima Y, et al (1995) Qualitative comparison of carbon dioxide-induced change in cerebral near-infrared spectroscopy versus jugular venous oxygen saturation in adults with acute brain disease. Crit Care Med 23:1734-1738

24. Skippen P, Seear M, Poskitt K, et al (1997) Effect of hyperventilation on regional cerebral blood flow in head-injured children. Crit Care Med 25:1402-1409

25. Croughwell ND, Newman MF, Blumenthal JA, et al (1994) Jugular bulb saturation and cognitive dysfunction after cardiopulmonary bypass. Ann Thorac Surg 58:1702-1708

26. Sapire KJ, Gopinath SP, Farhat G, et al (1997) Cerebral oxygenation during warming after cardiopulmonary bypass. Crit Care Med 25:1655-1662

27. Hänel F, von Knobelsdorff G, Werner C, Schulte am Esch J (1998) Hypercapnia prevents jugular bulb desaturation during rewarming from hypothermic cardiopulmonary bypass. Anesthesiology 89:19-23

28. Patel RL, Turtle MR, Chambers DJ, et al (1996) Alpha-stat acid-base regulation during cardiopulmonary bypass improves neuropsychologic outcome in patients undergoing coronary artery bypass grafting. J Thorac Cardiovasc Surg 111:1267-1279

29. Souter MJ, Andrews PJD, Alston RP (1998) Propofol does not ameliorate cerebral venous oxyhemoglobin desaturation during hypothermic cardiopulmonary bypass. Anesth Analg 86:926-931

30. Nakajima T, Kuro M, Hayashi Y, et al (1992) Clinical evaluation of cerebral oxygen balance during cardiopulmonary bypass: on-line continuous monitoring of jugular venous oxyhemoglobin saturation. Anesth Analg 74:630-635

31. Kadoi Y, Saito S, Goto F, Fujita N (2002) Slow rewarming has no effects on the decrease in jugular venous oxygen hemoglobin saturation and long-term cognitive outcome in diabetic patients. Anesth Analg 94:1395-1401

32. Ellis RJ, Wisniewski A, Potts R, et al (1992) Reduction of flow rate and arterial pressure at moderate hypothermia does not result in cerebral dysfunction. J Thorac Cardiovasc Surg 103:549-554

33. Linden J van der, Priddy R, Ekroth R, et al (1991) Cerebral perfusion and metabolism during

profound hypothermia in children. A study of middle cerebral artery ultrasonic variables and cerebral extraction of oxygen. J Thorac Cardiovasc Surg 102:103-114

34. von Knobelsdorff G, Brauer P, Tonner PH, et al (1997) Transmyocardial laser revascularization induces cerebral microembolization. Anesthesiology 87:58-62

35. Zarzuelo R, Castaneda J (1995) Differences in oxygen content between mixed venous blood and cerebral venous blood for outcome prediction after cardiac arrest. Intensive Care Med 21:71-75

36. Rivers EP, Paradis NA, Martin GB, et al (1991) Cerebral lactate uptake during cardiopulmonary resuscitation in humans. J Cereb Blood Flow Metab 11:479-484

37. Gopinath SP, Valadka AB, Uzura M, Robertson CS (1999) Comparison of jugular venous oxygen saturation and brain tissue PO2 as monitors of cerebral ischemia after head injury. Crit Care Med 27:2337-2345

38. Stocchetti N, Paparella A, Bridelli F, et al (1994) Cerebral venous oxygen saturation studied with bilateral samples in the internal jugular veins. Neurosurgery 34:38-44

39. Matta BF, Lam AM (1997) The rate of blood withdrawal affects the accuracy of jugular venous bulb oxygen saturation measurements. Anesthesiology 86:806-808

40. Gayle MO, Frewen TC, Armstrong RF, et al (1989) Jugular venous bulb catheterization in infants and children. Crit Care Med 17:385-358

Intracranial and cerebral perfusion pressure management in traumatic brain injury

J.A. MYBURGH

Medicine exists to entertain doctors while nature cures the disease – Voltaire

Historical perspective

Advances in the understanding of the pathophysiology of traumatic brain injury have influenced clinical management. In 1783, the Monro-Kelly doctrine, outlining the asymptotic relationship between intracranial pressure (ICP) and volume was defined. The concept of exhausted intracranial elastant reserve is as valid today, particularly when reviewing past, current, and new therapies for traumatic brain injury.

Intracranial pressure

Fifty years ago, pioneering work by Guillaume and Janny [1] identified intra-cranial hypertension as the prime pathophysiological entity in traumatic head injury. In 1960, Lundberg [2] described continuous measurement and ventricular drainage in patients with head injury. So began an era of pioneering work that focussed on treatments aimed at the reduction of ICP. Treatments such as osmotherapy, hyperventilation, steroids, hypothermia, barbiturate coma, and decompressive craniectomy were applied with varying degrees of enthusiasm to heterogeneous groups of head-injured patients by clinicians. Despite these efforts, the all-cause mortality of traumatic brain injury remains distressingly high; the financial, social, and emotional impact of disabled survivors on the community is substantial.

Almost entirely, the efficacy and effectiveness of these treatments have not been subjected to scientific evaluation. There were, and continue to be, many valid and practical reasons for the lack of evidence-based treatment. The focus of researchers in traumatic brain injury has been directed at reproducible head injury models with definable primary outcomes. This resulted in intensive study of the cellular mechanisms of primary head injury, predominantly in animal models. Unfortunately, the translation of positive results from these phase II studies into clinical trials has not been forthcoming [3-5]. Essentially, there are many confounding variables in the clinical scenario that make conducting a randomized controlled trial of a clinical intervention (let alone a single neuro-modulating agent) analysing the outcome of traumatic brain injury logistically extremely difficult. These variables include case-mix variation between centres, assessment and standardization of the initial injury, controlling for the degree of secondary insult and lead time bias before appropriate resuscitation, degree of extracranial injuries, standardization of resuscitation, intensive care protocols, monitoring thresholds and operative interventions, and quantification of outcomes. Given the caseload of even the largest neurotrauma centres, multi-centred studies are required to adequately power such studies [6].

The Traumatic Coma Databank

Towards the end of the last millennium, a number of epidemiological studies highlighted marked differences in practices within and between major trauma centres in the developed world [7-9]. Despite these differences, mortality remained in excess of 30%, even in major specialist centres [10].

In 1993, data from the Traumatic Coma Databank (TCDB) highlighted the impact of secondary brain insults on outcome from traumatic brain injury [11, 12]. These insults were defined as any injury occurring after the primary injury and are characterized by a reduction in cerebral substrate utilization. They include hypoxia, hypotension, hypocapnia, abnormal deviations in temperature, osmolality and blood glucose. Indeed, raised ICP due to reversible causes may be regarded as a secondary insult. Importantly, most of these secondary insults, particularly systemic hypotension occurring at any stage from injury, from resuscitation through subsequent intrahospital stay were independently associated with increased mortality and worse functional outcome [12-14]. The data from the TCDB provided some of the most-compelling data to date about treatment and prevention options for traumatic brain injury.

Based on the TCDB data, many of the time-honoured "brain-specific" treatments have become increasingly questioned [15]. Whilst there may be a physiological or pharmacological basis for the efficacy of some of these treatments, the associated adverse systemic effects, particularly resultant hypotension, reduce the utility of these treatments, particularly when applied in a non-specific manner. For example, the empirical use of mannitol during resuscitation of head-injured patients is ubiquitous and is regarded as first-line treatment [16]. However, the associated diuresis, particularly when administered to patients with concomitant alcohol, may precipitate hypovolaemia and hyperosmolality, and potentiate hypotension in a polytraumatized patient. Subsequent fluid management is complicated, and the effects of the injudicious use of mannitol may last for several hours, often associated with secondary insults.

The Brain Trauma Foundation guidelines

In 1996 and 2000, the first and second editions of the Brain Trauma Foundation guidelines were published [17, 18]. Using evidence-based medicine principles, comprehensive reviews of 14 key areas of assessment and management of severe head injury were identified.

Standards

Of these areas, only three areas had sufficient class I evidence upon which to base evidence-based standards of practice. These standards applied to the role of hyperventilation, steroids, and seizure prophylaxis, recommending against the routine use of the first two and for a limited period (initial 10 days) for the third. These recommended standards have had little impact on overall practice. The use of hyperventilation and steroids had significantly decreased before the development of the Brian Trauma Foundation guidelines. This is a reflection of the paucity of class I evidence in clinical traumatic brain injury.

Guidelines

Guidelines, based on class II evidence, were developed for seven areas: recommendations for integrated trauma systems, indications for brain-specific resuscitation, ICP monitoring [including computed tomography (CT) classification of injury], thresholds and treatment of ICP, nutritional support, and critical pathways. Essentially, these guidelines emphasized the need for rigorous and prompt resuscitation, early quantification of injury using standardised Glasgow Coma Scores and CT classifications and "good" intensive care. The importance of maintenance of systemic and cerebral perfusion pressures was emphasized and the use of "brain-specific" treatments was recommended within this context. Cerebral perfusion pressures (CPPs) of >70mmHg were advocated, and thus a change in emphasis from reducing ICP to increasing CCP was mandated. These guidelines have direct application to the management of the head-injured patient, primarily in the initial phases of management – i.e., from time of injury, through resuscitation and into the initial period in intensive care.

Options

Treatment options, based on class III evidence, were developed for the following areas: osmotherapy, barbiturate coma, chronic hyperventilation, decompressive craniectomy, and hypothermia. It appeared that the Brain Trauma Foundation initiatives fell short of providing evidence-based instruction for the patient with refractory intracranial hypertension further down the time course after injury. Consequently, ICP-based treatments became less-important and CCP-based treatments were advocated.

ICP versus CPP treatments

Based on the Brain Trauma Foundation guidelines, management strategies for traumatic brain injury have therefore undergone a paradigm shift.

ICP treatments

ICP-based treatments have focussed on maintaining an ICP < 20 mmHg at all stages of management [19]. The use of "ICP-specific" treatments include mechanical methods, such as drainage of cerebrospinal fluid and decompressive craniectomy. Medical therapies include osmotherapy, hyperventilation, barbiturate coma, hypothermia, neuromuscular blockade, and cerebral volume regulation. The evidence for the use of all of these strategies is lacking [20]. However, a reasonable physiological rationale exists for the use of some if not all of these treatments in specific situations.

The Monro Kelly doctrine states that, due to the non-compliant skull and dura, small increases in intracranial volume result in sharp increases in ICP (Fig. 1). Applying the doctrine clinically would suggest that therapies or strategies directed at reducing intracranial volume would be most effective. To this aim, supratentorial drainage of cerebrospinal fluid remains the most-effective method of reducing intracranial volume and thereby ICP. For this reason, transduction of external ventricular drainage is recommended as the method of choice for measuring ICP [21].

Changing the elastant relationship within the cranial vault by decompressive craniectomy is another effective method of reducing ICP. Whilst this has been a surgical option for many years, it has been invariably applied as a late manoeuvre in patients with refractory intracranial hypertension. Outcomes have varied, although the role of early decompressive craniectomy in patients at risk of developing intracranial hypertension has increased and is currently the subject of renewed study [22-24].

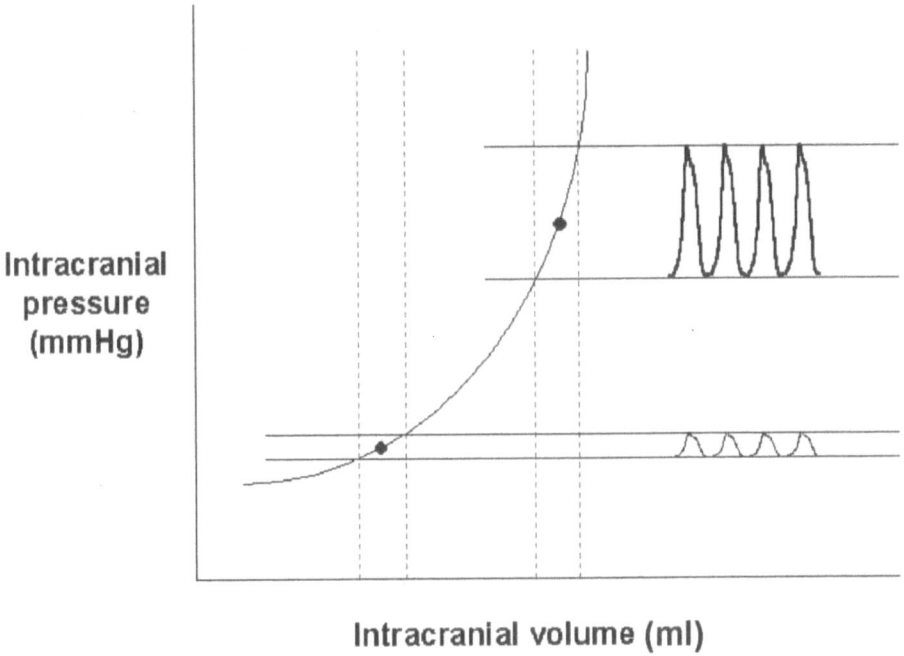

Intracranial
pressure
(mmHg)

Intracranial volume (ml)

Fig. 1 Conceptual relationship between intracranial pressure and intracranial volume

The principles of cerebral volume regulation for intracranial hypertension are based on the hypothesis that traumatic cerebral oedema is related to alteration in the Starling forces of the brain [25]. This strategy is directed at reducing cerebral hydrostatic pressure. This is achieved by reducing mean arterial pressure, using antihypertensive agents such as clonidine and metoprolol, and increasing vascular tone with dihydroergotamine. Preliminary studies of this technique (cerebral volume regulation or "Lund therapy") have demonstrated significant reductions in ICP without compromising cerebral blood flow [26]. Importantly, this strategy is commenced after initial resuscitation is complete and the patient stabilized. To date, there are no definitive outcome studies [27].

On the basis of current evidence, the use of chronic hyperventilation is not recommended for the treatment or prevention of raised ICP. Whilst hypocapnia is the most-effective medical method for reducing ICP, it is invariably associated with cerebral tissue ischaemia and hypoxia. However, advocates of "optimized hyperventilation" directed at reducing or minimizing cerebral hyperaemia claim that hyperventilation is an effective method for controlling ICP. Cruz [28] published a longitudinal series of patients (n=178) in whom "optimized" hyperventilation, titrated to derived parameters measured from jugular bulb oximetry, resulted in a significant reduction in overall mortality compared with a historically matched cohort. Due to significant methodological limitations of this series, the conclusion from this study that this management strategy results in better outcomes than when CPP is managed requires some circumspection [29].

CPP treatments

CPP-based treatments focus on maintaining a CPP >70mmHg at all stages. CPP (calculated as the difference between mean arterial pressure and ICP) may be maintained equally by augmenting mean arterial pressure, whilst reducing or controlling ICP. However, most CPP-based algorithms are directed at augmentation of mean arterial pressure. This includes the early and liberal use of inotropes (such as adrenaline, noradrenaline, and dopamine), vasopressors (such as phenylephrine or metaraminol), induced normo- or hypervolaemia, normocapnia, and nursing the patient flat [30].

Although this approach was regarded by some as novel, the principle of CPP-based treatment has been around for some time. Rosner et al. [31] described their practice of aggressive augmentation of CPP in a longitudinal series of 93 patients in whom CPP was maintained >90 mmHg by infusions of noradrenaline or phenylephrine. These patients were compared with a historical cohort of similar patients. Lower mean ICPs (determined by quadratic logarithm analysis) and improved Glasgow Outcome Scores in the CPP group were demonstrated. However, these results should be interpreted with some caution due to the intervention bias and weak comparative methodology. Nevertheless, this non-randomized, retrospective study indicated a potential role for CPP-based treatment in traumatic brain injury without demonstrably adverse effects on ICP.

Importantly, a targeted CPP threshold of 70 mmHg using the strategies outlined above may artefactually increase ICP. Consequently, thresholds for "acceptable" ICP using CPP-based therapies have increased to 20 – 30 mmHg [19]. However, the distinction between actual intracranial hypertension due to cerebral oedema and raised ICP due to medical therapies remains difficult.

Comparative studies

An attempt to determine whether there was a true difference in outcome between CPP- and ICP-based treatment strategies was attempted by Robertson et al. [32]. In this study, two groups of patients (n=189) with severe head injury (defined as a motor component of the Glasgow Coma Score within 48 h) were randomized (in a block randomization fashion) to receive either CPP- or ICP--based treatment. The principle difference between the two groups related to prescribed targets of mean arterial pressure (>90 vs. >70 mmHg), CPP (>70 vs. >50 mmHg), arterial carbon dioxide tension (35-40 vs. 25-30 mmHg), and pulmonary artery occlusion pressure (15 vs. 10 mmHg). The study was underpowered to determine differences in outcome (defined by Glasgow Outcome Score), and primary endpoints were adjusted to determine the incidence of secondary insults (defined as episodes of sustained jugular venous desaturation <50%). CPP was maintained at significantly higher levels in the CPP group. There was no statistically significant difference in mean ICP; nor was there a difference in the incidence of refractory intracranial hypertension between the groups. The frequency and duration of episodes of jugular venous desaturation was significantly lower in the CPP group. Whilst there was no difference in the incidence of delayed intracranial haematomas between the groups, there was a higher incidence of pulmonary oedema [attributed to acute respiratory distress syndrome (ARDS)] in the CPP group. No differences in 6-month Glasgow Outcome Scores were demonstrated. This study concluded that secondary ischaemic insults caused by systemic factors after severe head injury were prevented with a targeted CPP-based management protocol.

Although no benefit in outcome was demonstrated, potential adverse effects of this management strategy, i.e., "ARDS," may offset these beneficial effects. Although this study had major methodological flaws, the conclusions were interesting in drawing attention to the potential adverse effects. Whilst the cause of "ARDS" was probably due to fluid overload caused by aggressive fluid loading to achieve a target pulmonary artery occlusion pressure, this highlights one of the pitfalls of protocol-driven treatment strategies. Indeed, this conclusion is concordant with anecdotal reports of patients receiving very large doses of inotropes to achieve prescribed CPPs. This is particularly alarming if this occurs in patients with underlying cardiac or renal disease.

Clearly, it is difficult to prove whether there is any difference between CPP- and ICP-based treatment strategies. In fact, attempting to show such a difference is focussing on the wrong priority. It appears that although the current emphasis on CPP is valid and stems from the best (albeit limited) published evidence to date, reduction of ICP is an equally important factor.

Targeted therapy revisited

As outlined above, the absence of evidence-based strategies reduces the treatment options available to clinicians to an "intention-to-treat" approach. Clearly aspects of ICP-based treatments are required and are appropriate, as is the maintenance of CPP. An appraisal of current treatment strategies therefore requires a reapplication of basic principles. These include a revision of principles of physiological measurement, pathophysiological processes, and integration of these factors to the clinical situation.

Measurement of ICP

The physiological basis of treatment of traumatic brain injury has focussed on ICPs and elastance. This may in part represent the historical developments outlined, but also underscores the limitations of physiological measurement in clinical practice.

Measurement of ICP is predicated on the principle that raised ICP is the fundamental pathological process in head injury, and that reducing the "number" will result in better outcomes. ICP is also used as a surrogate index of cerebral blood flow. Unfortunately, neither of these tenets have been proven.

Firstly, accuracy of measurement is critical. This requires a system that is stable over time and may be zero-calibrated. The development of solid-state intraparenchymal systems (e.g., strain gauge Codman of fibreoptic Camino systems) has facilitated the (bedside) insertion of ICP monitors. Although high-fidelity waveforms are produced, these systems cannot be calibrated once inserted and are subject to significant drift after 5 days. Furthermore, the ability to drain cerebrospinal fluid is lost if these systems are used exclusively. For these reasons, ventricular drainage remains the optimal and recommended method of ICP monitoring [21].

Secondly, ICP must be interpreted within the clinical context. The concomitant use of catecholamines to augment CPP may artefactually increase ICP; surges in ICP may result from sympathetic swings and fluctuation in sedation levels. Simply prescribing and treating a number is simplistic and potentially dangerous. Changes in trends of ICP should be interpreted rather than absolute values. These changes should also be assessed in accordance with associated CT scan images.

Thirdly, the reliance of ICP monitoring to reflect cerebral blood flow has been predicated on the premise that cerebral blood flow will be maintained at a constant rate in the presence of changing CPP (cerebral autoregulation). This is an outdated hypothesis and has been invalidated with the recognition of the vulnerability of the cerebral circulation to hypotension. The inability to measure cerebral blood flow at the bedside has been a major factor in using ICP monitoring as a surrogate measurement. Labour-intensive techniques such as Xe^{133} measurements and laser flowmetry remain the domain of selected research centres. Indirect measurements such as transcranial Doppler and jugular venous oximetry have broader utilization, but have limitations [33]. A generally applicable, calibrated, bedside cerebral blood flow monitor remains elusive.

Cerebral blood flow/perfusion pressure relationships

Despite inadequacies and limitations of routine, bedside clinical measurement of cerebral blood flow, changes in cerebral blood flow following traumatic brain injury are increasingly recognized as important determinants in the pathophysiological process.

Traumatic brain injury is associated with disruption of cerebral autoregulation, in particular myogenic (pressure) autoregulation [34]. Over a range of systemic blood pressures, cerebral blood flow is linearly dependent. Although cerebral hypoperfusion associated with systemic hypotension is well recognized, cerebral hyperaemia associated with increased systemic blood pressures probably occurs equally as often (Fig. 2). These theoretical zones of hypoperfusion and hyperaemia are the clinically relevant zones where secondary brain injury may potentially occur [35, 36].

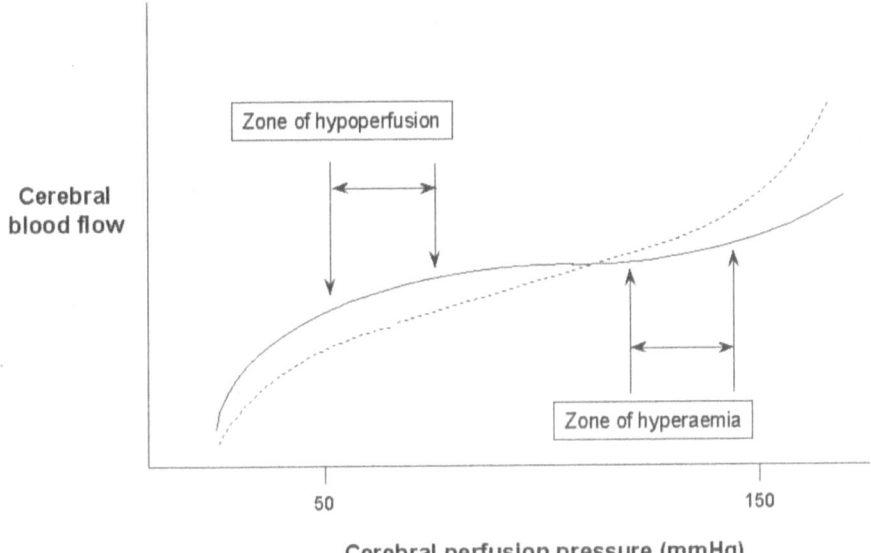

Fig. 2 Conceptual relationship between cerebral blood flow and cerebral perfusion pressure. *Solid line* represents normal physiological relationship; *dashed line* represented altered autoregulation following traumatic brain injury

Cerebral blood flow/perfusion pressure relationships change over time. These may be due to absolute changes in cerebral blood flow induced by the head injury and due to recovery of cerebral autoregulatory function.

Abnormal patterns of cerebral blood flow occur at various time intervals following injury. In a seminal article, Bouma et al. [37] described changes in cerebral blood flow in the first 48 h following traumatic brain injury in a cohort of 186 patients. Cerebral blood flow, measured using Xe^{133}, was significantly reduced in the initial 12 h following injury and associated with cerebral ischaemia, measured by transcranial Doppler. This phenomenon was independent of systemic hypotension and attributed to the primary injury.

The concept of mapping cerebral blood flow over time following injury was explored further by Martin et al. [36]. Using a similar technique to Bouma et al. [37], phases in cerebral blood flow and associated degree of ischaemia were determined from time of injury to 15 days post injury in a series of 313 patients. Three distinct phases of cerebral blood flow were identified (Fig. 3).

An initial period of hypoperfusion, essentially similar to the patterns identified by Bouma et al. [37], was detected in the majority of patients in the first 24 h. A subset of patients developed a consequent phase of cerebral hyperaemia up to 5 days post injury, with a nadir of hyperaemia occurring at 72 h. Thereafter,

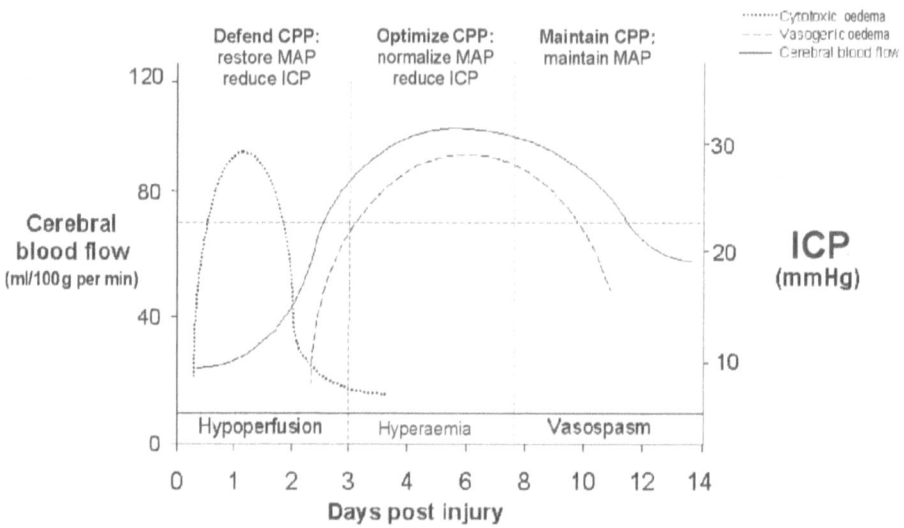

Fig. 3 Conceptual changes in cerebral blood flow and intracranial pressure (*ICP*) over time following traumatic brain injury (*CPP* cerebral perfusion pressure, *MAP* mean arterial pressure)

a syndrome of normal to low cerebral blood flow-associated vasospastic transcranial Doppler patterns was identified in a further subset, suggestive of prolonged cerebral vasospasm.

A pathological basis exists for each of these phases, which may explain associated changes in ICP and may provide a platform upon which to target appropriate therapies.

"Time-based" targeted therapy

Applying the principles outlined by Bouma et al. [37] and Martin et al. [36] and integrating the physiological basis of ICP- and CPP-based therapies, a novel approach based on evolution of the injury may be developed.

The hypoperfusion phase (0 – 72 h)

Pathological process

Cerebral blood flow is reduced in the first 72 h following injury, with resultant global and regional ischaemia. Intrinsic mechanisms for this process include neurohumoral vasoconstriction, intravascular thrombosis, extrinsic microvascular compression due to glial swelling, mass lesion, and traumatic subarachnoid haemorrhage [36, 37]. Extrinsic mechanisms include extracranial injuries, associated hypovolaemia, and iatrogenic factors, such as the injudicious use of mannitol or hyperventilation. During this phase, myogenic autoregulation is markedly impaired and cerebral blood flow is essentially directly dependent on systemic blood pressure. Resultant neuronal ischaemia may result in "cytotoxic" cerebral oedema with associated increased ICP.

Potential secondary insults

During this phase, the patient is most vulnerable to a number of life-threatening insults. These must be constantly and promptly sought for, assessed, and corrected. These insults include absolute hypotension (recognizing that hypertensive patients may be "hypotensive" with normal blood pressures), hypoxia from any cause, hypovolaemia, ventilator-induced hypocapnia, delay in CT scan, and detection of evacuable mass lesions. Surgery for non-life- or non-limb-threatening injuries is associated with secondary hypoxic and hypotensive insults [38,39].

Targeted therapy

The principles outlined in the Brain Trauma Foundation guidelines essentially apply to this phase. Treatment is focussed around the maintenance of adequate systemic blood pressure. This includes prompt resuscitation, accurate measurement of systemic blood pressure, and where indicated ICP. Once ICP monitoring is in place, systemic blood pressure must be assiduously maintained during this phase, so that CPP is maintained ≥70 mmHg.

Control of ICP is directed at maintaining adequate CPP, with the assumption that restoration of cerebral perfusion to the ischaemic brain will result in improvement in cytotoxic oedema. Drainage of cerebrospinal fluid and prompt evacuation of mass lesions are the most-effective methods of reducing ICP during this period.

During this phase, medical therapies directed at raised ICP such as osmotherapy or hyperventilation should only be used if CPP is maintained at an appropriate level and the patient is adequately monitored.

Jugular bulb oximetry may have a limited role in this phase. Jugular venous desaturations (<50-55%) most probably represent cerebral oligaemia, and the prevention of these episodes is associated with improved outcomes [32,40].

Extracranial surgery should be limited to life- or limb-threatening injuries only. This includes fixation of closed long bone fractures until the patient is stabilized. Patients undergoing prolonged early surgery should have ICP or jugular bulb oximetry in situ.

Assessment of adequacy of the response to augmentation of CPP is made by ICP trends, CT scan appearance, and where possible, neurological assessment.

The hyperaemic phase (3-7 days)

Pathological process

The development of cerebral hyperaemia represents two processes. Firstly, this may be the clinical expression of an ischaemia-reperfusion injury mediated through inflammatory mediators. This is associated with cellular hyperglycolysis, vasoplegia and absolute increases in cerebral blood flow (>55 ml/100g per min). This has been described in 20%-32% of patients [36].

Secondly, autoregulatory recovery begins during this period and the effects of associated therapies directed at augmenting cerebral blood flow/perfusion pressure may result in an "iatrogenic" hyperaemia. These include catecholamines (adrenaline, noradrenaline, and dopamine), mannitol and post-hypocapnic vasodilation (in patients receiving hyperventilation). Hyperaemia may result in raised ICP due to vasogenic cerebral oedema.

Potential secondary insults

These relate primarily to the iatrogenic factors outlined above. However, another important source of "hyperaemia" may be due to baseline drift of ICP measured by non-zero calibration monitors.

Targeted therapy

The diagnosis of cerebral hyperaemia is difficult. These patients are characterized by those who develop progressive intracranial hypertension after 3 days. Initial strategy is directed at ensuring accurate measurement of ICP and quantifying parenchymal changes on CT appearance.

Catecholamine-induced hyperaemia should be suspected in patients who require progressively increasing doses of catecholamines (e.g., >40 µg/min of adrenaline or noradrenaline) to attain a prescribed CPP of 70 mmHg. This phenomenon is due to tachyphylaxis to prolonged catecholamine infusions and may be responsible for iatrogenically increasing ICP. If CT appearance is unchanged, CPP targets may be lowered (50-60 mmHg) in order to use lower doses of inotropes. This exercise may be facilitated by jugular venous saturation monitoring or transcranial Doppler to provide an index of adequate cerebral blood flow for the lower CPP. Whilst the incidence and frequency of jugular venous desaturation is associated with adverse outcomes, so too have high jugular venous saturations. These data suggest that hyperaemia is a potentially preventable secondary insult [41].

If patients continue to have raised ICP, strategies directed at reducing ICP should be considered. In this context, "anti-hyperaemic" strategies such as cerebral volume regulation ("Lund" therapy), early decompressive craniectomy, low-dose barbiturates, and possibly "optimized" hyperventilation or hypothermia may have potential, effective roles.

The vasospastic phase

In a small cohort of patients (10%-15%), particularly those with severe primary and secondary injuries or those with significant traumatic subarachnoid haemorrhage, a vasospastic phase characterized by typical cerebral blood flow patterns may persist. This phase represents a complex of cerebral hypoperfusion due to arterial vasospasm, post-traumatic hypometabolism, and impaired autoregulation [36].

Cerebral angiography and transcranial Doppler are frequently used to diagnose vasospasm, although false positives and negatives exist with both techniques, and the true incidence of clinically significant vasospasm is uncertain [42].

Treatment options remain limited. Calcium antagonists, such as nimodipine, have not been shown to be effective in traumatic subarachnoid haemorrhage [43]. Strategies that have been used in aneurysmal subarachnoid haemorrhage such as "triple H" therapy (induced hypertension, hypervolaemia, and haemodilution) or chemical angioplasty have not been evaluated in traumatic subarachnoid haemorrhage and are not recommended.

Conclusion

The management of traumatic brain injury remains difficult. Unfortunately, significant improvements in outcomes in patients who reach hospital are unlikely to be demonstrated, as this is largely determined by the severity of the primary injury. The initiatives of the Traumatic Coma Databank and Brain Trauma Foundation have focussed our attention on the early phases of management, much akin to the initiatives of the Advance Trauma Life Support guidelines. Prevention of secondary insults are the priority in these patients and it is likely that these initiatives will greatly benefit both patient and clinician alike.

However, blindly applying management guidelines to all patients may negate these early benefits. The time has come to move away from artificially separated concepts of ICP- versus CPP-based strategies. These should be considered in parallel and applied to an individual patient, rather than making the patient fit into an all-encompassing treatment algorithm. A paradigm shift from a "set and forget" philosophy to one of "titration against time" to achieve appropriate therapeutic targets is now required.

References

1. Guillaume J, Janny P (1951) Manometrie intracranienne continue. Interpret phisiopatologique et clinique de la methode. Press Med 59:953-955
2. Lundberg N (1960) Continuous recording and control of ventricular fluid pressure in neurosurgical practice. Acta Psychiatr Scand 36:1-193
3. Maas AI, Steyerberg EW, Murray GD, et al (1999) Why have recent trials of neuroprotective agents in head injury failed to show convincing efficacy? A pragmatic analysis and theoretical considerations. Neurosurgery 44:1286-1298
4. Teasdale GM, Maas A, Iannotti F, et al (1999) Challenges in translating the efficacy of neuroprotective agents in experimental models into knowledge of clinical benefits in head injured patients. Acta Neurochir [Suppl] (Wien) 73:111-116
5. Narayan RK, Michel ME, Ansell B et al (2002) Clinical trials in head injury. J Neurotrauma 19:503-557
6. Dickinson K, Bunn F, Wentz R, et al (2000) Size and quality of randomised controlled trials in head injury: review of published studies. BMJ 320:1308-1311
7. Stocchetti N, Penny KI, Dearden M, et al (2001) Intensive care management of head-injured

patients in Europe: a survey from the European brain injury consortium. Intensive Care Med 27:400-406

8. Kay A, Teasdale G (2001) Head injury in the United Kingdom. World J Surg 25:1210-1220

9. Nell V, Brown DS (1991) Epidemiology of traumatic brain injury in Johannesburg--II. Morbidity, mortality and etiology. Soc Sci Med 33:289- 296

10. Fearnside MR, Cook RJ, McDougall P, Lewis WA (1993) The Westmead Head Injury Project. Physical and social outcomes following severe head injury. Br J Neurosurg 7:643-650

11. Chesnut RM, Marshall LF, Klauber MR, et al (1993) The role of secondary brain injury in determining outcome from severe head injury . J Trauma 34:216-222

12. Chesnut RM (1995) Secondary brain insults after head injury: clinical perspectives. New Horiz 3:366-375

13. Chesnut RM (1997) Avoidance of hypotension: conditio sine qua non of successful severe head-injury management. J Trauma 42:S4-S9

14. Chesnut RM, Marshall SB, Piek J, et al (1993) Early and late systemic hypotension as a frequent and fundamental source of cerebral ischemia following severe brain injury in the Traumatic Coma Data Bank. Acta Neurochir [Suppl] (Wien) 59:121-125

15. Chesnut RM (1997) Guidelines for the management of severe head injury: what we know and what we think we know. J Trauma 42:S19-S22

16. Myburgh JA, Lewis SB (2000) Mannitol for resuscitation in acute head injury: effects on cerebral perfusion and osmolality. Crit Care Resusc 2:344-353

17. Brain Trauma Foundation (1996) Guidelines for the management of severe head injury. J Neurotrauma 13:639-734

18. The Brain Trauma Foundation (2000) Management and prognosis of severe head injury. J Neurotrauma 17:457-627

19. The Brain Trauma Foundation. The American Association of Neurological Surgeons. The Joint Section on Neurotrauma and Critical Care. (2000) Intracranial pressure treatment threshold J Neurotrauma 17:493-495

20. The Brain Trauma Foundation. The American Association of Neurological Surgeons. The Joint Section on Neurotrauma and Critical Care. (2000) Critical pathway for the treatment of established intracranial hypertension. J Neurotrauma 17:537-538

21. The Brain Trauma Foundation. The American Association of Neurological Surgeons. The Joint Section on Neurotrauma and Critical Care. (2000) Recommendations for intracranial pressure monitoring technology. J Neurotrauma 17:497-506

22. Taylor A, Butt W, Rosenfeld J et al (2001) A randomized trial of very early decompressive craniectomy in children with traumatic brain injury and sustained intracranial hypertension. Childs Nerv Syst 17:154-162

23. Guerra WK, Piek J, Gaab MR (1999) Decompressive craniectomy to treat intracranial hypertension in head injury patients. Intensive Care Med 25:1327-1329

24. Kunze E, Meixensberger J, Janka M et al (1998) Decompressive craniectomy in patients with uncontrollable intracranial hypertension. Acta Neurochir [Suppl] (Wien) 71:16-18

25. Grande PO, Asgeirsson B, Nordstrom CH (1997) Physiologic principles for volume regulation of a tissue enclosed in a rigid shell with application to the injured brain. J Trauma 42:S23-S31

26. Asgeirsson B, Grande PO, Nordstrom CH (1994) A new therapy of post-trauma brain oedema based on haemodynamic principles for brain volume regulation. Intensive Care Med 20:260-267

27. Eker C, Asgeirsson B, Grande PO, et al (1998) Improved outcome after severe head injury with a new therapy based on principles for brain volume regulation and preserved microcirculation. Crit Care Med 26:1881-1886

28. Cruz J (1998) The first decade of continuous monitoring of jugular bulb oxyhemoglobinsaturation: management strategies and clinical outcome. Crit Care Med 26:344-351

29. Chesnut RM (1998) Hyperventilation versus cerebral perfusion pressure management: time to change the question. Crit Care Med 26:210-212

30. The Brain Trauma Foundation. The American Association of Neurological Surgeons. The Joint

Section on Neurotrauma and Critical Care. (2000) Guidelines for cerebral perfusion pressure. J Neurotrauma 17:497-506

31. Rosner MJ, Rosner SD, Johnson AH (1995) Cerebral perfusion pressure: management protocol and clinical results. J Neurosurg 83:949-962

32. Robertson CS, Valadka AB, Hannay HJ, et al (1999) Prevention of secondary ischemic insults after severe head injury. Crit Care Med 27:2086-2095

33. Macmillan CS, Andrews PJ (2000) Cerebrovenous oxygen saturation monitoring: practical considerations and clinical relevance. Intensive Care Med 26:1028-1036

34. Mascia L, Andrews PJ, McKeating EG, et al (2000) Cerebral blood flow and metabolism in severe brain injury: the role of pressure autoregulation during cerebral perfusion pressure management. Intensive Care Med 26:202-205

35. Lang EW, Chesnut RM (1995) Intracranial pressure and cerebral perfusion pressure in severe head injury. New Horiz 3:400-409

36. Martin NA, Patwardhan RV, Alexander MJ, et al (1997) Characterization of cerebral hemodynamic phases following severe head trauma: hypoperfusion, hyperemia, and vasospasm. J Neurosurg 87:9-19

37. Bouma GJ, Muizelaar JP, Choi SC, et al (1991) Cerebral circulation and metabolism after severe traumatic brain injury: the elusive role of ischemia. J Neurosurg 75:685-693

38. McKee MD, Schemitsch EH, Vincent LO, et al (1997) The effect of a femoral fracture on concomitant closed head injury in patients with multiple injuries. J Trauma 42:1041-1045

39. Jaicks RR, Cohn SM, Moller BA (1997) Early fracture fixation may be deleterious after head injury. J Trauma 42:1-5

40. Gopinath SP, Robertson CS, Contant CF, et al (1994) Jugular venous desaturation and outcome after head injury. J Neurol Neurosurg Psychiatry 57:717-723

41. Macmillan CS, Andrews PJ, Easton VJ (2001) Increased jugular bulb saturation is associated with poor outcome in traumatic brain injury. J Neurol Neurosurg Psychiatry 70:101-104

42. Martin NA, Doberstein C, Zane C, et al (1992) Posttraumatic cerebral arterial spasm: transcranial Doppler ultrasound, cerebral blood flow, and angiographic findings. J Neurosurg 77:575-583

43. The European Study Group on Nimodipine in Severe Head Injury (1994) A multicenter trial of the efficacy of nimodipine on outcome after severe head injury. J Neurosurg 80:797-804

Essential cerebral monitoring when resources are limited

W. VIDETTA

The pathophysiological mechanisms occurring in cerebral ischemia are multiple, complex, and incompletely understood [1]. Different processes like raised intracranial pressure (ICP), derangements in cerebral blood flow (CBF), and brain hypoxia may be transient and last only a few minutes [1-3]. Methods for assessing brain function in an uninterrupted fashion have attracted increased clinical attention [4-6], particularly those that can be adapted for bedside monitoring.

The aim of monitoring neurocritical patients is to provide facilities for early detection of secondary insults [7]. In this way, monitoring alerts the physician that something is going wrong. It gives a chance for taking or indicating new therapeutics before the effect of secondary brain insults and secondary brain damage is clinically evident, and provides objective parameters on which therapeutic interventions can be based and their effectiveness evaluated.

In severe traumatic brain injury (sTBI) patients, ICP might be increased in more than a half [8]. The highest value of ICP reached and the duration of intracranial hypertension (ICH) strongly correlate with an increased morbidity and mortality [9]. Indications for ICP monitoring are still being debated [10,11]. Jugular venous oxygen saturation (SjvO2) and near infrared spectroscopy (NIRS) are new tools to detect episodes of cerebral ischemia as early as possible, in an attempt to provide treatment before the development of permanent damage [5,12-15].

Lately, the development of transcranial Doppler (TCD) ultrasonography offered a noninvasive means to evaluate the basal cerebral arteries flows. All this monitoring information and data from regional cerebral monitoring can be used to guide medical management. Surveys from United States [16], Europe [17], United Kingdom and Ireland [18], and Argentina (unpublished data) indicated that there is a considerable variation in the monitoring and management of TBI patients. Essential cerebral monitoring when resources are limited is discussed.

Monitoring brain injury

Routine clinical checks of Glasgow Coma Scale (GCS) and pupils remain important in all neurocritical patients, particularly in patients with head injury. Accurate determination of the full GCS is not always possible because of opioids, sedation and paralysis, facial lesions, and intubation, but, when possible, at least the best motor score should be recorded. Monitoring ICP, cerebral perfusion pressure (CPP) and SjvO$_2$ provides information regarding the intracerebral system as a whole [19]. Clinical signs cannot be used to detect neurological deterioration in the sedated and paralyzed patient. Imaging studies can predict the occurrence of ICH [20] but cannot measure it. Measuring ICP directly is the only known way to calculate both ICP and CPP. It is widely accepted that there are no reliable clinical signs of increasing ICP in TBI until dilated pupils indicate cerebral herniation. Electrical monitoring through the measurement of evoked potentials, assessing the integrity of sensor and motor pathways, may provide diagnostic and prognostic information. Also, an electroencephalogram can be useful to detect seizure activity. New regional monitoring became available recently.

ICP monitoring

ICP is currently the main parameter monitored in acute neurological patients. Its use is more frequent in head-injured patients but it is common in other diseases (intracerebral haemorrhage, subarachnoid haemorrhage, etc.) that could affect the normal ICP range. Severe TBI patients developed intracranial hypertension frequently (50-75%). ICP monitoring provides information on the likelihood of cerebral herniation and allows calculation of CPP. ICP of ≥ 20 mmHg and CPP <60 mmHg correlate strongly with outcome after TBI. Several studies [9,21-25] showed that, under conditions of aggressive ICP management, the probability of a good outcome is inversely proportional to the maximum ICP reached and the percentage of monitored time spent at levels > 20 mmHg.

Therapies for lowering ICP and/or increasing CPP can be aggressive, but it is part of an overall management that includes ICP monitoring. In the light of several studies [8,21-31] showed, four arguments favor ICP monitoring : (1) there is a very strong correlation between successful ICP management and low rates of mortality and morbidity, (2) ICP monitoring can be used to minimize the eventual risk of the agents commonly used to treat ICH, (3) ICP monitoring provides early warning signs of ICH or herniation in patients whose neurological examination is limited, (4) ICP monitoring is required to manage accurately CPP as a major means of avoiding secondary insults. Such considerations support the position that monitoring and treatment of ICP while maintaining

CPP should be strongly considered as a routine part of the overall treatment of patients with severe TBI [32].

In a developing country, Argentina, the survey (unpublished data) indicated that in only 33% of hospitals was ICP monitored in >90% of severe TBI patients. It is therefore surprising that ICP has not become more widely used in Argentine units. Hence, in most hospitals where the ICP survey was performed, ICH is treated empirically. It may be under or over-utilized. Several reasons may play a role in the low utilization and indication of ICP monitoring: (1) ICP monitoring is labor intensive (implying a great responsibility), (2) requires trained physicians and nurses, (3) limited resources, (4) inadequate number of neurosurgeons and neurocritical care physicians, (5) lack of knowledge about ICP monitoring and management modalities of TBI, (6) theoretical risks of insertion of ICP catheter, and (7) nihilist attitude in the face of TBI patients.

In developing countries, the resources are limited. Sometimes, economic crises have a powerful and negative impact on the health system making the situation worse. At present, Argentina's health services are struggling as the social security system limitations depend on several factors [33]. This is a partial explanation. Limited economic resources may explain why solid-state devices are used in a small proportion of potential TBI patients who need ICP monitoring, but it cannot explain why other cheaper methods, like fluid-coupled systems, are not used. The recommended general strategy is simple: (1) to assess the needs, (2) to evaluate personnel skills, (3) to have anticipated costs of ICP monitoring in the proper intensive care unit (ICU), and (4) to match them with ICP monitoring system in ICU [34]. Having limited resources, with multi-purpose ICUs with a specialized area and trained medical and nursing personnel who frequently monitor ICP, fluid-coupled systems may be the choice. These systems have higher overall system accuracy despite the complexity of maintaining the ICP monitoring device and transducer system.

To summarize, ICP monitoring with cheap devices can be done when ICP monitoring is indicated. Its disadvantages are: (1) it demands more trained staff, (2) greater care, (3) higher infection risk, (4) inadequate reading when the ICP ≥ 30-35 mmHg when placed in the subdural space. The most-important advantages are: (1) low cost, (2) it provides the necessary information about ICP, (3) CPP can be calculated, (4) the information can be used for control, follow-up, and eventually to make a decision in patients with moderate or severe TBI.

Jugular venous oxygen saturation

Several studies during the last 2 decades have demonstrated the potential utility of continuously monitoring $SjvO_2$ in the ICU after TBI [5,6,14,35-40] to provide new therapeutic approaches for severely head-injured patients. The technique of continuous $SjvO_2$ measurement, although artefact prone, yields important real-time data about the state of brain oxygenation in severely head-injured patients at risk for cerebral ischemia [41-44]. Monitoring of $SjvO_2$ is commonly used to judge the adequacy of cerebral oxygenation because it provides an assessment of the overall balance between cerebral metabolism and CBF [45]. The role of posttraumatic hyperemia in the development of raised ICP has important patho-physiological and therapeutic implications [41,42].

Calculations of oxygen and glucose concentrations on samples drawn from internal jugular bulb have been performed in other studies [40,43]. Consequently, cerebral venous blood samples for oxygen saturation monitoring, as well as for all other derived calculations, are usually obtained from unilateral jugular bulb catheterization. However, as recently demonstrated, marked differences can occur in patients with head injuries, especially in cases of unilateral lesions [44]. There are concerns about the most-appropriate side for monitoring [44]. In head-injured patients, CBF is often heterogeneous in different areas of the brain [45,46]. In this setting, the major problem is that therapeutic procedures, based on information obtained from unilateral jugular bulb catheterization, may be dangerous to the contralateral hemisphere [44].

Previous studies [7,38,47] have emphasized a worse outcome in patients in whom a reduced CBF and episodes of reduced $SjvO_2$ were found. A greater than normal $SjvO_2$ is often interpreted as indicating that the CBF is more than adequate to satisfy cerebral metabolic requirements. Cormio et al. [42] pointed out the possibility that, in many cases, this interpretation may be incorrect and that an elevated $SjvO_2$ should not be automatically equated with hyperaemia. An elevated $SjvO_2$ appears to be a heterogeneous condition. If the cause of the high $SjvO_2$ is primarily an increase in CBF and not a major decrease in cerebral metabolic rate of oxygen ($CMRO_2$), the outcome is generally favourable. However, if the cause of the high $SjvO_2$ is a decrease in the $CMRO_2$, especially to 1.5 ml/100 g per min, the outcome is usually poor. The cause of the reduced $CMRO_2$ is either an alteration in cerebral oxygen extraction capabilities or the presence of ischemic regions in the brain. Patients with such symptoms are often older and have severe ICH.

Latronico et al. [48], in a recent published study, pointed out that intermittent $SjvO_2$ monitoring is a low-sensitivity method compared with continuous $SjvO_2$ monitoring by means of fiberoptic devices. Surprisingly, the frequency of $SjvO_2$ < 50%, which modified the management, was only 3.4% of all observations.

This observation was explained in part by the low sensitivity of the 8-h interval adopted. These findings are controversial. A possible criticism of intermittent $SjvO_2$ monitoring is the potential for missing critical periods of cerebral ischemia, which could be detected with continuous monitoring. Despite this obvious disadvantage, the intermittent method has not been replaced. On the other hand, the accuracy of continuous monitoring is far from optimal, good-quality data are obtained only 40-60% of the time.

Hyperventilation has been used routinely as the first line of treatment or as a prophylactic therapy following sTBI [49]. Studies assessing hyperventilation-associated CBF reduction have raised issues regarding the safety and efficacy of induced hypocapnia. These considerations have their basis in the cerebral effects of hypocapnia, and are well covered in the literature [50,51]. During the first hours and days after injury, global and regional CBF are critically reduced. Marion and Bouma [52] found that there is significant regional heterogeneity in CO_2 vasoresponsivity, and that regional loss of normal CO_2 vasoresponsivity is much more common than global estimates have suggested. There is evidence demonstrating that hyperventilation can be a double-edged sword [50]. Hyperventilation has a much greater effect on CBF than on ICP [28]. The potential for hyperventilation to cause cerebral ischemia has been addressed by several studies [50,53], demonstrating that hyperventilation was the second most-common cause of jugular venous oxygen desaturation. Gopinath et al. [37] found that the incidence and duration of jugular venous desaturation significantly correlated with adverse neurological outcomes at 3 and 6 months. In the present survey, we found that hyperventilation was used in 95% of referral centers. In about 51% of the units it was used at $PaCO_2$ levels > 30 mmHg and in 49% it was used with a $PaCO_2$ level between 25 and 30 mmHg. Since many hospitals were not using ICP monitoring, hyperventilation was frequently used empirically and potentially overused.

In Argentina, the survey of critical care management of severe TBI patients (unpublished data) indicated that $SjvO_2$ was used in 46 ICUs (49.4%), almost in an intermittent way. Fifteen units (28.84%) used hyperventilation without cerebral oxygen monitoring, and in 7 of these units (13.46%) hyperventilation was used in 100% of patients with TBI. The frequent usage of hyperventilation persists despite less cerebral oxygen monitoring. There are several reasons for the low utilization and indication of $SjvO_2$ monitoring: (1) people are unconvinced of the importance of oxygen saturation, because of the difficulties in interpretation resulting from the mixture of potential regions of the brain with increased use as well as those with decreased use, (2) there are no widely available co-oximeters, (3) the low sensitivity of the method means a reduced number of critical detectable episodes, depending on the frequency of sampling.

When the resources are limited, the ICU director has to choose what kind of monitor to use. The choice for neurocritical care is based on the money included in the budget for a neurocritical care monitor or for sophisticated ventilators. Otherwise, intermittent SjvO$_2$ monitoring is plausible. Intermittent SjO$_2$ monitoring by jugular bulb blood sampling through common vascular catheters is easier, inexpensive, and samples can be reliably analyzed using available co-oximeters.

Essential monitoring, ICP and CPP, has been a key issue for the management of severe TBI (advocated as the main part of the approach to the management of severe TBI) [9,10]. Multimodality monitoring is therefore recommended for such patients [4]. So, jugular bulb oxyhemoglobin saturation monitoring has a place, bearing in mind the limitations of each modality, continuous or intermittent, as well as the controversies about what each measure means at any given time in brain-injured patients.

Transcranial Doppler ultrasonography

Transcranial Doppler (TCD) ultrasonography is a noninvasive method of assessing flow velocity in the basal cerebral arteries [54]. TCD measures the blood velocity, not flow, and therefore the CBF is only estimated if vessel diameter is constant, but it seems to reflect properly the changes in CBF. Many ICUs use TCD for neuromonitoring [55]. TCD has been proposed as a noninvasive method to: (1) detect vasospasm [56], (2) estimate CPP and ICP in head-injured patients [57], (3) assess autoregulation and thus CBF [58,59], (4) confirm cerebral death [60], (5) monitor during neurosurgery, (6) detect emboli during endarterectomy [61], and (7) detect intracranial aneurysms [62]. TCD is not accepted worldwide. There is a disadvantage in that it is a subjective measure and an expert is needed for this task. The data provided by TCD is more useful in the setting of vasospasm and brain death. TCD is not a priority when resources are limited.

Conclusions

Neurocritical monitoring is a fundamental requirement to understand intracranial physiopathology. Some monitoring systems are more accepted than others and yield more basic information. When resources are limited, it is possible to use devices that allow basic monitoring, such as ICP, and at the same time monitor PPC and, less frequently, cerebral oxygenation through intermittent SjvO$_2$ monitoring. Nevertheless, with these systems, probably cheaper catheters will be used. This can vary depending on the resource availability at a given time. This kind of situation is frequent in developing countries, where economic stability is an exception and public health usually is not a priority and must face basic challenges. Cultural factors and educational levels also have to be taken into account for all people involved in the health process.

References

1. Sjeso BK (1992) Pathophysiology and treatment of focal cerebral ischaemia. I and II. J Neurosurg 77:169-84;337-354
2. Macpherson P, Graham DI (1973) Arterial spasm and slowing of the cerebral circulation in the ischaemia of head injury J Neurol Neurosurg Psychiatry 48:560-564
3. Marion DW, Darby J, Yonas H (1991) Acute regional cerebral blood flow changes caused by severe head injuries. J Neurosurg 74:407-414
4. Kirkpatrick PJ, Czosnyka M, Pickard JD (1996) Multimodal monitoring in neurointensive care J Neurol Neurosurg Psychiatry 60:131-139
5. Fortune JB, Feustel JP, Weigle CGM, et al (1994) Continuous measurement of jugular venous oxygen sauration in response to transient elevations of blood pressure in head-injured patients. J Neurosurg 80:461-468
6. Cruz J (1988) Continuous versus serial global cerebral hemometabolic monitoring: applications in acute brain trauma. Acta Neurochir [Suppl] (Wien) 42:35-39
7. Robertson CS, Contant CF, Gokaslan ZL (1992) Cerebral blood flow, arteriovenous oxygen difference, and outcome in head injured patients. J Neurol Neurosurg Psychiatry 55:594-603
8. Marmarou A, Anderson RL, Ward JD, et al (1991) Impact of ICP instability and hypotension on outcome in patients with severe head trauma. J Neurosurg [Suppl] 75:S59-S66
9. Bullock R, Chesnut R, Clifton G, et al (1996) Guidelines for the management of severe head injury J Neurotrauma 13:639-734
10. Maas AI, Dearden M, Teasdale GM, et al (1997) EBIC guidelines for management of severe head injury in adults: European Brain Injury Consortium. Acta Neurochir (Wien) 139:286-294
11. Sheinberg M, Kanter MJ, Robertson CS, et al (1992) Continuous monitoring of jugular venous oxygen saturation in head injured patients. J Neurosurg 76:212-217
12. Robertson CS, Contant CF, Narayan RK et al (1992) Cerebral blood flow, AVDO$_2$, and neurologic outcome in head injury patients. J Neurotrauma 9 [Suppl1]:S349-S358
13. Bouma GJ, Muizelaar JP, Choi SC, et al (1991) Cerebral circulation and metabolism after severe traumatic brain injury: the elusive role of ischemia. J Neurosurg 75:685-693
14. Cruz J (1993) On-line monitoring of global cerebral hypoxia in acute brain injury: relationship to intracranial hypertension. J Neurosurg 79:228-233
15. Prough DS, Pollard V (1995) Cerebral near-infrared spectroscopy: ready for prime time? Crit Care Med 23:1624-1626
16. Ghajar J, Hariri RJ, Narayan RK, et al (1995) Survey of critical care management of comatose, head-injured patients in the United States. Crit Care Med 23:560-567
17. De Deyne C, De Jong R (2000) Euro-Neuro 1998 survey on the management of severe head injury Eur J Anesthesiol 17 [Suppl 18]:3-5
18. Matta B, Menon D (1996) Severe head injury in the United Kingdom and Ireland: a survey of pratice and implications for management. Crit Care Med 24:1743-1748
19. Maas AI, Dearden M, Servadei F, et al (2000) Current recommendations for neurotrauma. Curr Opin Crit Care 6:281-292
20. Marshall LF, Bowers-Marshall S, Klauber MR, et al (1991) A new classification of head injury based on computerized tomography. J Neurosurg 75 [Suppl]:S14-S20

21. Rosner M, Rosner SD, Johnson AH (1995) Cerebral perfusion pressure: management protocol and clinical results. J Neurosurg 83:949-962
22. Marshall LF, Becker DP, Bowers SA, et al (1983) The National Traumatic coma Data Bank. 1. Design, purpose, goals and results. J Neurosurg 59:276-284
23. Kauffmann AM, Cardoso ER (1992) Aggravation of vasogenic cerebral edema by multiple-dose mannitol. J Neurosurg 77:584-589
24. Marshall L, Smith R, Shapiro H (1979) The outcome with aggressive treatment in severe head injuries. II. Acute and chronic barbiturate administration in the management of head injury. J Neurosurg 50:26-30
25. Mendelow AD, Teasdale GM, Russell T, et al (1985) Effect of mannitol on cerebral blood flow and cerebral perfusion pressure in human head injury. J Neurosurg 63:43-48
26. Smith HP, Kelly DL Jr, McWhorter JM, et al (1986) Comparison of mannitol regimes in patients with severe head injury undergoing intracranial monitoring. J Neurosurg 65:820-824
27. Muizelaar JP, Marmarou A, Ward JD, et al (1991) Adverse effects of prolonged hyperventilation in patients with severe head injury: a randomized clinical trial. J Neurosurg 75:731-739
28. Cold GE (1989) Does acute hyperventilation provoke cerebral oligoemia in comatose patients after acute head injury? Acta Neurochir (Wien) 96:100-106
29. Changaris DG, Mc Graw CP, Richardson JD, et al (1987) Correlation of cerebral perfusion pressure and Glasgow Coma Scale to outcome. J Trauma 27:1007-1013
30. Miller JD (1987) ICP monitoring – current status and future directions. Acta Neurochir (Wien) 85:80-86
31. Hsiang JK, Chesnut RM, Crisp CB, et al (1994) Early, routine paralysis for intracranial pressure control in severe head injury; is it necessary? Crit Care Med 22:1471-1476
32. Lang EW, Chesnut RM (1995) Intracranial pressure and cerebral perfusion pressure in severe head injury. New Horiz 3:400-409
33. Arie S (2002) Argentina running out of medical supplies. BMJ 324:192
34. Tobin MJ (ed) (1997) Principles and practice of intensive care monitoring. McGraw-Hill Professional Publishing
35. Andrews PJ, Dearden NM, Miller JD (1991) Jugular bulb cannulation: description of a cannulation technique and validation of a new continuous monitor. Br J Anaesth 67:553-558
36. Garlick R, Bihari D (1987) The use of intermittent and continuous recordings of jugular venous bulb oxygen saturation in the unconscious patient. Scand J Clin Lab Invest 47 [Suppl 188]:47-52
37. Gopinath SP, Robertson CS, Contant CF, et al (1994) Jugular venous desaturation and outcome after head injury. J Neurol Neurosurg Psychiatry 57:717-723
38. Cruz J, Jaggi JL, Hoffstad OJ (1993) Cerebral blood flow and oxygen consumption in acute brain injury with acute anemia: an alternative for the cerebral metabolic rate of oxygen consumption? Crit Care Med 21:1218-1224
39. Jakobsen M, Enevoldsen E (1989) Retrograde catheterization of the right internal jugular vein for serial measurements of cerebral venous oxygen content. J Cereb Blood Flow Metab 9:717-720
40. Nemoto EM, Hoff JT, Severinghaus JW (1974) Lactate uptake and metabolism by brain during hyperlactatemia and hypoglycemia. Stroke 5:48-53
41. Kelly D, Kordestain RK, Martin NA et al (1996) Hyperemia following taumatic brain injury: relationship to intracraneal hypertension and outcome. J Neurosurg 85:762-771
42. Cormio M, Valadka AB, Robertson CS (1999) Elevated jugular venous oxygen saturation after severe head injury. J Neurosurg 90:9-15
43. Cruz J, Hoffstad OJ, Jaggi JL (1994) Cerebral lactate-oxygen index in acute brain injury with acute anemia: assessment of false versus true ischemia. Crit Care Med 22:1465-1470
44. Stocchetti N, Paparella A, Bridelli F, et al (1994) Cerebral venous oxygen saturation studied with bilateral samples in the internal jugular veins. Neurosurgery 34:38-44
45. Raichle ME, Grubb RL Jr, Gado MH (1976) Correlation between regional cerebral blood flow and oxidative metabolism. In vivo studies in man. Arch Neurol 33:523-526

46. Metz C, Holzschuh M, Bein T, et al (1998) Monitoring of cerebral oxygen metabolism in the jugular bulb: reliability of unilateral measurements in severe head injury. J Cereb Blood Flow Metab 18:332-343
47. Kelly DF, Martin NA, Kordestani RK (1997) Cerebral blood flow as a predictor of oucome following traumatic brain injury. J Neurosurg 86:633-641
48. Latronico N, Beindorf AE, Rasulo FA, et al (2000) Limits of intermittent jugular bulb oxygen saturation monitoring in the management of severe head trauma patients. Neurosurgery 46:1131--1138
49. Marion DW, Firlik A, Mc Gaughlin MR (1995) Hyperventilation therapy for severe traumatic brain injury. New Horiz 3:439-447
50. Obrist WD, Langfitt TW, Jaggi JL, et al (1984) Cerebral blood flow and metabolism in comatose patients with acute head injury. J Neurosurg 61: 241–253
51. Fortune JB, Feustel PJ, deLuna C, et al (1995) Cerebral blood flow and blood volume in response to O_2 and CO_2 changes in normal humans. J Trauma 39:463-472
52. Marion DW, Bouma GJ (1991) The use of stable xennon-enhanced computed tomgraphic studies of cerebral blood flow to define changes in cerebral carbon dioxide vasoresponsivity caused by severe head injury. Neurosurgery 29:869-873
53. Olsen KS, Madsen PL, Borme T, Schmidt JF (1994) Evaluation of a 7.5 French pulmonary catheter for continuous monitoring of cerebral venous oxygen saturation. J Neurosurg Anesthesiol 6:233-238
54. Aaslid R, Markwalder TM, Nornes H (1982) Non-invasive transcranial Doppler ultrasound recording of flow velocity in basal cerebral arteries. J Neurosurg 50:570-577
55. Castillo MÁ del (2001) Monitoring neurologic patients in intensive care. Curr Opin Crit Care 7:49-60
56. Jarus-Dziedzic K, Zub W, Wronski J, et al (2000) The relationship between cerebral blood flow velocities and the amount of blood clots in computed tomography after subarachnoid haemorrhage. Acta Neurochir (Wien) 142:309-318
57. Czosnyka M, Matta BF, Smielewski P et al (1998) Cerebral perfusion pressure in head injured patients: a noninvasive assessment using transcranial doppler ultrasonography. J Neurosurg 88:802-808
58. Florence G, Seylaz J (1989) Rapid autoregulation of cerebral blood flow: a laser-doppler flowmetry study. J Cereb Blood Flow Metab 9:515-522
59. Lam JMK, Hsiang JNK, Poon WS (1997) Monitoring of autoregulation using laser doppler flowmetry in patients with head injury. J Neurosurg 86:438-445
60. Hassler W, Steinmets H, Gawlowski J (1988) Transcranial doppler ultrasonography in raised intracranial pressure and intracranial arrest. J Neurosurg 68:745-751
61. Halsey JH, McDowell HA, Gelman S (1986) Transcranial Doppler and rCBF compared in carotid endarterectomy. Stroke 17:1206-1208
62. Turner CL, Kirkpatrick PJ (2000) Detection of intracranial aneurysms with unenhanced and echo contrast enhanced transcranial power Doppler. J Neurol Neurosurg Psychiatry 69:489-495

Therapeutic hypothermia

C.K Spiss, U.M. Illievich, A. Bacher

Core temperature varies not only interindividually and diurnally, but also between different parts of the body. Nevertheless body core temperature is precisely controlled between set points triggering thermoregulatory responses in the healthy awake individual. The temperature range not triggering thermoregulatory responses is approximately 0.2°C in un-anaesthetized humans. During anaesthesia this temperature range increases because physiological thermoregulatory responses normally triggered by hypothermia do not occur (e.g., behavioural changes, shivering), or at lower temperatures (vasoconstriction). Therefore, if normothermia is not actively maintained, general anaesthesia may lead to unintentional low body temperature. In contrast to accidental hypothermia is deliberate hypothermia, which has been used as a therapeutic adjunct for a variety of medical procedures.

Topical hypothermia as anaesthetic has been applied for decades, and deep global hypothermia is established as the principal cerebroprotective technique for circulatory arrest procedures. However, the use of deep hypothermia in neurosurgical procedures has been restricted by the need for extracorporeal circulation and postoperative/post-bypass complications [1].

Of greater immediate relevance than the use of deep hypothermia for neurosurgical procedures has been the realization that small decreases in brain temperature can reduce ischaemia-induced neurological injury [2]. Secondary brain injury after trauma is also markedly affected by changes in brain temperature. In contrast to mild hypothermia that can ameliorate ischaemia-induced brain injury, hyperthermia, even if delayed, may worsen neurological outcome after neurotrauma [3]. These findings, if the results can be generalized to humans, are of considerable interest, because they suggest that levels of hypothermia easily obtainable in the operating room or the intensive care unit may reduce the consequences of cerebral ischaemia or secondary brain injury after trauma. Interestingly this concept is not always applied, since untreated increases in temperatures up to 38°C and more in hospitalized patients at risk (successful resuscitation after cardiac arrest, subarachnoid haemorrhage, traumatic closed-head injury) have been reported [4].

Temperature measurement

Since brain temperature is not easily measured in humans, various other measurement sites have been studied. Since the jugular vein is anatomically close to the brain and transports venous return of the brain, blood temperature of this site was thought to reflect brain temperature. Furthermore, catheterization of the jugular bulb is routinely utilized for metabolic function measurements of the brain in head-injured patients. However, simultaneous measurements of brain, jugular venous blood, and body core temperatures in patients with severe head injuries showed that brain temperature is on average 1.1°C higher (-0.30°C to 2.1°C) than body core temperature. This difference between brain and body core temperature increases with low cerebral perfusion pressures, and decreases with high dose barbiturates. Interestingly, jugular venous blood and body core temperatures are similar; therefore, jugular venous blood temperature reflects body, not brain temperature [5]. Considering intracerebral temperature gradients, especially under intraoperative conditions, knowledge of the relationship between surface temperatures and temperatures taken at standard sites is essential. Due to the cooling rate of the exposed cerebral cortex, brain temperature during surgery is approximately half a degree lower than oesophageal temperature. Tympanic temperature reflects oesophageal temperature changes adequately. Similarly, except during periods of rapid temperature changes, bladder temperature reflects oesophageal temperature. For clinical use, oesophageal, tympanic, and bladder temperature are also sufficient to assess brain surface temperature during surgery [6]. In contrast to conditions during surgery, in patients with traumatic brain injury core temperature underestimates brain temperature [7].

Temperature management

Although body core temperature typically decreases more than 1°C during the first hours of general anaesthesia, active cooling is usually necessary if core temperature must be rapidly reduced. Methods used to reduce brain temperature during animal experiments include packing in ice, fanning, partial immersion in cold water, nasopharyngeal cooling, and cardiopulmonary bypass. These methods are theoretically applicable in humans, although packing in ice will build up extreme temperature gradients that at least irritate skin, and immersion is difficult under clinical conditions. Rapid reduction of core temperature can be facilitated by administration of refrigerated IV fluids, circulating water mattresses, forced air cooling, and extra-corporeal means.

IV administration of refrigerated (1-6°C) of 5% albumin (5 ml/kg) over 3-5 min after surface cooling to 34°C reduces core temperature approximately 0.6°C. To achieve maximal effectiveness, refrigerated fluids must be administered very rapidly (100 ml/min) to avoid heat gains in standard IV tubing [8]. Administration of refrigerated fluids is limited by cardiovascular side effects.

If the patient is placed on a circulating water mattress, the relatively small area of skin surface contact limits the effectiveness of cooling by this device. Additionally, the exposed area is not as well perfused, since the pressure of the body weight is applied to it [9].

In controlling body core temperature, forced air cooling has the advantage of cooling a large skin area, but seems to be even more effective when used in combination with circulating water mattress cooling. Active core cooling using an extra-corporeal heat exchanger may circumvent the rather slow induction speed and temperature drifts ("after drop") observed with surface cooling techniques. In a series of eight patients with severe traumatic brain injuries, a heat exchanger was connected via a pressure-controlled roller pump to a percutaneously introduced double-lumen cannula in the femoral vein. Cooling was initiated at a cooling speed of 3.5°C/h and hypothermia was maintained within 0.1°C at 32°C brain temperature for 48 h. Using this technique, brain temperature of 32°C was achieved within 1 h and 53 min (±1 h and 21 min) after induction of cooling. Although this is an invasive technique and platelet count decreased during treatment, no clinical bleeding complications or problems resulting from extra-corporeal circulation occurred [10]. A recent publication on a newer, more-sophisticated device for intravascular cooling (Cool Line catheter and Cool Gard cooling device, Alsius, Irvine, Calif., USA) showed a very high efficacy and safety in 51 patients with severe intracranial disease (intracranial haemorrhage, head trauma, hypoxic encephalopathy, and stroke) in prophylactically controlling the body temperature (E. Schmutzhard, et al., Crit Care Med, in press). The Cool Gard system circulates temperature-controlled sterile saline through small balloons mounted on the tip of the Cool Line catheter. The patient's blood is gently cooled as it passes over the balloons. The Cool Gard system responds to temperature probes measuring the patient's core temperature and adjusts the temperature of circulating sterile saline in the Cool Line catheter.

Pathophysiology

The classic mechanism proposed for neuronal protection by hypothermia, the reduction of oxygen and glucose consumption by a parallel reduction of the rates of enzymatic reactions subserving metabolism, has been challenged for mild and moderate hypothermia. Experimentally, focal and global cerebral ischaemia are markedly affected by small changes in brain temperature. Mild *hypo*thermia ameliorates and mild *hyper*thermia exacerbates ischaemic-induced neuronal injury [11]. In contrast to deep hypothermia, during which low temperature protects the tissue by reducing the rates of enzymatic reactions, CMR suppression alone cannot explain the cerebral protective effect of mild and moderate hypothermia. Mechanisms involved include reduction of ischaemia induced excitatory neurotransmitter increase [12], effects on ion homeostasis and membrane permeability, recovery of post-ischaemic protein synthesis [13], prevention of protein kinase C downregulation [14], and the consumption of free radical scavengers in the brain tissue.

Mild hypothermia is neuroprotective in models of focal and global ischaemia, as well as in models of traumatic brain injury. It appears that hypothermia affects not only many steps in the ischaemic cascade, but also suppresses several components of secondary brain injury after traumatic brain injury, including hypermetabolism and inflammation.

Hypothermia and traumatic brain injury

In a first study Marion et al. [15] randomly assigned 40 patients with a severe closed head injury (GCS 3–7) to either a normothermic or a hypothermic group. Hypothermic patients were cooled to 32°-33°C (brain temperature) within 10 h of injury for the following 24 h and then rewarmed over 12 h. Hypothermia significantly reduced intracranial pressure (ICP) (40%) and cerebral blood flow (26%) during the cooling period, and neither parameter showed a significant rebound after rewarming. Three months after injury, 12 patients in the hypothermic group had moderate, mild, or no disabilities versus 8 patients in the normothermic group. Systemic complications were similar in both groups. The authors conclude that therapeutic hypothermia (32°C) after severe closed head injury is a safe procedure, and a trend toward better outcome in hypothermic patients indicates a limitation of secondary brain injury [15].

Shiozaki et al. [16] used a different approach. The patients in this study were only included if intracranial hypertension was refractory to all conventional treatment modalities, including high-dose barbiturate therapy. Then patients were divided into two groups: 16 patients received mild hypothermia and 17 patients served as a normothermic control group. Mild hypothermia significantly reduced ICP and therefore increased cerebral perfusion pressure (CPP). Eight patients (50%) in the hypothermia group and 3 (18%) in the control group survived. These results suggest that mild hypothermia is an effective method of controlling traumatic intracranial hypertension in patients in whom conventional ICP therapy was infective [16].

Clifton et al. [17] randomized 46 patients with severe brain injury (GCS 4–7) to either standard normothermic management or to management with systemic hypothermia at 32-33°C. Surface cooling was initiated within 6 h of injury and maintained for 48 h. There were no cardiac or coagulopathy related complications, and the incidence of seizures was significantly lower in the hypothermia group. Mean Glasgow Outcome Scale (GOS) score at 3 months after injury showed an increase of 16% in the good recovery/moderate disability category compared with severe disability/vegetative/dead [17].

This study was followed by a randomized, controlled trial, in which Marion et al. [18] compared the effects of moderate hypothermia and normothermia in 82 patients with severe closed head injuries (GCS 3-7). The patients assigned to hypothermia were cooled to 33°C within 10 h of injury and kept at 32-33°C for 24 h. A specialist in physical medicine and rehabilitation unaware of the treatment randomization evaluated the patients 3, 6, and 12 months by applying the GOS. At 12 months, 62% of the patients in the hypothermia group and 38% in the normothermia group had favorable outcomes (moderate, mild, or no disabilities). However, hypothermia did not improve the outcome in the patients with coma scores of 3-4 on admission. Among the patients with scores of 5-7, hypothermia was associated with significant improved outcomes at 3 and 6 months, although not at 12 months. The authors concluded that treatment with moderate hypothermia for 24 h in patients with severe traumatic brain injury and coma scores of 5-7 on admission expedited neurological recovery and may have improved outcome [18].

This study has been criticized mainly for two reasons [19]. First, although the authors reported that the causes and severity of injury were similar in the hypothermia and normothermia groups, on basis of the computed tomography (CT) class the patients in the hypothermic group were favoured. Marion [20] responded that CT-defined severity of injury has never been validated as an independent measure of outcome. There are numerous examples (e.g., epidural haematoma, diffuse hypoxic brain injury) where the initial CT appearance is not predictive of the neurological outcome [20]. Second, patients in the normothermic group were allowed to reach temperatures as high as 38.5°C before they were cooled to 37°C. Therefore, the reported beneficial effect of hypothermia might have been the effect of avoiding detrimental effects of hyperthermia.

Based on these results, a multicenter trial "National Acute Brain Injury Study: Hypothermia (NABIS-H)" was launched [21]. Finally 392 patients were enrolled in the study. Because the outcome after 6 months showed no differences regarding morbidity and mortality, a subgroup analysis was performed. It showed a higher mortality rate if the patient was more severely injured (GCS 3-4) and experienced a higher percentage of hours of hypotension [mean arterial pressure (MAP) 70 mmHg] during treatment. Additionally, ICP was not reduced in these patients. Therefore, the study was stopped by the NIH. However, the general conclusion that hypothermia is of no advantage in head-injured patients may not be drawn from these results. The principal investigator, Clifton published a critical appraisal where he searched for the reasons for this apparently negative outcome of NABIS-H [22]. One of the reasons could be that hypothermia was maintained for only 48 h after trauma. Our clinical experience shows that severe increases in ICP and thereby critical decreases in CPP very often occur later and last for longer during intensive care in such patients. At this time the danger of secondary ischaemia is high, but in NABIS-H patients were already normothermic. Further, cooling might have been initiated far too late (8.4±3.6 h after trauma) to be effective during primary cerebral ischaemia. There was also a lack of difference in core temperature during this time between the control group and the treatment group since the control group was also subjected to mild hypothermia during emergency resuscitation and transport to the hospital. Additionally, there were no standardized treatment protocols regarding the important physiological variables MAP, CPP, and $PaCO_2$. Sedation was only performed with (low) doses of morphine and the patients were immobilized with muscle relaxation rather than adequate sedoanalgesia. Due to these facts, the NIH will fund a second study after selection of competent study centers based on track records and a test phase.

It seems that a beneficial effect of mild hypothermia can be achieved in younger patients with a GCS of 5-8 and elevated ICP of 20-40 mmHg, but is less effective in most severely injured patients (GCS 3-4) or patients without increased ICP. The increased risks of medical side effects in hypothermic elderly patients leads to a poor outcome, therefore outweighing the benefits of hypothermia.

Hypothermia and stroke

Although clinical studies to date have not been able to prove indisputably (small sample size, methodological problems, and the complexity of the underlying mechanism) that hypothermia is effective as brain protective therapy, several animal models have demonstrated neuroprotection of mild and moderate hypothermia in trauma and ischaemia. Results from animal models in which hyperthermia worsened and hypothermia improved the effects of cerebral ischaemia led to the prospective non-interventional study by Reith et al. [23]. The possible beneficial effects of mild hypothermia in other cerebral pathologies besides head trauma, like cerebral ischaemia due to stroke, were investigated in 390 stroke patients admitted within 6 h of stroke. Interest focused on the relationship of body temperature on admission and initial stroke severity, infarct size, mortality, and outcome. Other covariates (age, gender, stroke severity on admission, body temperature, infections, leukocytosis, diabetes, hypertension, atrial fibrillation, ischaemic heart disease, smoking, previous stroke, and co-morbidity) were included in the analysis. The results led to the conclusion that there is an association between body temperature and initial stroke severity, infarct size, mortality, and outcome.

Because this study was only non-interventional and a causal relationship was not proven, Schwab et al. [24] initiated a pilot study on the efficacy, feasibility, and safety of induced moderate hypothermia in the therapy of patients with acute severe middle cerebral artery infarction and increased ICP. Moderate hypothermia was induced in 25 patients with severe ischaemic stroke in the middle cerebral artery (MCA) territory within 14 h of stroke by external cooling. Patients were kept between 33 and 34°C body temperature for 2-3 days, and ICP, CPP, and brain temperature were monitored continuously. In all patients intraparenchymatous brain temperature exceeded body core temperature. This temperature gradient varied interindividually and over the measurement period. Outcome at 4 weeks and 3 months after stroke was analyzed with the Scandinavian Stroke Scale (SSS) and the Barthel index; 14 patients survived the hemispheric stroke (56%). Neurological outcome according to the SSS score was 29 (range 25-37) 4 weeks after stroke and 38 (range 28-48) 3 months after stroke. During hypothermia, elevated ICP values could be significantly reduced. Herniation caused by a secondary rise in ICP after rewarming was the cause of death in all remaining patients.

Similar to the traumatic brain injury studies Schwab et al. [24] were able to reduce elevated ICP (mean initial ICP 20 mmHg) by applying hypothermia. In space-occupying MCA infarction, fatal outcome was reported by the same institution in 80% of the patients with standard treatment. The hypothermic patients also fulfilled the criteria of a space-occupying MCA infarction. However, the mortality rate in the hypothermic patients was only 44%. This impressive reduction of the mortality of 80% in the historic control to 44% using hypothermia unfortunately does not prove the effectiveness of hypothermic therapy, but is a striking argument for a prospective randomized trial.

Since ICP seems to be of such a great importance to avoid herniation, it may be hypothesized that a combination therapy of hypothermia and surgical ICP reduction by early decompressive carniotomy is the most-effective treatment regimen in patients with hemispheric stroke, at least in younger patients. Preliminary results showed that mortality could be reduced to only 16% [25].

Hypothermia and cardiopulmonary resuscitation

Early this year results of two randomized clinical trials in Australia and Europe showed a neurological benefit of mild therapeutic hypothermia in survivors of out-of-hospital cardiac arrest. In the Australian study (n=77 patients who remained comatose after restoration of spontaneous circulation), 49% of those treated with hypothermia were discharged compared with 26% of the control patients (P=0.046) [26]. In this study, hypothermia was associated with a lower cardiac index, higher systemic vascular resistance, and hyperglycaemia. There was no difference in the frequency of adverse events. In the European multi-center study guided by the Emergency Department of the University of Vienna, 136 patients were included. Of the hypothermia group, 55% had a favourable outcome compared with 39% in the normothermic group. Additionally, the mortality at 6 months was 41% in the hypothermic group compared with 55% in the normothermic group [27]. The target temperatures in these two studies were between 32 and 34°C maintained for 12 and 24 h, respectively. In patients who have been successfully resuscitated after out-of-hospital cardiac arrest due to ventricular fibrillation, therapeutic mild hypothermia increased the rate of favorable neurological outcome and reduced mortality. Nevertheless, further experimental and clinical data are of great interest to finally establish this rather simple therapy for such patients. Safar and Kochanek [28] recommended the use of mild hypothermia in survivors of cardiac arrest as early as possible, and for at least 12 h [28].

Hypothermia and myocardial infarction

The safety and tolerability of hypothermia as adjunctive therapy to limit infarct size have been observed in pre-clinical animal studies and in phase I clinical studies involving human volunteers with acute myocardial infarction (AMI). Catheter-based induction of systemic hypothermia in animal models of myo-cardial infarction (MI) has demonstrated cardioprotective effects including decreased infarct size, preserved microvascular flow, and maintained cardiac output [29, 30].

Recently, a pilot study examining the feasibility of endovascular cooling during primary percutaneous cardiac intervention (PCI) demonstrated trends in reduced infarct volume, with no increase in haemodynamic instability or cardiac dysrhythmias [31]. Among 42 AMI patients presenting within 6 h of symptom onset, randomization to endovascular cooling (Radiant Medical, Redwood City, Calif., USA) as an adjunct to primary PCI resulted in a 78% reduction in median infarct size by Tc-99m sestamibi SPECT imaging (14.7% with control vs. 6.1% with hypothermia, P=0.375). No significant adverse events (bradyarrhythmias, in particular) were observed in the cooling group, whose mean target core temperature was 33.2°C assessed by nasoesophageal monitoring. Nine patients experienced mild episodic shivering, requiring an increase in pharmacotherapy in 4 patients and a small increase in target core temperature in 5 patients. Importantly, door-to-balloon times were similar in the cooling group, reaffirming the practical application of this therapy in contemporary practice. Finally, if proven effective, the design of trials employing this therapy has been proposed for other AMI treatment algorithms (e.g., fibrinolytic therapy, facilitated PCI).

During myocardial ischaemia, dysregulation of cellular metabolism in addition to reperfusion injury contributes to myocardial injury and cell death that extends in a wavefront pattern from the epicenter of necrosis. The mechanism of cardioprotection associated with hypothermia is believed to occur through downregulation of cardiac myocyte metabolism, thereby limiting the area of myocardium at risk. The data from these studies form the scientific and clinical rationale for the application of systemic hypothermia in reperfusion strategies for AMI.

References

1. Williams M, Rainer W, Fieger H, et al (1991) Cardiopulmonary bypass, profound hypothermia, and circulatory arrest for neurosurgery. Ann Thorac Surg 52:1069-1074
2. Busto R, Dietrich WD, Globus MY et al (1987) Small differences in intraischemic brain temperature critically determine the extent of ischemic neuronal injury. J Cereb Blood Flow Metab 7:729-738
3. Dietrich WD, Alonso O, Halley M, et al (1996) Delayed posttraumatic brain hyperthermia worsens outcome after fluid percussion brain injury: a light and electron microscopic study in rats. Neurosurgery 38:533-541
4. Albrecht RF 2nd, Wass CT, Lanier WL (1998) Occurrence of potentially detrimental temperature alterations in hospitalized patients at risk for brain injury. Mayo Clin Proc 73:629-635
5. Rumana CS, Gopinath SP, Uzura M, et al (1998) Brain temperature exceeds systemic temperature in head-injured patients. Crit Care Med 26:562-567
6. Schuhmann MU, Suhr DF, Gosseln HH v., et al (1999) Local brain surface temperature compared to temperatures measured at standard extracranial monitoring sites during posterior fossa surgery. J Neurosurg Anesthesiol 11:90-95
7. Henker RA, Brown SD, Marion DW (1998) Comparison of brain temperature with bladder and rectal temperatures in adults with severe head injury. Neurosurgery 42:1071-1075

8. Baumgardner JE, Baranov D, Smith DS, et al (1999) The effectiveness of rapidly infused intravenous fluids for inducing moderate hypothermia in neurosurgical patients. Anesth Analg 89:163-169

9. Kurz A, Kurz M, Poeschl G, et al (1993) Forced-air warming maintains intraoperative normothermia better than circulating-water mattresses. Anesth Analg 77:89-95

10. Piepgras A, Roth H, Schurer L, et al (1998) Rapid active internal core cooling for induction of moderate hypothermia in head injury by use of an extracorporeal heat exchanger. Neurosurgery 42:311-317

11. Minamisawa H, Nordstrom CH, Smith ML, et al (1990) The influence of mild body and brain hypothermia on ischemic brain damage. J Cereb Blood Flow Metab 10:365-374

12. Busto R, Globus MY, Dietrich WD, et al (1989) Effect of mild hypothermia on ischemia-induced release of neurotransmitters and free fatty acids in rat brain. Stroke 20:904-910

13. Widmann R, Miyazawa T, Hossmann KA (1993) Protective effect of hypothermia on hippocampal injury after 30 minutes of forebrain ischemia in rats is mediated by postischemic recovery of protein synthesis. J Neurochem 61:200-209

14. Cardell M, Boris MF, Wieloch T (1991) Hypothermia prevents the ischemia-induced translocation and inhibition of protein kinase C in the rat striatum. J Neurochem 57:1814-1817

15. Marion DW, Obrist WD, Carlier PM, et al (1993) The use of moderate therapeutic hypothermia for patients with severe head injuries: a preliminary report. J Neurosurg 79:354-362

16. Shiozaki T, Sugimoto H, Taneda M, et al (1993) Effect of mild hypothermia on uncontrollable intracranial hypertension after severe head injury. J Neurosurg 79:363-368

17. Clifton GL, Allen S, Barrodale P, et al (1993) A phase II study of moderate hypothermia in severe brain injury. J Neurotrauma 10:263-271

18. Marion DW, Penrod LE, Kelsey SF, et al (1997) Treatment of traumatic brain injury with moderate hypothermia. N Engl J Med 336:540-546

19. Hartung J, Cottrell JE (1998) Statistics and hypothermia. J Neurosurg Anesthesiol 10:1-4

20. Marion DW (1998) Response to "Statistics and hypothermia". J Neurosurg Anesthesiol 10:120-123

21. Clifton GL, Miller ER, Choi SC, et al (2001) Lack of effect of induction of hypothermia after acute brain injury. N Engl J Med 344:556-563

22. Clifton GL, Choi SC, Miller ER, et al (2001) Intercenter variance in clinical trials of head trauma--experience of the National Acute Brain Injury Study: hypothermia. J Neurosurg 95:751-755

23. Reith J, Jorgensen HS, Pedersen PM, et al (1996) Body temperature in acute stroke: relation to stroke severity, infarct size, mortality, and outcome. Lancet 347:422-425

24. Schwab S, Schwarz S, Spranger M, et al (1998) Moderate hypothermia in the treatment of patients with severe middle cerebral artery infarction. Stroke 29:2461-2466

25. Steiner T, Ringleb P, Hacke W (2001) Treatment options for large hemispheric stroke. Neurology 57:S61-S68

26. Bernard SA, Gray TW, Buist MD, et al (2002) Treatment of comatose survivors of out-of-hospital cardiac arrest with induced hypothermia. N Engl J Med 346:557-563

27. The Hypothermia after Cardiac Arrest Study Group (2002) Mild therapeutic hypothermia to improve the neurologic outcome after cardiac arrest. N Engl J Med 346:549-556

28. Safar PJ, Kochanek PM (2002) Therapeutic hypothermia after cardiac arrest. N Engl J Med 346:612-613

29. Dae MW, Gao DW, Stillson CA, et al (2000) Profound reduction of myocardial infarct size and preservation of microvascular flow by mild endovascular hypothermia (abstract). Circulation

30. Dae MW, Gao DW, Stillson CA, et al (2001) Effects of mild endovascular hypothermia on infarct size and cardiac output in acute myocardial infarction (abstract). Circulation

31. Dixon SR, Whitbourn RJ, Schaer GL, et al (2001) Systemic hypothermia as an adjunct to primary angioplasty for acute myocardial infarction: results of a safety and feasibility study (abstract). Circulation

ADEQUACY OF CEREBRAL PERFUSION IN THE EARLY PHASES AFTER ACUTE DAMAGE

Strategies to maintain cerebral perfusion pressure during rescue and transport

W. Videtta, G. Domeniconi

Traumatic brain injury (TBI) accounts for a substantial portion of the morbidity and mortality caused by all types of trauma, significantly contributing to more than half of trauma-related deaths. It is the most-frequent cause of mortality and morbidity in those aged up to 45 years, not only in the Western world, but also in developing countries [1-3]. It is also the leading cause of loss of years of productive life. The cost to American society is over 40 billion dollars annually [4]. Neurotrauma is a serious public health problem, demanding continuing efforts in the areas of prevention and treatment [5].

Secondary brain injury of extracranial origin affects the outcome in head--injured patients. A distinctive feature of head injury is the brain's vulnerability to ischemia. The extents of hypoxemia and hypotension suffered by the patient with a TBI are usually underestimated in the pre-hospital phase. Hypotension affects directly cerebral perfusion pressure (CPP) and diminishes cerebral blood flow (CBF).

The treatment of TBI often begins in the field by emergency medical service specialists. This care is continued while en route to the hospital [2]. The pre--hospital assessment and treatment is the critical first link in providing appropriate care for these individuals with severe brain injuries [6]. This paper will focus on CCP and the relationship with other cerebral and systemic variables during the pre-hospital phase.

Head injury during the pre-hospital phase: the scope of the problem

The secondary brain damage of extracranial origin influence the outcome. The biological basis of secondary traumatic brain damage is now well understood [7]. Injured neurons have heightened susceptibility to the effect of hypoxemia and cerebral hypoperfusion [1] and are vulnerable to damage by the high concentrations of neurotransmitters and toxic metabolites that accumulate in their extracellular environment after injury, [9,10]. Neuronal swelling, oedema, and cerebral hyperaemia from carbon dioxide retention are combined to raise the intracranial pressure (ICP) and lower the CPP, which is the main determinant of CBF when head injury has impaired the ability of the cerebral circulation to autoregulate in response to fluctuations in systemic blood pressure. The situation can only be worse if the ICP is further raised by a hematoma or by swelling, or if the CPP is further reduced by extracranial blood loss. The resulting positive feedback loop rapidly causes irreversible clinical deterioration if CPP and oxygenation are not quickly improved. A direct line can thus be traced from adverse events at the neuronal level to the early clinical management of the patient [7].

The pathophysiological understanding and the therapeutic management of head trauma have undergone dramatic changes in the past 2 decades [11]. There is evidence that secondary ischemic brain injury, occurring before and during hospitalization for TBI, contributes to morbidity and mortality [12]. To a great extent, advances in the physiological management of patients with head injuries have depended on the availability of improved physiological monitoring devices, enhancing our understanding of both systemic and cerebral hemodynamic changes [11].

One central concept is that all neurological damage does not occur immediately at the time of impact (primary injury), but evolves over the ensuing minutes, hours, and days. This secondary brain injury can increase mortality and worsen disability. In recognition of this potentially treatable injury, the guidelines for the management of severe head injury were developed for in-hospital care in 1995 using scientific, evidence-based methodology [4], based on consensus and expert opinion [13], or based on scientific support plus consensus and expert opinion [14, 15]. Evidence, consensus, and/or expert opinion to support early assessment, treatment, and transport to appropriate facilities of these severe head injury patients has been compiled and used in a systematic way to formulate guidelines in the pre-hospital setting in few publications [5, 15].

The cerebral variables of greatest interest are the neurological examination, ICP, CPP, and cerebral venous saturation. The systemic variables of greatest interest are blood pressure, PaO_2, $PaCO_2$, serum glucose, oxygen delivery, and body temperature [11]. The pre-hospital phase is pragmatically useful because it is associated with different intensities of monitoring, but also to the quick changes that occur in the cerebral circulation over the first hours after TBI [11].

CCP during the rescue and transport

One of the most-controversial areas of TBI is the management of CPP. CPP is the difference between the mean arterial blood pressure (MABP) and the ICP. CPP cannot be calculated because ICP cannot be monitored during the pre--hospital phase. CPP and ICP cannot be adequately assessed by physical examination. CPP calculation cannot be done because ICP is not monitored, but in some cases, MABP is available. Therefore, the CPP approximation is only empiric and is based on an indirect relationship with systemic variables like systolic blood pressure (SBP) or MABP.

What is the systolic or the mean blood pressure threshold during the rescue and transport?

Abundant evidence is available on the deleterious effects of a low blood pressure (< 90 mmHg systolic) and of hypoxia (arterial oxygen tension < 60 mmHg), and, conversely, that stabilization of blood pressure during resuscitation improves outcome [16]. Hypotension was defined as a single measure < 90 mmHg [17]. Systolic and diastolic blood pressure (DBP) should be measured using the most-accurate system available under the circumstances, as often as possible.

The value of 90 mmHg as a systolic pressure threshold for hypotension has arisen in a rather arbitrary fashion, and it is more of a statistical than a physiological parameter [17]. Given the evidence on the influence of CPP on outcome, it is possible that SBP significantly higher than 90 mmHg [5], 110 mmHg [14, 15], or equal to 120 mmHg [13] would be achieved and maintained during the pre-hospital and resuscitation phase as soon as possible, but no studies have been performed to corroborate this. The importance of MABP, as opposed to systolic pressure, should also be stressed, not only because of its role in calculating CPP, but due to the lack of a consistent relationship between systolic and MABP. The calculation based on systolic values is unreliable. It may be valuable to maintain mean arterial pressure considerably above those represented by systolic pressures of 90, 110, or 120 mmHg throughout the patient's course. Hence, there is no established threshold for systolic or mean blood pressure.

Early in the 1970s and 1980s studies published by Miller et al. [18, 19] established that secondary brain injuries occurring during the early posttraumatic period were primary determinants of outcome. Investigations into the data from the Traumatic Coma Data Bank (TCDB) confirmed these early suggestions using a large, multicenter prospectively collected database [17]. There were five statistically significant independent outcome predictors such as age, intracranial computed tomographic diagnosis, Glasgow Coma Scale (GCS) score, pupillary reactivity, and presence or absence of pre-hospital hypotension (defined as one or more recordings of a SBP ≤ 90 mmHg). The only predictor more amenable to therapeutic modification is the occurrence of hypotension. Patients who were hypotensive at the time of admission had twice the mortality and a significant increase in morbidity when compared with patients who were normotensive. The concomitant presence of hypoxia and hypotension upon admission resulted in a 75% mortality.

The influence of secondary brain injuries, particularly hypotension, on outcome from severe TBI has recently been confirmed in other retrospectively [20, 21] and prospectively collected data sets [22, 23]. In 1993, Fearnside et al. [22] conducted a prospective study of 315 severe head-injured patients admitted consecutively to a single center and investigated pre-hospital and in-hospital predictors of outcome. Hypotension (SBP < 90 mmHg) was an independent predictor of increased mortality and morbidity. In 1996, Stocchetti et al. [23] carried out a prospective study of data collection at the accident scene from 50 severely head-injured patients rescued by helicopter. Blood pressure or oxygen saturation measurements were classified as above or below a certain threshold. This study revealed that 55% had an oxygen saturation less than 90% measured at the scene prior to intubation. Of the 28 patients who were hypoxemic, 13 did not have associated hypotension. There was a significant (P < 0.005) association between arterial desaturation and poor outcome. Low pre-hospital blood pressures or oxygen saturations were associated with worse outcomes.

One of the most-important strategies to maintain an adequate CPP "in a blind fashion" seems to be avoiding hypotension at the level determined for each emergency medical system. According to the wide variety of literature regarding hypotension, it is better to define this in terms of SBP and at a level 90 mmHg.

How to improve the CPP through improving systemic variables?

The pre-hospital phase is the first and the most-critical interval in determining the ultimate outcome after clinical TBI. Critical to the outcome of acute head injury, there are rapid interventions to prevent secondary brain damage [11]. Hypotension or hypoxaemia, alone or in combination, occur in 57% of comatose patients with head injuries from the time of injury through resuscitation [17]. Due to impaired cerebral autoregulation after trauma, hypovolaemic hypotension that would not otherwise reduce CBF may lead to brain ischaemia. Thus, prompt application of basic or advanced life support, i.e., tracheal intubation, positive pressure ventilation with oxygen, and intravenous fluid resuscitation, may limit secondary hypoxic brain damage. Concerns that adequate fluid resuscitation results in increased ICP after head injury appear to be unfounded [24,25]. On a purely physiological basis, it is reasonable to argue that the cerebral circulation is so pressure dependent immediately after TBI that even short-term support with vasopressors might be defensible [11].

The greatest concern regarding early, aggressive haemodynamic support is the possibility that restoration of blood pressure in hypotensive trauma patients could aggravate haemorrhage from systemic injuries. In experimental models of uncontrolled haemorrhage, increasing blood pressure increased bleeding and may have adversely influenced mortality [26]. In patients with penetrating truncal trauma, Bickell et al. [27] reported that immediate, pre-hospital resuscitation did not improve mortality in comparison with resuscitation initiated only at hospital arrival. However, because hypotensive patients with TBI will usually be victims of blunt vehicular trauma and will have associated non-penetrating injuries, and the beneficial effect of permissive hypotension in an exsanguinating head injury patient would be overwhelmed by the devastating effects of hypotension upon an injured brain, these data are not directly relevant.

One of the promising intervention is small-volume resuscitation with hypertonic saline solutions. Evidence from experimental studies [28, 29] demonstrates that hypertonic saline solutions, with or without added colloid, increase blood pressure, decrease ICP, and reduce brain water in areas in which the blood-brain barrier is intact. In trauma patients with SBP $\leq$ 100 mmHg, Vassar et al. [30] compared 250 ml of lactated Ringer's solution with 7.5% saline in 6.0% dextran 70 (HSD) for pre-hospital resuscitation. In the subset of patients with severe head injury (53 of 186 patients), 32% of those who received HSD survived, versus only 16% of the patients who received lactated Ringer's solution (P = 0.04). In a subsequent, randomized multi-center study, Vassar et al. [31] compared the effects of 250 ml of 7.5% sodium chloride with and without 6% and 12% dextran 70 with 250 ml of lactated Ringer's solution for the pre-hospital resuscitation of hypotensive trauma patients. A small subgroup of patients with GCS but without severe anatomical injury seemed to benefit most from resuscitation with 7.5% saline [31].The beneficial effects of hypertonic resuscitation could be due to reduction in ICP or, more likely, to rapid increases in SBP in comparison with comparable volumes of isotonic solutions. These findings are not conclusive.

Restoration of effective gas exchange is equally important. Although pre-hospital monitoring of PaO_2 and $PaCO_2$ is not currently performed in most ambulances and helicopters, the adverse effects of hypoxaemia and hypercarbia are sufficient determinant. Hypoxaemia and hypercarbia cause vasodilation and increase ICP and lower CPP, respectively. Neither will be optimally effective under the conditions of emergency transport. Pulse oximetry will often not be effective in patients who are being moved or who are severely hypoperfused. Capnography will be less effective than in healthy patients; however, in those patients where the monitoring is effective, early warning of abnormal gas exchange may be life-saving [11].

Although serum glucose is not customarily measured in the pre-hospital phase, clinicians should recognize the hazards of inadvertently aggravating hyperglycaemia. Iatrogenic hyperglycemia can limit the effectiveness of fluid resuscitation by inducing an osmotic diuresis and, in animals, may aggravate ischaemic neurological injury [32]. Although associated with worse outcome in both ischaemic [33] and traumatic [34] brain injury in humans, separation of cause and effect is difficult because hyperglycemia constitutes a hormonally mediated response to more-severe injury [33].

During pre-hospital stabilization and transport, especially if accompanied by vigorous fluid resuscitation, body temperature typically decreases. From the perspective of the brain, mild hypothermia may be protective. Preliminary clinical data suggested that the possibility of therapeutic hypothermia during intensive care of patients with head injuries might improve neurological outcome in survivors [35,36], but this was not confirmed in the last trial [37].

Conclusions

After TBI, an adequate CPP is necessary, but not enough to guarantee that CBF is adequate. The available clinical studies suggest that a CPP of 60 mmHg provides an adequate perfusion pressure for the majority of adult TBI patients, based on measures of global CBF and cerebral oxygenation, but it is not possible to measure the perfusion pressure in the field. Thus, the most-prudent strategy to achieve and maintain an adequate CPP and guarantee an adequate CBF in the pre-hospital phase is to avoid hypotension and to achieve a SBP of 90 – 120 mmHg or a MABP close to 90 – 100 mmHg when available. A reliable threshold for SBP or MABP should be established. The optimal choice of fluids and volume for resuscitation of patients with TBI is not known. Much more work is needed for this controversial aspect of management of TBI patients.

References

1. Kraus JF (1987) Epidemiology of head injury. In: Cooper PR (ed) Head injury. Williams and Wilkins, Baltimore, pp 1-19
2. Valadka AB, Pepe PE (1999) Prehospital management. In: Marion DW (ed) Traumatic brain injury. Thiemes Medical Publishers, New York, pp 55-65
3. Baethmann A, Eriskat J, Stoffel M, et al (1998) Special aspects of severe head injury: recent developments. Curr Opin Anaesthesiol 11:193-200
4. Bullock R, Chesnut RM, Clifton C, et al (1996) Guidelines for the management of severe head injury. J Neurotrauma 13:643-734
5. Gabriel EJ, Ghajar J, Jagoda A, et al (2002) Guidelines for prehospital management of traumatic brain injury. J Neurotrauma 19:111-174
6. Baxt WG, Moody P (1987) The impact of advanced prehospital care on the mortality of severely brain-injured patients J Trauma 27:365-369
7. Gentleman D, Dearden M, Midgley S, Maclean D (1993) Fortnightly review: guidelines for resuscitation and transfer of patients with serious head injury. BMJ 307:547-552
8. Ishige N, Pitts LH, Hashimoto T, et al (1987) Effect of hypoxia on traumatic brain injury in rats. 1. Changes in neurological function, electroencephalograms, and histopathology. Neurosurgery 20:848-853
9. Faden AI, Demediuk P, Panter SS, Vink R (1989) The role of excitatory amino-acids and NMDA receptors in traumatic brain injury Science 244:798-800
10. Desalles AAF, Kontos HA, Becker DP, et al (1986) Prognostic significance of ventricular CSF lactic acidosis in severe head injury J Neurosurg 65:615-624
11. Prough DS, Lang J (1997) Therapy of patients with head injuries: key parameters for management. J Trauma 42:10S-18S
12. Chesnut RM (1995) Secondary brain insults after head injury: clinical perspectives New Horiz 3:366-375
13. Maas AI, Dearden M, Teasdale GM, et al (1997) EBIC-guidelines for management of severe head injury in adults European Brain Injury Consortium. Acta Neurochir (Wien) 139:286-294
14. Procaccio F, Stocchetti N, Citerio G, et al (2000) Guidelines for the treatment of adults with severe head trauma. II. Criteria for medical treatment. J Neurosurg Sci 44:11-18
15. Procaccio F, Stocchetti N, Citerio G, et al (2000) Guidelines for the treatment of adults with severe head trauma. I. Initial assessment; evaluation and pre-hospital treatment; current criteria for hospital admission; systemic and cerebral monitoring. J Neurosurg Sci 44:1-10
16. Marmarou A, Anderson RL, Ward JD, et al (1991) Impact of ICP instability and hypotension on outcome in patients with severe head trauma. J Neurosurg 75:S59-S66
17. Chesnut RM, Marshall LF, Klauber MR, et al (1993) The role of secondary brain injury in determining outcome from severe head injury. J Trauma 34:216-222
18. Miller JD, Sweet RC, Narayan R, Becker DP (1978) Early insults to the injured brain. JAMA 240:439-442
19. Miller JD, Becker DP (1982) Secondary insults to the injured brain. J R Coll Surg Edinb 27:292-298
20. Gentleman D (1992) Causes and effects of systemic complications among severely head injured patients transferred to a neurosurgical unit. Int Surg 77:297-302
21. Hill DA, Abraham KJ, West RH (1993) Factors affecting outcome in the resuscitation of severely injured patients. Aust N Z J Surg 63:604-649
22. Fearnside MR, Cook RJ, McDougall P, McNeil RJ (1993) The Westmead Head Injury Project outcome in severe head injury: a comparative analysis of pre-hospital, clinical and CT variables. Br J Neurosurg 7:267-269
23. Stocchetti N, Furlan A, Volta F (1996) Hypoxemia and arterial hypotension at the accident scene in head injury. J Trauma 40:764-767
24. Schmoker JD, Schackford SR, Wald SL, Pietropaoli JA (1992) An analysis of the relationship

between fluid and sodium administration and intracranial pressure after head injury J Trauma 33:476-481

25. Zornow MH, Prough DS (1995) Fluid management in patients with traumatic brain injury. New Horiz 3:488-498
26. Gross D, Landau EH, Klin B, Krausz MM (1990) Treatment of uncontrolled hemorrhagic shock with hypertonic saline solution Surg Gynecol Obstet 170:106-112
27. Bickell WH, Wall MJ Jr, Pepe PE, et al (1994) Immediate versus delayed fluid resuscitation for hypotensive patients with penetrating torso injuries. N Engl J Med 331:1105-1109
28. Hartl R, Schurer L, Goetz C, et al (1995) The effect of hypertonic fluid resuscitation on brain edema in rabbits subjected to brain injury and hemorrhagic shock. Shock 3:274-279
29. Schmoker JD, Zhuang J, Shackford SR (1991) Hypertonic fluid resuscitation improves cerebral oxygen delivery and reduces intracranial pressure after hemorrhagic shock. J Trauma 31:1607--1613
30. Vassar MJ, Perry CA, Gannaway WL, Holcroft JW (1991) 7.5% sodium chloride/dextran for resuscitation of trauma patients undergoing helicopter transport. Arch Surg 126:1065-1072
31. Vassar MJ, Fischer RP, O'Brien PE, et al (1993) A multicenter trial for resuscitation of injured patients with 7.5% sodium chloride: the effect of added dextran 70. Arch Surg 128:1003-1011
32. Lanier WL, Stangland KJ, Scheithauer BW, et al (1987) The effects of dextrose infusion and head position on neurologic outcome after complete cerebral ischemia in primates: examination of a model. Anesthesiology 66:39-48
33. Longstreth WT Jr, Diehr P, Cobb LA, et al (1986) Neurologic outcome and blood glucose levels during out-of-hospital cardiopulmonary resuscitation Neurology 36:1186-1191
34. Lam AM, Winn HR, Cullen BF, Sundling N (1991) Hyperglycemia and neurological outcome in patients with head injury. J Neurosurg 75:545-551
35. Marion DW, Obrist WD, Carlier PM, et al (1993) The use of moderate therapeutic hypothermia for patients with severe head injuries: a preliminary report. J Neurosurg 79:354-362
36. Clifton GL, Allen S, Barrodale P, et al (1993) A phase II study of moderate hypothermia in severe brain injury. J Neurotrauma 10:263-271
37. Clifton GL, Miller ER, Choi SC et al (2001) Lack of effect of induction of hypothermia after acute brain injury. N Engl J Med 344:556-563

The systemic and cerebrovascular effects of inotropes and vasopressors

J.A. MYBURGH

Inotropes and vasopressors form the cornerstone for pharmacological support of the circulation. The principle aim of these drugs is to restore inadequate systemic and regional perfusion to physiological levels in conditions of circulatory failure. These drugs are increasingly used to augment the circulation in situations where the circulation is ostensibly normal, with the specific aim of increasing or improving regional perfusion. This strategy has been used for many years and has been directed at the prevention or amelioration of acute renal failure, hepatic insufficiency, and acute brain syndromes. Regarding the latter, inotropes and vasopressors have been used in the management of neurological conditions, such as traumatic brain injury and aneurysmal subarachnoid haemorrhage.

Definitions

Inotropic agents are defined as drugs that act on the heart by increasing the velocity and force of myocardial fibre shortening. The resultant increase in contractility results in increased cardiac output and blood pressure. The most commonly used drugs are pharmaceutical preparations of the naturally occurring catecholamines: adrenaline, noradrenaline, and dopamine.

Vasopressors are drugs that have a predominantly vasoconstrictive action on the peripheral vasculature, both venous and arterial. These drugs are primarily used to increase mean arterial pressure. Commonly used drugs include phenylephrine and metaraminol.

The distinction between these two groups of drugs is often confusing. Many of the commonly used agents, such as the catecholamines, have both inotropic and variable effects on the peripheral vasculature that include venoconstriction, arteriolar vasodilatation, and constriction.

For the purposes of this discussion, inotropes and vasopressors will considered as equivalent groups of vasoactive drugs.

Characteristics of the ideal vasoactive drug are shown in Table 1.

Table 1 Characteristics of the ideal inotrope

The ideal inotrope
Increases contractility

Increases mean arterial pressure
     Increases cardiac output
     Improves regional perfusion

No increase in myocardial oxygen consumption

Avoidance of tachycardia
     Non arrhythmogenic
     Maintenance of diastolic blood pressure

Does not develop tolerance
Titratable
Rapid onset   Rapid termination of action
Compatible with other drugs
Non-toxic
Cost-effective

Pharmacology

Vasoactive agents may be classified according to their chemical structure and biosynthesis, cellular action, or pharmacodynamic effects. Although pharmacodynamic effects are the most useful from a clinical perspective, an appreciation in developments in the cellular biology of these drugs is important to understand the applicability and potential shortfalls of these drugs in acute neurological syndromes.

Classification

Sympathomimetic amines are the most frequently used vasoactive agents in the intensive care unit and include the naturally occurring catecholamines dopamine, noradrenaline, and adrenaline. Synthetic sympathomimetics are derivatives of dopamine and include dobutamine, isoprenaline, and dopexamine. Phenylephrine and metaraminol are synthetic direct-acting agonists that are selective venous and arterial vasoconstrictors. These synthetic agents have similar pharmacokinetics to catecholamines.

Biosynthesis

The biosynthesis of the endogenous catecholamines is shown in Fig. 1. Catecholamines consist of an aromatic ring attached to a terminal amine by a carbon chain. The configuration of each drug is important for determining affinity to respective receptors.

Dopamine is hydroxylated to form noradrenaline, which is the predominant peripheral sympathetic chemotransmitter in humans, acting at all adrenergic receptors. The release of noradrenaline from sympathetic terminals is controlled by re-uptake mechanisms mediated via α_2 receptors and augmented by adrenaline released from the adrenal gland at times of stress. Noradrenaline is converted to form adrenaline that is subsequently metabolized in liver and lung. [1]

All catecholamines have very short biological half-lives (1-2 min). A steady-state plasma concentration is achieved within 5-10 min after the start of a

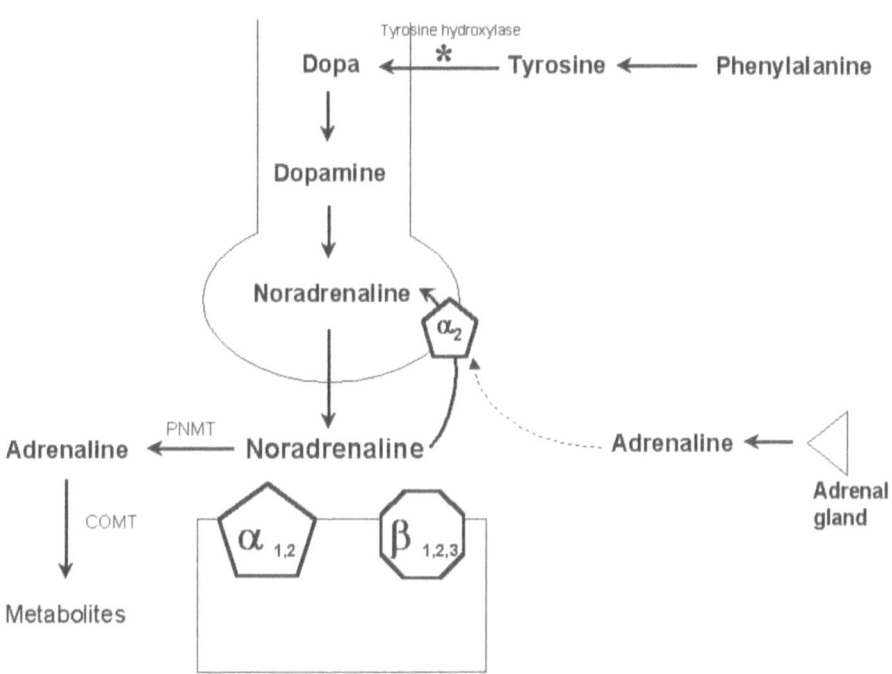

Fig. 1 Biosynthesis of catecholamines in sympathetic terminals (* rate limiting step by tyrosine hydroxylase, *PNMT* phenethanolamine-N-methyltransferase, *COMT* catechol-*o*-methyl-transferase)

constant infusion. This allows rapid titration of drug to a clinical endpoint such as mean arterial pressure.

Adrenaline and noradrenaline infusions produce blood concentrations similar to those produced endogenously in shock states, whereas dopamine infusions produce much higher concentrations than those naturally encountered. Dopamine may exert much of its effect by being converted to noradrenaline, thus bypassing the rate-limiting (tyrosine hydroxylase) step in catecholamine synthesis.

The synthetic catecholamines are derivatives of dopamine. These agents are characterized by increased length of the carbon chain, which confers affinity for β-receptors. Dobutamine is a synthetic derivative of isoprenaline. These agents have relatively little affinity for α-receptors due to the configuration of the terminal amine, which differs from the endogenous catecholamines.

Adrenaline, noradrenaline, and isoprenaline all have hydroxyl groups on the β carbon atom of the side chain, and this is associated with 100-fold greater potency than dopamine or dobutamine [1]. Phenylephrine and metaraminol are direct acting α_2-agonists that are selective vasoconstrictors, both venous and arterial, with minimal β activity.

Receptor biology

Agonists bind to populations of adrenergic receptors, largely divided into α- and β-subgroups. Further subgroups of α (α_{1A}, α_{1B}, α_{2A}, α_{2B}, α_{2C}) and β-receptors (β_1, β_2, and β_3) have been identified. [2]

Signal transduction from agonist-receptor occupation to the effector cell is modulated by conformational changes in G proteins associated with these receptors [3]. Under the additional influence of second messengers such as nitric oxide, endothelin, and eicosanoids, these conformational changes promote the release of calcium from intracellular stores and increase membrane calcium permeability [4]. Subsequent phosphorylation of substrate proteins via protein kinases triggers a cascade of events that leads to specific cardiovascular effects. [2]

This complex agonist-receptor-effector relationship is responsible for homeostatic mechanisms, such as physiological responses to stress and autoregulation.

The activity and function of this system is dynamic and may be markedly influenced by pathological states. This may result in qualitative changes in the agonist-receptor-effector organ relationship (desensitization), where receptors no longer respond to physiological or pharmacological sympathetic stimulation to the same extent [5]. Quantitative changes, such as reduced receptor density, receptor sequestration, and enzymatic uncoupling (downregulation), may also result in impaired responses. [6] Both desensitization and downregulation occurs in patients receiving prolonged infusions of high-dose catecholamines. This is commonly seen in patients with traumatic brain injury and subarachnoid haemorrhage where these drugs are used to augment cerebral perfusion pressure.

Pharmacodynamic effects

Vascular responsiveness is mediated via adrenergic receptors: α mechanisms predominantly cause vasoconstriction (both arterial and venous), β mechanisms, specifically β_2-receptors, mediate vasodilatation.

Alpha-adrenergic mechanisms have an increasingly important role in the failing or downregulated circulation [7]. This applies at both myocardial and peripheral vascular levels

The systemic and regional effects of any of these agents will vary greatly between patients and within individuals at different times. Adequacy of response is often unpredictable and depends on the aetiology of circulatory failure and systemic co-morbidities. In some patients, dramatic responses to small doses may occur, whilst in others, large doses of inotropes may be required to support the failing circulation.

The classification of sympathomimetic agents into α- and β-agonists based on the above structure/function relationships is only a crude predictor of systemic effects.

Adrenaline, noradrenaline and dopamine are all predominantly β-agonists at low doses, with increasing α effects becoming evident as the dose is increased. The synthetic catecholamines are all predominantly β-agonists, whilst synthetic vasoconstrictors act predominantly on α_2-receptor populations.

Applications of vasoactive agents

The recognition of the importance of defending cerebral perfusion pressure in acute brain syndromes such as traumatic brain injury and aneurysmal subarachnoid haemorrhage has resulted in a marked increase in the use of vasoactive agents in these patients. This has developed in the absence of definitive outcome-based studies of the use of these drugs in these conditions. There are no studies that have demonstrated the benefit of one inotrope over another or combination of inotrope(s). Consequently, there is marked variation in the selection, use, and role of vasoactive agents in acute brain syndromes.

Applying the pharmacological and physiological principles outlined above in conjunction with available animal and clinical data, it is possible to formulate an approach to the use of these drugs in acute brain syndromes.

Systemic effects of vasoactive agents

These drugs act on all regions where the adrenergic system predominates. Clearly, the main effect is on the cardiovascular system, which has direct applicability to strategies directed at augmenting cerebral perfusion.

Cardiovascular physiology

The predominant effects of inotropes on the cardiovascular system are increased systemic blood pressure, cardiac output, and venous return. This is achieved by increasing stroke volume of the ejecting ventricle by increased myocardial contractility and associated increase in cardiac output. The latter may be further increased by associated increases in heart rate. Importantly, cardiac output is controlled by the peripheral vasculature that is as energetic at returning blood to the heart as the heart is at pumping blood to the periphery [8-10]. The effects of vasoactive agents on the peripheral vasculature are predominantly on the venous circulation, augmenting and increasing return from the capacitance venous system, rather than specific arteriolar vasoconstriction. Both the arterial and venous systems are integrated under complex neurohormonal influences.

The cardiovascular system is not a homogenous pump-driven system through conduits of uniform length and resistance. Consequently, the oft-used extrapolation of Ohm's law (which states that perfusion pressure is proportional to cardiac output and systemic vascular resistance) to describe or assess haemodynamic function is invalid. The use of derived indices such as systemic vascular resistance to assess the effects of a particular drug on vascular function is dubious. Right atrial pressure is a more-accurate measurement of venous return and tone than systemic vascular resistance [10]. Similarly, calculated global oxygen delivery and consumption measurements, using the Fick principle, are frequently used as surrogate indices of global metabolic activity. Oxygen delivery and consumption are surrogate measurements of cardiac output and arterial oxygen tension. Oxygen extraction ratio, using derived oxygen delivery and consumption, are invalidated by mathematical coupling.

Given the limitations of physiological measurement of cardiovascular function and the physiological complexities of the system, comparative studies between vasoactive agents are confounding.

Physiological studies

Few studies directly comparing the physiological, systemic and regional effects of vasoactive agents have been performed. In an ovine preparation, the effects of equivalent ramped infusions of adrenaline and noradrenaline (0-60 µg/min) and dopamine (0-60 µg/kg/min) on systemic haemodynamic and oxygenation variables were determined [11]. These effects are shown in Fig. 2.

All three drugs produced equivalent and significant increases in mean arterial pressure and cardiac output from baseline. Systemic vascular resistance initially decreased from baseline and approached baseline levels as doses were increased. These observed changes in systemic vascular resistance would not occur if the assumptions of Ohm's law were valid. In comparison, the effects of the three catecholamines on right atrial pressure (as an index of venous

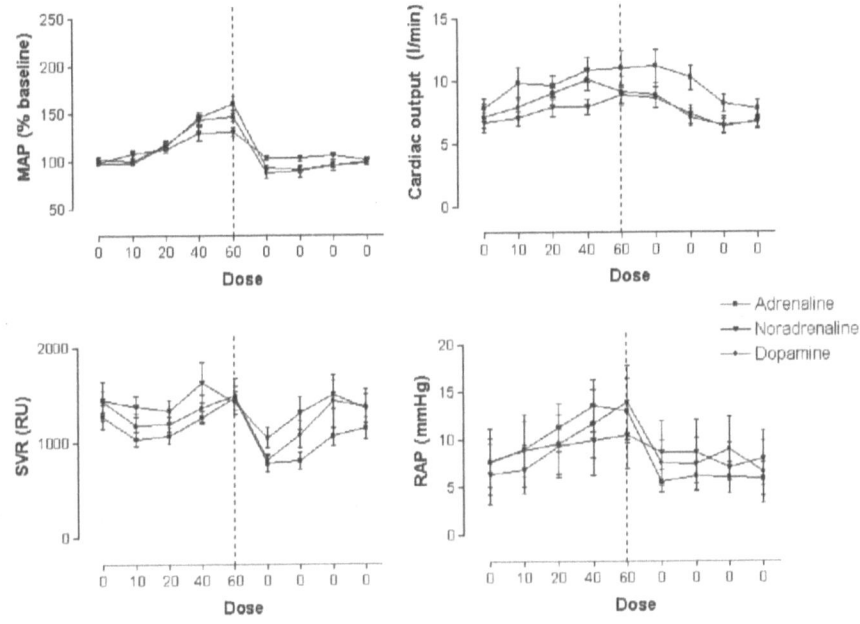

Fig. 2 Clockwise from top left: comparisons of the effects of adrenaline, noradrenaline, and dopamine infusions on mean arterial pressure (*MAP*, expressed as percentage change from baseline), cardiac output (l/min), systemic vascular resistance (*SVR*, resistance units), and right atrial pressure (*RAP*, mmHg). Dose refers to 5-min intervals in µg/min for adrenaline and noradrenaline, µg/kg per min for dopamine during infusion followed by a 20-min washout period. Data are expressed as mean ± SEM

return) showed equivalent and significant increases in right atrial pressure as doses were increased. The effects of the catecholamines on the peripheral vasculature were more accurately represented by changes in right atrial pressure than systemic vascular resistance [10].

Changes in oxygen delivery mirrored changes in cardiac output: equivalent effects with adrenaline, noradrenaline, and dopamine were demonstrated. No significant changes from baseline were demonstrated in oxygen consumption and extraction, suggesting that mathematical coupling produced an equivocal result.

Pathological studies

Despite established use in clinical practice, selection of a particular agent is predicated on purported physiological effects, clinical dogma, and experience, and applied to a particular clinical scenario.

For example the cardiovascular effects of septic shock are complex and range from a hyperdynamic, vasodilated state to one of increasing myocardial failure and paralysis of the peripheral vasculature (vasoplegia) [12-14]. The latter represents inability of the venous circulation to respond to endogenous or exogenous catecholamines with resultant venous pooling. Noradrenaline was considered to be a potent vasoconstrictor agent used to reverse vasoplegia, but potentially caused renal and splanchnic ischaemia. However, an increasing body of literature now supports the use of noradrenaline and adrenaline as first line agents in the septic syndrome and septic shock by effectively defending cardiac output, mean arterial pressure, and thereby tissue perfusion [15-19]. Systemic vascular resistance was not demonstrated to be significantly altered by catecholamine infusions in septic shock [20]. Despite widespread recent use, the efficacy of dobutamine and isoprenaline in septic shock is questionable and appears to add little to the efficacy of noradrenaline or adrenaline when used in combination [21].

The use of noradrenaline has changed significantly over this period and is now regarded by most clinicians as a first-line drug for the defence of blood pressure [16,17]. This change in practice has occurred in the absence of controlled trials; rather due to the recognition of augmenting failing endogenous systems, using the synthetic form of the predominant endogenous catecholamine. However, it is likely that adrenaline is equieffective with a similar profile, although there are no studies to affirm this hypothesis.

Given a degree of pharmacological equivalence in the septic shock literature, it is tempting to apply these data to patients with normal cardiovascular systems who are receiving vasoactive agents to augment systemic blood pressure. There are no human studies addressing this issue and the answer is best provided in animal studies.

In summary, it appears that under physiological conditions, the endogenous catecholamines produce equivalent haemodynamic effects, predominantly increasing systemic blood pressure. From a teleological and physiological perspective, it would appear that noradrenaline is the drug of choice under these conditions. Under pathological conditions, a similar profile is probable, although there are no outcome-based studies that demonstrate an attributable benefit of one vasoactive agent over another.

Cerebrovascular effects of vasoactive agents

Augmentation of regional blood flow and perfusion has been intensely studied over the last 20 years. Strategies directed at optimizing regional circulation in the kidney and gut have been analyzed with variable results. The recognition that maintenance of adequate systemic haemodynamics is the principle factor in optimizing regional circulation has led to a reductionist philosophy. The lack of effect of "renal dose" dopamine in preventing acute renal failure is an example of this development [22].

Cerebrovascular physiology

Regarding the cerebral circulation, two factors make the application of a reductionist view, i.e., "keep the blood pressure up and the brain will perfuse," somewhat simplistic.

Firstly, the brain is an efficient autoregulator. Cerebral blood flow is maintained at a constant rate over a range of changing perfusion pressures. Autoregulatory systems are complex and involve a number of myogenic (pressure) and metabolic systems [23]. Cerebral vasoregulation is under the influence of complex neurohumoral systems such as nitric oxide, endothelin, eicosanoids, vasopressin, endogenous neuropeptides, and cellular elements, such as perivascular pH, cellular oxygen tension, and carbon dioxide. Secondly, the blood--brain barrier forms an anatomical and metabolic barrier to systemic drugs. The access of vasoactive agents to the cerebral vasculature is regulated by factors such as lipid solubility and exposure to metabolic enzyme systems within the blood-brain barrier [24,25].

Under physiological conditions, catecholamines do not normally cross the blood-brain barrier. This is an integral mechanism in maintaining cerebral autoregulation. However, this effect may be altered by changes in blood-brain barrier permeability, induced either by systemic physiological perturbations or by associated pathophysiological or pathological conditions.

The direct effect of catecholamines on the cerebral circulation under physiological and pathophysiological conditions remains contentious, due to variability of experimental models and methods of measurement of cerebrovascular mechanics.

Physiological studies

In animal models, catecholamine-induced hypertension with adrenaline [26], dopamine [27], and phenylephrine [28] has been demonstrated to alter the morphology of the blood-brain barrier. This has been attributed to changes induced by the associated hypertension the upper autoregulatory threshold exceeded and by alterations in blood-brain barrier permeability.

There are few studies quantifying and comparing the effects of catecholamines on cerebrovascular mechanics. In an early study, King et al. [29] compared the effects of adrenaline (using doses of 6-22 µg/min) and noradrenaline (19-73 µg/min) on cerebral blood flow, measured using the nitrous oxide method, in awake, human volunteers. Induced hypertension with adrenaline was associated with increased cerebral blood flow that was attributed to increased cerebral metabolism. Noradrenaline was associated with decreased cerebral blood flow that was attributed to increased cerebrovascular resistance in the absence of demonstrable changes in metabolism.

In a physiological ovine preparation, the effects of infusions of exogenous catecholamines on cerebral blood flow (measured by continuous sagittal sinus Doppler) [30], intracranial pressure and cerebral perfusion pressure ($CMRO_2$) were determined [11]. Adrenaline and noradrenaline (0-60 µg/min) and dopamine (0-60 µg/kg/min) were administered by ramped infusion to achieve sustained systemic hypertension (Fig. 2). The effects on cerebrovascular mechanics and metabolism are shown in Fig. 3.

Dopamine significantly increased cerebral blood flow and intracranial pressure in a dose dependent manner without demonstrable changes in calculated cerebrovascular resistance or $CMRO_2$. The effects of dopamine on cerebral blood flow and intracranial pressure were significantly greater than adrenaline, which increased cerebral blood flow, albeit to a lesser extent and noradrenaline, which did not. Of the three catecholamines, noradrenaline had the least effect on cerebrovascular mechanics, despite inducing an equivalent systemic effect to dopamine and noradrenaline, suggesting little or no direct effect on the cerebral circulation. This study demonstrated that in a directly comparative model, catecholamine-induced hypertension was associated with changes in cerebrovascular mechanics that were independent of calculated cerebral metabolic rate for oxygen. The variance between this study and the earlier study of King et al. [29] may be explained by the difference in doses used – a standardized infusion over a dose range using a continuous method of cerebral blood flow measurement compared with disparate doses in different individuals.

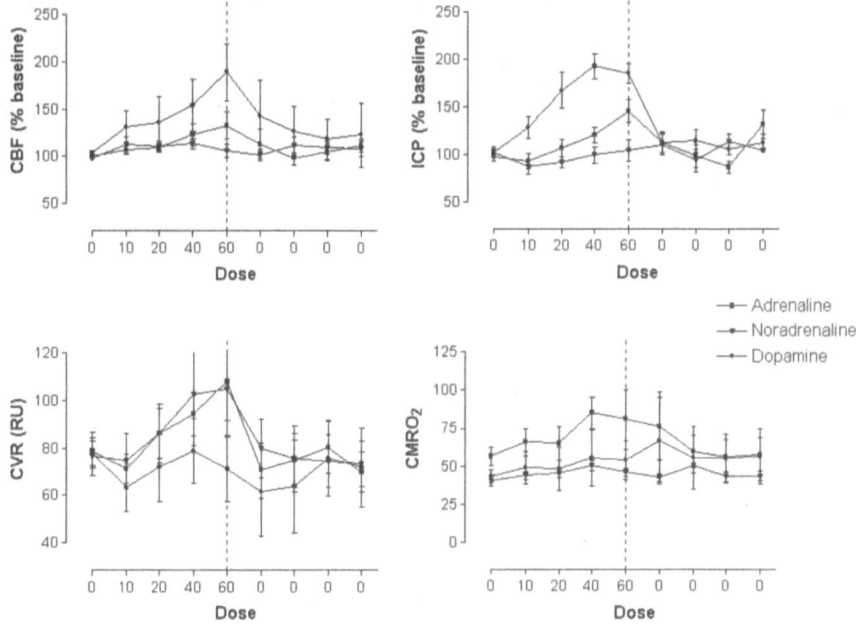

Fig. 3 Clockwise from top left: comparisons of the effects of adrenaline, noradrenaline, and dopamine infusions on cerebral blood flow (*CBF*, expressed as percentage change from baseline), intracranial pressure (*ICP*), cerebrovascular resistance (*CVR*, resistance units), and cerebral metabolic rate for oxygen (*CMRO₂*). Dose refers to 5-min intervals in µg/min for adrenaline and noradrenaline, µg/kg per min for dopamine during infusion, followed by a 20-min washout period. Data are expressed as mean ± SEM

Cerebrovascular resistance is a derived index that is prone to cumulative measurement errors and should be interpreted with circumspection when assessing cerebrovascular changes.

Dopamine exerted a more-pronounced effect on cerebral blood flow and intracranial pressure once upper autoregulatory thresholds were exceeded. This implies that dopamine was either able to cross the blood-brain barrier at lower concentrations or that there may be a direct effect of dopamine on the cerebral circulation. Selective transmission of dopamine may occur across the natural defects in the blood-brain barrier, such as the posterior pituitary gland or pineal gland that have specific dopaminergic receptors, or via non-adrenergic central neural mechanisms [31, 32]. This may be compounded by high circulating concentrations of catecholamines (either endogenous or exogenous) that may also open the morphological barrier, by inducing an acute rise in systemic blood pressure [24, 33].

The effect of catecholamines such as adrenaline, noradrenaline, and dopamine on blood-brain barrier permeability has been demonstrated in a number of experimental models, including labelled albumin leakage [34] and Evans blue [35]. The effects of catecholamines on cerebral blood flow and metabolism were demonstrated using various methods of cerebral blood flow measurement including ^{14}C ethanol [36], quantitative autoradiography [33], and hydrogen clearance techniques [37]. A consistent finding in these studies was that blood-brain barrier permeability was altered by induced hypertensive stimuli [33, 38], particularly by dopamine and adrenaline [26]. This phenomenon has been implicated in the pathogenesis of hypertensive encephalopathy [39].

Pathological studies

There is therefore a sound physiological basis for the direct cerebrovascular effects of vasoactive agents under certain conditions. Induced hypertension with catecholamines is a relatively uncommon clinical situation, although these drugs are increasingly being used in acute brain syndromes to augment cerebral perfusion pressure.

Pathological changes in cerebral autoregulation and blood-brain barrier permeability, induced by conditions such as traumatic brain injury and subarachnoid haemorrhage, render the cerebral circulation more vulnerable to vasoactive agents than the associated induced hypertension.

There are few studies analyzing these effects under pathological conditions. Noradrenaline, adrenaline, dopamine, and phenylephrine have been used to augment cerebral perfusion pressure, although there is no conclusive evidence to recommend one drug over another. [40]

In an early comparative study of hypertension-induced changes in blood-brain barrier permeability by phenylephrine, adrenaline, and noradrenaline in rats, Tsai et al. [28] demonstrated direct effects of these vasoactive agents on cerebral blood flow, cerebral perfusion pressure and intracranial pressure. These rats were anaesthetized by urethane, which is associated with direct changes in blood-brain barrier permeability. Concomitantly administered drugs, such as volatile and intravenous anaesthetics, to head-injured patients receiving vasoactive agents provide a high potential for alterations in cerebrovascular function [41-43].

Similarly, there are few human studies comparing vasoactive agents in pathological conditions. Catecholamines and vasoconstrictors have been used for years as first-line drugs to increase cerebral perfusion pressure. Rosner et al. [44] described their practice of using phenylephrine and or noradrenaline to aggressively augment cerebral perfusion pressure in a longitudinal series of 93 patients in whom cerebral perfusion pressure was maintained > 90 mmHg [44]. These patients were compared with a historical cohort of similar patients. Lower mean intracranial pressures (determined by quadratic logarithm analysis) and improved Glasgow Outcome Scores in the test group were demonstrated. However, these results should be interpreted with some caution due to the intervention bias and weak comparative methodology. Nevertheless, this non-randomized, retrospective study indicated a potential role for cerebral perfusion pressure-based treatment in traumatic brain injury without demonstrably adverse effects on intracranial pressure.

A small study by Biestro et al. [45] compared the effects of dopamine, noradrenaline, methoxamine, and dopamine plus methoxamine on cerebral perfusion pressure and intracranial pressure in a series of head-injured patients. Noradrenaline and dopamine plus methoxamine were equally effective in increasing cerebral perfusion pressure without demonstrable increases in intracranial pressure.

In a recent study, Ract and Vigue [46] compared the effects of dopamine and noradrenaline, using a cross-over design, in 19 head-injured patients. For the same mean arterial pressure, intracranial pressure was significantly greater with dopamine than with noradrenaline. This was not associated with changes in indirect measurements of cerebral blood flow with jugular venous saturation or transcranial Doppler. This small human study is in accordance with the physiological studies outlined, suggesting that, in traumatic brain injury which is associated with altered cerebral autoregulation and blood-brain barrier permeability, dopamine has more-pronounced effects on the cerebral circulation.

Clinical applications

The use of vasoactive agents in acute brain syndromes is therefore based to an intention-to-treat basis, according to the associated clinical scenario. There is a paucity of human, physiological and pathophysiological outcome-based evidence to direct therapy. However, some conclusions may be drawn from the evidence that is available, coupled with advances in the understanding of pathophysiological mechanisms.

Traumatic brain injury

In traumatic brain injury, cerebral hypoperfusion is associated with adverse outcome, particularly in the early phases of management [47]. This has resulted in the increased use of drugs such as adrenaline, noradrenaline, dopamine, and phenylephrine to augment or maintain systemic blood pressures at near-normal levels. This is now part of standard practice and is endorsed by the Brain Trauma

Foundation guidelines [48-50]. It probably matters little which agent is used, provided appropriate monitoring is in place and those reversible causes of hypotension are promptly excluded and treated.

However, vasoactive agents to augment cerebral perfusion pressure in traumatic brain injury must be used with circumspection, particularly in the latter phases of management. During recovery of initial cerebral hypoperfusion or oligaemia, a subset of patients is vulnerable to the development of an ischaemia-reperfusion injury [51]. This is characterized by cerebral hyperae-mia, which may be compounded by vasoactive agents such as noradrenaline or dopamine. In this situation, cerebral perfusion pressure targets should be reassessed, ideally using a measurement of cerebral blood flow in an attempt to minimize iatrogenically induced hyperaemia. For this hypothetical reason, based on the comparative physiological studies outlined above, noradrenaline would be the drug of choice and dopamine avoided.

Subarachnoid haemorrhage

Augmentation of cerebral blood flow by induced hypertension, hypervolaemia, and haemodilution ("HHH" therapy) to treat cerebral vasospasm associated with aneurysmal subarachnoid haemorrhage is a strategy that has been advo-cated for 20 years. However, there is little evidence that "HHH" therapy either reverses vasospasm or improves outcome for aneurysmal subarachnoid hae-morrhage [52]. Indeed, the use of vasoactive agents to increase cerebral blood flow in these patients may be associated with adverse outcomes due to cerebral hyperaemia and ischaemia, particularly with dopamine [27]. Furthermore, "HHH" therapy is associated with an increased rate of medical compilations that may be in part due to the injudicious use of inotropes in these patients [53]. For similar reasons outlined above, noradrenaline would appear to be drug of choice, if this strategy is employed. However, this should be used with great circumspection.

Inotropes and vasopressors are integral drugs in the armamentarium of intensivists, anaesthetists, emergency physicians, and surgeons for the pharma-cological support of the circulation. Despite their established role and wide-spread use, there is little unequivocal evidence upon which clinical practice may be based. A reappraisal of the physiological and pharmacological principle of these drugs in various clinical situations is warranted, as are randomized controlled trials directed at determining efficacy and effectiveness.

References

1. Runciman WB, Morris JL (1993) Adrenoceptor agonists. In: Feldman AC et al (eds) Mechanisms of drugs in anaesthesia. Arnold, London, pp 262-291
2. Insel PA (1996) Seminars in medicine of the Beth Israel Hospital, Boston. Adrenergic receptors--evolving concepts and clinical implications. N Engl J Med 334:580-585
3. Bohm M, Flesch M, Schnabel P (1996) Role of G-proteins in altered beta-adrenergic responsiveness in the failing and hypertrophied myocardium. Basic Res Cardiol 91 [Suppl 2]:47-51
4. Hajjar RJ, Muller FU, Schmitz W, et al (1998) Molecular aspects of adrenergic signal transduction in cardiac failure. J Mol Med 76:747-755
5. Kompa AR, Gu XH, Evans BA, Summers RJ (1999) Desensitization of cardiac beta-adrenoceptor signaling with heart failure produced by myocardial infarction in the rat. Evidence for the role of Gi but not Gs or phosphorylating proteins. J Mol Cell Cardiol 31:1185-1201
6. Silverman HJ, Penaranda R, Orens JB, Lee NH (1993) Impaired beta-adrenergic receptor stimulation of cyclic adenosine monophosphate in human septic shock: association with myocardial hyporesponsiveness to catecholamines. Crit Care Med 21:31-39
7. Hwang KC, Gray CD, Sweet WE, et al (1996) Alpha 1-adrenergic receptor coupling with Gh in the failing human heart. Circulation 94:718-726
8. Jacobsohn E, Chorn R, O'Connor M (1997) The role of the vasculature in regulating venous return and cardiac output: historical and graphical approach. Can J Anaesth 44:849-867
9. Guyton AC, Lindsay AW, Kaufmann BN (1955) Effect of mean circulatory filling pressure and other peripheral circulatory factors on cardiac output. Am J Physiol 180:463-468
10. Magder S (1998) More respect for the CVP. Intensive Care Med 24:651-653
11. Myburgh JA, Upton RN, Grant C, Martinez A (1998) A comparison of the effects of norepinephrine, epinephrine, and dopamine on cerebral blood flow and oxygen utilisation. Acta Neurochir [Suppl] (Wien) 71:19-21
12. MacKenzie IM (2001) The haemodynamics of human septic shock. Anaesthesia 56:130-144
13. Carpati CM, Astiz ME, Rackow EC (1999) Mechanisms and management of myocardial dysfunction in septic shock. Crit Care Med 27:231-232
14. Magder S, Vanelli G (1996) Circuit factors in the high cardiac output of sepsis. J Crit Care 11:155-166
15. LeDoux D, Astiz ME, Carpati CM, Rackow EC (2000) Effects of perfusion pressure on tissue perfusion in septic shock. Crit Care Med 28:2729-2732
16. Nasraway SA (2000) Norepinephrine: no more "leave 'em dead"? Crit Care Med 28:3096-3098
17. Tordoff SG, Thompson JL, Williams AW (2000) Noradrenaline as a vasoactive agent in septic shock. Intensive Care Med 26:648
18. Martin C, Papazian L, Perrin G, et al (1993) Norepinephrine or dopamine for the treatment of hyperdynamic septic shock? Chest 103:1826-1831
19. Martin C, Viviand X, Leone M, Thirion X (2000) Effect of norepinephrine on the outcome of septic shock. Crit Care Med 28:2758-2765
20. Moran JL, O'Fathartaigh MS, Peisach AR, et al (1993) Epinephrine as an inotropic agent in septic shock: a dose-profile analysis. Crit Care Med 21:70-77
21. Martin C, Viviand X, Arnaud S, et al (1999) Effects of norepinephrine plus dobutamine or norepinephrine alone on left ventricular performance of septic shock patients. Crit Care Med 27:1708-1713
22. Bellomo R, Chapman M, Finfer S, et al (2000) Low-dose dopamine in patients with early renal dysfunction: a placebo-controlled randomised trial. Australian and New Zealand Intensive Care Society (ANZICS) Clinical Trials Group. Lancet 356:2139-2143
23. Paulson OB, Strandgaard S, Edvinsson L (1990) Cerebral autoregulation. Cerebrovasc Brain Metab Rev 2:161-192
24. Hardebo JE, Owman C (1980) Barrier mechanisms for neurotransmitter monoamines and their precursors at the blood-brain interface. Ann Neurol 8:1-31

25. MacKenzie ET, McCulloch J, O'Kean M. et al (1976) Cerebral circulation and norepinephrine: relevance of the blood-brain barrier. Am J Physiol 231:483-488

26. Sokrab TE, Johansson BB, Tengvar C. et al (1988) Adrenaline-induced hypertension: morphological consequences of the blood-brain barrier disturbance. Acta Neurol Scand 77:387-396

27. Darby JM, Yonas H, Marks EC, et al (1994) Acute cerebral blood flow response to dopamine--induced hypertension after subarachnoid hemorrhage. J Neurosurg 80:857-864

28. Tsai ML, Lee CY, Lin MT (1989) Responses of cerebral circulation produced by adrenoceptor agonists and antagonists in rats. Neuropharmacology 28:1075-1080

29. King BD, Sokoloff L, Wechsler R (1951) The effects of l-epinephrine and l-norepinephrine upon cerebral circulation and metabolism in man. J Clin Invest 31:273-279

30. Ludbrook GL, Upton RN, Grant C, Grey EC (1994) An ultrasonic doppler venous outflow method for the continuous measurement of cerebral blood flow in conscious sheep. J Cereb Blood Flow Metab 14:680-688

31. Teasdale G, McCulloch J (1977) Effect of stimulation of dopaminergic receptors upon local cerebral blood flow. Acta Neurol Scand [Suppl] 64:98-99

32. okote H, Itakura T, Nakai K, et al (1986) A role of the central catecholamine neuron in cerebral circulation. J Neurosurg 65:370-375

33. Tuor UI, Edvinsson L, McCulloch J (1986) Catecholamines and the relationship between cerebral blood flow and glucose use. Am J Physiol 251:H824-H833

34. Ben Menachem E, Johansson BB, Svensson TH (1982) Increased vulnerability of the blood-brain barrier to acute hypertension following depletion of brain noradrenaline. J Neural Transm 53:159-167

35. Suzuki R, Nitsch C, Fujiwara K, Klatzo I (1984) Regional changes in cerebral blood flow and blood-brain barrier permeability during epileptiform seizures and in acute hypertension in rabbits. J Cereb Blood Flow Metab 4:96-102

36. Johansson B, Hardebo JE (1982) Cerebrovascular permeability and cerebral blood flow in hypertension induced by gammahydroxybutyric acid. An experimental study in the rat. Acta Neurol Scand 65:448-457

37. MacKenzie ET, Strandgaard S, Graham DI, et al (1976) Effects of acutely induced hypertension in cats on pial arteriolar caliber, local cerebral blood flow, and the blood-brain barrier. Circ Res 39:33-41

38. Ekstrom-Jodal B, Larsson LE (1982) Effects of dopamine of cerebral circulation and oxygen metabolism in endotoxic shock: an experimental study in dogs. Crit Care Med 10:375-377

39. Tamaki K, Sadoshima S, Baumbach GL, et al (1984) Evidence that disruption of the blood-brain barrier precedes reduction in cerebral blood flow in hypertensive encephalopathy. Hypertension 6:I75-I81

40. Kroppenstedt SN, Stover JF, Unterberg AW (2000) Effects of dopamine on posttraumatic cerebral blood flow, brain edema, and cerebrospinal fluid glutamate and hypoxanthine concentrations. Crit Care Med 28:3792-3798

41. Olsen KS, Henriksen L, Owen-Falkenberg A, et al (1994) Effect of 1 or 2 MAC isoflurane with or without ketanserin on cerebral blood flow autoregulation in man. Br J Anaesth 72:66-71

42. Stephan H, Sonntag H, Schenk HD, Kohlhausen S (1987) [Effect of Disoprivan (propofol) on the circulation and oxygen consumption of the brain and CO2 reactivity of brain vessels in the human]. Anaesthesist 36:60-65

43. Chi OZ, Anwar M, Sinha AK, et al (1992) Effects of isoflurane on transport across the blood-brain barrier. Anesthesiology 76:426-431

44. Rosner MJ, Rosner SD, Johnson AH (1995) Cerebral perfusion pressure: management protocol and clinical results. J Neurosurg 83:949-962

45. Biestro A, Barrios E, Baraibar J, et al (1998) Use of vasopressors to raise cerebral perfusion pressure in head injured patients. Acta Neurochir [Suppl] (Wien) 71:5-9

46. Ract C, Vigue B (2001) Comparison of the cerebral effects of dopamine and norepinephrine in severely head-injured patients. Intensive Care Med 27:101-106

47. Chesnut RM (1997) Avoidance of hypotension: conditio sine qua non of successful severe head-injury management. J Trauma 42:S4-S9
48. The Brain Trauma Foundation. The American Association of Neurological Surgeons. The Joint Section on Neurotrauma and Critical Care (2000) Resuscitation of blood pressure and oxygenation. J Neurotrauma 17:471-478
49. The Brain Trauma Foundation. The American Association of Neurological Surgeons. The Joint Section on Neurotrauma and Critical Care (2000) Hypotension. J Neurotrauma 17:591-595
50. The Brain Trauma Foundation. The American Association of Neurological Surgeons. The Joint Section on Neurotrauma and Critical Care (2000) Guidelines for cerebral perfusion pressure. J Neurotrauma 17:497-506
51. Martin NA, Patwardhan RV, Alexander MJ, et al (1997) Characterization of cerebral hemodynamic phases following severe head trauma: hypoperfusion, hyperemia, and vasospasm. J Neurosurg 87:9-19
52. Oropello JM, Weiner L, Benjamin E (1996) Hypertensive, hypervolemic, hemodilutional therapy for aneurysmal subarachnoid hemorrhage. Is it efficacious? No. Crit Care Clin 12:709-730
53. Solenski NJ, Haley EC Jr, Kassell NF, et al (1995) Medical complications of aneurysmal subarachnoid hemorrhage: a report of the multicenter, cooperative aneurysm study. Participants of the Multicenter Cooperative Aneurysm Study. Crit Care Med 23:1007-1017

Awake craniotomy

M. KLIMEK

For decades general anaesthesia with endotracheal intubation has been the anaesthesiological standard procedure for the resection of brain tumors. Vital parameters are controlled, intubation provides a safe airway especially during surgical procedures in the head/neck region, drugs used ensure analgesia and suppression of vegetative reactions. Immobilization is easy even with the patient in an atypical position. Furthermore the anaesthesiologist may control the intracranial pressure and the acid-base state of the patient by mechanical ventilation. At the same time these aspects ensure optimal working conditions for the neurosurgeon.

However, the intraoperative monitoring of any functional lesion to the central nervous system is severely inhibited by general anaesthesia. Some drugs suppress neuronal activity and some higher cortical brain functions (e.g., speech) cannot be monitored except by awakening the patient.

After widespread introduction of microsurgery and brain imaging techniques, the development of function-controlled neurosurgery demands a novel anaesthetic approach. Function-controlled neurosurgery has yet more potential, although neurosurgeons already can perform procedures thought impossible 10 years ago [1]. However, from the historical point of view it is not a new invention, but one can talk about a renaissance of the function-controlled neurosurgery [2-4].

The anaesthesiologist plays an important part in function-controlled neurosurgery, enabling maximum safety and a minimum discomfort to the patient without using drugs or measures that make functional monitoring impossible [5].

In this paper the implications of function-controlled neurosurgery (e.g., awake craniotomy with speech monitoring for resection of a brain tumour) for the anaesthesiological management of the patient will be described. Possible pitfalls and the author's personal experience will be discussed. Of importance, most published literature is about the choice of drugs and complications of awake craniotomy. There is little about how to perform awake craniotomy, and it is hoped to fill this gap a little.

Definition

Awake craniotomy is a misleading term, because the patient is not awake during craniotomy. However, the patient is awake during resection of tumour, so that the term "brain tumour resection with intraoperative neuropsychological monitoring in awake patients" better covers what is done. Also the terms "monitored anaesthesia care" or "monitored conscious sedation" are used for this kind of procedure and can also be considered as a synonym. For practical reasons we continue to use "awake craniotomy" for this procedure. Surgical treatment of drug-resistant seizures is also performed as awake craniotomy. However, this review on awake craniotomy will focus on surgery of intracranial neoplasms.

Selection of patients

Speech monitoring is useful in all patients with speech impairment due to the tumour or with tumours close to the speech area. In cases where speech function recovered during preoperative steroid treatment, the awake tumour resection with speech monitoring may be very beneficial. By positron emission tomography with speech activation an overlap of the tumour and speech areas can be determined preoperatively. In the same way, other higher cortical function (e.g., calculation, directed movement) can be monitored if necessary in relation to the site of the tumour.

Besides these pathological-anatomical aspects, there are several more virtues of awake craniotomy. The conscious and awake patient can communicate with the surgeon and can retain more speech function, although a less-radical resection of the tumour might be the consequence. A complete resection (R0) of malignant brain tumours is almost impossible, regardless of the surgical or anaesthesiological approach.

Perioperatively, the intracranial pressure and the risk of bleeding should not be increased. The surgery must be performed in the supine or semi-lateral position. Sitting or prone positions are not suitable for awake craniotomy. Other unsuitable patients are those with expectable difficult intubation (e.g., severe Morbus Bechterew, orofacial malformation). Early discussion between neurosurgeon, anaesthesiologist, neuropsychologist, and patient about each individual procedure is essential.

Preoperative anaesthesiological visit

It is highly desirable that the preoperative visit and anaesthesia should be performed by the same anaesthesiologist. One must know the patient in order to provide optimal intraoperative medical and psychological guidance. With good reason Pasquet [3] uses the term "vocal anaesthesia" to describe such intraoperative care for the patient. This implicates another aspect of the preoperative visit: the patient must have a chance to become familiar with his anaesthesiologist.

Procedures must me explained to the patient in detail [7-9]. The following aspects demand special attention:
- shaving of the head
- covering with surgical drapes
- intraoperative sounds of the monitoring devices and surgical instruments
- long period of lying flat
- feeling of cold
- immobilization of the head with tape
- insertion of tubes and lines, especially of the urinary catheter
- temporary loss of neuropsychological function during electrical stimulation or due to brain oedema
- possibility of pain

The patient may hear some irritating remarks and should be forewarned. The summarized message to the patient should be: "We are prepared for almost all possible events and are able to deal with any discomfort. Please, tell us, what you want us to do; but you may not be able to move or find a more-comfortable position."

In case of complications, general anaesthesia and endotracheal intubation must be performed. The patient must be informed about such course of events and of other risks of the procedure. The need to abstain from smoking, eating, and drinking before surgery should be explained.

The neurosurgeon and the neuropsychologist pay separate preoperative visits. The neuropsychologist explains the intraoperative speech monitoring and runs his tests once (e.g., Aachener aphasie test in case of monitoring of speech function). During this test the ability of the patient to recognize images without glasses and to talk without dentures can be estimated.

Premedication

On the evening before surgery, lorazepam (1.5 - 2.0 mg for an average adult) is a good choice, owing to its anxiolytic action. For immediate preanaesthetic medication, piritramide (7.5 mg) combined with promethazine (50 mg), intra-muscularly, are the author's drugs of choice half an hour before starting the induction. Choice of premedication agents is based on the idea that the evening before surgery the patient has no other need than having a peaceful night, provided there is no preoperative pain or vegetative instability. On the day of surgery, the opioid drug piritramide provides a basic analgesia during the induction and the trepanation. The antihistaminic, mild neuroleptic prometha-zine provides agreeable sedation, antiemetic effect, and vegetative stability. Benzodiazepines should be avoided on the day of surgery, because their effect on vigilance is unpredictable and may interfere with the management of intravenous sedation and make speech monitoring unreliable. In patients with stomach complaints, additional preoperative metoclopramide (10 mg) and ranitidine (50 mg) are useful. All dosages are for an average adult. Most of the regular drug intake is continued, especially anticonvulsants.

Induction of anaesthesia

The anaesthesiological measures during the induction for awake craniotomy take about 20 min more than for usual general anaesthesia; extra time is needed for additional local anaesthesia for all insertions. If a wake-up test is performed, the procedure takes an additional 10 - 20 min.

After obtaining baseline values of standard monitoring, venous access is established through the skin weal of mepivacaine 1.0 %. Oxygen is applied via a nasal catheter (flow 4 l/min) and sedation with propofol is started. The patient should tolerate all invasive procedures, be comfortable, and breath sufficiently. This can be achieved by a single bolus of 40 - 100 mg propofol, continued by an infusion-rate of 2-3.5 mg/kg per hour, aiming at effect-controlled titration. In patients using anticonvulsants or other enzyme-inducing drugs, require-ments for propofol may be much higher.

Nasopharyngeal airway (Wendl tube) is placed to keep the airways open. From the start of propofol sedation and during the whole procedure, emergency intubation must be possible without delay: drugs ready in syringes, adequate endotracheal tube and the laryngoscope. A prophylactic laryngoscopy to check the airway anatomy during the sedation period can not be recommended, because the low degree of sedation means a high risk of regurgitation and aspiration. Especially in the beginning of the individual learning curve, the anaesthetist's threshold to switch over to general anaesthesia should be low.

When sedation is well established, arterial blood pressure cannula (radial artery) and central venous catheter are placed under local anaesthesia. Placement of all tubes and connections should be checked carefully to avoid discomfort to the patient. If necessary, at the place of the connection of the arterial line an additional subcutaneous mepivacaine infiltration can be performed.

With monitoring and access lines in place, one can proceed with infusion of 50 mg ranitidine to prevent excessive gastric acidity and 40 mg dexamethasone for optimal control of brain oedema. Also, infusion of 20-40 mmol potassium chloride may be useful to substitute preexisting deficiency. Furthermore, antibiotic prophylaxis is administered. Then the patient's scalp is prepared and the urinary catheter is placed.

Even with the patient seemingly asleep, all procedures are communicated to him. Uncontrolled movements may subside after an extra bolus of 20 - 30 mg propofol.

A wake-up test following the placement of all tubes and lines is advisable for all those patients who show severe adverse movements. The propofol infusion is stopped and the patients are observed for degree of agitation, especially of uncontrolled head movements during the wake-up period. All patients who were calm during this wake-up test showed the same peaceful behaviour during the intraoperative wake-up procedure.

Anaesthesiological management during awake craniotomy

Period of trepanation

After the wake-up test the patient is transferred awake to the operating theatre to get accustomed to the surroundings, the sounds, and the drapes. Patients may actively help positioning themselves for the procedure. Then another bolus of propofol is injected and sufficient sedation should be achieved before local infiltration analgesia of the scalp and periosteum.

The patient's head is not immobilized with the mayfield clamp, but is taped on a ring and upholstered with additional pads, when necessary. A slight elevation of the patient's head and avoidance of extreme torsion of the cervical spine are strongly recommended [10, 11]. Most tumours afflicting the speech function are localized in the frontotemporal lobe. A semi-lateral position of the body and a certain side-rotation of the head are required for the surgical access. The underlying ear may be pressurized in this position, which must be avoided [2]. Careful upholstering must be carried out, to provide a warm and comfortable position for the patient. The legs should be strapped by a belt and the arms by broad strips of tape, which are placed over the upholstering pads, to avoid damage by uncontrolled movements.

One surgical drape should be placed along the brows and lifted, so that the patient has a free view towards his feet. This drape can be dropped over the open skull and an emergency intubation can be performed without contaminating the surgical field.

The surgical field is infiltrated with 40 ml 0.375 % bupivacaine with or without adrenaline (1:200,000). The resulting volume is sufficient for local anaesthesia of the surgical field. Long-acting local anaesthetic drugs are preferable [6].

The need for sedation during trepanation shows a high interindividual variability and dosage should be effect adjusted. In our patients, 0 - 650 mg propofol per hour was needed. Sedation is continued until the end of the preparation of the dura mater. Girvin [7, 8] showed that the dura preparation becomes less painful with an increasing distance to the sphenoid wings and the meningeal vessels. Afterwards the intraoperative wake-up period starts.

During trepanation repeated checks of arterial blood gases are needed to exclude hypercapnia. Regularity and frequency of breathing along with pulse oximetry must be monitored all the time.

General aspects of the intraoperative guidance and management

The intraoperative wake-up period should be managed with minimal stimulation to the patient. One can address the patient just by words, no tactile stimuli should be used. If the patient reacts adequately, he is informed about the actual situation. Messages are: "We are in the operating theatre, up to now everything went fine, we can see the tumour". The patient is asked whether there are any troubles (dryness of the mouth, positioning). Then the first pictures for the speech monitoring are presented to check the visibility in the new surrounding (side-rotated head, operating room lights, blankets around the head).

The intraoperative guidance of the patient requires repeated dialogue between the patient, the neuropsychologist, the neurosurgeon, and the anaesthesiologist. The patient should be informed about the course of the procedure, that all vital parameters monitored are fine, he should be congratulated for successfully naming the objects during the aphasia test period, and should be asked about any discomfort, which might be reduced.

Furthermore, a sidetracking dialogue between the neuropsychologist and the patient should continue all the time. Some music in the operation theatre might be played, depending on the patient's wishes. Headphones limit the patient's ability to communicate and one rather refrains from using them.

During the surgical procedure some additional medication may be necessary, like mannitol for prophylaxis and/or treatment of brain oedema. Phenytoin is usually administered prior to the electrical stimulation to reduce the occurrence of seizures [12]. When focal or general seizures do occur the topical application of a few millilitres of ice-cold saline on the surface of the brain in the irritated area has proven effective.

Additional ondansetron or metoclopramide are required in patients who report nausea. In these patients the dura mater of the temporobasilary area and small dura vessels were irritated, which induced the trigeminal nerve-mediated nausea. By irritation of the trigeminal structures, vagal reactions with severe bradycardia may also occur. Therefore atropine sulphate should be available immediately, but a prophylactic injection of atropine might be better. In any case the surgeon must be warned to stop irritating these fields as soon as possible.

Urapidil is useful to control hypertensive systolic blood pressures not associated with pain. Tramadol and metamizole are efficient to combat increasing headache or lower back pain towards the end of the procedure. In order to alleviate dryness of the mouth and thirst, compresses soaked in water are suitable to suck on.

Severe complications, like major bleeding, excessive brain oedema, grand--mal seizures, vomiting, or venous air embolism, would demand emergency intubation and general anaesthesia. Fortunately, in the author's series of more than 50 awake craniotomies with a mean duration of 331 min from induction to end of the procedure, no such major complication occurred.

Neuopsychological and neurophysiological monitoring

Before the surgeon starts to cut into a certain area of the brain, he electrically stimulates underlying structures. During the electrical stimulation the patient is asked to name the pictures, which are shown to him by the neuropsychologist (e.g., "This is a helicopter!"). If naming is successful, the surgeon may cut into this area, if not, he should not do so. In addition to the speech function, motor function may be tested, too (e.g., "Move your right hand!"). Some sophisticated projection machines help to check the correctness of the patient's answer, and measure the latency between presentation of the picture and the answer, which may provide additional neurophysiological information.

It is essential to warn the patient prior to electrical stimulation and so to avoid the situation where the patient is shocked by a sudden loss of ability to speak, but will be reassured to know it is a temporary functional disorder and not permanent damage. It must be stressed that in most patients stimulation of areas influenced the patient's ability to speak.

The procedure of awake craniotomy demands from all involved to be careful with verbal remarks. Certainly, the result of the intraoperative histopathological examination should not be announced audibly. Signs at the doors of the theatre to remain silent will be helpful [8].

Haemostasis and closure of the wound

After resection of the tumour, there is no more need to continue speech monitoring. The patient is informed about the successful course of the procedure and is re-sedated again by an additional bolus of propofol, followed by a continuous infusion. In case of signs of pain during the wound closure, the wound may be infiltrated again by the local anaesthetic.

Postoperative period

The propofol infusion is discontinued immediately after closing of the wound and the patient is transferred awake to the intensive care unit for further observation. Safe transfer to the ward follows the morning after. An immediate postoperative transfer of the patient to the general ward or even early discharge home seem possible sometimes, but is not advisable for safety reasons [13].

A postoperative check-up of speech function by the neuropsychologist is a must. Sometimes a transient worsening of neuropsychological functions is attributed to focal oedema at the operative site and subsequently disappears. Such a transient postoperative deficit is seen in about one-third of the patients [14]. Worsening deficits or decreasing vigilance are alarming signs, indicating postoperative intracranial bleeding, and emergency computed tomography scan should be performed. Postoperative pain can be successfully relieved by i.v. administration of tramadol or metamizol, or a combination of both.

Postoperative nausea and vomiting seem to occur much less frequently following awake craniotomy than after general anaesthesia for intracranial procedures [15].

Awake craniotomy: ongoing debate

In addition to the aforementioned practical aspects of awake craniotomy, two more subjects of ongoing discussion are of interest, management of free airway and of analgesia.

Management of free airway

We have satisfactory experience with minimally invasive administration of supplemental oxygen with either oxygen probe or through the nasal airway. Some experts perform more-invasive airway management. There are reports on awake craniotomy with a laryngeal mask, which also enables the patient to speak or vocalize and supposedly offers partial protection against aspiration during deep sedation [16]. The laryngeal mask has also been temporarily removed during the tests [17]. There is also a case report of mechanical ventilation via a nasal airway, which can be considered as a modified mask-ventilation technique [18]. Moreover, some authors report a successful intubation-extubation-reintubation regimen [19].

In some places brief general anaesthesia on day 1 enables trepanation and placement of stimulation electrodes, and on day 2 brain mapping is done using these electrodes on the awake patient. Later on, the surgeon proceeds, again with general anaesthesia. This technique certainly provides maximal airway safety. Unfortunately, the functional evaluation of some deeper brain structures cannot be done by this technique.

Management of sedation and analgesia

Before propofol, neuroleptic agents were drugs of choice in the management of epilepsy surgery on (half) awake patients. From spinal cord surgery it is known that an asleep-awake-asleep technique can be done with almost all available anaesthetic drugs [20]. Propofol is nowadays the cornerstone for sedation [21,22]. Importantly, propofol does not interfere with electrocortico-graphic recording [23]. Many authors use opioids in addition to propofol, but most have reported short periods of unacceptable respiratory depression [24, 25]. As of now, it appears that there is still much to learn about anaesthesia for awake craniotomy. Finding the right dosage for safe, adequate, and smooth sedation in each individual patient is the most-demanding part of the procedure [26]. Promising patient-controlled sedation with propofol has already been reported [27,28]. However, if the patient does not recover as fast as expected, one should remember to use physostigmine. Physostigmine can be used to antagonize a postanaesthetic central anticholinergic syndrome, but also has opioid analgesia-enhancing properties and antagonizes residual opioid-induced respiratory depression and somnolence [29]. Its use can be recommended when patients do not recover as fast as might be expected. If injected in such a state, one is able to differentiate between narcotic hangover and a possible early intracranial bleeding [30].

Conclusions

Awake craniotomy is quite possible and can be performed safely. All depends on selection of patients and preoperative instructions. Possible pitfalls of this procedure must be borne in mind. High patient acceptance and satisfaction are guaranteed, because some of the temporo-parietal lesions may otherwise be inoperable [31-33]. However, one cannot consider awake craniotomy as a standard approach for most supratentorial tumours. Namely because perioperative mortality rate of 1% seems to be higher than for procedures under general anaesthesia [34]. The long-term outcome of the patients who suffered from severe complications related to the technique will determine its value for the future. Nevertheless, one can expect that anaesthetic technique for awake craniotomy will continue to develop along with technical advancement of intraoperative imaging or robot-assisted surgery [35]. According to a recent study of computer-guided awake craniotomy, in the majority of patients a greater than 90% reduction of tumour mass was achieved, which is very encouraging. However, the overall future of surgery for glioma and the development of associated anaesthetic techniques will remain uncertain until the effect of cytoreduction on patient outcome is elucidated [36].

References

1. Schmid UD, Gall C, Schröck E, et al (1995) Function-controlled neurosurgery. Neurophysiologic and neuropsychological monitoring during surgery of the nervous system. Nervenarzt 66:582-595
2. Feindel W (1986) Electrical stimulation of the brain during surgery for epilepsy - historical highlights. Intern Anesthesiol Clin 24:75-87
3. Pasquet A (1986) Combined regional and general anesthesia for craniotomy and cortical exploration. II. Anesthetic considerations. Reprint of a lecture given 1953. Intern Anesthesiol Clin 24:12-20
4. Penfield W (1986) Combined regional and general anesthesia for craniotomy and cortical exploration. I. Neurosurgical considerations. Reprint of a lecture given 1953. Intern Anesthesiol Clin 24:1-11
5. Varkey GP (1986) Introduction to "Anesthetic considerations for craniotomy in awake patients." Intern Anesthesiol Clin 24:15-21
6. Manninen P, Contreras J (1986) Anaesthetic considerations for craniotomy in awake patients. Intern Anesthesiol Clin 24:157-174
7. Girvin JP (1986) Resection of intracranial lesions under local anesthesia. Intern Anesthesiol Clin 24:133-155
8. Girvin JP (1986) Neurosurgical considerations and general methods for craniotomy under local anesthesia. Intern Anesthesiol Clin 24:89-114
9. Trop D (1986) Conscious-sedation analgesia during neurosurgical treatment of epilepsies - practice at Montreal Neurological Institute. Intern Anesthesiol Clin 24:75-83
10. Mavrocordatos P, Bissonnette B, Ravussin P (2000) Effects of neck position and head elevation on intracranial pressure in anaesthetized neurosurgical patients: preliminary results. J Neurosurg Anesthesiol 12:10-14

11. Rolighed Larsen JK, Haure P, Cold GE (2002) Reverse Trendelenburg position reduces intra-cranial pressure during craniotomy. J Neurosurg Anesthesiol 14:16-21
12. Ojemann GA (1986) Mapping of neuropsychological language parameters at surgery. Intern Anesthesiol Clin 24:115-131
13. Blanshard HJ, Chung F, Manninen PH, et al (2001) Awake craniotomy for removal of intracranial tumour: considerations for early discharge. Anesth Analg 92:89-94
14. Danks RA, Aglio LS, Gugino LD, et al (2000) Craniotomy under local anesthesia and monitored conscious sedation for the resection of tumours involving eloquent cortex. J Neuro-oncol 49:131-139
15. Manninen PH, Tan TK (2002) Postoperative nausea and vomiting after craniotomy for tumor surgery: a comparison between awake craniotomy and general anesthesia. J Clin Anesth 14:279-283
16. Shinokuma T, Shono S, Iwakiri S, et al (2002) Awake craniotomy with propofol sedation and a laryngeal mask airway: a case report. Masui 51:529-531
17. Fukaya C, Katayama Y, Yoshino A, et al (2001) Intraoperative wake-up procedure with propofol and laryngeal mask for optimal excision of brain tumour in eloquent areas J Clin Neurosci 8:253-255
18. Weiss FR, Schwartz R (1993) Anaesthesia for awake craniotomy. Can J Anaesth 40:1003
19. Huncke K, van de Wiele B, Fried I, et al (1998) The asleep-awake-asleep anesthetic technique for intraoperative language mapping. Neurosurgery 42:1312-1317
20. McCann ME, Brustowicz RM, Bacsik J, et al (2002) The bispectral index and explicit recall during intraoperative wake-up test for scoliosis surgery. Anesth Analg 94:1474-1478
21. Drader KS, Craen RA (1997) Anaesthetic considerations for awake craniotomy. Curr Opin Anaesthesiol 10:311-314
22. Johnson KB, Egan TD (1998) Remifentanil and propofol combination for awake craniotomy: Case report with pharmacokinetic simulations. J Neurosurg Anesthesiol 10:25-29
23. Soriano SG, Eldredge EA, Wang FK, et al (2000) The effect of propofol on intraoperative electrocorticograph and cortical stimulation during awake craniotomies in children. Pediatr Anaesth 10:29-34
24. Hans P, Bonhomme V, Born JD, et al (2000) Target-controlled infusion of propofol and remifentanil combined with bispectral index monitoring for awake craniotomy. Anaesthesia 55:255-259
25. Gignac E, Manninen PH, Gelb AW (1993) Comparison of fentanyl, sufentanil and alfentanil during awake craniotomy for epilepsy. Can J Anaesth 40:421-424
26. Berkenstadt H, Perel A, Hadani M, et al (2001) Monitored anesthesia care using remifentanil and propofol for awake craniotomy. J Neurosurg Anesthesiol 13:246-249
27. Sahjpaul RL (2000) Awake craniotomy: controversies, indications and techniques in the surgical treatment of temporal lobe epilepsy. Can J Neurol Sci 27:S55-S63
28. Herrick JA, Craen JA, Gelb AW, et al (1997) Propofol sedation during awake craniotomy for seizures: patient-controlled administration versus neurolept analgesia. Anesth Analg 84:1285--1291
29. Schneck HJ, Tempel G, Hundelshausen B von (1988) Pharmacologic modification of vigilance in the postnarcotic phase - naloxone or physostigmine? Anasth Intensivther Notfallmed 23:209--213
30. Rupreht J, Jupa V (1980) Physostigmine in the differential diagnosis of coma after neurosurgery. Acta Anaesthesiol Belg 31:71-74
31. Danks RA, Rogers M, Aglio LS, et al (1998) Patient tolerance of craniotomy performed with the patient under local anesthesia and monitored conscious sedation. Neurosurgery 42:28-36
32. Danks RA, Aglio LS, Gugino LD, et al (2001) Craniotomy under local anesthesia and monitored conscious sedation for the resection of tumors involving eloquent cortex. J Neurooncol 49:131-139
33. Black PM, Ronner SF (1987) Cortical mapping for defining the limits of tumour resection. Neurosurgery 20:914-919
34. Tylor MD, Bernstein M (1999) Awake craniotomy with brain mapping as the routine surgical

approach to treating patients with supratentorial intraaxial tumours: a prospective trial of 200 cases. J Neurosurg 90:35-41

35. Lanier WL (2001) Brain tumor resection in the awake patient. Mayo Clin Proc 76:670-672
36. Meyer FB, Bates LM, Goerss SJ, et al (2001) Awake craniotomy for aggressive resection of primary gliomas located in eloquent brain. Mayo Clin Proc 76:677-687

Fast-track neuroanaesthesia

M. KLIMEK

When performing a Medline-Request with the subjects "fast-track" and "neuroanaesthesia" in the title of any publication, one gets no results. The question is whether this is due to the fact that almost everybody is already practicing fast-track neuroanaesthesia and nobody thinks it to be worthy to publish, or whether this is due to the fact that this technique is much more unpopular and much more unscientific than one might expect?! This review will summarize the current published knowledge on this topic together with the personal experience of the author.

What is fast-track neuroanaesthesia?

Patients should be extubated, if they are in a stable cardiorespiratory state, free from residual relaxation, and have a body temperature of >35°C. If one considers these aspects, there is no early or late extubation, but only a good and right one [1,2]. However, to meet these criteria, anaesthesia must be performed in a special manner, to be able to extubate a patient within the 1 h after an intracranial procedure. This anaesthesiological regimen, which enables early extubation (and avoids the possible pitfalls of this technique), can be called fast-track neuroanaesthesia.

Why perform fast-track neuroanaesthesia?

In the early postoperative period there are contradictory demands on the state of the neurosurgical patient. On the one side there is the neurosurgical demand for early on-line neurological evaluation, on the other side there is the anaesthesiological demand for a stable haemodynamic and respiratory status of the patient. All types of stress should be avoided, to maintain a low intracranial pressure (ICP) and to avoid the risk of intracranial bleeding caused by hypertension.

An already awake patient will show a decrease of vigilance and new neurological deficits due to an increase of ICP by bleeding or oedema much earlier than a sedated and ventilated patient will develop an anisocoria or vegetative signs of an increased ICP. So the computed tomography (CT) diagnosis and treatment of a possible intracranial bleeding can be started faster. On the other hand prolonged sedation and mechanical ventilation have some risks of their own (pneumonia, barotrauma, pneumothorax etc.) [1].

From cardiosurgical patients it is known that early extubation decreases the time on the intensive care unit (ICU) and the costs of treatment. So, fast-track neuroanaesthesia can increase the efficacy of a neurosurgical department and optimize the use of financial and ICU resources [3-5].

When not to perform fast-track neuroanaesthesia?

It must be stated that not all intracranial procedures can be followed with an early extubation. In the following conditions a prolonged postoperative period of sedation and ventilation is recommended [1, 2, 6]:
- pre-existing reduced level of consciousness
- severe traumatic brain injury
- large brain tumour with extended zone of oedema
- infratentorial lesions close to the brainstem
- extended intracerebral bleeding
- poor general condition (ASA > III)
- impressive intraoperative swelling of the brain
- significant vasospasm after intracranial vascular surgery
- following procedures in the sitting position

What are possible dangers of fast-track neuroanaesthesia?

There are some general pathophysiological aspects, which must be taken into consideration when performing fast-track neuroanaesthesia in selected patients. When there is prolonged action of opioids or other sedative drugs, postoperative hypoventilation may occur leading to hypoxia and hypercapnia, which may severely increase the ICP.

The neurosurgical procedure is also a trauma, which can lead to a postoperative brain oedema and an excessive increase in ICP, which makes re-intubation mandatory. However, due to the microsurgical technique, this risk has been markedly reduced during the last decades.

A sedated and ventilated patient can be kept in a stable condition after a neurosurgical procedure for hours, so that haemodynamic changes due to stress and/or pain, coughing or other vegetative reactions do not occur, at least during sedation and ventilation.

Therefore, when planning to fast-track in neuroanaesthesia, one should ensure a smooth wake-up period and avoid excessive haemodynamic changes and coughing. However, this "smoothening" should not lead to a respiratory depression with hypoventilation and the need for re-intubation.

How to smoothen early recovery from intracranial procedures?

How to prevent stress and haemodynamic instability during extubation?

The first postoperative hour is a period of intense stress for neurosurgical patients. There is a stress response to pain, discomfort caused by lines and tubes, shivering with or without hypothermia, and other external stimulating factors. This stress response is associated with an increase in blood pressure, heart rate, oxygen consumption, and stress hormone blood levels. It takes about 1 h for blood pressure and heart rate to normalize after extubation, and the important factor is that removing the stress factor, the tube, causes an additional increase in both by laryngeal and tracheal stimulation [7].

Intravenous lidocaine and filling the cuff with lidocaine were most successful in prevention of coughing and sore throat [8]. In another study, alkalinized lidocaine was superior to normal lidocaine [9]. Contrary to this no difference was found between topically applied lidocaine and 0.9% NaCl solution when using a especially designed LITA tube for laryngeal instillation of topical anaesthestics above and below the cuff via an additional pilot tube [10]. However, there are other results showing a 75% suppression of coughing by this technique [11].

Concerning suppression of the haemodynamic response to extubation there are also some reports about the use of cardiovascular drugs. A combination of verapamil 0.1 mg/kg i.v. and lidocaine 1 mg/kg i.v. has turned out to be effective [12]. Other groups showed useful effects of a combination of 0.2 mg/kg diltiazem i.v. and 1.0 mg/kg lidocaine i.v. or an infusion of esmolol (200 µg/kg per min) [13, 14].

Clonidine, which can be used to block the stress reaction on intubation when given i.v. at a dosage of 3 µg/kg preoperatively, due to its long half-life time also blunts the haemodynamic response to extubation [15]. The same was found for dexmedetomidine 2 µg/kg i.v. [16]. However, an undesirable decrease of mean arterial pressure and of cerebral perfusion pressure may occur when using these agents and should be corrected [17].

Also, when using antihypertensive agents, one should always bear in mind that cerebral vasodilation must be avoided, because it leads to an increase in cerebral blood volume, which might increase the ICP. Therefore the use of alpha- and beta-blocking agents is recommended to treat hypertensive blood pressure in neurosurgical patients [18].

Considering stress factors during extubation it should be recalled that endotracheal suctioning can cause a short mean increase in ICP of 15 mmHg and much higher in some patients [19-22]. This stress can also be reduced by the use of topical or systemic lidocaine or opioids, but in first line the indication for endotracheal suctioning must be taken very carefully. We recommend endotracheal suctioning only in deep sedation. Oropharyngeal suctioning of the awake patient can be performed without provoking coughing or a greater haemodynamic response.

However, recent data from Bruder et al. [23] show that cerebral hyperaemia might be a general reaction of the body on awakening after neurosurgical procedures, because it happens independently of the anaesthetic technique used and independently of haemodynamic or ventilatory changes.

How to prevent shivering?

About 40% of patients recovering from general anaesthesia with a body temperature of less than 36.5 °C shiver [24]. Shivering is associated with an enormous increase in oxygen consumption to the two- to four-fold the baseline value [25-28]. To prevent shivering, the maintenance of a normal body temperature is the first rule. However, in some neurosurgical procedures moderate hypothermia is used intraoperatively for brain protection and the active warming during surgical closure will not lead to normothermia until the end of the procedure [29]. In such patients, awakening and extubation should be delayed until normothermia is almost reached.

Besides maintaining ambient temperature and warming air blankets some drugs have turned out to be effective in preventing shivering by altering the temperature threshold: clonidine 2-5 µg/kg i.v., meperidine 0.2-0.5 mg/kg i.v, nefopam 0.1-0,15 mg/kg i.v. and tramadol 2mg/kg i.v., as well as physostigmine 0.02 mg/kg i.v., dexamethasone 0.6 mg/kg i.v., or urapidil 0.2-0.5 mg/kg i.v. [30-36]. For urapidil these data are inconsistent [37].

How to manage postoperative analgesia?

Pain causes an increase in oxygen consumption and release of catecholamines, especially noradrenaline [38, 39]. Although intracranial surgery is not considered to be as painful as, e.g., abdominal surgery, a postoperative regimen for pain treatment should be established. This regimen depends closely on the anaesthetics used intraoperatively, especially opiods. Patients who were on remifentanil require postoperative analgesics earlier than patients receiving fentanyl [40]. In a recent study it was shown that paracetamol alone is not sufficient in treating the postoperative pain after intracranial surgery, and the addition of opioids like tramadol, nalbuphine, or codeine (usually administered i.m.), oxycodone or morphine is recommended [41-43]. Local infiltration of the wound by the neurosurgeon or placing a skull block can be useful measures in reducing postoperative pain.

Clonidine enhances the effects of opioids, offers haemodynamic stability, prevents shivering, and this author prefers the combination of clonidine 2 µg/kg i.v. at induction of anaesthesia in combination with fentanyl 0.25 mg i.v. at induction and 0.25 mg i.v. at placement of the Mayfield clamp. Remifentanil is used for the rest of the procedure (0.01-0.02 mg/kg per hour) and a second dose of clonidine (75 µg) and fentanyl (0.15 mg) are injected, if necessary, when the procedure lasts longer than 4 h.

Early or delayed recovery?

Bruder et al. [44] failed to demonstrate that delayed recovery attenuates metabolic and hemodynamic changes due to waking up after intracranial surgery. Early recovery of consciousness and extubation were associated with fewer cardiovascular and metabolic changes than a delayed recovery of 2 h. One possible explanation might be that in the early postoperative period higher residual blood levels of opioids and sedative drugs are still present [44].

Where to extubate?

Another aspect that must be taken into consideration is the place of extubation. Is the patient extubated in the operating room (OR) or in the recovery? Is there a longer transport of the patient from OR to ICU and can the patient be adequately monitored during this transport? Is it preferable for the patient to stay in the recovery room for the 1st hour after extubation, before transfer to the ICU? Decisions depend on the local circumstances of the hospital. Is there a well-equipped recovery room? Are there anaesthesiologically trained doctors on the ICU? Can the patient easily be transferred from the OR table to a bed?

Considering such factors, it is recommended that the anaesthesiologist supervise the patient as long as possible and that transportation is done with complete monitoring [6].

In short, smooth recovery after intracranial procedures should be supervised by the anaesthesiologist. Disturbances like hypothermia, severe pain, shivering, coughing, and haemodynamic instability can be (at least partially) prevented and treated early. So fast-track neuroanaesthesia becomes safe and feasible.

Can the use of antagonists be recommended to achieve fast recovery?

Neostigmine

The use of neostigmine to antagonize residual neuromuscular block seems to be useful, if needed. Fawcett et al. [45] reported that the increase in cerebrospinal fluid pressure after administration of neostigmine following cerebral aneurysm surgery is lower than the increase in cerebrospinal fluid pressure (CSFP) caused by an increase of P_aCO_2 from 4 to 5 kPa, which is due to hypoventilation caused by a residual neuromuscular block (increase of CSFP +0.7 kPa after neostigmine vs. +6.1 kPa after hypoventilation) [45].

Flumazenil

The use of flumazenil to antagonize benzodiazepines can not be recommended. In patients with head injury, flumazenil induced a marked increase of ICP. In patients undergoing craniotomy for supratentorial tumours, no influence on cerebral blood flow was found [46-48]. Additionally, the short half-life time of flumazenil makes a resedation possible and the antiepileptic action of benzodiazepines is antagonized. There is no evidence that the GABA receptor effects of propofol can be antagonized by flumazenil [49]. However, considering context-sensitive half-life time kinetics of propofol and knowing the interactions with the opioids, the dosage of propofol can easily be adjusted, so that no delay of awakening follows propofol infusion, especially when a target-controlled infusion method is used [50-52].

Naloxone

The decision to fast-track in neuroanaesthesia should be taken before the induction of anaesthesia. Due to some intraoperative problems it may happen that a patient, initially planned to be fast-tracked, must undergo prolonged sedation. The opposite will almost never happen. It occurs rarely that higher doses of long-acting opioids are used in a patient who unexpectedly can be extubated according to the fast-track protocol. In such a case, administration of naloxone may be an option. For remifentanil the half-life-time remains unchanged over the time of the procedure. Nevertheless, the pharmacodynamic and pharmakokinetic interactions of opioids with propofol should be considered to avoid unnecessary naloxone administration [50-52].

Whenever naloxone is used, severe withdrawal reactions may ensue, with hemodynamic impairment caused by a too-rapid awakening, pain, and nausea. A resedation may occur as well. Therefore, the use of naloxone in fast-track neuroanaesthesia cannot be recommended.

What are typical problems of the early postoperative period?

Psychomotor recovery

It is known that low doses of fentanyl and midazolam can provoke otherwise compensated neurological disturbances in 30% of patients and aggravate an existing neurological deficit in more than 70% [53]. Minimal impairment of the remaining functioning neurons in patients with limited neuronal reserve produces an exaggerated response. Therefore, mild psychomotor deficits found immediately after fast-track neuroanaesthesia should not lead to immediate diagnostic measures. A wait-and-see strategy can be recommended for the 1st hour. Having used propofol and remifentanil in a target-controlled manner, there will be a rapid improvement of the psychomotor function in the absence of structural damage caused by the disease or by the procedure. Other factors inducing delayed recovery must be considered, too, including postoperative hypothermia, location of the lesion in the frontal lobe, hangover effects of long-acting benzodiazepines, sedative side-effects of antiemetic drugs, or postoperative brain swelling.

Nausea and vomiting

A surprisingly high incidence of 38% nausea and vomiting after neurosurgical procedures has been reported [54]. However, the authors state that patients after brain tumour surgery have a lower incidence of postoperative complications than after spine or brain vascular surgery. This author's experience is that nausea and vomiting are not a major problem after intracranial surgery and that they can be easily treated, if necessary.

Intracranial haematoma

About 1% of the neurosurgical patients develop a major intracranial hematoma postoperatively. This occurs mostly within the first 12 h after surgery and is followed by quite a poor outcome in about 50% of patients [55-57]. Coagulation disorders, emergency surgery, and postoperative hypertension are the most-important risk factors for postoperative intracranial haematoma. Postoperative hypertension can be caused by an increased ICP (Cushing reflex) and therefore should not be treated too aggressively to avoid too low cerebral perfusion pressure with ischaemic lesions. Repeated neurological examination is the best monitoring of intracranial haematoma, and a progressively decreasing Glasgow Coma Score must lead to an emergency CT scan.

Seizures

Postoperative epileptic seizures can be related to cerebral bleeding, cerebral oedema, or hypoxia. They must be controlled immediately by injecting benzo-diazepines or barbiturates (0.1 mg/kg midazolam i.v. or 1-1.5 mg/kg thiopental i.v.) followed by a phenytoin loading scheme. There is no evidence that prophy-lactic phenytoin before supratentorial surgery is useful. Preoperative anticonvul-sant treatment should be continued perioperatively. Early postoperative seizures should be taken seriously and an emergency CT scan is indicated.

Silent aspiration

During procedures in the posterior fossa, lesions of the cranial nerves may occur. Lesions of the cranial nerves IX, X, and XII may impair swallowing, which may lead to early silent aspiration, hypoxia, and pneumonia. Patency of the airway is additionally related to the function of the cranial nerves V and VII, which may be damaged by procedures in the cerebellopontine angle. To be sure of adequate function of these nerves, extubation should only be performed in patients with an intact gag reflex, who are able to follow verbal commands and breathe spontaneously with an adequate respiratory rate and tidal volume. In doubtful cases fiberoptic evaluation of swallowing and the upper airways might be helpful [6].

Laryngeal swelling

After long-lasting procedures with extreme flexion of the head, a swelling of the airway mucosa might be seen [58]. This is most probably due to impaired venous or lymphatic drainage and will normalize after repositioning of the head within less than 24 h. This hazard must be taken into consideration, because early extubation in such patients may be followed by severe dyspnea, re-intubation may be impossible and tracheostomy must be performed.

How to manage recovery?

As stated above, the decision whether a patient will be able to undergo fast-track neuroanaesthesia must be taken already before the procedure and must be re-evaluated at the end of the procedure. In general, fast-track neuroanaesthesia is the procedure of choice for otherwise healthy patients undergoing uncomplicated surgery, who are normothermic at the end of the procedure. Opioids and sedative drugs should be used sparingly during surgical closure, an emergency syringe of anaesthetic for the case of too early awakening should be kept. Stimuli like prolonged fixation in the Mayfield clamp or endotracheal suctioning should be minimized. Lidocaine i.v. should be used before extubation. Beta-blocking agents or urapidil should be kept available to treat hypertensive reactions. Esmolol has the most-adequate pharmacokinetic profile, but the personal experience of the anaesthesiologist with longer-acting drugs like metoprolol or clonidine might be a good reason to use them. Following remifentanil as the only opioid, a postoperative analgesic regimen should be established early. Extra oxygen for the early postoperative period should be administered after extubation. Monitoring of ECG, blood pressure, and oxygen saturation should be continued. Neurological examination should be performed as early as possible and well recorded as a baseline.

What to do in case of doubt?

If in doubt whether to fast-track, there is the possibility to use the technique of the "neurological window" by stopping the sedative drugs and allowing the patient to awaken. The neurological examination of the intubated patient is performed and depending on the findings of the examination the decision is taken whether the patient can be extubated or must be resedated. Severe haemodynamic changes may be seen during this period, and careful monitoring of the patient is recommended. If the patient is to be kept sedated, a second evaluation after 1-2 h can be carried out.

Principal aspects of fast-track neuroanaesthesia

Fast-track neuroanaesthesia
- is **desirable**. It enables early clinical monitoring of the patient and early treatment of postoperative complications.
- is **possible** without antagonists, when short-acting anaesthetic agents are used.
- is **feasible** and **safe**, when performed by a skilled anaesthesiologist in cooperative patients undergoing uncomplicated surgical procedures and when contraindications are recognized.
- is an **interdisciplinary challenge**. The neurosurgeon evaluates the surgical site (swelling, bleeding, nerve damage), the anaesthesiologist evaluates the cardiorespiratory function and the consciousness. Both must agree to fast-track.
- leads **to cost reduction**. This might be expected, but it is still strongly recommended, that patients after intracranial procedures are monitored in an ICU or high-care unit for the first postoperative night [59].
- is **appreciated** by patients, relatives, and by the neurosurgeons.

References

1. Thees C, Schramm J, Frenkel C (1998) Early extubation after intracranial procedures: pro. Anasthesiol Intensivmed Notfallmed Schmerzther 33:334-336
2. Börner U, Klimek M (1998) Early extubation after intracranial procedures: contra. Anästhesiol Intensivmed Notfallmed Schmerzther 33:336-337
3. Cheng DHC, Karski J, Peniston C, et al (1996) Early tracheal extubation after coronary artery bypass graft surgery reduces costs and improves resource use. Anesthesiology 85:1300-1310
4. Dehnen-Seipel H (1993) Early extubation after cardiac surgery: pro. Anästhesiol Intensivmed Notfallmed Schmerzther 28:248-250
5. Lee JH, Kim KH, van Heckeren DW, et al (1996) Cost analysis of early extubation after coronary bypass surgery. Surgery 120:611-617
6. Bruder N, Ravussin P (1999) Recovery from anesthesia and postoperative extubation of neurosurgical patients: a review. J Neurosurg Anesthesiol 11:282-293
7. Ravussin P, Tempelhoff R, Modica PA, et al (1991) Propofol vs. thiopental-isoflurane for neurosurgical anesthesia: comparison of hemodynamics, CSF pressure and recovery. J Neurosurg Anesthesiol 3:85-95
8. Soltani HA, Aghadavoudi O (2002) The effect of different lidocaine application methods on postoperative cough and sore throat. J Clin Anesth 14:15-18
9. Estebe JP, Dollo G, Le Corre P, et al (2002) Alkalinization of intracuff lidocaine improves endotracheal tube-induced emergence phenomena. Anesth Analg 94:227-230
10. Andrzejowski J, Francis G (2002) The efficacy of lidocaine administered via the LITA tracheal tube in attenuating the extubation response in beta-blocked patients following craniotomy. Anaesthesia 57:399-401
11. Diachun CA, Tunink BP, Brock-Utne JG (2001) Suppression of cough during emergence from general anesthesia: laryngotracheal lidocaine through a modified endotracheal tube. J Clin Anesth 13:447-451

12. Mikawa K, Nishina K, Takao Y, et al (1997) Attenuation of cardiovascular responses to tracheal extubation: comparison of verapamil, lidocaine, and verapamil-lidocaine combination. Anesth Analg 85:1005-1010
13. Fujii Y, Saitoh Y, Takahashi S, et al (1999) Combined diltiazem and lidocaine reduces cardiovascular responses to tracheal extubation and anesthesia emergence in hypertensive patients. Can J Anaesth 46:952-956
14. Lim SH, Chin NM, Tai HY, et al (2000) Prophylactic esmolol infusion for the control of cardiovascular responses to extubation after intracranial surgery. Ann Acad Med Singapore 29:447-451
15. Zalunardo MP, Zollinger A, Spahn DR, et al (2000) Preoperative clonidine attenuates stress response during emergence from anesthesia. J Clin Anesth 12:343-349
16. Lawrence CJ, De Lange S (1997) Effects of a single pre-operative dexmedetomidine dose on isoflurane requirements and peri-operative haemodynamic stability. Anaesthesia 52:736-744
17. Favre JB, Gardaz JP, Ravussin P (1995) Effect of clonidine on ICP and on the hemodynamic responses to nociceptive stimuli in patients with brain tumors. J Neurosurg Anesthesiol 7:159--167
18. Van Aken H, Cottrell JE, Anger C, et al (1989) Treatment of intraoperative hypertensive emergencies in patients with intracranial disease. Am J Cardiol 63:43C-47C
19. Brucia J, Rudy E (1996) The effect of suction catheter insertion and tracheal stimulation in adults with severe brain trauma. Heart Lung 25:295-303
20. Donegan MF, Bedford RF (1980) Intravenously administered lidocaine prevents intracranial hypertension during endotracheal suctioning. Anesthesiology 52:516-518
21. White PF, Schlobohm RM, Pitts LH, et al (1982) A randomized study of drugs for preventing increases in intracranial pressure during endotracheal suctioning. Anesthesiology 57:242-244
22. Miller KA, Harkin CP, Bailey PL (1995) Postoperative extubation. Anesth Analg 80:149-172
23. Bruder N, Pellissier D, Grillot P, et al (2002) Cerebral hyperemia during recovery from general anesthesia in neurosurgical patients. Anesth Analg 94:650-654
24. Just B, Delva E, Camus Y, et al (1992) Oxygen uptake during recovery following naloxone. Relationship with intraoperative heat loss. Anesthesiology 76:60-64
25. Bay J, Nunn JF, Prys-Roberts C (1968) Factors influencing arterial pO_2 during recovery from anesthesia. Br J Anaesth 40:398-407
26. Ralley FE, Wynands JE, Ramsay JG, et al (1988) The effect of shivering on oxygen consumption and carbon dioxide production in patients rewarming from hypothermic cardiopulmonary bypass. Can J Anaesth 35:332-337
27. Rodriguez JL, Weissman C, Damask MC, et al (1983) Morphine and postoperative rewarming in critically ill patients. Circulation 68:1238-1246
28. MacIntyre PE, Pavlin EG, Dwersteg JF (1987) Effect of meperidine on oxygen consumption, carbon dioxide production, and respiratory gas exchange in postanesthesia shivering. Anesth Analg 66:751-755
29. Baker KZ, Young WL, Stone G, et al (1994) Deliberate mild intraoperative hypothermia for craniotomy. Anesthesiology 81:361-367
30. Alfonsi P (2001) Postanaesthetic shivering: epidemiology, pathophysiology, and approaches to prevention and management. Drugs 61:2193-2205
31. Bilotta F, Pietropaoli P, La Rosa I, et al (2001) Effects of shivering prevention on haemodynamic and metabolic demands in hypothermic postoperative neurosurgical patients. Anaesthesia 56:514-519
32. Mathews S, Al Mulla A, Varghese PK, et al (2002) Postanaesthetic shivering - a new look at tramadol. Anaesthesia 57:394-398
33. Zhang Y, Wong KC (1999) Anesthesia and postoperative shivering: its etiology, treatment and prevention. Acta Anaesthesiol Sin 37:115-120
34. Piper SN, Suttner SW, Schmidt CC, et al (1999) Nefopam and clonidine in the prevention of postanaesthetic shivering. Anaesthesia 54:695-699

35. Yared JP, Starr NJ, Hoffmann-Hogg L, et al (1998) Dexamethasone decreases the incidence of shivering after cardiac surgery: a randomized, double-blind, placebo-controlled study. Anesth Analg 87:795-799

36. Schwarzkopf KR, Hoff H, Hartmann M, et al (2001) A comparison between meperidine, clonidine and urapidil in the treatment of postanesthetic shivering. Anesth Analg 92:257-260

37. Piper SN, Fent MT, Rohm KD et al (2001) Urapidil does not prevent postanesthetic shivering: a dose-ranging study. Can J Anaesth 48:742-747

38. Breslow MJ, Parker SD, Franck SM, et al (1993) Determinants of catecholamine and cortisol responses to lower extremity revascularization. The PIRAT study group. Anesthesiology 79:1202-1209

39. Rutberg H, Hakanson E, Anderberg B, et al (1984) Effects of the extradural administration of morphine, or bupivacaine, on the endocrine response to upper abdominal surgery. Br J Anaesth 56:233-238

40. Guy J, Hindman BJ, Baker KZ, et al (1997) Comparison of remifentanil and fentanyl in patients undergoing craniotomy for supratentorial space-occupying lesions. Anesthesiology 86:514-524

41. Verchere E, Grenier B, Mesli A, et al (2002) Postoperative pain management after supratentorial craniotomy. J Neurosurg Anesthesiol 14:96-101

42. Jeffrey HM, Charlton P, Mellor DJ, et al (1999) Analgesia after intracranial surgery: a double--blind, prospective comparison of codeine and tramadol. Br J Anaesth 83:245-249

43. Stoneham MD, Cooper R, Quiney NF, et al (1996) Pain following craniotomy: a preliminary study comparing PCA morphine with intramuscular codeine phosphate. Anaesthesia 51:1176--1178

44. Bruder N, Stordeur JM, Ravussin P, et al (1999) Metabolic and hemodynamic changes during recovery and tracheal extubation in neurosurgical patients: Immediate versus delayed recovery. Anesth Analg 89:674-678

45. Fawcett WJ, Chung RA, Fairley CJ, et al (1995) The effect of reversal of myoneural blockade on cerebrospinal fluid pressure following cerebral aneurysm surgery. Eur J Anaesthesiol 12:591- 595

46. Knudsen L, Cold GE, Holdgard HO, et al (1991) Effects of Flumazenil on cerebral blood flow and oxygen consumption after midazolam anaesthesia for craniotomy. Br J Anaesth 67:277-280

47. Fleischer JE, Milde JH, Moyer TP, et al (1988) Cerebral effects of high-dose midazolam and subsequent reversal with Ro 15-1788 in dogs. Anesthesiology 68:234-242

48. Chiolero RL, Ravussin P, Anderes JP, et al (1988) The effects of midazolam reversal by Ro 15-1788 on cerebral perfusion pressure in patients with severe head injury. Intensive Care Med 14:196-200

49. Fan SZ, Liu CC, Yu HY, et al (1995) Lack of effect of flumazenil on the reversal of propofol anaesthesia. Acta Anaesthesiol Scand 39:299-301

50. Vuyk J (2001) Clinical interpretation of pharmacokinetic and pharmacodynamic propofol-opioid interactions. Acta Anaesthesiol Belg 52:445-451

51. Vuyk J (1999) Drug interactions in anaesthesia. Minerva Anestesiol 65:215-218

52. Vuyk J (1997) Pharmacokinetic and pharmacodynamic interactions between opioids and propofol. J Clin Anesth 9[Suppl]:23S-26S

53. Thal GD, Szabo MD, Lopez-Bresnahan M, et al (1996) Exacerbation or unmasking of focal neurologic deficits by sedatives. Anesthesiology 85:21-25

54. Manninen PH, Raman SK, Boyle K, et al (1999) Early postoperative complications following neurosurgical procedures. Can J Anaesth 46:7-14

55. Palmer JD, Sparrow OC, Ianotti F (1994) Postoperative hematoma: a 5-year survey and identification of avoidable risk factors. Neurosurgery 35:1061-1064

56. Taylor WA, Thomas NW, Wellings JA, et al (1995) Timing of postoperative intracranial hematoma development and implications for the best use of neurosurgical intensive care. J Neurosurg 82:48-50

57. Kalfas IH, Little JR (1988) Postoperative hemorrhage: a survey of 4992 intracranial procedures. Neurosurgery 23:343-347

58. McAllister RG (1974) Macroglossia - a positional complication. Anesthesiology 40:199-200
59. Kelly DF (1994) Neurosurgical postoperative Care. Neurosurg Intensive Care 5:789-819

LUNG

Interaction between ventilation and pulmonary circulation

G. Hedenstierna

The cardiac output and the distribution of lung blood flow are both affected by the ventilation, whether it is spontaneous or mechanically administered and whether a positive end-expiratory pressure (PEEP) has been applied externally or has been produced intrinsically by interrupted expiration. This chapter will describe the distributions of lung perfusion and of ventilation. Effects of increasing the airway and alveolar pressures, as during positive pressure ventilation and the application of PEEP will be discussed.

Distribution of lung blood flow

The blood flow through the lung is governed by the driving pressure and the vascular resistance. If these are unevenly distributed, then perfusion may also be uneven. The mechanisms behind an uneven distribution of lung blood flow have become a controversial subject during recent years. Thus, the previously generally accepted explanation of a gravitational orientation of perfusion, as demonstrated in the pioneering work of West [1], has been challenged by others who propose a "fractal" distribution with gravity playing a minor role only [2]. Here we will first deal with the "gravitational" concept, and then proceed to the "fractal" one.

Gravitational distribution of lung blood flow

Pulmonary artery pressure increases down the lung, an effect of the hydrostatic pressure that builds up on the way from the top to bottom of the lung. This pressure increases by 1 cmH$_2$O per cm distance down the lung (or 0.74 mmHg/cm vertical distance, blood has a density close to 1 or 1.04). This causes a pressure difference in the pulmonary arterial vessels between apex and base (upright position) or from the anterior to the posterior side (supine position) of some 11-15 mmHg, depending on the size of the lung. There is thus less driving pressure to the top of the lung. Since the mean pulmonary artery pressure is approximately 12 mmHg at the level of the heart, it may approach zero in the apex of the lung in the upright position. Moreover, if alveolar pressure is increased, as during positive pressure ventilation, it may exceed that in the pulmonary artery, and compress the pulmonary capillaries. No blood will then flow through the vessels. This part of the lung is called zone I. If arterial and capillary pressure exceeds alveolar pressure, as it will further down the lung because of the addition of hydrostatic pressure, a blood flow will be established. The perfusion pressure will be arterial minus alveolar pressure, as long as the latter pressure exceeds that of the pulmonary veins. This is different from the systemic circulation, where perfusion pressure is arterial minus venous pressure. Moreover, the increasing pulmonary arterial pressure down the lung and the constant alveolar pressure increase the perfusion pressure down this part of the lung, called zone II. Blood flow therefore increases down this zone. Further down the lung, both arterial and venous pressures exceed that in the alveoli, so that perfusion pressure is arterial minus venous pressure. This part of the lung is called zone III. Since both arterial and venous pressures increase to the same extent down zone III, hydrostatic pressure adding to both sides, perfusion pressure does not increase down the zone. However, perfusion increases downwards, albeit less than the increase in zone II. The explanation proposed is that the increasing vascular pressure dilates the vessels down the lung, and by this means reduces the vascular resistance [1].

A few years after these initial observations, it was noticed that blood flow decreased in the bottom of the lung, so a zone IV had to be added to the model of lung perfusion [1]. This called for a new explanation that suggested that an increasing interstitial pressure down the lung pressed on the extra-alveolar vessels and made them narrower. The vertical distribution of blood flow could accordingly be explained by the influence of gravitation on vascular, alveolar and interstitial pressures.

The homogeneity of blood flow distribution has also been tested during zero or micro-gravity shuttle flights with the NASA Space Lab. Using indirect techniques, based on an analysis of the variation of expired gas concentrations that are synchronous with the heart beats ("cardiogenic oscillations"), more--uniform lung blood flow distribution was recorded [3]. However, some inhomogeneity still persisted.

Non-gravitational inhomogeneity of blood flow distribution

In dog experiments, groups at the Mayo Clinic and subsequently in Seattle noticed that the vertical lung blood flow distribution was rather even, and did not change when position was altered between supine and prone [2]. This led the Seattle group to conclude that gravity was of minor importance in determining perfusion distribution. The same group also showed that the perfusion at a given vertical level is unevenly distributed on that horizontal plane, with an inhomogeneity that far exceeded that in the vertical direction. In carefully repeated experiments they could reproduce the same pattern of inhomogeneity. This suggests that there are morphological and/or functional differences between lung vessels that also, and perhaps more importantly than gravity, determine blood flow distribution. In their hypothesis, they postulate that blood flow in the lung varies between lung regions, and that the variation becomes larger the smaller the lung unit under study. This could explain the failure to find a non-gravitational inhomogeneity of blood flow in early studies with poorer resolution of the techniques used.

Other groups have also suggested an uneven distribution of blood flow, that can not be explained by gravity with more blood going to the core of the lung and less to the periphery [4]. A longer distance to the peripheral bed was suggested as an explanation, causing larger vascular resistance to the periphery. However, others found less difference between central and peripheral lung regions. The application of a PEEP in anaesthetized and mechanically ventilated dogs forced perfusion of the lung towards the periphery [5]. As always, the reliability of the techniques used is critical. It seems as if the spatial distribution of blood flow, as measured by single photon emission computed tomography, suffers from reconstruction artefacts, a technique that has been used in some studies. Still others have used microsphere techniques and have measured the distribution in excised lungs. Although it may suffer from other limitations, one may conclude that enough evidence has accumulated to support a non-gravitational inhomogeneity of lung perfusion.

Distribution of ventilation

The air that is inspired will not be evenly distributed in the lung. During quiet breathing, most gas goes to the lower, dependent regions, i.e., basal, diaphragmatic areas in the upright or sitting position, and to dorsal units in the supine position [6]. This also means that the lower, left lung will receive most of the air if the subject is in the left lateral position, and the right lung is preferentially ventilated in the right position. The reason for this seemingly gravitational orientation of something as light as gas is the combined effect of the curved pressure-volume relationship of the lung tissue and the increasing pleural pressure down the lung.

Firstly, the curved pressure-volume curve, typical for an elastic tissue, means that with increasing lung volume more and more pressure is required to inflate the lung by a given volume increment. Secondly, the increasing pleural pressure, at constant alveolar pressure all over the lung, causes transpulmonary pressure to decrease from top to bottom of the lung. In the upright position, apical lung regions are exposed to a higher transpulmonary pressure than dependent, basal ones. Thus, upper and lower lung regions are positioned at different levels of the pressure-volume curve. During an inspiration, pleural pressure is lowered and causes lower lung regions to inflate more than upper ones, for a similar change in transpulmonary pressure (it is assumed that pleural pressure changes uniformly in the pleural space) [6]. Thus, in the healthy subject, ventilation goes preferentially to the basal regions. The pleural pressure gradient is oriented in a vertical, gravitational direction, and that is why ventilation distribution changes with body position. What causes the pleural pressure gradient? The major factor is the weight of the lung itself, less lung tissue exerting a pressure at a level higher up in the thoracic cavity than at a lower lung level. This pressure is mediated in all directions, as well as to the pleural space. The specific density of an air-filled and perfused lung is on an average approximately 0.3, and this causes the pleural pressure to increase by 0.3 cmH$_2$0 per cm vertical distance. If the lung is heavier, as when it is suffering from oedema, the pleural pressure gradient will increase, as does the vertical difference in alveolar size. If weight is reduced or eliminated, as in zero or micro-gravity, there should be no vertical pleural pressure gradient, and lung expansion as well as gas distribution should be more even. This was studied during flights in the NASA Space Lab that showed more-homogeneous ventilation [7]. However, some inhomogeneity persisted, indicating that non-gravitational factors also contribute to the ventilation distribution. These may be uneven convectional and diffusional flows in small lung units [8].

It also seems as if the vertical pleural pressure gradient is smaller in the prone position compared with the supine [9]. This seems to be due to the weight of the heart that is compressing the dependent parts of the lung in the supine position, permitting the non-dependent regions to expand. In the prone position, the heart is resting on the sternum with no or minor effect on the shape of the lung. The only force that can distort the shape of the lung is the weight of the lung itself. This may result in more even distribution of inspired gas in the prone position.

With increasing flow rate, regional differences in airway resistance (and in lung tissue and possibly to some extent chest wall resistance) will play an increasing role in determining the gas distribution. Since the lung tissue, both alveoli and airways, is more expanded in upper regions than in lower, resistance to gas flow is less in the upper part of the lung. This results in a change in the distribution pattern, with more gas going to upper units [10]. At a flow of 0.3 l/s, two-thirds of ventilation went to the lower half of the lung, as assessed by isotope technique, and when inspiratory flow was increased to 4-5 l/s, distribution between the upper and lower half of the lung was even. This is advantageous for optimizing the gas transfer in the lung, as for example during exercise, since the alveolar-capillary surface area will be more efficiently used.

Airways become narrower during expiration. If the expiration is deep enough, airways in dependent regions will eventually close. The volume above residual volume (RV) at which airways begin to close during an expiration is called closing volume (CV) and the sum of RV and CV is called closing capacity (CC) [11]. Airway closure is a normal physiological phenomenon and is the effect of an increasing pleural pressure during the expiration. When pleural pressure becomes "positive" (or, rather, above atmospheric) it will exceed the pressure inside the airway that is just or nearly atmospheric at low flow rate. The higher outside than inside pressure will compress the airway and close it. Since pleural pressure is higher in dependent regions than higher up, closure of airways begins in the bottom of the lung. The crucial point is thus the creation of a "positive" pleural pressure. In young subjects it may not occur until they have expired to RV. However, with increasing age, pleural pressure becomes "positive" at higher and higher lung volume, and at an age of 65-70 years airway closure may occur above functional residual capacity (FRC) [11]. This means that in elderly subjects dependent lung regions are intermittently closed during the breath. These regions will re-open during inspiration, when the lung volume exceeds the CC. The impediment of ventilation that the closure of airways causes seems to be the major explanation as to why arterial oxygenation decreases with age.

Airway closure will play an even greater role in the supine position. This is because FRC is reduced, whereas CC is not affected by body position. Closure of airways may occur above FRC at an age of 45-50 years, and in the 70-year-old subject airways may be continuously closed if closing capacity exceeds FRC plus the tidal volume.

Interactions of ventilation and lung blood flow

Two major factors that influence both cardiac output and the distribution of lung blood flow are intrathoracic pressure and vascular volume load. A rise in intrathoracic pressure as during positive pressure ventilation compared with spontaneous breathing, and the application of a PEEP impedes the venous

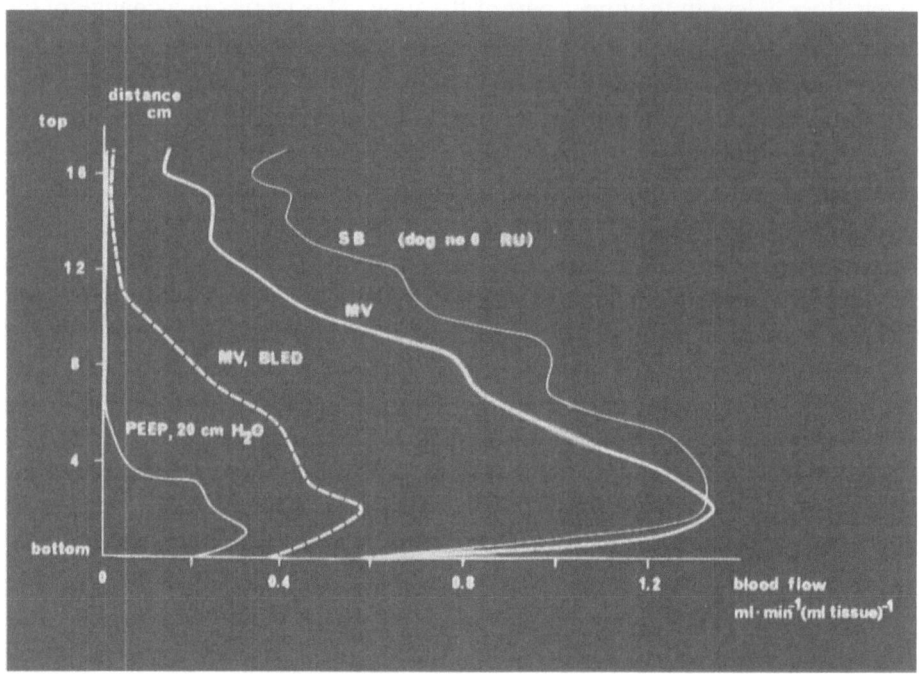

Fig 1 Gravitational distribution of lung blood flow in awake and subsequently anaesthetized dogs. Note the increase in blood flow down the lung. The vertical gradient of blood flow is slightly increased with mechanical ventilation and dramatically augmented by a positive end-expiratory pressure (PEEP) of 20 cmH$_2$O. With PEEP, total lung blood flow is also markedly reduced. Note also that hypovolemia not only decreases total blood flow but enhances the vertical gradient, causing a perfusion that goes preferentially to the bottom of the lung. Redrawn from [18]

return to the right atrium and thus lowers the right ventricular reload. Moreover, the rise in intrathoracic pressure increases pleural pressure and reduces the transmural pulmonary vascular pressure. This raises the right ventricular after-load. During the 1960s, coronary angiography was performed during anaesthesia, after the application of a continuous positive airway pressure of 40 cmH$_2$O. This high pressure effectively stopped venous return to the right heart and slowed down heart rate. This slightly embarrassing procedure was undertaken in order to improve the imaging quality of the angiography, but can be used as an example of how intrathoracic pressure can affect cardiac output.

The drop in cardiac output on application of PEEP is also well known to all working in anaesthesia and intensive care. Moreover, the more-recent techniques of allowing spontaneous breathing during ongoing mechanical ventilation (BiPAP, APRV) result in significantly higher cardiac output [12].

The other important determinant of cardiac output is volume load. It is well known that hypovolemia, e.g., after bleeding, and loss of vessel tone, as in septic shock, cause a low cardiac output, an effect of reduced preload of both right and left ventricles. Moreover, the effect of increased intrathoracic pressure on cardiac output will be more marked with a low volume load than with normal or high volume. Thus, there is a strong need for simple techniques to evaluate the volume status in patients undergoing mechanical ventilation or those given ventilatory support with increased intrathoracic pressure. A large majority (93%) of intensive care physicians use central venous pressure recording for assessing volume status and 58% pulmonary artery wedge pressure [13]. However, neither technique provides sufficient information and cannot distinguish between patients who would benefit from further volume loading and those who would not. Even more-sophisticated measures like right ventricular and diastolic volume that can be measured by termodilution, or the assessment of left ventricular and diastolic dimensions by echocardiography, are poor predictors of the responsiveness to fluid therapy. More successful as a predictor of the volume loading therapy has been the measurement of right atrial pressure during inspiration. A fall by more than 2 mmHg suggests a good response to volume loading [14]. A problem is that many patients in the intensive care unit are not breathing spontaneously.

During mechanical ventilation with a positive pressure inflation, there is a decrease in right ventricular preload during inspiration and that reduces the stroke volume of the right heart. After a lag time corresponding to 2-3 heart beats, the left ventricular preload will be reduced, causing a decrease in the stroke volume of the left heart that coincides with the expiration. Systemic arterial pressure will therefore vary over the respiratory cycle and this systolic pressure variation (SPV) can be used to assess volume load and effects of fluid replacement therapy. The SPV is frequently divided into two components (delta up and delta down) [15].

When PEEP is applied, cardiac output is not only reduced because of impeded venous return but the perfusion of the lung is also affected. The increased intrathoracic pressure reduces transmural pulmonary artery pressure, and more so in upper lung regions than in dependent areas. The latter is an effect of the increasing hydrostatic pressure down the lung. This results in a downward shift of the lung blood flow, so that dependent lung regions, as a percentage of cardiac output, are more perfused than without PEEP. This may have implications for the oxygenation of blood by two opposing mechanisms. Firstly, PEEP as part of recruitment maneuver opens up collapsed lung tissue, and this will reduce shunt and improve oxygenation. Secondly, the downward shift of blood flow increases blood flow in persistently collapsed lung regions. The net effect will depend on how much collapsed lung was opened up and to what extent blood flow is shifted downwards [16]. PEEP does not improve oxygenation in routine anaesthesia and Hewlett et al. [17] warned against its indiscriminate use as early as 1974. The redistribution of lung blood flow by positive pressure ventilation and of PEEP are shown in Fig. 1 (redrawn from [18]).

A concept was proposed almost 20 years ago where patients with acute respiratory distress syndrome (ARDS) were treated in the lateral position with the application of PEEP solely to the dependent lung via a double lumen and the bronchial catheter, and ventilation of the two lungs with similar tidal volumes [19]. The hypothesis was, before computed tomographic scan studies in ARDS patients had been performed, that the pathology of the lung was localized in dependent lung regions and that re-expansion efforts of lung tissue therefore should be directed to dependent regions. Moreover, it was assumed that the application of PEEP solely to the dependent lung would force blood flow upwards, so that perfusion of each lung in the lateral position would be similar, hence the similar tidal volumes to both lungs. The effect of PEEP to the dependent lung on perfusion can be seen in Fig. 2 [20]. In this example an

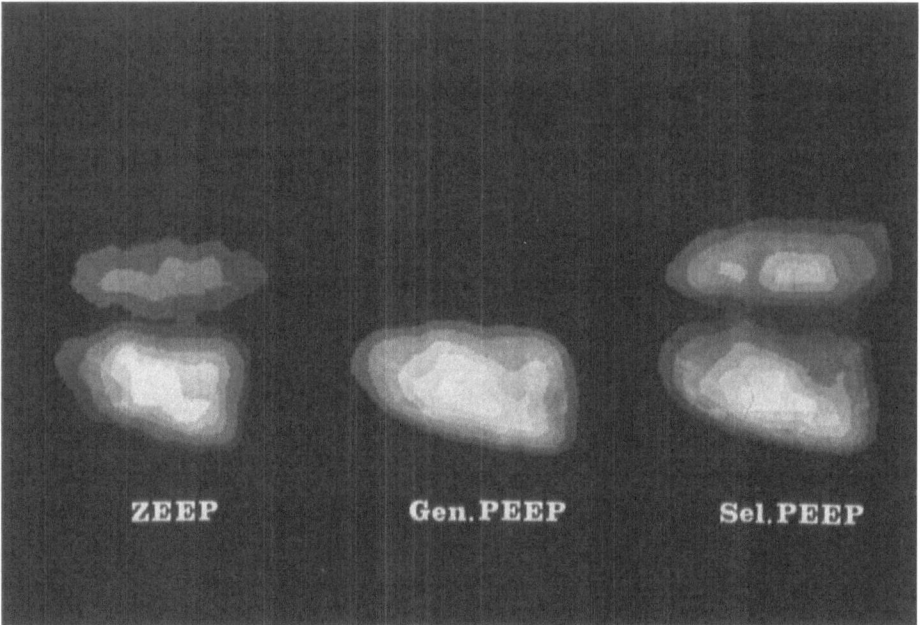

Fig 2 Lung perfusion assessed by isotope technique in an anaesthetized patient in the lateral position. Note the larger perfusion of the dependent lung during ventilation with zero end-expiratory pressure and the further shift of blood flow to the dependent lung during ventilation with a PEEP of 10 cmH$_2$O. With PEEP in this particular patient, almost no blood flow goes to the upper lung! During independent lung ventilation with PEEP of 10 cmH$_2$O solely to the dependent lung, and equal distribution of ventilation to the lungs, lung blood flow is equal in the two lungs. From [20]

anaesthetized patient was ventilated on his side, and with zero end-expiratory pressure, approximately two-thirds of the perfusion went to the dependent lung. When a PEEP of 10 cmH$_2$O was applied, almost all perfusion was distributed to the dependent lung (average result of 10 patients in that study was 80% perfusion of the dependent lung). Finally, when a selective PEEP of 10 cmH$_2$O was applied to the dependent lung and ventilation was similar in two lungs, perfusion was evenly distributed between upper and lower lung. The technique, independent lung ventilation with selective PEEP, showed impressive improvement in oxygenation of blood in healthy subjects and patients with early acute lung insufficiency [19]. However, the results were modest in severe and long--standing ARDS. The poor effect may reasonably be attributed to non-recruitable consolidated tissue in the dependent lung with the selective PEEP.

In conclusion, the distribution of lung blood flow and of ventilation are both affected by gravitational forces, but also by non-gravitational mechanisms that are not yet fully elucidated. Ventilation will have an influence on the distribution of perfusion. Two important factors in this respect are intrathoracic pressure and vascular filling (or volume load).

References

1. West JB (1977) Blood flow. In: West JB (ed) Regional differences in the lung. Academic Press, New York, pp 85-165
2. Glenny RW, Lamm WJ, Albert RK, et al (1991) Gravity is a minor determinant of pulmonary blood flow distribution. J Appl Physiol 71:620-629
3. Prisk GK, Guy HJ, Elliott AR, et al (1994) Inhomogeneity of pulmonary perfusion during sustained microgravity on SLS-1. J Appl Physiol 76:1730-1738
4. Hakim TS, Lisbona R, Dean GW (1987) Gravity-independent inequality in pulmonary blood flow in humans. J Appl Physiol 63:1114-1121
5. Hedenstierna G, White F, Wagner PD (1979) Spatial distribution of pulmonary blood flow in the dog with PEEP ventilation. J Appl Physiol 47:938-946
6. Milic-Emili J, Henderson JAM, Dolovich MB, et al (1966) Regional distribution of inspired gas in the lung. J Appl Physiol 21:749-759
7. Guy HJ, Prisk GK, Elliott AR, et al (1994) Inhomogeneity of pulmonary ventilation during sustained microgravity as determined by single-breath washouts. J Appl Physiol 76:1719-1729
8. Crawford AB, Makowska M, Paiva M, et al (1985) Convection- and diffusion-dependent ventilation maldistribution in normal subjects. J Appl Physiol 59:838-846
9. Ganesan S, Lai-Fook SJ (1989) Finite element analysis of regional lung expansion in prone and supine positions: effect of heart weight and diaphragmatic compliance. Physiologist 32:191
10. Bake B, Wood L, Murphy B, et al (1974) Effect of inspiratory flow rate on regional distribution of inspired gas. J Appl Physiol 37:8-17
11. Leblanc P, Ruff F, Milic Emili J (1970) Effects of age and body position on "airway closure" in man. J Appl Physiol 28:448-451
12. Putensen C, Mutz NJ, Putensen-Himmer G, et al (1999) Spontaneous breathing during ventilatory support improves ventilation-perfusion distributions in patients with acute respiratory distress syndrome. Am J Respir Crit Care Med 159:1241-1248

13. Boldt J, Lenz M, Kumle B (1998) Volume replacement strategies on intensive care units. Results from a postal survey. Intensive Care Med 24:147-151
14. Magder S, Georgiadis G, Cheong T (1992) Respiratory variations in right atrial pressure predict the response to fluid challenge. J Crit Care 7:76-86
15. Preisman S, Pfeiffer U, Lieberman N, et al (1997) New monitors of intravascular volume: a comparison of arterial pressure waveform analysis and the intrathoracic blood volume. Intensive Care Med 23:651-657
16. Hedenstierna G (2000) Anesthesia and gas exchange. In: Roca J, Rodriguez-Roisin R, Wagner PD (eds) Pulmonary and peripheral gas exchange in health and disease. Dekker, pp 177-198
17. Hewlett AM, Hulands GH, Nunn JF, et al (1974) Functional residual capacity during anaesthesia. Br J Anaesth 46:495-503
18. Hedenstierna G, White FC, Mazzone R, et al (1979) Redistribution of pulmonary blood flow in the dog with positive end-expiratory pressure ventilation. J Appl Physiol 46:278-287
19. Baehrendtz S, Hedenstierna G (1984) Differential ventilation and selective positive end-expiratory pressure. Effects on patients with acute bilateral lung disease. Anesthesiology 61: 511-517
20. Hedenstierna G, Baehrendtz S, Klingstedt C, et al (1984) Ventilation and perfusion of each lung during differential ventilation with selective PEEP. Anesthesiology 61:369-376

Acute respiratory distress syndrome: strategies to improve gas exchange

D. Chiumello, P. Pelosi, D. D'Onofrio

Since its first description, more than 25 years ago [1], the acute respiratory distress syndrome (ARDS) has received more attention than any single entity in critical care medicine. The syndrome consists of an acute, severe alteration in lung structure and function, characterized by severe hypoxemia, low respiratory system compliance, low functional residual capacity and diffuse radiographic infiltrates, along with increased lung endothelial and alveolar epithelial permeability.

Thus intrapulmonary shunt and ventilation perfusion imbalances cause life--threatening hypoxemia. Moreover, high work of breathing from increased dead space and reduced respiratory compliance may cause further ventilatory failure. The main supportive care of ARDS is mechanical ventilation. By stabilizing respiration, mechanical ventilation allows us to buy time for administration of treatment for the underlying cause of ARDS (antibiotic or surgical) and for the evolution of the natural healing process. On the other hand it has been recognized that mechanical ventilation per se can be injurious to the lung, due to excessive pressures/volumes, excessive opening and collapses forces, and potentially self-induced lung inflammation. Arterial oxygenation can be supported by different methods, but it is not yet completely clear which of them are linked with less ventilator-associated lung injury. These strategies can be briefly summarized as "mechanical strategies", involving the ventilatory setting, or "pharmacological strategies", involving administration of drugs potentially improving oxygenation. These strategies can be different in the early compared with the late stages of ARDS, due to the important morphological changes occurring with the progression of the disease.

Lung structure in ARDS in the early phase

Lung injury may originate from a direct insult on the lung ("direct insult") or pulmonary lesions that result from an acute systemic inflammatory response ("indirect insult"). In the direct insult, pulmonary epithelium is subjected to an initial injury, with activation of alveolar macrophages and the inflammatory network, which leads to pulmonary inflammation. In the indirect insult, the pulmonary lesions may originate from extrapulmonary foci, such as peritonitis, pancreatitis, and various abdominal diseases. The subsequent lesions of the alveolar-endothelial barrier cause an increase in the vascular permeability, with an increased interstitial and alveolar edema. The distribution of edema is quite uniform throughout the lung parenchyma, suggesting that the vascular permeability defect should also be evenly distributed [2]. As the total mass of the ARDS lung is more than twice that of the normal lung, the lung progressively collapses under its own weight. The ARDS lung is uniformly affected by the primary disease, and edema accumulates uniformly, as a sponge immersed in water. The gas spaces are restricted by edema and the total gas content decreases. The increased hydrostatic forces progressively compress the lung regions along the vertical axis, and the gas is progressively squeezed out from the dependent regions, with formation of compression atelectasis.

This is why ARDS is characterized by radiographic densities, primarily located in the dependent regions, i.e., the vertebral ones in supine position (Fig.1) [3]. Using computed tomographic (CT) analysis of the regional expiratory limb of the pressure–volume (PV) curve, we found that the upper lung regions are always open, while the middle and lower lung regions present a progressive higher closing pressure [4].

Other mechanisms than the superimposed pressure due to the gravitational forces in an edematous "heavy" lung [5] have been found responsible for the presence of atelectasis-dependent lung, such as (1) the weight of the heart [6,7], (2) the possible increase in the abdominal pressure [8], and (3) the possible deficit of surfactant [9].

Thus, the ARDS lung is composed of normally inflated lung regions, consolidated lung regions and collapsed atelectatic recruitable lung regions. The normally inflated lung regions are primarily distributed in the non-dependent lung regions. The collapsed-atelectatic lung regions are distributed along the vertical gradient from non-dependent to dependent lung, and their amount likely depends on the severity of the disease and edema formation, the shape of the thoracic cage, and the shape of the heart. Finally the consolidated lung regions are evenly distributed throughout the lung parenchyma. Both the atelectatic and consolidated lung regions represent, if perfused, the main cause of hypoxemia and pulmonary shunt. However, it is noteworthy that in ARDS,

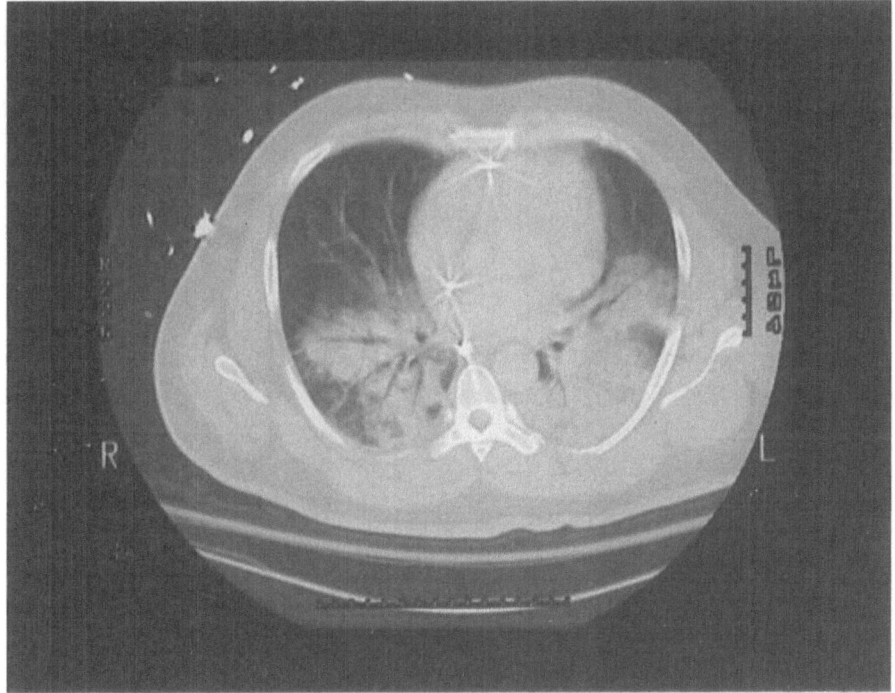

Fig. 1 A typical computed tomographic (CT) scan characterized by radiographic densities, primarly located in the dependent regions in an acute respiratory distress syndrome (ARDS) patient

despite the generalized vasoconstriction, collapsed lung regions are appropriately underperfused compared with the inflated regions.

Effects of tidal volume and positive end-expiratory pressure on lung structure

During mechanical ventilation and tidal volume breath, a considerable part of the lung continuously collapses and decollapses, especially if positive end--expiratory pressure (PEEP) is not enough to keep the lung open at end expiration (Fig. 2). This phenomenon occurs often in the most-dependent lung regions, where compression atelectasis is prevalent. With higher PEEP levels, the reopening-collapsing tissue is decreased, because the amount of collapsed tissue at end-expiration is reduced. The mechanisms underlying the effectiveness of PEEP in early ARDS relate to the presence of compression atelectasis formed under the action of hydrostatic forces. It follows that to prevent the

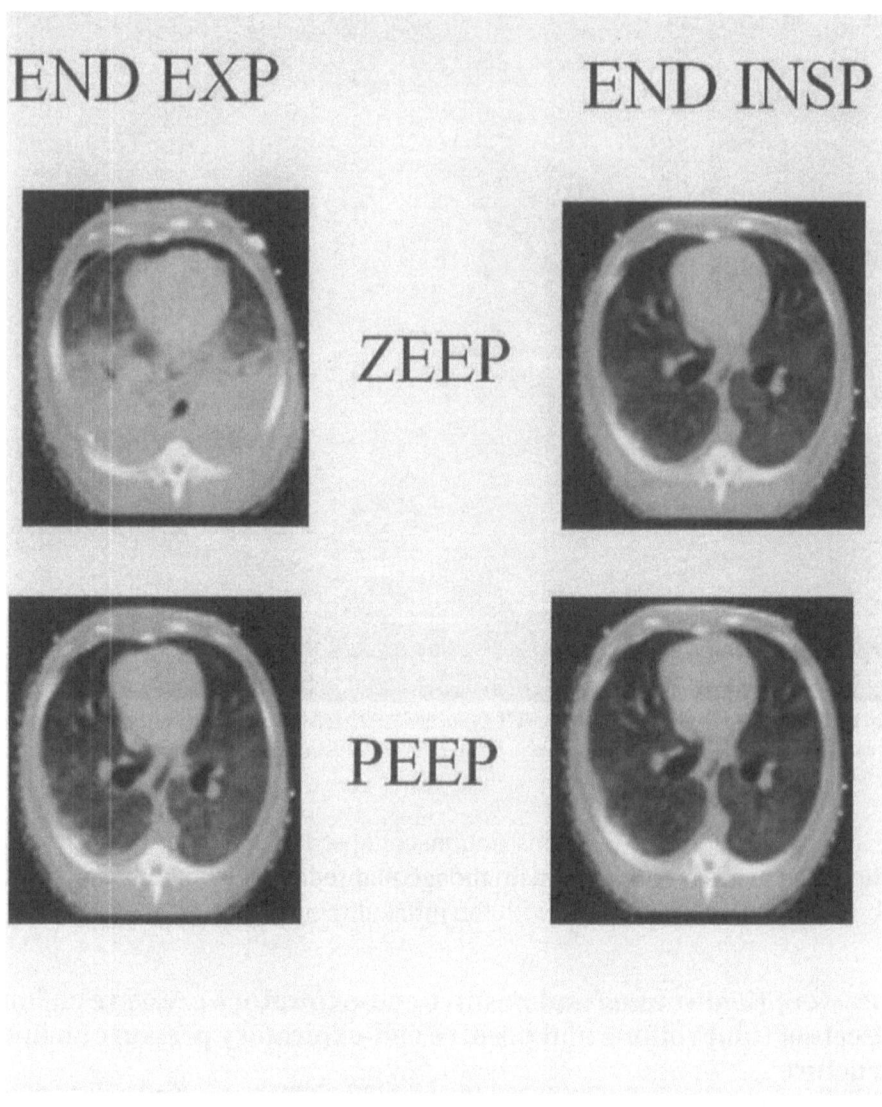

Fig. 2 CT scans at end-expiration and end-ispiration at ZEEP and PEEP, in the oleic acid model of lung injury in dog

collapse of a given pulmonary unit must be at least equal or higher than the hydrostatic forces acting over that unit. As the hydrostatic forces increase along the ventral-dorsal axis in the supine position, the ideal PEEP should also increase along the same axis [5,10,11]. Consequently, the ideal PEEP to keep open the most-dependent lung regions is excessive in the non-dependent lung, where overdistension occurs [4].

Effects of recruitment on lung structure

From the law of La Place we know that a critical opening pressure has to be overcome before the lung volume is augmented, the prerequisite for the recruitment and stabilization of collapsed lung areas. There fore, the goal of an inspiratory pressure increase is to determine this critical opening pressure. Several factors determine the elevated pressure needed to open up previously collapsed alveoli: (1) the absence or reduction in surfactant [12]; (2) the reduced size of the alveoli to be reopened [5]; (3) the increased regional pleural pressure gradient in the most-dependent part of the lung, i.e., a lower transpulmonary pressure at the same alveolar pressure [13]; (4) the weight of the heart on the most-dependent part of the lung [6,14]; (5) the reduction in the chest wall compliance, often due to an increase in the intra-abdominal pressure [15-17]. Thus the transmural pressure required to open atelectasis in the supine position may be high even at 30-35 cmH_2O (i.e., 50-60 cmH_2O in the respiratory system under particular conditions).

Several approaches have been used to perform recruitment maneuver, such as the application of continuous positive airway pressure of 35-40 cmH_2O for 40 s [18], intermittent higher tidal volumes [19], intermittent higher PEEP [20], and extended sigh [21].

In our opinion, the adequate recruitment maneuver depends on the patient's characteristics and few rules should be observed. First, we should consider that the "potential" for recruitment is low in primary ARDS and large in secondary ARDS [17]. Second, it must be borne in mind that the actual opening pressure is the transpulmonary pressure, which strictly depends on the elastances of the lung and chest wall.

In fact, TP = Paw*[EL/(EL+EW)]

In which TP is the transpulmonary pressure, Paw is the applied airway pressure, EL is the elastance of the lung, and EW is the elastance of the chest wall. Under normal conditions EL equals EW, and the TP would be approximately 50% of the applied pressure to the airways. In primary ARDS, EL is greater than EW, while in secondary ARDS the opposite applies [17]. It follows that, to reach the same transpulmonary pressure, a higher Paw is necessary in secondary ARDS. Indeed for the same applied airway pressure the potential risk of the recruitment maneuver would be barotrauma in primary ARDS (high transpulmonary pressure) and hemodynamic derangement in secondary ARDS (high pleural pressure).

Mechanical determinants of lung injury

High pressure - high volume (barotrauma-volotrauma)

Barotrauma has been attributed to mean airway pressure, peak pressure, or PEEP. High airway pressure was first considered as the major determinant of lung injury, causing the passage of alveolar air to the extraalveolar space [22]. A number of animal [23-26] and human studies [27, 28] documented a high association between the incidence of barotrauma and high inspiratory peak pressures. The consequent damage was called barotrauma, which includes interstitial emphysema [29], pneumomediastinum [29], pneumothorax [22], and gas embolism [26]. In the late stages of acute lung injury (ALI)/ARDS the use of high airway pressure treatment was associated with the appearance of emphysema-like lesions [30-33].

However, the concept of barotrauma was challenged by Dreyfuss et al. who underlined the importance of the high volumes (i.e., volotrauma) instead of the high pressures in inducing lung injury. Pressures alone may be an important risk only to the extent that they reflect or influence the transalveolar pressure, thus alveolar distension [25, 34, 35]. In an animal model, high tidal volume caused severe lung edema, not observed in animals ventilated with the same high airway pressure, but lower tidal volume. Previous work also showed that the use of high volumes caused an increase of lung permeability [36] and lung edema [37].

In our opinion barotrauma and volotrauma are two aspects of the same phenomenon: the abnormal increase of transpulmonary pressure, which is the distending force of the lung. The high airway pressure per se does not cause barotrauma, if the transpulmonary pressure is normal, due to an increase of chest wall elastance. In fact, in Dreyfuss' experiments the pleural pressure was likely increased by the chest wall binding [38]. On the other hand, the high volume per se does not induce lung damage when the transpulmonary pressure is in the normal range, as when ventilating with large tidal volume lungs with an elevated functional residual capacity.

Intratidal collapse and decollapse (shear stress trauma, atelectrauma)

More recently several papers reported lung damage resulting from continuous collapse and decollapse of some lung regions throughout the ventilatory cycle. In fact, during inspiration most of the lung regions open up as the inspiratory pressure is sufficient to overcome the regional opening pressure. During expiration, if PEEP is inadequate, part of the lung (usually the dependent regions) undergoes collapse [11]. The damaging effect of the shear forces generated by the cycling collapse and decollapse has been theoretical quantified by Mead et al. [39] and subsequently demonstrated in experimental [40] and clinical settings [41].

Inflammatory agents (biotrauma)

Besides the macroscopic effects of high volume-pressure ventilation (volotrauma-barotrauma), injurious forms of mechanical ventilation resulted in inflammatory response (i.e., biotrauma) [42]. This has been shown first in an ex vivo lung model [43], and subsequently in an in vivo model [44]. The inflammatory mediators released may lead to distal organ damage [45,46] and predispose to multiorgan failure [35].

However, Ricard et al. [47], using mechanical ventilation with high tidal volume in healthy rats, was unable to detect in the lung or in the blood any inflammatory mediators. Similar results were obtained in patients without previous lung injury, in which high tidal volumes for 1 h did not cause consistent changes in the blood of a variety of inflammatory mediators [48]. Thus the role of proinflammatory cytokines in the pathogenesis of ventilator-induced lung injury is still questionable [49].

Reduced tidal volume to improve oxygenation and to avoid baro-volutrauma

Hickling et al. [50] first focused on the potential benefit of tidal volume reduction, disregarding the consequent hypercapnia (i.e., hypercapnia permissive), showing retrospectively a significant decrease of mortality, relative to the expected, in 50 ARDS patients . However, the hypercapnia may be a problem in intracranial pathology [51], severe pulmonary hypertension [52], and congestive heart failure [53].

In 1998, based on experts opinions, it was suggested that the airway plateau pressure should be limited between 30 and 40 cmH_2O or a transpulmonary pressure below 25-30 cmH_2O [54]. However, three randomized controlled trials did not find any benefit in the clinical outcome comparing tidal volumes ranging between 7 and 10.7 ml/kg [55-57]. However, in early 2000, the ARDS network showed a 22% decrease in mortality when ALI/ARDS patients were ventilated with 6 ml/kg compared with 12 ml/kg [58]. Several explanations have been proposed to explain the difference in outcome in these different trials. Among these are the tidal volume differences tested, the study power, the treatment of respiratory acidosis, and the presence of intrinsic PEEP. Eisner et al. [59] in the ARDS network database found that 6 ml/kg tidal volume ventilation was equally effective in subgroups of patients with different risk factors for ARDS. Based on these results, it has been recommended that 6 ml/kg tidal volume ventilation should be broadly applied to ARDS patients [60,61]. Its actual implementation in routine ARDS management is under investigation in the centers who participated in the study. Interestingly, it was found that patients ventilated with reduced tidal volumes showed worse oxygenation in the 1st week of mechanical ventilation compared with the large tidal volume group. However, after the 1st week a dramatic inversion was found, with patients in the reduced tidal volume group showing a rapid, marked, and substantial increase in oxygenation compared with the other group. This was likely due to the fact that the protective ventilation produces results later, but these effects are extremely important in determining the final outcome.

However, the mandatory use of 6 ml/kg of tidal volume is, in our opinion, questionable. In fact while we know that 12 ml/kg tidal volume increased mortality compared with 6 ml/kg, we do not know the effects of the intermediate tidal volume ventilation (i.e., 8-10 ml/kg) Interestingly, in a post hoc analysis of a randomized clinical trial in ALI/ARDS, we found that the mortality was similar at whatever tidal volume below 12 ml/kg, while the mortality sharply increased with tidal volume equal or greater than 12 ml/kg [62].

The safe use of intermediate tidal volume instead of 6 ml/kg is not clinically irrelevant, as the 6 ml/kg implies an increased use of sedative or muscle relaxant agents to adapt the patient to the ventilator and carries potential harmful effects, such as progressive atelectasis and derecruitment [63]. Indeed, in our opinion, while the mechanical ventilation with high tidal volume must be banded, intermediate ventilation (i.e., 8-10 ml/kg of tidal volume) should be reconsidered. If in a given patient 8-10 ml/kg ventilation results in a transpulmonary pressure or airway pressure within the safe range, we do not see any reason for 6 ml/kg ventilation, with its potential complications.

PEEP to improve oxygenation and to avoid collapse and decollapse (atelectrauma-biotrauma)

Besides avoiding high-volume and pressure ventilation, the other cornerstone to improve oxygenation and avoid ventilator-associated lung injury is the application of PEEP [64]. This was stated by Lachmann [12] who focused on the concept of opening the lung (i.e., recruit the lung) and keeping it open (i.e., avoid the derecruitment). PEEP: (1) prevents derecruitment and maintains open at end expiration previously collapsed lung regions, thus reducing the amount of non-ventilated or poorly ventilated but perfused lung tissues; (2) reduces the amount of tissue continuously collapsing and decollpasing during tidal breaths, likely reducing atelectrauma and biotrauma [41].

Different methods have been proposed to select at the bedside the "optimal" PEEP level. The "optimal PEEP" level is the level of PEEP at which the least amount of collapsed tissue is maintained at end-expiration with least interefe-rence with regional overdistension and hemodynamics.

PV curve

For PEEP selection, the PV curve has been widely used since the 1970s [65, 66]. The traditional view suggests that the PV curve, in its inspiratory limb, is the expression of three phenomena: (1) the lower part up to the inflection point reflects recruitment zone, (2) the straight line reflects normal inflation zone, (3) the upper inflection point reflects the overdistension zone [67]. According to this model, Amato et al. [18], in a randomized clinical trial, setting the PEEP 2 cmH$_2$O above the lower inflection point and limiting the airway plateau pressure to 40 cmH$_2$O, found a significant increase in survival at 28 days compared with a control group [18]. Ranieri et al. [41] using the same technique for PEEP selection, were able to decrease a variety of proinflammatory media-tors in ARDS patients.

However, the use of the inspiratory limb of the PV curve for PEEP selection appears at least questionable. Venegas et al. [68], based on theory [68], and Hickling [69, 70], with a mathematical model, suggested that the recruitment occurs throughout the entire inspiratory limb of the PV curve. In CT analysis of the PV curve we were not able to find differences in the recruitment across the lower inflection point [67] and more recently we found both in animal [13] and in ARDS patients [71] that recruitment is an inspiratory phenomenon occurring along the entire inspiratory limb of the PV curve, well above the lower inflection point. Indeed the bulk of data suggest that setting the PEEP (i.e., controlling the derecruitment) according to the inspiratory limb of the PV curve does not have a solid physiological basis.

The positive results obtained by Amato et al. [18] and Ranieri et al. [41], setting the PEEP above the inflection point, may be simply explained by the higher PEEP applied in the treatment compared with the control group.

Gas exchange trial

Another easy method to perform to select the "optimal PEEP" at the bedside is the gas exchage trial. Usually different PEEP levels from 5 to 20 cmH₂O are randomly applied or applied in a given order (increasing or decreasing) and gas exchange is measured. Both changes in oxygenation (PaO_2) and carbon dioxide ($PaCO_2$) are evaluated. An increase in oxygenation likely reflects the amount of aerated tissue present at end expiration, or the amount of collapsed non--aerated tissue that has been maintained open at end expiration [72]. We usually consider as a positive response to the gas exchange trial an improvement in oxygenation of at least 10-15 mmHg (whatever inspired oxygen fraction is used). However, we have to consider the behavior of $PaCO_2$. The value of $PaCO_2$ is not usually considered when a PEEP trial is performed. However, we believe that a change in $PaCO_2$ (at constant minute ventilation) may be more informative than changes in oxygenation. We have to bear in mind that a change in oxygenation of 40 mmHg (i.e., form 60 to 100 mmHg) causes a change in oxygen content similar to the change in carbon dioxide content of 5 mmHg (i.e., from 40 to 45 mmHg). Our hypothesis is that when carbon dioxide decreases during the PEEP test, this likely means prevalent alveolar recruitment, no change in balance between recruitment and overdistension, and finally even small increases in $PaCO_2$ likely indicate prevalent overdistension (or at least the amount of overdistension that we have to pay) compared with the amount of recruitment. Thus we believe that when a gas exchange trial is performed, both oxygenation and carbon dioxide changes have to be taken into account to optimize the selection of PEEP.

Respiratory mechanics trial

Other authors have suggested using the respiratory mechanics to select PEEP [16, 73]. The best compliance of the respiratory system should indicate the level of PEEP at which the lung is maintained more open [74]. An alternative mode to select PEEP by using respiratory mechanics has been suggested by Ranieri et al. [75] using the pressure time curve during constant flow ventilation, and analyzing the shape of the curve. This interesting approach, however, has not yet been validated in the clinical setting. New forms of continuous monitoring of collapse and decollapse, as with electrical impedance tomography, are still at the experimental stage [76].

   We also believe that, when present, improvements in respiratory compliance likely indicate more open lung relative to overdistension, no changes or no overdistension, or an equal relationship between opening and overdistension, and finally reduction in respiratory compliance, a prevalent overdistension.

However, this method is limited by the fact that not always does respiratory compliance really parallel changes in aeration and if so these changes are small and poorly sensitive. Moreover, the respiratory compliance may not be representative of the lung mechanical behavior in the presence of altered chest wall compliance, as found in patients with abdominal surgical respiratory related problems [15, 16] or in obese patients [77].

Oxygen transport

Other authors [15,78] proposed setting "optimal PEEP" by considering mainly its effects on oxygen delivery. In other words they proposed considering as the main effect of PEEP the interaction between the level of oxygenation and its effects on hemodynamics. This approach has the advantage that it is relatively integrated between gas exchange and hemodynamics. However, its limiting factor is that it is possible to reach acceptable oxygen delivery (greater than 600 ml O_2/min) even with relatively low levels of PEEP that we know do not optimize alveolar opening [11]. In other words, with this method a safe oxygenation is likely, but it is very likely that the collapse and decollapse of the alveolar units continues to occur.

Selection of "optimal PEEP" – an integrated approach

Recently, an integrated approach to select "optimal PEEP" has been proposed using: (1) oxygenation and respiratory mechanics; (2) lung morphology by chest X-ray and /or CT scan, respiratory mechanics, and oxygenation.

Oxygenation and respiratory mechanics

An interesting integrated approach of gas exchange and respiratory mechanics has been proposed by Bohm and Lachmann [79] and recently investigated in animal [13,80,81] and human studies [71]. It consists of opening up the lung (increasing plateau and PEEP levels) and then keep the lung open (progressively decreasing the PEEP levels).

First the ventilatory setting should be switched from volume to pressure control mode. The level of the previous inspiratory plateau pressure on volume control could serve as a guide to find the appropriate plateau pressure for pressure control ventilation. Otherwise, the plateau pressure during volume control ventilation minus 5 cmH₂O could be chosen. The levels of PEEP may initially be the same as in the first mode. With an inspiratory/expiratory ratio equal to 1:1, both PEEP levels and plateau inspiratory pressures are successively incremented in steps of 3-5 cmH₂O. Rarely, levels of 20/60 cmH₂O for PEEP and plateau inspiratory pressure are necessary. During the process of opening the lungs, the PaO_2 helps to guide this effort, because it is the only parameter that reliably correlates with the amount of the lung tissue that participates in gas exchange. Moreover, a more than proportional increase in the size of the tidal volume following an increase in airway pressure also indicates alveolar recruitment. It is important during the maneuver (opening procedure) to maintain a sufficient intravascular volume. It may be necessary to administer fluids and give inotropic support to the right heart. This type of hemodynamic support will be superfluous at lower airway pressures.

If a further increase in airway pressure does not result in a parallel increase in PaO_2, plateau inspiratory pressures can be carefully reduced, because now reopened alveoli are present, which, to keep open, no longer require such high intrapulmonary pressures. The PaO_2 should, however, remain high despite the reduction in airway pressures, just until the critical level of pressure is reached at which the least-compliant parts of the lungs starts to collapse. Should this occur, the inspiratory pressures should be increased to the previously determined values for a short period. The lung tissue is yet again fully recruited and the pressures should then be reduced to levels that are safely above the closing pressure, usually 2-3 cmH_2O.

Oxygenation, respiratory mechanics, and lung morphology

Another integrated approach has been suggested by Rouby et al. [82] by using respiratory mechanics and lung morphology. Briefly, the authors performed a chest X-ray or CT scan at PEEP 5 cmH_2O. If they showed a diffuse loss of aeration (diffuse and bilateral hyperdensities "white lungs"), they performed a PV curve to determine the upper inflection point and subsequently a PEEP trial at 10, 15, 20, and 25 cmH_2O, with a pressure limitation at 2 cmH_2O lower than the upper inflection point. If the morphological study shows bilateral hyperdensities predominating in the lower lobes, they suggest performing a PEEP trial at 5, 8, 10, and 12 cmH_2O. The optimal PEEP level is defined as the PEEP allowing the highest PaO_2 and $SatO_2$ at the lowest FiO_2, If the optimal PEEP level is not reached and it does not allow reduction of FiO_2 below 0.5, other supports are used, such as the prone position, inhaled nitric oxide, an almitrine trial, and finally extracorporeal membrane oxygenation.

All these reccomendations for selecting the "optimal PEEP" levels consider the hypothesis that PEEP is not only useful to improve oxygenation, maintaining open previously collapsed alveoli, but also that PEEP is a "therapeutic" strategy to avoid collapse and decollapse of the alveolar units, preventing ventilator-associated lung injury, such as atelectrauma and biotrauma. However, it is also possible that keeping the lung "closed", avoiding recruitment (as in lobar pneumonia), is not dangerous and may be beneficial. Experimental studies showed that keeping part of the lung closed resulted in a decrease of lung damage compared with the control [83,84]. In our opinion we should be ready to consider and study this prospective, and in line with this extracorporeal assistance should be reconsidered [85].

Other ventilatory strategies proposed to improve oxygenation and minimize ventilator-associated lung injury

Among controlled mechanical ventilation strategies, alternative strategies have been proposed. Although the physiological basis for the lung protective strategy has been well established, several questions are still open. As the tidal volume is harmful, we may expect a decrease in lung injury using high-frequency oscillation (HFO) or high-frequency ventilation (HFV). In fact it has been shown that HFV compared with the conventional mechanical ventilation resulted in lower production of inflammatory mediators [86]. Unfortunately these kinds of ventilations did not show any benefit in clinical practice [87]. However, the PEEP levels used in these studies were likely inadequate. To define the role of HFV and HFO in lung protective strategy, appropriate trials are needed [88].

Another possible improvement would be the intermittent use of higher tidal volume (sigh). When the airway pressure is intermittently increased to 45 cmH_2O, maintaining the tidal volume in the safe range, two possible advantages have been demonstrated. First, the "sigh" ventilation may prevent the development of reabsorption atelectasis, supplying a fresh gas to lung regions with low ventilation/perfusion ratio; second, in case of atelectasis development the "sigh" may act as a recruitment maneuver [19].

Among assisted methods, airway pressure release ventilation and bilevel positive airway pressure have been proposed. All allow unrestricted spontaneous breathing at any time during of the respiratory cycle while the machine periodically switches between two levels of positive airway pressure. Compared with total control mechanical ventilation, unrestricted spontaneous breathing superimposed on mechanical ventilation results in an improvement in the oxygenation parameters by an improvement in V/Q matching (decrease in intrapulmonary shunt and dead space) in ARDS animals [89] and in humans [90]. The diaphragmatic contraction improves the ventilation of dependent part of the lungs (redistribution of ventilation to less-aerated areas, with a reduction in the pulmonary shunt). Moreover, as spontaneous breathing decreases mean intrathoracic pressure, venous return increases and so does the cardiac output and oxygen delivery.

Hence, unrestricted spontaneous breathing superimposed on mechanical ventilation may improve ventilation of the dependent lung zones and may recruit underventilated or collapsed areas. Interestingly these effects are not observed during pressure support ventilation (PSV), a form of mechanical assistance of each inspiratory effort. The spontaneous inspiratory activity during mechanically assisted breaths during PSV is probably not sufficient to improve the ventilation of the dependent parts of the lung and to decrease the intrathoracic pressure significantly. Anyway the PSV has been shown to allow the same oxygenation as controlled mechanical ventilation, with much less need of sedation [91].

Another form of assisted mechanical ventilation that has been proposed to improve oxygenation in ARDS is proportional assist ventilation [92]. Like other modes of positive pressure ventilation, proportional assist ventilation elevates airway pressure during inspiration. Unlike other modes, the inspiratory airway pressure assistance varies directly with patient effort [93]. This allows breath- -to-breath variations in inspiratory flow and tidal volume, as with pressure support but the magnitude of the pressure assistance increases with patient effort. Moreover, the inspiratory assistance can be customized to the elastance and resistance properties of each patient's respiratory system. This mode of ventilation is most favorable for breathing comfort and for reducing unnecessary work of breathing. Studies in ARDS have shown that proportional assist ventilation can imrove oxygenation compared with conventional mechanical ventilation [94].

In conclusion, assisted modes of mechanical ventilation can be useful to improve oxygenation in ARDS, perhaps similar to or even better than conventional methods. Moreover, they need much less sedation and curarization. However, these encouraging physiological results have not been paralleled by large clinical studies indicating the effective superiority of these techniques compared with conventional mechanical ventilation.

Prone position to improve oxygenation and reduce ventilator-associated lung injury

Prone positioning leads to substantial improvement in arterial oxygenation in approximately 65-75% of ARDS patients [62,95,96]. There is little information to predict which patients will respond positively to prone positioning. However, the improvements in some patients are quite striking, allowing substantial reduction in the inspiratory oxygen fraction required and levels of PEEP. The mechanisms by which the prone position improves oxygenation have been investigated experimentally. It has been shown [97] that improved ventilation to previously dependent (dorsal) regions occurs in the prone position. The same it has been shown in humans [98]. In the supine position, pleural pressures are higher near the most-dependent part of the lung due to hydrostatic pressures [5,13]. Higher pleural pressures reduce transmural pressures of the dependent bronchioles and alveoli, contributing together with other factors to the tendency for atelectasis in these zones. In the prone position, pleural pressures appeared more uniform, allowing some dorsal regions to open up and participate in ventilation and gas exchange.

However, the redistribution in alveolar inflation and ventilation has to be paralleled by relatively no change or more-uniform distribution of perfusion to explain the improvement in oxygenation. Most of the data of lung perfusion in the prone position arise from experimental work, and direct evidence on ALI/ARDS patients is lacking. The experimental data suggest that the gravitational model does not apply in the prone position. In fact, Glenny et al. [99] showed that in the prone position the gravitational gradient is reduced with a more-homogeneous distribution of blood flow, i.e., similar blood flow in the dependent and non-dependent lung regions [99].

Thus in ALI/ARDS patients the prone position may cause a more-homogeneous distribution of perfusion, relatively unaffected by the gravity. In conclusion, the available evidence suggests that the perfusion does not dramatically change when changing the position [97].

Ventilation-induced lung injury is now widely recognized as a major problem in the management of acute respiratory failure [100]. The use of high transpulmonary pressure (i.e., ventilation with high tidal volumes or high pressures) by overstretching the alveoli can cause epithelial and endothelial disruptions and induce lung edema. Failure to apply adequate PEEP levels can further increase the shear forces resulting from the repeated airspace opening and closing. When ALI/ARDS patients are in the supine position, the airspace opening and closing, the largest alveolar volumes excursion, and the smallest end expiratory alveolar volumes are preferentially distributed in the dorsal regions, due to the more-positive pleural pressure and to the lower regional functional residual capacity. The prone position, by reducing the gravitational gradient of pleural pressure, can increase the transpulmonary pressure and the regional functional residual capacity. Moreover, it can limit the shear forces and the alveolar volume excursions in the dorsal regions. Similarly, the prone position, causing a more-homogeneous pulmonary blood flow distribution, may limit the capillary stress and reduce the lung edema.

Recent animal data showed that in the prone position, either in healthy subjects or in a lung injury model, the lung edema and the severity of histological abnormalities were less severe in the prone compared with the supine position [101-103]. Moreover, in the supine position the lung edema and the histological abnormalities were higher in the dorsal regions, while in the prone position the distribution of lung edema and histological abnormalities was more uniform between the dorsal and the ventral regions. Moreover, it has been shown that the prone position may also reduce the incidence of pneumothorax [104]. In conclusion, the use of the prone position besides improving the gas exchange, can limit the ventilation-induced lung injury [105].

Besides the effect of the prone position on arterial oxygenation, its effects on outcome are still under investigation. In a multicenter trial, 305 ALI/ARDS patients were randomized to be kept prone for at least 6 h per day for a period of 10 days [62]; 152 patients were assigned to the prone group and 152 to the supine (control) group. The mortality did not differ significantly between the prone and the supine group at the end of the 10-day study period (21% vs. 25%), at the time of discharge from intensive care (50% vs. 48%), or at 6 months (62% vs. 59%). In a post hoc analysis, a significantly lower 10-day mortality rate was found in the prone group than in the supine group in the patients with the lowest PaO_2/F_IO_2 ratio (< 88 mmHg), with the highest Simplified Acute Physiologic Score (> 49) and the highest tidal volume (> 12 ml/kg).

These negative results could be explained by a true lack of effect of the prone position on outcome or alternatively by: (1) an inadequate statistical power, (2) the short length of the prone position; an average of only 7.0 h/day, meaning that the patients were supine for more than 70 % for each day, (3) the limitation of prone position to only 10 days.

However, considering these potential limitations, we believe that, at present, the prone position with this protocol should not be used in all kinds of ALI/ARDS patients, but limited, as suggested by the post hoc analysis, only to the most-severe case of respiratory failure [106].

Two categories of ARDS patients have been poorly investigated: the trauma and brain-injured patients, since in this case the prone position is still considered inadequate or even potentially dangerous. Recently, several studies showed the utility of the prone position to improve arterial oxygenation in trauma patients with severe respiratory failure. In these studies, different types of trauma patients were enrolled, such as multiple trauma, blunt chest trauma, abdominal trauma, and multiples fractures. The prone position was safe, well tolerated, and caused only minor complications, such as swelling and edema of the face and pressures sores. Moreover, in one study the trauma patients with ARDS were treated for at least 20 consecutive h/day in the prone position (mean 8±4 days spent in the prone position) without any significant side effects [107]. Patients with intracranial pressure (ICP) > 25 mmHg, despite adequate treatment, and unstable cervical spine fractures were excluded.

Brain-injured patients have an increased risk of extracerebral organ dysfunctions, mainly pulmonary dysfunction [108]. Brain-injured patients are characterized by an increased risk of developing ventilator-associated pneumonia (30-50% compared with 20% of the normal population) [66, 67]. Several studies indicate that pulmonary dysfunctions after brain injury may significantly increase the intensive care stay, the mortality and worsen the neurological outcome [109]. The prone position has not usually been considered in brain-injured patients because of the fear of possible negative effects on brain perfusion and ICP.

Obviously, strict exclusion criteria should be considered when the prone position is used: (1) presence of an unstable brain situation (unstable ICP and/or ICP higher than 20-25 mmHg despite adequate treatment); (2) evidence of ischemia, as indicated by a low jugular oxygen saturation levels (below 55-60 mmHg). Furthermore, in this particular type of patient we have to consider: (1) an adequate level of sedation; (2) a careful positioning of the patient with an antitrendelemburg position (the head and trunk at 20°) with a good alignment of the cervical with the thoracic spine; (3) in the more-severe brain-injured patients monitoring of ICP and jugular oxygen saturation are preferable; (4) a careful clinical monitoring of the nervous component is necessary (in particular, the pupillary diameter in the acute phases of positioning and overall neurological status in the daily clinical assessment).

We recently investigated the effect of a short period of prone positioning in a randomized controlled study of severe brain-injured patients sedated and paralyzed with acute respiratory failure due to ventilator-associated pneumonia [110]. The patient during the prone position markedly improved the arterial oxygenation within 4 h and maintained the improvement in arterial oxygenation 24 h later in the supine position. No significant increase in ICP was found during the prone position and no patients experienced an increase in ICP greater than 25 mmHg. Although these are very preliminary data, obtained in a relatively small population over a short period of time, they suggest that the prone position in brain-injured patients: (1) can be safely used; (2) improves oxygenation and the improvement is maintained for at least 24 h while the patient is repositioned in the supine position; (3) if accurately performed, with a moderate duration and carefully monitored, does not negatively affect the brain perfusion and ICP.

At present it is still unknown when ALI/ARDS patients should be turned prone [111]. We suggest the early phase of the disease and to try to maximally recruit the lung by recruitment maneuvers (i.e., sighs or sustained inflations).

There are no guidelines suggesting how long the prone position should be maintained to attain the maximal beneficial effect on respiratory function. Experiences from the literature suggest that most of the improvement occurs rapidly in only a few minutes after turning prone. However, a continuous increase in arterial oxygenation can be still present even after 6 h of the prone position [62].

In some responder patients, the gain in arterial oxygenation is partially maintained when returning supine (i.e., persistent responders), while other responder patients suddenly lose the gain when returning supine (i.e., non--persistent responders) [112]. A possible explanation is that in the persistent responders the recruited lung volume in the prone position is better maintained in the supine position compared with the non-persistent responders.

So in the persistent responders a strategy of repeated supine-prone cycles could be useful, avoiding the complication of a prolonged time in the prone position. In non-persistent responders we suggest increasing the length of time in the prone position, to decrease the risk of severe hypoxemia when returning supine.

Recruitment maneuver and PEEP during the prone position

The CT scan studies in supine ALI/ARDS patients showed that the presence of lung collapse not only along a vertical gradient (i.e, ventral to dorsal) but also along a cephalo to caudal axis. The recruitment maneuvers are recommended as a useful tool to reopen the collapsed lung regions and to improve arterial oxygenation. However, the recruitment maneuver in the supine position, besides reopening the dorsal regions (i.e., collapsed ones), will also overdistend those already open. The prone position, by reducing the pleural pressure gradient, can increase the transpulmonary pressure in the dorsal regions. This property of the prone position causes a higher lung recruitment of the dorsal regions and higher arterial oxygenation improvement when the recruitment maneuver is applied in the prone compared with the supine position. This has been shown in the experimental setting and in ALI/ARDS patients [19, 113].

The PEEP is one of the most-important tools to increase the arterial oxygenation in severe respiratory failure. The PEEP, by opposing the critical closing pressure (i.e., superimposed pressure), can maintain the lung open at end expiration. Several data suggest that the PEEP in the prone position can cause a more-homogeneous distribution of pulmonary blood flow compared with the supine position [114]. Due to the lower closing pressures and a more-favorable pulmonary blood distributions in the prone position, lower PEEP levels are likely necessary to reach the same increase in the arterial oxygenation compared with the supine position [113, 115].

CT scan showed that the ventral regions remain aerated at lower PEEP levels in the prone position, while the dorsal regions previously collapsed in the supine position became aerated. The same dorsal regions to remain aerated in supine positions need higher PEEP levels, and this can cause an overdistension of the ventral regions.

Indeed, the prone position compared with the supine position can ameliorate the beneficial effect of a recruitment maneuver to increase the arterial oxygenation and requires lower PEEP levels to maintain this increase.

Inhaled nitric oxide

Inhaled nitric oxide (NO) acutely improves oxygenation by dilating pulmonary vessels supplying ventilated alveolar units and improving V/Q matching [116]. It may reduce pulmonary arterial hypertension. Its short half-life in blood (around 100 ms)[117] means that vascular effects are limited to the pulmonary circulation. The combination of rapid clinical improvement in some patients and lack of perceived risks has led to the widespread adoption of inhaled NO in ARDS. Three prospective controlled trials of efficacy have recently been completed. The first was a placebo-controlled, blinded phase II trial of 177 patients, randomized to control or one of five treatment groups according to dosage, with therapy maintained for up to 28 days or until improvement criteria were fulfilled [118]. Transient improvements in oxygenation were detected at all doses of NO over days, but no difference in mortality was found. There was only a suggestion of an outcome difference in the number of patients successfully weaned from ventilation on day 28, when a post hoc subgroup analysis showed that the group receiving 5 ppm NO had significantly more survivors than the control group. A smaller recent pilot study (30 patients) reflected these results [119], with no difference in 30-day mortality and a non-significant higher number of patients alive and successfully weaned from ventilation in the trial period.

Interestingly, the results of a recent prospective, double-blinded, randomized French phase III study of inhaled NO for ARDS in 208 patients also demonstrated no effect on mortality or the duration of mechanical ventilation [120].

In another recent study [121], the authors examined the ability to reduce oxygen fraction and so minimize the intensity of ventilation in patients on inhaled NO. No significant difference was shown in the ability of inhaled NO to reduce aggressive mechanical ventilation.

Overall all these studies suggest little benefit from long-term administration of NO in ARDS. Recent published systematic historical data from Scandinavia showed no evidence of benefit in patients administered NO over a 3-year period [122].

Some authors have taken the view that NO should not be administered outside the context of controlled trials, or even that there is no place for further trials

[123]. Inhaled NO is certainly efficacious in the short term and may have a place as rescue therapy, offering a window of stability for further investigation (for example bronchoscopy), interhospital retrieval, or transfer for high-resolution CT. In this context, it should be noted that none of the studies seemed to show any benefit in initial doses above 5-10 ppm and that, in other work, only 54% of patients showed a reproducible response, even in the acute phase [124]. A long-term supportive role is more difficult to sustain, especially given the risk of toxicity and the need to monitor inspired nitrogen dioxide levels and methemoglobin.

Other authors proposed that other inhaled pulmonary vasodilators (for example nebulized prostacyclin) may be equally efficient compared with NO, easier to administer, but much more expensive [125].

Inhaled NO and the prone position

NO has been shown to be beneficial in ALI/ARDS patients to increase the arterial oxygenation [126-128]. When NO is inhaled in the prone position it causes a greater improvement in arterial oxygenation than either treatment used alone. The improvement in the arterial oxygenation can allow a faster reduction of the inspired oxygen fraction, with a possible benefit in decreasing the oxygen toxicity. Furthermore, the combination of the prone position and inhaled NO could decrease the necessary dose of NO, so reducing the accumulation of toxic proinflammatory degradation products, such as nitrogen dioxide.

The effects of NO may be different in primary and secondary ARDS. Rialp et al. [127] found, in the prone position, an improvement in the arterial oxygenation with NO only in primary ARDS.

However, all the studies to date have evaluated only the short-term effects of inhaled NO combined in the prone position. Hence further studies are necessary to evaluate the real benefits of this fascinating dual therapy in the outcome of ALI/ARDS patients.

Conclusions

In conclusion, our knowledge of the pathophysiology of ARDS has dramatically increased in these last years, allowing a better tailoring of the clinical management of these patients. In early ARDS, hypoxemia is a characteristic factor, mainly due to the presence of atelectatic and consolidated lung areas that are non ventilated but relatively well perfused. Moreover, it has been emphasized that the amount of ventilable aerated lung tissue is markedly reduced. On the other hand, it has been recognized that mechanical ventilation can seriously negatively affect the lung (ventilator-associated lung injury) by several mechanisms (barotrauma/volutrauma, atelectrauma, biotrauma). The main goal is to improve oxygenation without increasing the iatrogenic effects caused by mechanical ventilation.

We have different methods now to achieve this goal that have been investigated in several experimental and clinical trials. Some of these methods are related to the ventilatory setting, while others are related to drug administration. Among the methods related to the ventilatory setting, those found really effective are: (1) to reduce tidal volume; (2) to apply PEEP to reduce the amount of non-aerated atelectatic lung; (3) to apply the prone position, at least in more severely hypoxemic patients. On the other hand, drug administration by using inhaled NO has not been really effective.

References

1. Ausbaugh DG, Bigelow DB, Petty TL, et al (1967) Acute respiratory distress in adults. Lancet: 319-323
2. Sandiford P, Province MA, Shuster DP (1995) Distribution of regional density and vascular permeability in the adult respiratory distress syndrome. Am J Respir Crit Care Med 151:737-742
3. Gattinoni L, Mascheroni D, Torresin A, et al (1986) Morphological response to positive end-expiratory pressure in acute respiratory failure. Intensive Care Med 12:137-142
4. Gattinoni L, D'Andrea L, Pelosi P, et al (1993) Regional effects and mechanism of positive end expiratory pressure early adult respiratory distress syndrome. JAMA 269:2122-2127
5. Pelosi P, D'Andrea L, Vitale G, et al (1994) Vertical gradient of regional lung inflation in adult respiratory distress syndorme. Am J Respir Crit Care Med 149: 8-13
6. Albert RM, Hubmayr RD (2000) The prone position eliminates compression of the lungs by the heart. Am J Respir Crit Care Med 16: 1660-1665
7. Malbuisson LM, Brush CJ, Puybasset L, et al (2000) Role of the heart in the loss of aeration characterizing lower lobes in acute respiratory distress syndrome. Am J Respir Crit Care Med 161:2005-2012
8. Froese AB, Bryan AC (1974) Effects of anesthesia and paralysis on diaphragmatic mechanics in man. Anesthesiology 41:242-254
9. Vasquez de Anda GF, Lachmann RA, et al (2001) Treatment of ventilation induced lung injury with exogenous surfactant. Intensive Care Med 3:559-565
10. Puybasset L, Curiel P, Chao N, et al (1998) A computed tomography scan assessment of regional lung volume in acute lung injury. Am J Respir Crit Care Med 198:1644-1655
11. Gattinoni L, Pelosi P, Crotti S, et al (1995) Effects of positive end expiratory pressures on regional distribution of tidal volume and recruitment in adult respiratory distress syndrome. Am J Respir Crit Care Med 151:1807-1814
12. Lachmann B (1992) Open up the lung and keep the lung open. Intensive Care Med 18:319-322
13. Pelosi P, Golden A, Mc Kibben A, et al (2001) Recruitment and derecruitment during acute respiratory failure: an experimental study. Am J Resp Crit Care 164: 122-130
14. Malbouisson LM, Busch CJ, Puybasset L, et al (2000) Role of the heart in the loss of aeration characterizing lower lobes in acute respiratory distress syndrome. CT Scan ARDS Study Group. Am J Respir Crit Care Med 161:2005-2012
15. Pelosi P, Cereda M, Foti G, et al (1995) Alterations of lung and chest wall mechanics in patients with acute lung injury: effects of positive end-expiratory pressure. Am J Respir Crit Care Med 152:531-537

16. Ranieri VM, Brienza N, Santostasi S, et al (1997) Impairment of lung and chest wall mechanics in patients with acute respiratory distress syndrome: role of abdominal distension. Am J Respir Crit Care Med 156:1082-1091

17. Gattinoni L, Pelosi P, Suter PM, et al (1998) Acute respiratory distress syndrome caused by pulmonary and extrapulmonary disease. Different syndromes ? Am J Respir Crit Care Med 158: 3-11

18. Amato MBP, Barbas CSV, Medeiros DM, et al (1998) Effect of a protective ventilation strategy on mortality in the acute respiratory distress syndorme. N Engl J Med 338:347-354

19. Pelosi P, Cadringher P, Bottino N, et al (1999) Sigh in acute respiratory distress syndrome. Am J Respir Crit Care Med 159:872-880

20. Foti G, Cereda M, Sparacino ME, et al (2000) Effects of periodic lung recruitment maneuvres on gas exchange and respiratory mechanics in mechanically ventilated acute respiratory distress syndrome (ARDS) patients. Intensive Care Med 26:501-507

21. Lim CM, Koh Y, Park W, et al (2001) Mechanistic scheme and effect of "extended sigh" as a recruitment maneuver in patients with acute respiratory distress syndrome: A preliminary study. Crit Care Med 29:1255-1260

22. Macklin MT, Macklin CC (1994) Malignant interstitial emphysema of the lungs and mediastinum as an important complication in many respiratory diseases and other conditions: an interpretation of the clinical literature in the light of laboratory experiment. Medicine (Baltimore) 23:281-352

23. Kolobow T, Moretti MP, Fumagalli R, et al (1987) Severe impairment in lung function induced by high peak airway pressure during mechanical ventilation. Am Rev Respir Dis 135: 312-315

24. Tsuno K, Prato P, Kolobow T (1990) Acute lung injury from mechanical ventilation at moderately high airway pressures. J Appl Physiol 69:956-961

25. Dreyfuss D, Saumon G (1998) Ventilator-induced lung injury. Lessons from experimental studies. Am J Respir Crit Care Med 157:294-323

26. Marini JJ, Culver BH (1989) Systemic gas embolism complicating mechanical ventilation in the adult respiratory distress syndrome. Ann Intern Med 110:699-703

27. Latorre F de, Tomasa A, Klamburg J (1977) Incidence of pneumothorax and pneumomediastinum in patients with aspiration requiring mechanical ventilatory support. Chest 72:141-144

28. Shnapp LM, Chin DP, Szaflarski N, et al (1995) Frequency and importance of barotrauma in 100 patients with acute lung injury. Crit Care Med 23:272-278

29. Lawrence RD (1974) Respirator induced pneumothorax and subcutaneous emphysema. Experimental overinflation of cadaver lungs. J Forensic Sci 19:548-556

30. Rouby JJ, Lherm T, Martin de Lassale E, et al (1993) Histologic aspects of pulmonary barotrauma in critically ill patients with acute respiratory failure. Intensive Care Med 7:369-371

31. Pelosi P, Crotti S, Brazzi L, et al (1996) Computed tomography in adult respiratory distress syndrome: what has taught us. Eur Respir J 5:1055-1062

32. Gattinoni L, Bombino M, Pelosi P, et al (1984) Lung structure and function in different stages of severe adult respiratory distress syndrome. JAMA 8:1772-1779

33. Goldstein I, Bughalo MT, Marquette CH, et al (2001) Mechanical ventilation induced airspace enlargement during experimental pneumonia in piglets. Am J Respir Crit Care Med 163: 958-964

34. Gillette MA, Hess D (2001) Ventilator induced lung injury and the evolution of lung protective strategies in acute respiratory distress syndrome. Respir Care 46:130-148

35. Slutsky AS, Tremblay L (1998) Multiple system organ failure: is mechanical ventilation a contributing factor ? Am J Respir Crit Care Med 157:1721-1725

36. Webb HH, Tierney DF (1974) Experimental pulmonary edema due to intermittent positive pressure ventilation with high inflation pressures. Protection by positive end expiratory pressure. Am Rev Respir Dis 110:556-565

37. Corbridge TC, Wood LDH, Crawford GP, et al (1990) Effects of large tidal volume and low PEEP in canine acid aspiration. Am Rev Respir Dis 142:311-315

38. Dreyfuss D, Soler P, Basset G, et al (1988) High inflation pressure pulmonary edema: respective effects of high airway pressure, high tidal volume and positive end-expiratory pressure. Am Rev Respir Dis 137:1159-1164

39. Mead J, Takishima T, Leith D (1970) Stress distribution in lungs: a model of pulmonary elasticity. J Appl Physiol 28:596-608
40. Muscedere JG, Mullen JB, Gan K, et al (1994) Tidal ventilation at low airway pressures can augment lung injury. Am J Respir Crit Care Med 149:1327-1334
41. Ranieri VM, Suter PM, Tortorella C, et al (1999) Effect of mechanical ventilation on inflammatory mediators in patients with acute respiratory distress syndrome. JAMA 282:54-61
42. International consensus conference in intensive care medicine: ventilator-associated lung injury in ARDS.(1999) Am J Respir Crit Care 160:2118-2124
43. Tremblay L, Valenza F, Ribeiro S, et al (1997) Injurious ventilatory strategies increase cytokines and c-fos m-RNA expression in an isolated lung model. J Clin Invest 99:944-952
44. Chiumello D, Pristine G, Slutsky AS (1999) Mechanical ventilation affects local and systemic citokines in an animal model of acute respiratory distress syndrome. Am J Respir Crit Care Med 160:109-116
45. Valenza F, Sibilla S, Porro GA, et al (2000) An improved in vivo rat model for the study of mechanical ventilatory support effects on organs distal to the lung. Crit Care Med 28: 3697-3704
46. Haitsma JJ, Uhlig S, Goggel R (2000) Ventilator induced lung injury leads to loss of alveolar and systemic compartmentalization of tumor necrosis factor alpha. Intensive Care Med 10: 1515-1522
47. Ricard JD, Dreyfuss D, Saumon G (2001) Production of inflammatory cytokines in ventilator induced lung injury: a reappraisal. Am J Respir Crit Care Med 163:1176-1180
48. Wrigge H, Zinserling J, Stuber F, et al (2000) Effects of mechanical ventilation on release of cytokines into systemic circulation in patients with normal pulmonary function. Anesthesiology 93:1413-1417
49. Ricard JD, Dreyfuss D (2001) Cytokines during ventilator induced lung injury: a word of caution. Anesth Analg 93:251-252
50. Hickling KG, Henderson SJ, Jackson R (1990) Low mortality associated with low volume pressure limited ventilation with permissive hypercapnia in severe adult respiratory distress syndrome. Intensive Care Med 16:372-377
51. Tasker RC, Peters MJ (1998) Combined lung injury, meningitis and cerebral edema: how permissive can hypercapnia be ? Intensive Care Med 24:616-619
52. Thorens JB, Jolliet P, Ritz M, et al (1996) Effects of rapid permissive hypercapnia on hemodynamics, gas exchange, and oxygen transport and consumption during mechanical ventilation for the acute respiratory distress syndrome. Intensive Care Med 22:182-191
53. Carvalho CRR, Barbas CSV, Medeiros DM et al (1997) Temporal hemodynamic effects of permissive hypercapnia associated with ideal PEEP in ARDS. Am J Respir Crit Care Med 156: 1458-1466
54. Artigas A, Bernard GR, Carlet J, et al (1998) The American-European consensus conference on ARDS. Intensive Care Med 24:378-398
55. Stewart TE, Meade MO, Cook DJ, et al (1998) Evaluation of a ventilation strategy to prevent barotrauma in patients at high risk for acute respiratory distress syndrome. N Engl J Med 338: 355-361
56. Brochard L, Roudot-Thoraval F, Roupie E, et al (1998) Tidal volume reduction for prevention of ventilator induced lung injury in acute respiratory distress syndrome. Am J Respir Crit Care 158:1831-1838
57. Brower RG, Shanholtz CB, Fessler HE, et al (1999) Prospective, randomized, controlled clinical trial comparing traditional versus reduced tidal volume ventilation in acute respiratory distress syndrome patients. Crit Care Med 27:1492-1498
58. The Acute Respiratory Distress Syndrome Network (2000) Ventilation with lower tidal volumes as compared with traditional tidal volumes for acute lung injury and the acute respiratory distress sydrome. N Engl J Med 342:1301-1308
59. Eisner MD, Thompson T, Hudson LD, et al (2001) Efficacy of low tidal volume ventilation in patients with different clinical risk factors for acute lung injury and the acute respiratory distress syndrome. Am J Respir Crit Care Med 164:231-236

60. Tobin MJ (2000) Culmination of an era in research on the acute respiratory distress syndrome. N Engl J Med 342:1360-1361
61. Brower RG, Warre LB, Berthiaume Y (2001) Treatments of ARDS. Chest 120:1347-1367
62. Gattinoni L, Tognoni G, Pesenti A, et al (2001) Effect of prone positioning on the survival of patients with acute respiratory failure. N Engl J Med 345:568-573
63. Richard JC, Maggiore SM, Jonson B, et al (2001) Influence of tidal volume on alveolar recruitment. Respective role of PEEP and a recruitment maneuver. Am J Respir Crit Care Med 163:1609-1613
64. Tobin MJ (2001) Advances in mechanical ventilation. N Engl J Med 344:1986-1996
65. Suter PM, Fairley HB, Isenberg M (1975) Optimum end expiratory airway pressure in patients with acute pulmonary failure. N Engl J Med 292:284-289
66. Falke KJ, Pontoppidan A, Kumar D (1972) Ventilation with end expiratory pressure in acute lung injury. J Clin Invest 51:2315-2323
67. Gattinoni L, Pesenti A, Avalli L, et al (1987) Pressure volume curve of total respiratory system in acute respiratory failure: a computed tomographic scan study. Am Rev Respir Dis 136:730-736
68. Venegas JG, Harris RS, Simon BA (1998) A comprehensive equation for the pulmonary pressure volume curve. J Appl Physiol 84:389-395
69. Hickling KG (1998) The pressure volume curve is greatly modified by recruitment. A mathematical model of ARDS lungs. Am J Respir Crit Care Med 158:194-202
70. Hickling KG (2001) Best compliance during a decremental but not incrememntal positive end expiratory pressure trial is related to open lung positive end expiratory pressure: a mathematical ,model of acute respiratory distress syndrome. Am J Respir Crit Care Med 163:69-78
71. Crotti S, Mascheroni D, Caironi P (2001) Recruitment and derecruitment during acute respiratory failure: a clinical study. Am J Respir Crit Care Med 164:131-140
72. Suter PM, Fairley HB, Isenberg MD (1978) Effect of tidal volume and positive end-expiratory pressure on compliance during mechanical ventilation. Chest 73:158-162
73. Gattinoni L, Pesenti A, Bombino M, et al (1988) Relationship between lung computet tomographic density, gas exchange and PEEP in acute respiratory failure. Anesthesiology 69:824-832
74. Sibilla S, Tredici S, Porro A, et al (2002) Equal increases in respiratory system elastance reflect similar lung damage in experimental ventilator-induced lung injury. Intensive Care Med 28: 196-203
75. Ranieri VM, Zhang H, Mascia L, et al (2000) Pressure time curve predicts minimally injurious ventilatory strategy in an isolated rat lung model. Anesthesiology 93:1320-1328
76. Kunst PWA, Bohm SH, Vazquez G et al (2000) Regional pressure volume curves by electrical impedance tomography in a model of acute0Nung injury. Crit Care Med 28:178-183
77. Pelosi P, Ravagnan I, Giurati G, et al (1999) Positive end-expiratory pressure improves respiratory function in obese but not in normal subjects during anesthesia and paralysis. Anesthesiology 91:1221-1231
78. Ranieri VM, Giuliani R, Cinnella G, et al (1993) Physiologic effects of positive end-expiratory pressure in patients with chronic obstructive pulmonary disease during acute ventilatory failure and controlled mechanical ventilation. Am Rev Respir Dis 147:5-13
79. Bohm S, Lachmann B (1996) Pressure control ventilation. Putting a mode into a perspective. Int J Intensive Care 4:45-55
80. Rimensberger PC, Cox PN, Frndova H, et al (1999) The open lung during small tidal volume ventilation: concepts of recruitment and "optimal" positive end-expiratory pressure. Crit Care Med 27:1946-1952
81. Rimensberger PC, Pristine G, Mullen BM, et al (1999) Lung recruitment during small tidal volume ventilation allows minimal positive end-expiratory pressure without augmenting lung injury. Crit Care Med 27:1940-1945
82. Rouby JJ, Lu Q, Goldstein I (2002) Selecting the right level of positive end-expiratory pressure in patients with acute respiratory distress syndrome. Am J Respir Crit Care Med 165:1182-1186
83. Rossi N, Kolobow T, Aprigliano M, et al (1998) Intratracheal pulmonary ventilation at low

airaway pressures in ventilatior-induce model of acute respiratory failure improves lung function and survival. Chest 114:955-957

84. Hickling KG, Timothy W, Laubscher K, et al (1998) Extreme hypoventilation reduces ventilator induced lung injury during ventilation with low positive end-expiratory pressure in saline-lavaged rabbits. Crit Care Med 26:1690-1697

85. Gattinoni L, Pesenti A, Bombino M, et al (1993) Role of extracorporeal circulation in adult respiratory distress management. New Horiz 4:603-612

86. Imai Y, Nokogawa S, Ito Y, et al (2001) Comparison of lung protection strategies using conventional and high frequency oscillatory ventilation. J Appl Physiol 4:1836-1844

87. HIFI Study Group (1989) High frequency oscillatory ventilation compared with conventional mechanical ventilation in the treatment of respiratory failure in preterm infants. N Engl J Med 320:88-93

88. Krishnan JA, Brower RG (2000) High frequency ventilation for acute lung injury and ARDS. Chest 118:795-807

89. Putensen C, Rasanen L, Lopez FA (1994) Ventilation perfusion distributions during mechanical ventilation with superimposed spontaneous breathing in canine lung injury. Am J Respir Crit Care Med 150:101-108

90. Putensen C, Mutz NJ, Putensen-Himmer G, Zinserling J (1999) Spontaneous breathing during ventilatory support improves ventilation perfusion distributions in patients with acute respiratory distress syndrome Am J Respir Crit Care Med 159:1241-1248

91. Cereda M, Foti G, Marcora B, et al (2000) Pressure support ventilation in patients with acute lung injury. Crit Care Med 28:1269-1275

92. Brower RG, Lorraine BW, Brithiaume Y, et al (2001) Treatment of ARDS. Chest 120: 1347-1367

93. Younes M (1992) Proportional assist ventilation: results of an initial clinical trial. Am Rev Respir Dis 145:114-120

94. Capra C (2001) Proportional pressure support in acute lung injury. In: Vincent JL (ed) Year book of Intensive care Medicine and Emergency Medicine, Sprinter-Verlag, Berlin Heidelberg New York, pp 434-435

95. Albert RK, Leasa D, Sanderson M, et al (1987) The prone position improves arterial oxygenation and reduces shunt in oleic acid induced acute lung injury. Am Rev Respir Dis 135:628-633

96. Pelosi P, Tubiolo D, Mascheroni D, et al (1998) Effects of the prone position on respiratory mechanics and gas exchange during acute lung injury. Am J Respir Crit Care Med 157:1-7

97. Lamm WJE, Graham MM, Albert RK (1994) Mechanism by which the prone position improves oxygenation in acute lung injury. Am J Respir Crit Care 150:184-193

98. Gattinoni L, Pelosi P, Vitale G, et al (1991) Body position changes redistribute lung computed tomographic density in patients with acute respiratory failure. Anesthesiology 74:15-23

99. Glenny RW, Lamm WJE, Albert RK, et al (1991) Gravity is a minor determinant of pulmonary blood flow distribution. J Appl Physiol 71:620-629

100. Gillette MA, Hess DR (2001) Ventilator induced lung injury and the evolution of lung protective strategies in acute respiratory distress syndrome. Respir Care 46:130-148

101. Broccard A, Shapiro RS, Schmitz LL, et al (2000) Prone position attenuates and redistibutes ventilator induced lung injury in dogs. Crit Care Med 28:295-303

102. Broccard A, Shapiro RS, Schmitz LL, et al (1997) Influence of prone position on the extent and distribution of lung injury in a high tidal volume oleic acid model of acute respiratory distress syndrome. Crit Care Med 25:16-27

103. Safar P, Agusto-Escarraga L (1959) Compliance in apneic anesthetized adults. Anesthesiology 20:283-289

104. Yamado HDL, Orii R, Suzuki S, et al (1997) Beneficial effects of the prone position on the incidence of barotrauma in oleic acid induced lung injury under continuous positive pressure ventilation. Acta Anaesthesiol Scand 4:701-707

105. Albert RK (1999) Prone position in ARDS: what do we know and what do we need to know. Crit Care Med 11:2574-2575

106. Slutsky AS (2001) The acute respiratory distress syndrome, mechanical ventilation and the prone position. N Engl J Med 345:610-611

107. Fridrich P, Krafft P, Hochleuthner H, et al (1996) The effects of long term prone positioning in patients with trauma induced adult respiratory distress syndrome. Anesth Analg 83:1206-1211

108. Mascia L, Andreus PJ (1988) Acute lung injury in head trauma patients. Intensive Care Med 24:1115-1116

109. Gruber A, Reinprect A (1998) Pulmonary function and radiographic abnormalities related to neurological outcome after aneurismal subaracnoid hemorrhage. J Neurosurg 88:28-37

110. Pelosi P, Colombo G, Gamberoni C, et al (2001) Acute respiratory failure in brain injured patients. Recent Res Dev Respir Crit Care Med 1:19-37

111. Albert RK (1997) The prone position in acute respiratory distress syndrome: where we are, and where do we go from here. Crit Care Med 25:1453-1454

112. Chatte G, Sab JM, Dubois JM, et al (1997) Prone position in mechanically ventilated patients with severe acute respiratory failure. Am J Respir Crit Care Med 155:473-478

113. Cakar N, Van der Kloot T, Youngblood M, et al (2000) Oxygenation response to a recruitment maneuver during supine and prone positions in an oleic acid induced lung injury model. Am J Respir Crit Care Med 161:1946-1956

114. Walther SM, Domino KB, Glenny RW, Hlastala MP (1999) Positive end-expiratory pressure redistributes perfusion to dependent lung regions in supine but not in prone lambs. Crit Care Med 27:37-45

115. Lim CM, Koh Y, Chin JY, et al (1999) Respiratory and haemodynamic effects of the prone position at two different levels of PEEP in a canine acute lung injury model. Eur Respir J 13: 163-168

116. Rossaint R, Falke KJ, Lopez F, et al (1993) Inhaled nitric oxide for the adult respiratory distress syndrome. N Engl J Med 328:399-405

117. Moncada S, Palmer RMJ, Higgs EA (1991) Nitric oxide: physiology, pathophysiology, and pharmacology. Pharmacol Rev 43:109-142

118. Dellinger RP, Zimmerman JL, Taylor RW, et al (1998) Effects of inhaled nitric oxide in patients with acute respiratory distress syndrome: results of a randomized phase II trial. Crit Care Med 26:15-23

119. Troncy E, Collet JP, Shapiro S, et al (1998) Inhaled nitric oxide in acute respiratory distress syndrome: a pilot randomized controlled study. Am J Respir Crit Care Med 157:1483-1488

120. Payen D, Vallet B, Group G (1999) Results of the French prospective multicentric randomized double blind placebo controlled trial on inhaled nitric oxide in ARDS. Intensive Care Med 25: S166

121. Michael JR, Barton RG, Saffle JR, et al (1998) Inhaled nitric oxide versus conventional therapy: effect of oxygenation in ARDS. Am J Respir Crit Care Med 157:1372-1380

122. Luhr O, Nathorst-Westfelt U, Lundin S, et al (1997) A retrospective analysis of nitric oxide inhalation in patients with severe acute lung injury in Sweden and Norway 1991-1994. Acta Anesthesiol Scand 41:1238-1246

123. Matthay MA, Pittet JF, Jayr C (1998) Just say NO to inhaled nitric oxide for the acute respiratory distress syndrome. Crit Care Med 26:15-23

124. Treggiari-Venzi M, Ricou B, Romand JA, et al (1998) The response to repeated inhaled nitric oxide inhalation is inconsistent in patients with acute respiratory distress syndrome, Anesthesiology 88:634-641

125. Putensen C, Hormann C, Kleinsasser A, et al (1998) Cardiopulmonary effects of aerosolized prostaglandin E1 and nitric oxide inhalation in patients with acute respiratory distress syndrome. Am J Respir Crit Care Med 157:1743-1747

126. Papazian L, Bregeon F, Caillot F, et al (1998) Respective and combined effects of prone position and inhaled nitric oxide in patients with acute respiratory distress syndrome. Am J Respir Crit Care Med 157:580-585

127. Rialp G, Betbese AJ, Marquez MP, Mancebo J (2001) Short term effects of inhaled nitric oxide and prone position in pulmonary and extrapulmonary acute respiratory distress syndrome. Am J Respir Crit Care Med 164:243-249
128. Borelli M, Lampati L, Vascotto E et al (2000) Hemodynamic and gas exchange response to inhaled nitric oxide and prone positioning in acute respiratory distress syndrome patients. Crit Care Med 28:2707-2712

Mechanical ventilation and the kidney

H. Burchardi, G. Kaczmarczyk

Mechanical ventilation increases intrathoracic pressures when compared with spontaneous breathing. During spontaneous inspiration intrapleural and intra-alveolar pressure decreases, and a pressure gradient in the airways generates inspiratory airflow. This mechanism also supports circulation: venous return is facilitated by the negative intrathoracic pressure as well as by the slightly positive intra-abdominal pressure generated by the downward diaphragm movement during spontaneous inspiration.

In mechanical ventilation, inspiration is generated by an artificial positive-pressure input into a closed airway system. This input causes positive pressures in the thorax as well as in the abdomen. Thus, there is no pressure gradient supporting venous return, and the heart is surrounded by a positive intrathoracic pressure. This totally different pressure distribution affects not only circulation but also the kidney.

As a result, the kidney's physiological reactions are considerably affected by mechanical ventilation. It has been well known for many years that during mechanical ventilation renal water elimination is restricted and sodium reabsorption is increased, and this effect is related to the intrathoracic pressure [1–7]. The degree of the influence may vary according to the ventilatory pattern used. Hemmer et al. [2] demonstrated in intensive care patients under mechanical ventilation that a reduction of airway pressure facilitated sodium and water excretion. Nevertheless, the fundamental difference between spontaneous breathing and mechanical ventilation remains relevant.

Intrathoracic pressure and circulation

An important primary mechanism during positive-pressure ventilation is the decrease in atrial filling resulting from the decrease in venous return. By this mechanism, atrial transmural pressures (i.e., difference between the pressures inside and outside the atria) decrease. The overall result is a decrease in cardiac

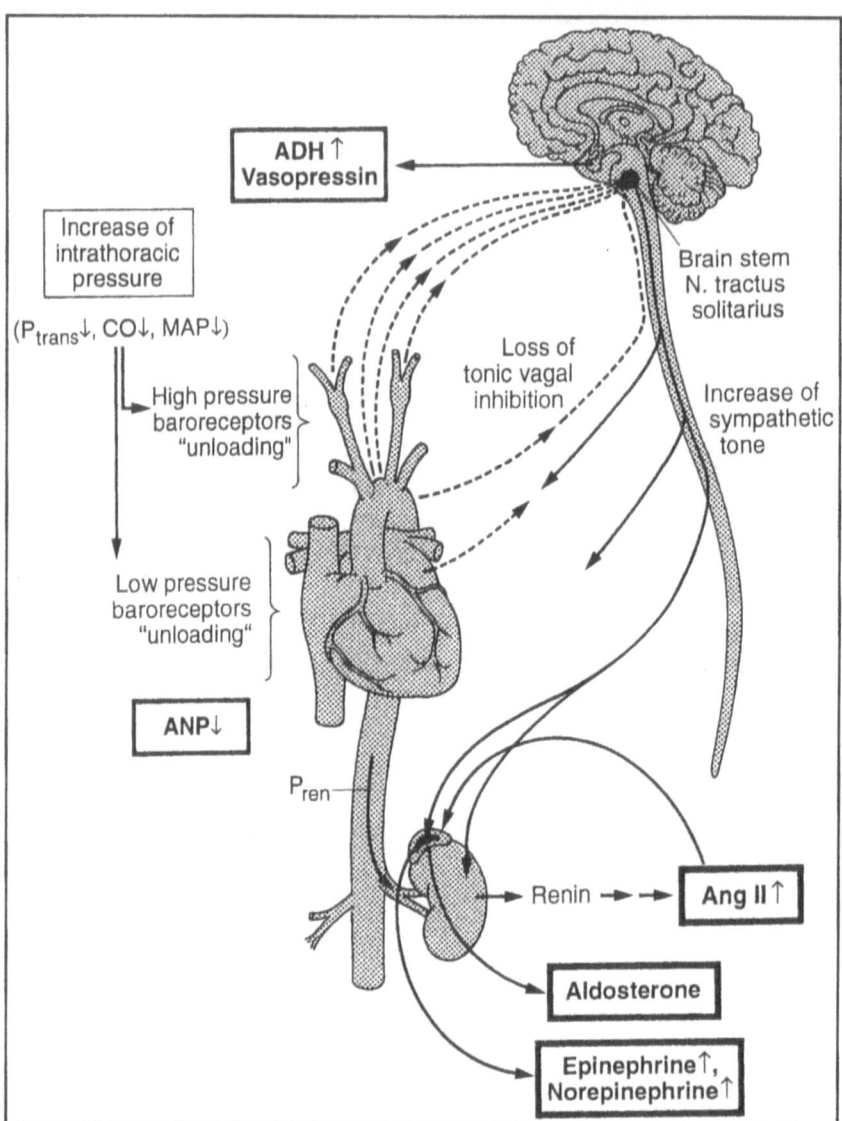

Fig. 1 The increase of intrathoracic pressure affects the kidney. Atrial transmural pressures (*Ptrans*), cardiac output (*CO*), and mean arterial pressure (*MAP*) decrease, followed by the unloading of low- and high-pressure baroreceptors and the increase of sympathetic activity and the loss of vagal inhibition through central connections. A decrease of renal perfusion, as well as an increase of renal nerve sympathetic activity, stimulate water and sodium reabsorptium and renal renin release. The formation of angiotensin II (*Ang II*) stimulates aldosterone production, resulting in a further decrease of water and sodium excretion. Circulating catecholamines are increased, as well as plasma concentrations of antidiuretic hormone (*ADH*). Atrial natriuretic peptide (*ANP*) may also be involved due to the decrease of atrial transmural pressures (modified with permission from Krebs and Kaczmarczyk [9])

output and a reduction in mean arterial perfusion pressure. These circulatory effects may already per se decrease water and sodium excretion. The decrease in atrial transmural pressure unloads the atrial receptors ("volume receptors") and stimulates various hormonal and sympathetic regulatory mechanisms, which again affect kidney reaction.

Thus, during positive-pressure ventilation, a variety of physical, hormonal, and neural changes occur that are primarily involved in the regulation of circulatory homeostasis. Because the kidney is an important target organ in this regulation, the renal effects are not due to a dysfunction but rather to an inevitable physiological renal response [8, 9].

Antidiuretic hormone changes

Secretion of the antidiuretic hormone (ADH) is controlled by osmotic and nonosmotic mechanisms. An increase in plasma osmolarity is a strong stimulus for ADH secretion. Nonosmostic stimuli for ADH are hypovolemia and hypotension. On the whole, the osmotic challenges are stronger than volume changes [10].

In the absence of osmotic changes, ADH release is increased by unloading of baroreceptors. The nonosmotic release of ADH is stimulated by afferent signals from arterial baroreceptors in the carotid sinus and aortic arch (high-pressure baroreceptors) as well as by volume receptors in the atria (low-pressure baroreceptors) [11]. Investigations, however, in animals with sinoaortic denervation or electrolytic destruction of medullary areas (nucleus tractus solitarius), known to process baroreceptor input, lead one to assume that other signals may also stimulate ADH release [12]. Input from other areas (such as renal afferent nerves) may also play a role. Osmotic changes may additionally potentiate nonosmotic ADH release.

The effects of mechanical positive-pressure ventilation on kidney reaction can clearly be deduced from these regulatory mechanisms. The decrease of cardiac output and mean arterial perfusion pressure causes an increase in plasma concentration of ADH (as well as renin). This has been shown in human as well as in animal experiments [2, 13]. A prerequisite condition for an adequate hormonal response is an intact hypothalamic perception of afferent inputs; patient with neurological disorders may not respond adequately to stimulation of ADH release during positive end-expiratory pressure (PEEP) [14]. Also the status of the extracellular volume plays an important role. The influence of positive-pressure mechanical ventilation on ADH release can be completely prevented by extracellular volume expansion [13]. In intensive care unit (ICU) patients, however, these effects can be obscured by numerous other afferent stimuli (e.g., stress, pain, nausea) which per se increase ADH release.

The increase in plasma ADH concentration results in several efferent mechanisms, including induction of thirst (obscured in ICU patients), decrease of urine volume, and (at higher ADH plasma concentrations) an increase in arterial blood pressure. Small changes in plasma ADH concentration apparently cannot be detected, although renal effects can already be shown [15].

Renin-angiotensin system

Activation of the renin-angiotensin system (RAS) results in the generation of angiotensin II, which stimulates renal sodium reabsorption and aldosterone release and which is a powerful vasoconstrictor.

A decrease in renal perfusion pressure stimulates renin release from the kidney via "renal baroreceptors" located in the juxtaglomerular cells near the afferent arterioles. Additionally, an increase in renal sympathetic nerve activity strongly stimulates renin release through renal alpha-adrenergic and beta-adrenergic receptors.

Furthermore, renal renin release is stimulated by delivery of sodium chloride to the macula densa and by high catecholamine levels; renin release is decreased by angiotensin II, ADH, and atrial natriuretic peptide (ANP) [16]. Dopamine, furosemide, and various nonneural mechanisms may also stimulate renal renin release [17, 18].

Renin catalyzes the conversion of angiotensinogen to the biologically inactive angiotensin I. During the pulmonary passage, angiotensin I is converted into the biologically active angiotensin II by the angiotensin-converting enzyme (ACE), which is located on pulmonary endothelial cells [19]. It has been supposed that angiotensin II generation may be impaired in pulmonary diseases [20]. ICU patients have high plasma renin activities and have been shown to convert angiotensin I to angiotensin II to a considerable extent [21].

During mechanical ventilation, the unloading of the baroreceptors, as well as the decrease in mean arterial blood pressure, leads to an increase in renal renin release. This increase has been shown in studies in patients [14, 22], as well as in animal experiments [23, 24]. The pressure-dependent renin release is a threshold phenomenon [25], which is probably modified by other factors affecting renal renin release, such as sympathetic nerve activity, extracellular volume expansion, and others. Generally, the RAS is powerful and fast acting in controlling 'normal' mean arterial blood pressure. Transient decreases in renal perfusion pressure (e.g., seconds to minutes after increasing intrathoracic pressure by PEEP) are able to stimulate the RAS.

Angiotensin II increases mean arterial blood pressure and induces thirst. Its well-known increase of renal tubular sodium and water reabsorption occurs fast and independently of aldosterone [26]. In conscious experimental animals, small increases in plasma angiotensin II concentrations decrease renal blood flow only, whereas higher concentrations of plasma angiotensin II decrease renal blood flow as well as glomerular filtration rate (GFR) [27]. It has been suggested that the endogeneous endothelium-derived relaxing factor modulates these angiotensin II effects [28]; thus, angiotensin II may still maintain GFR when renal blood flow slightly decreases. It may decrease GFR, however, when renal blood flow falls to a greater extent. The immediate and direct tubular actions of angiotensin II occur independently of aldosterone. When stimulated by angiotensin II, however, aldosterone additionally increases tubular sodium and water reabsorption. Diuretic therapy stimulates the RAS by intrarenal mechanisms.

Vasopressin

Increases of intrathoracic pressure are often associated with an increase of plasma vasopressin concentration [2, 23]. Vasopressin release is stimulated by reflexes generated by low-volume (atrial) and high-volume baroreceptors (carotid sinus and aortic arch). This release is apparently mediated by the status of the extracellular fluid volume [13]. Vasopressin has various effects on kidney reaction. It decreases the glomerular ultrafiltration coefficient, it decreases medullary blood flow, and it increases water reabsorption in the distal tubule.

Sympathetic outflow and renal nerve activity

The unloading of intrathoracic baroreceptors and the loss of vagal tone during ventilation with PEEP increases sympathetic activity and plasma catecholamine levels [29]. Renal sympathetic nerve activity induces renal vasoconstriction and increases tubular sodium and water reabsorption [30, 31], probably before renal blood flow and GFR decrease.

Bond and Lightfoot [24] have shown that renal nerves are involved in the mechanisms by which PEEP ventilation stimulates renal renin release. In healthy volunteers with continuous positive-pressure breathing of 12 mmHg, muscle sympathetic nerve activity on the peroneal nerve increased concomitantly with increased plasma renin levels, ADH, and plasma norepenephrine concentrations [32]. Data from patients are not yet available. Also, it is not known whether in patients an increase in intra-abdominal pressure and inferior vena cava pressure during mechanical ventilation with PEEP is involved, as has been shown in animals [33].

Under clinical conditions during mechanical ventilation, it is not possible to quantify the involvement of renal sympathetic nerves in renal sodium and water retention. In kidney transplant recipients, renal excretions seem to be related closely to perfusion pressure changes [34]. In standardized animal experiments, the renal nerves did not contribute to sodium and water retention during mechanical ventilation [35].

Atrial natriuretic peptide

An increase in atrial transmural pressure (e.g., by volume loading) is a strong stimulus for ANP release by atrial myocytes. The effects of ANP (mostly investigated by applying exogenous ANP and using extremely high infusion rates) include an increase in GRF (independent of renal blood flow), a decrease in tubular sodium reabsorption, and a decrease of renin release and aldostrone secretion. ANP also reduces mean arterial blood pressure and cardiac output; however, this in turn, stimulates renal renin release, which is attenuated by ANP. Thus, a complex control system of regulations and feedback mechanisms may mask the direct quantitative contribution of ANP on the kidney's response.

During mechanical positive-pressure ventilation right and left atrial pressures increase. Because of the increase in surrounding intrathoracic pressures, however, the resulting atrial transmural pressure decreases. It may therefore be expected that ANP release will decrease during mechanical ventilation. A decrease in ANP was shown by Frass et al. [36] in healthy volunteers breathing spontaneously with continuous positive airway pressure (CPAP), as well as in animals [37]. In many other studies in humans [22, 32, 38] as well as in animal experiments [38-40], however, no increase of ANP was found during positive-pressure mechanical ventilation. Among others, the magnitude of the decrease in atrial transmural pressure may play a role [41]. At present, it is not known to what extent a possible decrease of endogenous ANP may be involved in the decrease of water and sodium excretion during mechanical ventilation and PEEP. It is well established that an intravenous infusion of ANP at borderline physiological doses (5-10 ng/kg body weight per minute) decreases renal renin release and increases sodium and water excretion in patients [42].

Influence of extracellular volume expansion

The hemodynamic deterioration by PEEP ventilation can be compensated by extracellular volume expansion [3, 7]. It can be assumed that the atrial transmural pressure gradient decreases less at the same level of PEEP when extracellular volume loading is achieved. Experimental studies have shown the important role of extracellular volume expansion for the hormonal response to PEEP [13]. In volume-expanded animals, ADH, ANP, and aldosterone or renin activity were altered during ventilation with PEEP up to 20 cmH2O, whereas in the nonexpanded animals, plasma concentrations of ADH and aldosterone increased. It is suggested that ADH may play a role in the circulatory control mechanisms that maintain mean arterial pressure during PEEP ventilation when the extracellular volume is not expanded. Rossaint et al. [33], however, showed that even in volume-expanded animals an increase in renal venous pressure (inferior vena caval pressure) contributes to the decreases of renal water and sodium excretion during PEEP.

Influence of ventilatory patterns

Because the intrathoracic and intra-abdominal pressures play a key role in the influence of mechanical ventilation on the kidney, changes in ventilatory pattern may vary these effects considerably. Mean intrathoracic pressure is increased by augmenting tidal volume or PEEP (or both), by increasing the inspiratory-to-expiratory ratio (i.e., increasing inspiratory duration), or by any pulmonary hyperinflation (e.g., because of intrinsic PEEP in patients with chronic obstructive pulmonary disease). It has been well known for many years that ventilatory modes that partially allow spontaneous breathing ('ventilatory assist'), such as the intermittent mandatory ventilation, facilitate renal excretion [4, 5].

Today, modern ventilation strategies try to incorporate spontaneous breathing efforts, which may affect venous return to a lesser degree and may improve systemic circulation, cardiac output, and adequate renal excretion. Nothing is known yet whether the lower levels of sedation generally used for partial ventilatory support modes might affect renal response. An increase in renal sympathetic nerve activity stimulates renal sodium and water reabsorption [30]. Thus, at least stress and pain have to be avoided, because they may also stimulate ADH release. For an overview of the effects of anaesthesia on renal function see reference [43].

Acute hypercapnia and respiratory acidosis may stimulate the renin-angiotensin-aldosterone system and the release of ADH [44-46]. Carvalho et al. [47], however, investigated the effects of permissive hypercapnia (tidal volumes <

6 ml/kg and PEEP < 20 cmH$_2$O, set according to the lower inflexion point) in patients with acute respiratory distress syndrome, the initial hyperdynamic state due to the respiratory acidosis was only transient. Despite persistent hypercapnia systemic, hemodynamics stabilized after 36 h, and renal function was preserved. The direct effects of hypoxemia on renal function are complex and may include the loss of the ability to reabsorb sodium.

Inhibitory influences of positive-pressure ventilation on the kidney result in a water and sodium retention; this is a common observation during mechanical ventilation, such as with PEEP. Because pulmonary vascular permeability generally is increased in these critically ill patients, water retention can easily result in an increase in extracellular lung water, which deteriorates pulmonary oxygenation. Thus, some of the benefits of mechanical ventilation may partially be reduced if these effects on water balance are not carefully monitored.

References

1. Jarnberg PO, Villota ED de, Eklund J et al (1978) Effects of positive end-expiratory pressure on renal function. Acta Anaesthesiol Scand 22:508-514
2. Hemmer M, Viquerat CE, Suter PM, et al (1980) Urinary antidiuretic hormone excretion during mechanical ventilation and weaning in man. Anesthesiology 52:395-400
3. Priebe HJ, Heimann JC, Hedley-White J (1981) Mechanisms of renal dysfunction during positive end-expiratory pressure ventilation. J Appl Physiol 50:643-649
4. Steinhoff H, Falke K, Schwarzhoff W (1982) Enhanced renal function associated with intermittent mandatory ventilation in acute respiratory failure. Intensive Care Med 8:69-74
5. Steinhoff H, Kohlhoff RJ, Falke KJ (1984) Facilitation of excretory function and hemodynamics of the kidneys by intermittent mandatory ventilation. Intensive Care Med 10:59-64
6. Berry AJ, Geer RT, Marshall C, et al (1984) The effect of long-term controlled mechanical ventilation with positive end-expiratory pressure on renal function in dogs. Anesthesiology 61:406-415
7. Venus B, Mathru M, Smith RA, et al (1985) Renal function during application of positive end-expiratory pressure in swine: effects of hydration. Anesthesiology 62:765-769
8. Kaczmarczyk G (1994) Pulmonary-renal axis during positive-pressure ventilation. New Horiz 2:512-517
9. Krebs MO, Kaczmarczyk G (1996) Effects of mechanical ventilation on renal function. In: Dellinger RP (ed) Current topics in intensive care, vol. 3. Saunders, London pp 209-217
10. Dunn FL, Brennan TJ, Nelson AE, et al (1973) The role of blood osmoloality and volume in regulating vasopressin secretion in the rat. J Clin Invest 52:3212-3219
11. Share L (1976) Role of cardiovascular receptors in the control of ADH release. Cardiology 61[Suppl 1]:51-64
12. Schreihofer AN, Stricker EN, Sved AF (1994) Chronic nucleus tractus solitarius lesions do not prevent hypovolemia-induced vasopressin secretion in rats. Am J Physiol 267: R965-R973
13. Kaczmarczyk G, Jörres D, Rossaint R, et al (1993) Extracellular volume expansion inhibits antidiuretic hormone increase during positive end-expiratory pressure in conscious dogs. Clin Sci (Colch) 85:643-649
14. Payen D M, Farge D, Beloucif S, et al (1987) No involvement of antidiuretic hormone in acute antidiuresis during PEEP ventilation in humans. Anesthesiology 66:17-23

15. Baerwolff M, Bie P (1988) Effects of subpicomolar changes in vasopressin on urinary concentration. Am J Physiol 255:R940-R945
16. Katz SA, Malvin RL (1993) Renin secretion: control, pathways, and glycolysation. In: Robertson JI, Nicholls MG (eds) The renin-angiotensin-system. Mosby, London, pp 24.1
17. Mizoguchi H, Czau VJ, Siwek LG, et al (1983) Effect of intrarenal administration of dopamine on renin release in conscious dogs. Am J Physiol 244:H39-H45
18. Kopp U, DiBona GF (1984) Interaction between neural and nonneural mechanisms controlling renin secretion rate. Am J Physiol 246:F620
19. Skidgel RA, Erdös E (1993) Biochemistry of angiotensin I-converting enzyme. In: Robertson JI, Nicholls MG (eds) The renin-angiotensin-system. Mosby, London pp 10.1
20. Neilly JB, Clark CJ, Tweddel A, et al (1987) Transpulmonary angiotensin II formation in patients with chronic stable cor pulmonale. Am Rev Respir Dis 135:891-895
21. Wenz M, Steinau R, Gerlach H, et al (1997) Inhaled nitric oxide does not change transpulmonary angiotensin II formation in patients with acute respiratory distress syndrome. Chest 112:478-483
22. Riddervold F, Smiseth OA, Hall C, et al (1991) Endocrine responses to positive end-expiratory pressure ventilation in patients who have recently undergone heart surgery. Acta Anaesthesiol Scand 35:242-246
23. Bark H, Le-Roith D, Nyska M, et al (1980) Elevations in plasma ADH levels during PEEP ventilation in the dog: mechanisms involved. Am J Physiol 239:E474-E481
24. Bond GC, Lightfoot B (1983) Role of renal nerves in mediating the increased renin secretion during continuous positive-pressure ventilation. Proc Soc Exp Biol Med 173:104-108
25. Kirchheim H, Ehmke H, Persson P (1990) Role of blood pressure in the control of renin release. Acta Physiol Scand [Suppl] 173:40-47
26. Kaczmarczyk G, Marx M, Lee KE, et al (1984) Acute effects of angiotensin II in intact and adrenalectomized conscious dogs. J Physiol (Paris) 79:491-495
27. Keil J, Lehnfeld R, Reinhardt HW, et al (1989) Acute effects of angiotensin II on renal haemodynamics and excretion in conscious dogs. Renal Physiol Biochem 12:238-249
28. Ito S, Arima S, Ren YL, et al (1993) Endothelium-derived relaxing factor/nitric oxide modulates angiotensin II action in the isolated micro-perfused rabbit afferent but not efferent arteriole. J Clin Invest 91:2012-2019
29. Chernow B, Soldano S, Cook D, et al (1986) Positive end-expiratory pressure increases plasma catecholamine levels in non-volume loaded dogs. Anaesth Intensive Care 14:421-425
30. DiBona GF (1982) The function of renal nerves. Rev Physiol Biochem Pharmacol 94:75-181
31. Kopp U, DiBona GF (1993) Neural regulation of renin secretion. Semin Nephrol 13:543-551
32. Tanaka S, Sagawa S, Miki K, et al (1994) Changes in muscle sympathetic nerve activity and renal function during positive-pressure breathing in humans. Am J Physiol 266:R1220-R1228
33. Rossaint R, Krebs M, Förther J, et al (1993) Inferior vena caval pressure increase contributes to sodium and water retention during PEEP in awake dogs. J Appl Physiol 75:2484-2492
34. Jacob LP, Chazalet JJ, Payen DM, et al (1995) Renal hemodynamic and functional effect of PEEP ventilation in human renal transplantations. Am J Respir Crit Care Med 152:103-107
35. Boemke W, Krebs MO, Djalali K, et al (1998) Renal nerves are not involved in sodium and water retention during mechanical ventilation in awake dogs. Anesthesiology 89:942-953
36. Frass M, Popovic R, Hartter E, et al (1988) Atrial natriuretic peptide decrease during spontaneous breathing with continuous positive airway pressure in volume-expanded healthy volunteers. Crit Care Med 16:831-835
37. Kharasch ED, Yeo KT, Kenny MA, et al (1988) Atrial natriuretic factor may mediate the renal effects of PEEP ventilation. Anesthesiology 69:862-869
38. Teba L, Dedhia HV, Schiebel FG, et al (1990) Positive-pressure ventilation with positive end-expiratory pressure and atrial natriuretic peptide release. Crit Care Med 18:831-835
39. Kaczmarczyk G, Rossaint R, Altmann C, et al (1992) ACE inhibition facilitates sodium and water excretion during PEEP in conscious volume-expanded dogs. J Appl Physiol 73:962-967
40. Rossaint R, Jörres D, Nienhaus M, et al (1992) Positive end-expiratory pressure reduces renal

excretion without hormonal activation after volume expansion in dogs. Anesthesiology 77:700--708

41. Frass M, Watschinger B, Traindl O, et al (1993) Atrial natriuretic peptide release in response to different positive end-expiratory pressure levels. Crit Care Med 21:343-347

42. Andrivet P, Adnot S, Sanker S, et al (1991) Hormonal interactions and renal function during mechanical ventilation and ANF infusion in humans. J Appl Physiol 70:287-292

43. Burchardi H, Kaczmarczyk G (1994) The effect of anaesthesia on renal function. Eur J Anaesthesiol 11:163-168

44. Anderson RJ, Henrich WL, Gross PA, et al (1982) Role of renal nerves, angiotensin II, and prostaglandins in the antinatriuretic response to acute hypercapnic acidosis in the dog. Circ Res 50:294-300

45. Raff H, Roarty TP (1988) Renin, ACTH and aldosterone during acute hypercapnia and hypoxia in conscious rats. Am J Physiol 254:R431-R435

46. Chen HG, Wood CE (1993) The adrenocorticotropic hormone and arginine vasopressin responses to hypercapnia in fetal and maternal sheep. Am J Physiol 264:R324-R330

47. Carvalho CR, Barbas CS, Medeiros DM, et al (1997) Temporal hemodynamic effects of permissive hypercapnia associated with ideal PEEP in ARDS. Am J Respir Crit Care Med 156:1458-1466

Capnography and pulse oximetry

U. Lucangelo, G. Degrassi, M.L. Chierego

Capnography

The possible use of non-invasive monitoring (of great clinical significance) has given capnography a peculiar role in the assessment of the ventilatory function during anaesthesia. Such monitoring allows for constant display of CO_2 concentration expressed as a function either of time (conventional capnography) or end-tidal volume (volumetric capnography). Conventional capnograms can be divided into inspiratory and expiratory segments, the latter typically consisting of four phases.

The present paper reports on some situations which, unlike clinical routine, require careful interpretation of capnographic data, which should always be adequately contextualized.

Capnography under spontaneous ventilation

CO_2 monitoring today is crucial, not only under mechanical ventilation, but also postoperatively in spontaneously breathing patients. The possibility of monitoring the spontaneous ventilation pattern non-invasively is of considerable clinical value in the postoperative period, when breathing problems account for major causes of morbidity and mortality.

End-tidal CO_2 can be measured in spontaneously breathing patients in the following two ways:

- Using a catheter placed in the pharynx through the nose and connected to a side-stream analyser. Such procedure is well tolerated and supplies an adequate estimate of the patient's end-tidal CO_2 [1].
- Through a semirigid plastic mouthpiece connected to a combined sensor, which can estimate both CO_2 and end-tidal volume (CO_2SMO+ Novametrix CO_2SMO+, Novametrix Medical Systems, Wallinford, Conn., USA).

$P_{ET}CO_2$ monitoring aims at the early identification of alveolar hypoventilation and bronchospasm without resorting immediately to blood gas analysis [2].

It should be noted, however, that in healthy patients with minimal alveolar-arterial difference, the increased dead space – resulting from impaired ventilation/perfusion rate – makes the end-tidal CO_2 impossible to be correlated with the arterial PCO_2 value.

Capnography during the use of laryngeal mask airway

There is no substantial difference when end-tidal CO_2 is measured either via laryngeal mask airway (LMA) or via endotracheal tube (ETT) [3] in paediatric patients weighing more than 10 kg and undergoing general anaesthesia. Such correlation, however, disappears in subjects below 10 kg, who show higher values of LMA-measured end-tidal CO_2 compared with ETT measurements. One might assume that in this category of patients the use of LMA entails increased ratios between dead space and end-tidal volume, which might lead to alveolar hypoventilation. Such findings might also emerge during spontaneous breathing with LMA, in which $P_{ET}CO_2$ changes do not reflect $PaCO_2$ changes [4]. In spontaneously breathing adults, on the contrary, such differences do not appear, since $P_{ET}CO_2$ concentrations are practically identical whether measured via ETT or LMA [5]. A possible explanation of the different pattern between adults and paediatric subjects might lie in the different ventilation circuits used.

Capnography in paediatric settings

With a view to a proper interpretation of capnographic data in paediatric subjects, the following considerations should be borne in mind:

a. It is difficult to measure CO_2 in small babies ventilated at low end-tidal volumes and high respiration rates. When subjects weigh more than 12 kg, the expired gas sampling can be performed at the oral end of the ETT, as in adults. In children below 12 kg of weight, CO_2 has to be taken at the distal (tracheal) end of the tube by means of a special catheter [6].

b. Particularly important from the pathophysiological point of view is the effect of pulmonary development on the shape of the capnographic waveform. Pulmonary growth entails an increased number of acinar units with a resulting rise in alveolar surface and reduction of resistances to gas diffusion. The morphometric growth of the lung therefore lowers the CO_2 alveolar-arterial gradient with relative flattening and normalization of phase III [7]. Any interpretation of capnograms should therefore be correlated to the patient's age. Delayed stabilization of phase III could be a sign of silent pulmonary condition.

Capnography in neurosurgery

Capnography is commonly used to check CO_2 levels under anaesthesia for craniotomies and neurovascular procedures. Intraoperative manipulation of $PaCO_2$, though traditionally considered an integral part of neuro-anaesthesiological management, could induce unpredicted and deleterious effects on cerebral haemodynamics. In a normal brain, any mmHg of $PaCO_2$ change leads to a 2.5% variation in cerebral blood flow (CBF). A linear increase of CBF takes place when $PaCO_2$ rises within a range of 20-80 mmHg.

Intraoperative hypercapnia (leading to higher cerebral blood volume resulting from vasodilation) and deep hypocapnia (which might trigger brain ischaemia) should be susceptible to reliable exploration.

Reliability of $PaCO_2$-$P_{ET}CO_2$ gradient

Capnography supplies the estimated $PaCO_2$, while $P_{ET}CO_2$ generally underestimates $PaCO_2$. Several studies [8] have been carried out to assess the reliability of capnography. Considering that capnography has provided neuro-anaesthesiologists with a constant guide during intraoperative manipulation of $PaCO_2$, it is surprising to find so little interest in neurosurgical patients in the literature [9]. The first studies on neuro-anaesthesia were conducted by Russell et al. [10, 11, 12] and Isert [13], who detected an unexpectedly high $PaCO_2$-$P_{ET}CO_2$ gradient. Grenier [14] in 1998 evaluated the reliability of $P_{ET}CO_2$ as an estimate of $PaCO_2$ in neurosurgery exceeding 3 hours of duration. Isert and Grenier found a correct estimate of $PaCO_2$ by capnography only in 82% of cases. The difference was above 4 mmHg in 18% of cases. More than 25% of cases showed – in successive measurements – a changing gradient in the opposite direction; this feature was also reported by Russell and Graybeal in 18,4% of cases. The average gradient was 6±4 mmHg in Grenier, slightly above those found by Isert [13] (4±4 mmHg) and Sharma [15] (5±2 mmHg), as well as in comparison with the value indicated by Nunn and Hill [16] for surgery under general anaesthesia. The $PaCO_2$-$P_{ET}CO_2$ gradient has a complex nature [17] and is often unexpectedly high or even negative (4% of the measurements in Grenier). A negative gradient might be present in patients ventilated at low rates and high volumes [18], characterized by slow alveolar emptying with a long time constant. A negative gradient is found more frequently in Caesarean deliveries, in children, in laparoscopic interventions and after heart surgery.

Grenier [14] was the first to analyse the $PaCO_2$-$P_{ET}CO_2$ gradient in relation to the patient's position. It was 6±3 mmHg in supination, slightly less than in Russell and Graybeal [11, 12]. The gradient was higher (7±3 mmHg) in the lateral position, probably owing to an altered ventilation/perfusion ratio with increased alveolar dead space. In the sitting position the average gradient values were similar to those obtained in supination. The mechanisms involved, however, are different. When sitting, the patient undergoes haemodynamic changes caused by the reduced venous return, while the lung bases are adequately perfused, with an optimized ventilation/perfusion ratio. In the prone position, the residual functional capacity drops because of the abdominal pressure and the diaphragmatic excursion is limited.

The findings by Grenier [14] and Isert [13] suggest that capnography is inadequate for $PaCO_2$ monitoring. Blood gas analysis is indispensable in surgery exceeding 3 hours of duration [14]. According to Sharma [15], on the contrary, there is a constant relationship between $PaCO_2$ and $P_{ET}CO_2$, preserved over time. Sharma believes that $P_{ET}CO_2$ can be used as a reliable guidance of $PaCO_2$ even in interventions above 4 hours. Nunn and Hill [16], like Kerr [19] in 1996, suggested that during anaesthesia in healthy subjects (no pulmonary pathology) the ratio between the two concentrations remains so constant that $P_{ET}CO_2$ can be used as a continuous and indirect measurement of arterial CO_2.

Despite the conflicting indications about its accuracy, capnography remains an essential instrument for monitoring patients undergoing neurosurgery. It can identify life-threatening situations in the patient, intubation of the oesophagus, disconnection of ventilator, alveolar hypoventilation or pulmonary embolism.

Capnography in thoracic surgery

Capnography can be used during thoracic surgery for additional specific purposes:
1. Non-invasive monitoring of $PaCO_2$ during thoracic surgery
2. Evaluation of the shape of capnographic waveform during thoracic surgery
3. Evaluation of ventilation/perfusion ratio in both lungs (dual capnography)
4. Evaluation of the haemodynamic effects of CO_2 insufflation during thoracoscopy

Capnography for non-invasive monitoring of PaCO2 during thoracic surgery

The difference between arterial and end-tidal PCO_2 is closely linked to the presence of an underlying pulmonary condition. The surgical treatment of lung carcinoma is the most common indication for thoracotomy in adults. These patients are almost invariably smokers, with consequent bronchopneumopathy, and will therefore develop an increased $PaCO_2$-$P_{ET}CO_2$ gradient also in the supine position during anaesthesia.

In the study carried out by Werner et al. [21] on 17 patients, the average $PaCO_2$-$P_{ET}CO_2$ gradient was around 5 mmHg in supination with $PaCO_2$ at 28 mmHg and ventilation rate of 10/min.

The lungs receive an approximately equal share of ventilation when the patient is in supine position, whereas the ventilation of the upper lung is higher in the lateral position [21]. The pulmonary blood flow, however, depends on gravity and is therefore lower in the upper lung, which as a result shows a reduced $P_{ET}CO_2$. As demonstrated by Werner et al. [21], the $PaCO_2$-$P_{ET}CO_2$ was zero for the lower lung and 11 mmHg in the upper one.

In the light of the greater ventilation in the upper lung, one might assume that, if $P_{ET}CO_2$ were to be measured in the combined expirate of both lungs, the $PaCO_2$-combined $P_{ET}CO_2$ difference could be higher [20, 21].

The incision of the chest wall increases the average pulmonary arterial pressure [21], leading to higher elimination of CO_2 by the upper lung and lower physiological dead space homolaterally. The $PaCO_2$-$P_{ET}CO_2$ gradient of the upper lung therefore decreases whenever a surgical stimulus induces an augmentation of the average pulmonary arterial pressure.

Furthermore, the opening of the pleura amplifies the elimination of CO_2 by the upper lung, thus lessening the $PaCO_2$-$P_{ET}CO_2$ gradient. Retraction of the lung produces exactly the opposite effects. The gradient of the lower lung is not affected by these manoeuvres; it remains small-sized. If a combined monitoring of end-tidal CO_2 were applied, the $PaCO_2$-$P_{ET}CO_2$ difference would diminish once the pleura were opened and would build up again during retraction.

Single lung ventilation

When the ventilation of the upper lung is discontinued to carry out surgery, its perfusion does not end completely unless the pulmonary artery is clamped. As a result, a right to left shunt is created in the upper lung, leading to increased $PaCO_2$ and $PaCO_2$-$P_{ET}CO_2$ gradient. The latter, however, might not be any greater than the original combined two lung $PaCO_2$-$P_{ET}CO_2$ [20, 21].

Effects of prolonged expiratory manoeuvres on PaCO2-P_{ET}CO2 gradient during thoracotomy

Prolonged expiratory manoeuvres improve the predictive value of $PaCO_2$ from $P_{ET}CO_2$ [22], reducing the arterial-expiratory difference of PCO_2 especially during single lung ventilation.

The $ETCO_2$ value obtained through such manoeuvres during laparotomy and thoracotomy, however, hardly comes close to the $PaCO_2$ level, thereby suggesting that such manoeuvres should not be performed under anaesthesia to improve the predictive value of $PaCO_2$ from $P_{ET}CO_2$.

Difference between PaCO2 and P*et*ET2 after bilateral lung transplantation

The $PaCO_2$-$P_{ET}CO_2$ gradient and the $(PaCO_2$-$P_{ET}CO_2)/PaCO_2$ ratio (as a measure of the alveolar dead space) were evaluated in seven patients undergoing bilateral lung transplantation [23] (Table 1).

Table 1 $PaCO_2$-$P_{ET}CO_2$ gradient and $(PaCO_2$-$P_{ET}CO_2)/PaCO2$ ratio after bilateral lung transplantation

Variables		Time after lung transplantation			
Average (SD)	10 min	1 h	3 h	12 h	24 h
$PaCO_2$-$P_{ET}CO_2$ mmHg	16 (5)	14 (5)	9 (4)	6 (3)	5 (3)
$(PaCO_2$-$P_{ET}CO_2)/PaCO_2$		0.36 (0.13)	0.33 (0.13)	0.21 (0.12)	0.15 (0.07)	0.11 (0.06)

The evolution of the difference between $PaCO_2$ and $P_{ET}CO_2$ suggests the existence of a fast improvement of the ventilation/perfusion ratio. After 24 h the related concentrations were very close to the physiological intervals (4-5 mmHg).

A possible explanation might lie in the ischaemia-reperfusion damage of the microcirculation.

An impaired distribution of the pulmonary blood flow without alveolar perfusion might appear clinically as an alveolar dead space, as is typically the case immediately after lung transplantation. The normalization of the ventilation/perfusion mismatch which takes place in about 24 h suggests redistribution of pulmonary perfusion and restoration of microcirculation.

Evaluation of the capnographic waveform during thoracic anaesthesia

The following abnormal capnographic waveforms can be seen during thoracic anaesthesia:

1. Capnograms with increased phase III slope due to a large spread V/Q ratios, as in lung disease. The initial part of the slope is represented by areas which are well ventilated with high V/Q ratios (i.e., decreased CO_2 concentration), while the latter part is represented by areas which are poorly ventilated and with low V/Q ratios (i.e., increased CO_2 concentration) (Fig. 1).

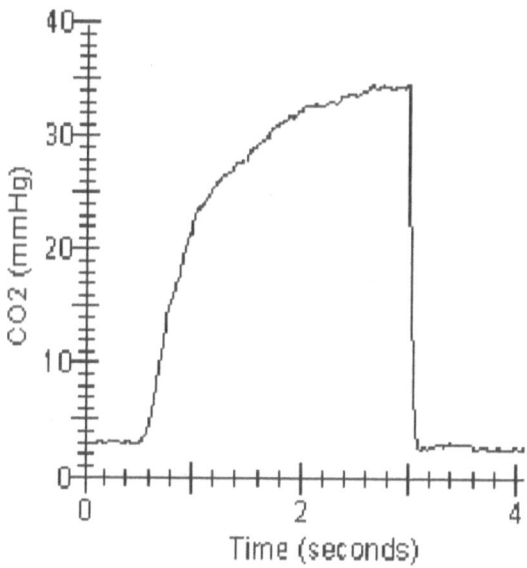

Fig. 1 Capnogram showing a significantly altered V/Q ratio

2. Biphasic capnogram: the phase III of the capnogram represents mixed alveolar gas at the CO_2 sampling site. Therefore, if the lungs have distinctly different V/Q ratios and exhalation time constants, then a 'biphasic' waveform can be seen, as in the lateral decubitus position [24] (Fig. 2). The upper lung (non-dependent) has a low airway resistance, high V/Q ratio (secondary to gravity dependent blood flow) and a low CO_2 concentration compared with the lower, dependent lung. The earlier part of the biphasic CO_2 waveform is due to the expired gases from the upper lung containing lower PCO_2 and the later part of the biphasic waveform is predominantly due to the expired gases containing high PCO_2 from the lower lung.

A similar capnogram can occur following a single lung transplant. Some patients with chronic obstructive pulmonary disease (COPD) may also display a slight biphasic expiratory plateau if they have, throughout both lungs, two distinct populations of alveoli with very different time constants. In this situation, rapidly exchanging alveolar spaces are overinsufflated during inspiration (their compliance is high) so that their CO_2 concentration is low, whereas slower exchanging alveoli empty only during the later part of exhalation, releasing a higher CO_2 content [24, 25].

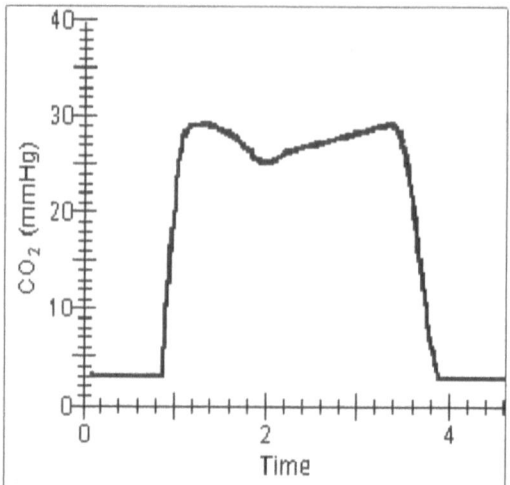

Fig. 2 Biphasic capnogram

3. Reverse phase III capnogram: occasionally seen in patients with emphy-
    sema. The slope of phase III can be reversed in patients with emphysema
    where there is marked destruction of alveolar capillary membranes and
    reduced gas exchange (Fig. 3).

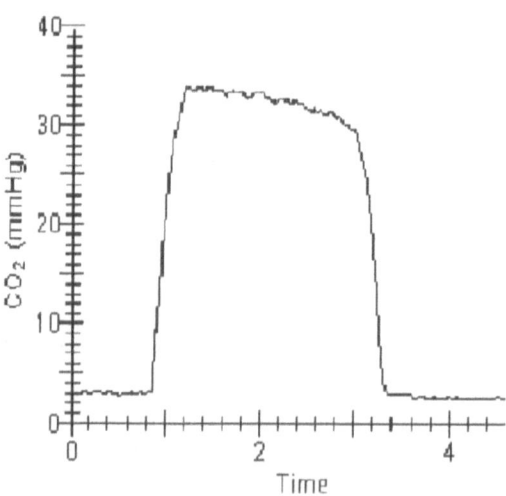

Fig. 3 The phase III of the capnogram can be occasionally reversed in patients with emphysema.

Dual lung capnography

Conventional capnography samples mixed expired gases from both lungs. When there is a pathophysiological defect in one lung, this approach would not be useful. Dual capnography overcomes this limitation by analysing gases from each lumen of a double-lumen tube (DLT) [26, 27].

Dual capnography can be achieved by using either two end-tidal CO_2 monitors to analyse CO_2 wave forms from each lumen of a DLT [26] or a device suggested by Bhavani-Shankar et al. [27]. Such a device has a three-way stopcock with connections to the two adapters that are interposed between each lumen and its corresponding limb on the Y-double-lumen tube adapter. This allows gas sampling from either each lung or two lungs simultaneously.

The standard method of $P_{ET}CO_2$ sampling via DLT (capnograms of individual lung obtained via interruption of ventilation to contralateral lung) can also reveal the ventilation/perfusion status of the lung. However, dual capnography allows the ventilation/perfusion status to be assessed in each lung of individuals who cannot tolerate one-lung ventilation long enough to reach a new steady state.

In the absence of a DLT, a fiber optic bronchoscope can be used to obtain $P_{ET}CO_2$ samples from each lung. It is possible, however, that bronchial sampling from one lung could be contaminated with expired gases from the contralateral lung, particularly when expired flow rate decreases to less than 150 ml/min (sampling flow rate of capnograph).

Such contamination, however, could be detected by analysing the shape of capnograms. Contamination is an unlikely factor in the presence of a normal shape of CO_2 waveforms from each lung [28]. Under these circumstances, therefore, a difference between the heights of the alveolar plateau of CO_2 waveforms from each lung suggests a difference between the V/Q ratio of the two lungs.

Uses of dual capnography:

1) Bronchospy is probably the best method to verify correct placement of double-lumen tubes. However, capnography can also be used to confirm correct DLT placement, detect malposition, unilateral obstruction or accidental displacement of a DLT [26].

   A major advantage of capnography is that it supplies continuous non-invasive monitoring. The correct placement of double-lumen tubes can also be verified by analysing the CO_2 waveform in each lung as well as during clamping and declamping in single lung ventilation. A change of CO_2 end-tidal concentration or waveform could give an early warning of a misplaced DLT or inadequate ventilation and elimination of CO_2 from the lungs.

2) Detection of perfusion defects secondary to thromboembolism, tumour, haemothorax: Bhavani-Shankar et al. [29] reported a case where a patient scheduled for right sided pneumonectomy was unable to tolerate single lung ventilation due to hypoxaemia and arterial blood gas analysis showed a large $PaCO_2$-$P_{ET}CO_2$ gradient. A dual capnography revealed the $PaCO_2$-$P_{ET}CO_2$ gradient more than twice as great in the left than in the right. Surgery was therefore restricted to pleurectomy and a further work-up via echocardiography and pulmonary angiogram later confirmed the presence of a large thrombus in the left pulmonary artery

Other uses include: to explain abnormal wave forms on capnograms, e.g., biphasic capnogram wave forms are seen in patients with single lung transplant [30]. Dual capnography could confirm the aetiology of biphasic capnogram by showing the individual characteristics of respective lungs.

Capnography in lateral decubitus under two-lung ventilation

The lateral decubitus position on two lung ventilation might induce the same modifications of V/Q ratio, of venous return and of dead space. The study by Pansard et al. [31] was one of the few studies, carried out in urological setting, which took into account the pathophysiological variations of this position. It showed an increased CO_2 alveolar arterial difference after positioning in lateral decubitus (7.9 mmHg), its progressive build-up during maintenance of anaesthesia (8.8 mmHg after 65 min and 8.9 mmHg after 85 min) and lower body temperature, whereas no significant haemodynamic modifications were recorded. These results are evidently related to the patient's position, which causes not only the typical modifications of V/Q ratio at pulmonary level, but also a diminished venous return as a consequence of the flexion of lower limbs. Once the intervention has been concluded with a return to the supine position, the alveolar-arterial gradient returns to the initial values.

There are still many factors which might affect the alveolar-arterial gradient during surgery, such as bleeding, mechanical ventilation, use of positive end-expiratory pressure, all of which testify to the undeniable clinical importance of arterial blood gas analysis during surgery in lateral decubitus.

Capnography in laparoscopy

Evaluation of PaCO₂-PₑₜCO₂ gradient and of capnographic curve in laparoscopy

Several studies have evaluated the reliability of $P_{ET}CO_2$ as an indicator of $PaCO_2$. Not always did $P_{ET}CO_2$ prove reliable. In 1990 Brampton and Watson [28] found that the arterial-alveolar gradient of CO_2 was not affected by the anaesthesiological method, duration of surgery or anaesthesia. During laparoscopy this gradient should remain constant with equal increase of both parameters. A wide variety of results, however, was found with stable, increased [32, 33], decreased [34, 35] or negative gradients. Bures [36] presented data with a constant or slightly decreased gradient. Bures did not detect higher gradients, but justified such findings in other authors [32, 33, 34] as the result of a possible augmentation [37] of alveolar dead space during insufflation. Lower cardiac output in the reverse Trendelenburg position and compressed lung bases in Trendelenburg might be the possible causes of the higher gradient. The gradient variability might be dependent on the failure to evaluate body temperature in the blood gas analysis reading. Blood gases have to be adjusted for body temperature to avoid overestimating $P_{ET}CO_2$. Bures showed that a 0.9° C fall induces an average 4.9 mmHg overestimate of the arterial alveolar gradient. The gradient might also be negative. Wahba and Mamazza [33] suggested that the upward slope of the capnographic curve might indicate a lack of homogeneity in the emptying of alveolar units or large exogenous CO_2 load or increased CO_2 elimination, as a result of the setting of ventilation parameters characterized by low respiration rate, large volumes and good alveolar perfusion. Wahba and Mamazza found decreased or negative gradients when $P_{ET}CO_2$ was higher than 41 mmHg during laparoscopic cholocystectomy. The gradient might fall because of extraperitoneal insufflation or might indicate the insufflation of high CO_2 volume. Several data suggest that substantial CO_2 load promotes a reversal of arterial alveolar gradient.

A negative arterial alveolar gradient is frequently seen in laparoscopy in paediatric subjects. $P_{ET}CO_2$ monitoring might lead to an overestimation of $PaCO_2$ with the risk of hyperventilating the patient. In the study by Laffon et al. [38] the evaluation of the gradient in 61 children undergoing laparoscopy showed the presence of negative gradients before and after peritoneal insufflation. There are no clear explanations in this respect.

Laparoscopic surgery during pregnancy is not frequent. Amos et al. [39] documented 4 foetal deaths in 7 pregnant women who underwent laparoscopy. Although Amos did not present data related to blood gas analysis in these patients, respiratory acidosis was described as a possible factor contributing to foetal loss. Cruz et al. [40] questioned the validity of capnography to estimate $PaCO_2$, after carrying out studies on pregnant ewes. The sheep showed foetal and maternal acidosis every time that insufflation was performed under capnographic monitoring alone. The study carried out by Bhavani-Shankar et al. [41] on 8 pregnant women did not show any difference of gradient during laparoscopy. This is in contrast with the results obtained by Cruz et al. [40] and Hunter et al. [42], where the gradient increased by 10 mmHg or so. The highest gradient observed among the patients in Bhavani-Shankar was 5.1 mmHg as against 16-25 mmHg observed by Cruz and Hunter in ewes. There are not many data in the literature on laparoscopy during pregnancy. Surgery is generally delayed if the patient's conditions make it possible. According to the data available, however, capnometric monitoring is reliable. Bhavani-Shankar reported about 23 parturients treated with laparoscopy, all of them successfully bringing pregnancy to term without problems.

During pelvic laparoscopy in the Trendelenburg position, a 20%-30% elevation of minute volume is necessary to maintain normocapnia [43]. Baraka [44, 45] suggests a 25% elevation. Wahba [43] increases minute ventilation by 12-16%. This solution cannot be applied to pneumopathic patients with previous episodes of severe respiratory acidosis during laparoscopy. As reported by several authors [44, 45] capnography is not reliable in these patients. Wahba does not consider $P_{ET}CO_2$ reliable for concentrations > 41 mmHg or in the presence of high volumes of insufflated CO_2. Wittgen does not regard $P_{ET}CO_2$ reliable for diagnosis of hypercapnia in patients with cardiorespiratory diseases.

Conclusions

The examples provided show that capnographic monitoring play a vital role even in the most complex clinical situations when haemodynamics and ventilation interactions cannot always be interpreted in a straightforward way. For this reason, a correct theoretical approach and a "reasoned" interpretation of information from expired CO_2 should lead anaesthesiologists to carry out a continuous critical review of the most subtle underlying pathophysiological mechanisms.

References

1. Se-Yuan Liu, Tai-shon Lee (1992) Accuracy of capnography in nonintubated surgical patients. Chest 102:1512-1515
2. Lenz G, Heipertz W, Epple E (1991) Capnometry for continuous postoperative monitoring of nonintubated, spontaneously breathing patients. J Clin Monit 7:245-248
3. Chhibber AK, Kolano JW, Roberts WA (1996) Relationship between end-tidal and arterial carbon dioxide with laryngeal mask airways and endotracheal tubes in children. Anaesth Analg 82:247-250
4. Spahr-Schopfer IA, Bissonnette B, Hartley EJ (1993) Capnometry and the pediatric laryngeal mask airway. Can J Anaesth 40:1038-1043
5. Hicks I, Soni N, Shephard J (1993) Comparison of end-tidal and arterial carbon dioxide measurements during anaesthesia with the laryngeal mask airway. Br J Anaesth 71:734-735
6. Badgwell JM, McLeod ME, et al (1987) End-tidal PCO_2 measurements sampled at distal and proximal ends of the endotracheal tube in infants and children. Anesth Analg 66:959-964
7. Ream RS, Schreiner MS, Neff JD, et al (1995) Volumetric capnography in children. Anesthesiology 82:64-67
8. Nunn JF (1987) Carbon dioxide. In: Nunn JF, (ed) Applied respiratory physiology. 3rd edn. London, Butterworth 207-234
9. Glenski J, Cucchiara R (1986) Transcutaneous O_2 and CO_2 monitoring of neurosurgical patients: detection of air embolism. Anesthesiology 64:546-550
10. Russell G, Graybeal J (1995) The arterial to end-tidal carbon dioxide difference in neurosurgical patients during craniotomy. Anesth Analg 81:806-810
11. Russell G, Graybeal J (1992) End-tidal carbon dioxide as an indicator of arterial carbon dioxide in neurointensive care patients. J Neurosurg Anesth 4:245-249
12. Russell G, Graybeal J, Stroudt J (1990) Stability of arterial to end-tidal PCO_2 during postoperative cardiorespiratory support. Can J Anaesth 37:560-566
13. Isert P (1994) Control of carbon dioxide levels during neuroanesthesia: current practice and an appraisal of our reliance upon capnography. Anaesth Intens Care 22:435-441
14. Grenier B, Verchére E, Mesli A, et al (1999) Capnography monitoring during neurosurgery: reliability in relation to various intraoperative positions. Anaesth Analg 88:43-48
15. Sharma S, Cruise C, McGuire G (1993) Stability of the arterial to end-tidal carbon dioxide gradient during anesthesia for prolonged neurosurgical procedures. Can J Anaesth 40:A37
16. Nunn JF, Hill DW (1960) Respiratory dead space and arterial to end-tidal CO_2 tension difference in anesthetized man. J Appl Physiol 15:383-389
17. Engoren M (1992) Evaluation of capnography to predict arterial CO_2 in neurosurgical patients. J Neurosurg Anesth 4:241-244
18. Fletcher R, Jonson B (1984) Deadspace and the single breath test for carbon dioxide during anaesthesia and artificial ventilation. Br J Anaesth 56:109-119
19. Kerr M, Zempsky J, Sereika S, et al (1996) Relationship between arterial carbon dioxide and end-tidal carbon dioxide in mechanically ventilated adults with severe head trauma. Crit Care Med 24:785-790
20. Fletcher R (1990) The arterio-end-tidal CO_2 difference during cardiothoracic surgery. J Cardiothorac Anesthesiol 4:105-117
21. Werner O. Malmkvist G, Beckman A, et al (1984) CO_2 elimination from each lung during endobronchial anaesthesia. Br J Anaesth 56:995-1001
22. Tavernier B, Rey D, Thevenin J, Triboulet P, Scherpereel P (1997) Can prolonged expiration manoeuvres improve the prediction of arterial PCO_2 from end-tidal PCO_2? Brit J Anaesth 78:536-540
23. Jellinek H, Hiesmayr M, Simon P, et al (1993) Arterial to end-tidal CO_2 tension difference after bilateral lung transplantation. Crit Care Med 21:1035-1040
24. Benumof JL (1995) Anesthesia For Thoracic Surgery. 2nd edn. Saunders, 245-250

25. Carlon GC, Ray C, Miodownik S, et al (1988) Capnography in mechanically ventilated patients. Crit Care Med 67:579-581
26. Shafieha MJ, Sit J, Kartha R, et al (1986) End Tidal CO_2 analyzers in proper positioning of the double lumen tubes. Anesthesiology 64: 844
27. Shankar KB, Moseley HSL, Kumar AY (1992) Dual end-tidal CO_2 monitoring and double lumen tubes. Can J Anaesth 39:100-101
28. Brampton WJ, Watson RJ (1990) Arterial to end-tidal carbon dioxide tension difference during laparoscopy. Magnitude and effect of anaesthetic technique. Anaesthesia 45:210-214
29. Shankar KB, Russell R, Aklog L, Mushlin P (1999) Dual capnography facilitates detection of a critical perfusion defect in an individual lung. Anesthesiology 90:302-304
30. Williams L, Scott Jellish W, Paul A (1991) Capnography in a patient after a single lung transplant. Anesthesiology 74:621-622
31. Pansard JL, Cholley B, Devilliers C, et al (1992) Variation in arterial to end-tidal CO_2 tension differences during anesthesia in the "kidney rest" lateral decubitus position. Anesth Analg 75:506-510
32. Ciofolo MJ, Clergue F, Seebacher J, et al (1990) Ventilatory effects of laparoscopy under epidural anesthesia. Anesth Analg 70:357-361
33. Wahba RWM, Mamazza J (1993) Ventilatory requirements during laparoscopic cholecystectomy. Can J Anaesth 40:206-210
34. Joris JL, Noirot DP, Legrand MJ, et al (1993) Hemodynamic changes during laparoscopic cholecystectomy. Anesth Analg 76:1067-1071
35. Puri GD, Singh H (1992) Ventilatory effects of laparoscopy under general anaesthesia. Br J Anaesth 68:211-213
36. Bures E, Fusciardi J, Lanquetot H, et al (1996) Ventilatory effects of laparoscopic cholecystectomy. Acta Anaesth Scand 40:566-573
37. Fizgerald SD, Andrus CH, Baudendistel LJ, et al (1992) Hypercarbia during carbon dioxide pneumoperitoneum. Am J Surg 163:186-190
38. Laffon M, Gouchet A, Sitbon P, et al (1998) Difference between arterial and end-tidal carbon dioxide pressures during laparoscopy in paediatric patients. Can J Anaesth 45:561-563
39. Amos JD, Schorr SJ, Norman PF, et al (1996) Laparoscopic surgery during pregnancy: a word of caution. Am J Surg 171:435-437
40. Cruz AM, Sutherland LC, Duke T (1996) Intraabdominal carbon dioxide insufflation in the pregnant ewe. Anesthesiology 85:1395-1402
41. Bhavani-Shankar K, Steinbrook R, Brooks D, et al (2000) Arterial to end-tidal carbon dioxide pressure difference during laparoscopic surgery in pregnancy. Anesthesiology 93:370-373
42. Hunter JG, Swanstrom L, Thornburg K (1995) Carbon dioxide pneumoperitoneum induces fetal acidosis in a pregnant ewe model. Surg Endosc 9:272-279
43. Tan PL, Lee TL, Tweed WA (1992) Carbon dioxide absorption and gas exchange during pelvic laparoscopy. Can J Anaesth 39:677-681
44. Baraka A, Jabbour S, Hammoud R, et al (1994) End-tidal carbon dioxide tension during laparoscopic cholecystectomy. Anaesthesia 49:304-306
45. Baraka A, Jabbour S, Hammoud R, et al (1994) Can pulse oximetry and end-tidal capnography reflect arterial oxygenation and carbon dioxide elimination during laparoscopic cholecystectomy. Surg Laparo Endosc 4:353-356

Pulse-oximetry

"On many occasions this instrument has detected anoxemia when observations of pulse, blood pressure, and color of the patient, and peripheral vascular tone have shown no abnormalities" [1].

Beginning in the early 1930s, considerable efforts were made to develop noninvasive optical techniques for accurate measurements of arterial oxygen saturation [2]. The development of pulse oximetry has been based on many people's contribution, during years of experimental and engineering antecedents. In 1935, Matthes [3, 4] built the first device that continuously measured human blood oxygen saturation by transilluminating ear tissue, but difficulties with calibration made it unwieldy. Glen Allen Millikan [5] coined the term "oximeter" to describe a lightweight device he used in aviation research. Its purpose was to assess the oxygenation of pilots flying at high altitude during the Second World War. After the war, Earl Wood [6] used it in the clinical setting to detect previously undiagnosed cyanosis [7]. The greatest step forward in the development of the modern pulse oximeter was made in 1974 by Aoyagi [8]. He recognized that the absorbency ratios of pulsations at different wavelengths varied with oxygen saturation. Aoyagi developed and marketed the first pulse oximeter in 1975, which was first used in health care in the United States in the mid to late 1980s. In 1986, pulse oximetry was recommended as a standard of care for basic intra-operative monitoring by the American Society of Anesthesiologists, as a device able to improve patient safety [9]. In 1988, the Society for Critical Care Medicine recommended that pulse oximetry be used to monitor patients undergoing oxygen therapy. Now it has become an essential tool in the current practice of emergency medicine [10].

Principles

The pulse oximeter is a useful monitoring device for evaluating the oxygen status of patients in a variety of clinical settings, enabling the detection of hypoxaemia before it can be detected by sight. It measures peripheral oxygen saturation, which is a close estimate of the saturation of arterial oxygen in haemoglobin (SaO_2), via a sensor which is usually clipped onto the patient's fingertip or earlobe (Fig. 6). The pulse oximeter consists of two light-emitting diodes (LEDs) and a photodetector, positioned precisely opposite the diodes (Fig. 2–3). The pulse oximeter is based upon two physical principles. First, the light absorbance of oxygenated haemoglobin is different from that of reduced haemoglobin at the oximeter's two wavelengths. Second, the absorbance at both wavelengths have a pulsatile component, which is the result of the fluctuating volume of arterial blood [11].

Taking these assumptions into consideration, one can derive SaO_2 by analyzing only the changes in absorbance caused by the pulsating arterial blood at red wavelength (typically 660 nm), where the absorbance of HbO_2 is less than that of Hb, and a second reference infrared wavelength (typically between 815 and 940 nm), where the absorbance of HbO_2 is slightly greater than that of Hb (Fig. 1).

The pulsatile component of the red and infrared photoplethysmograms is divided by the corresponding nonpulsatile component of the photoplethysmo-gram, which is composed of the light absorbed by tissue, nonpulsatile arterial blood, and venous blood (Fig. 4). The device operates on the principle of Beer's Law, which states that the concentration of an absorbing substance in solution can be determined from the intensity of light transmitted through that solution, given the intensity and wavelength of incident light, the transmission path-length, and the characteristic absorbance of that substance at a specific wave-length [12].

$$\frac{I_R}{I_T} = e^{-acd} \qquad [\text{equ 1}]$$

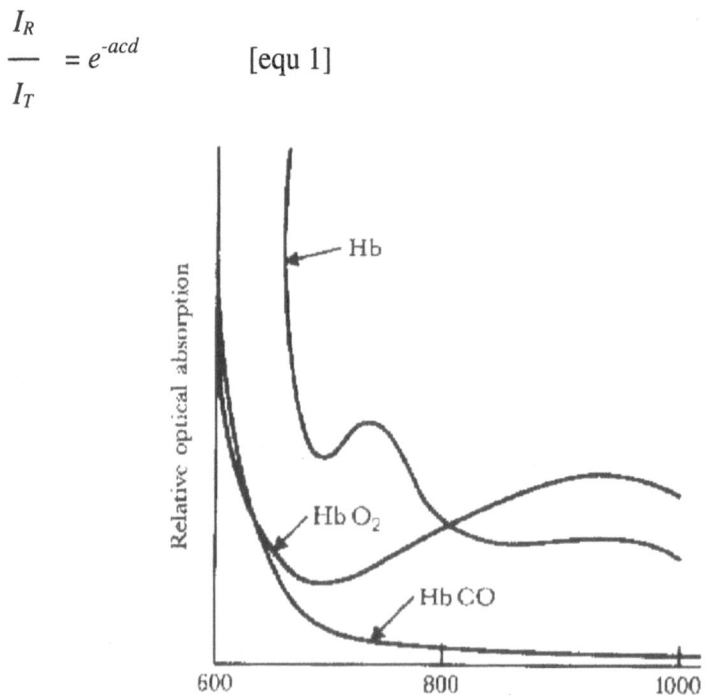

Fig. 1 Optical absorbance spectra of Hb, HbO_2 and HbCO in the visible and near-infrared wavelength region

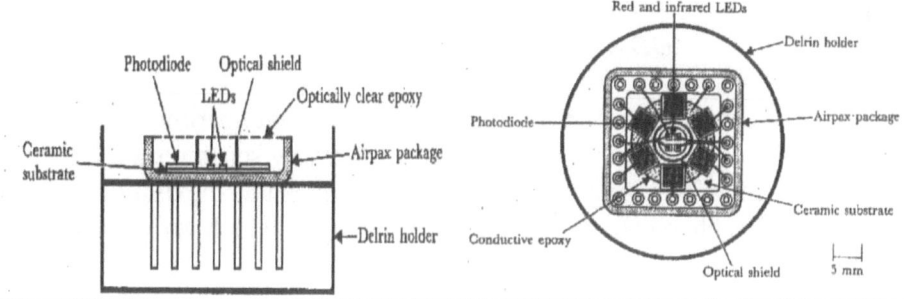

Fig. 2- 3 Pulse oximeter system

where I_R is the intensity of the received light, I_T is the intensity of the transmitted light, **a** is the absorption coefficient, **c** is the concentration of the absorbing molecule (Hb or HBO$_2$) and **d** is the thickness of the tissue.

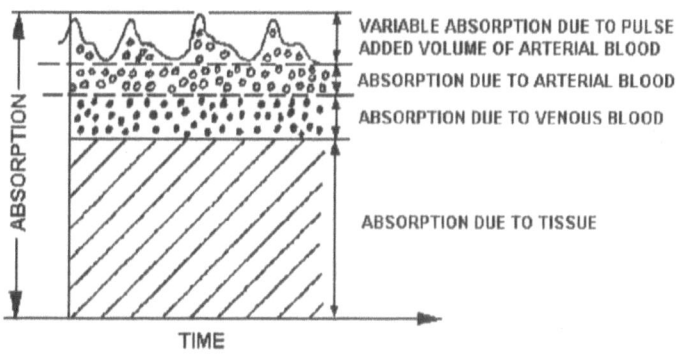

Fig. 4 Light absorption through living tissue

The term **acd** is known as the optical density (OD) of the tissue, and expressed as:

$$OD = \ln \left(\frac{I_T}{I_R} \right) = acd \ [equ\ 2]$$

In the case of pulse oximetery, OD is determined at two wavelengths and the SaO$_2$ is determined using the following relationship:

$$Sa(O2) = A - B \ \frac{OD_{660nm}}{OD_{990nm}} \qquad [equ\ 3]$$

where the coefficients A and B must be determined experimentally.

The device is also able to detect the heart beats by sensing the changes in the blood volume following systole. As more blood enters the tissue after each beat, absorption characteristics of the tissue changes, which is reflected in the I_R (Fig. 5).

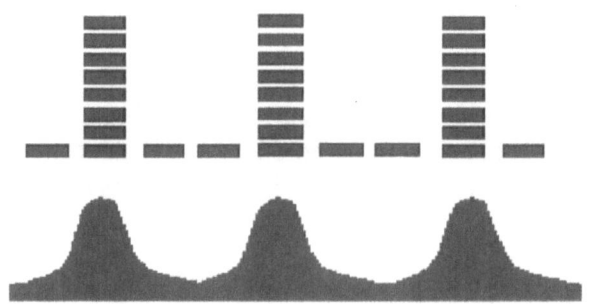

Fig. 5 Heart beat by sensing changes in blood volume

Indications

The pulse oximeter may be used in various clinical applications, including during anaesthesia, surgery, critical care, hypoxaemia screening, exercise, transport from the operating room to the recovery room and in emergency medicine [10].

Tab. 1 The most common uses of the pulse oximeter

- During general anaesthesia and recovery
- During IV conscious sedation or other procedures requiring monitoring of oxygenation status
- During mechanical ventilation
- Guidance for weaning from mechanical ventilation
- Guidance for determining therapeutic oxygen requirement
- Assessing oxygenation during sleep or exercise
- Assessing severity of illness, especially in the emergency department

Advantages of pulse oximetry

There are various makes and models of pulse oximeter available. Most provide a visual digital waveform display, an audible display of arterial pulsation and

Table 2 The advantages of pulse oximetry

- non-invasive
- simple to use
- continuous monitoring
- rapid response to significant desaturation

heart rate, and a variety of sensors to accommodate individuals regardless of age, size or weight (Fig. 6). The pulse oximeter is no substitute for arterial blood gas analysis, but can give clinicians an early warning of decreasing arterial oxyhaemoglobin saturation prior to the patient exhibiting clinical signs of hypoxia. Cyanosis occurs at a saturation of about 75% in normally perfused

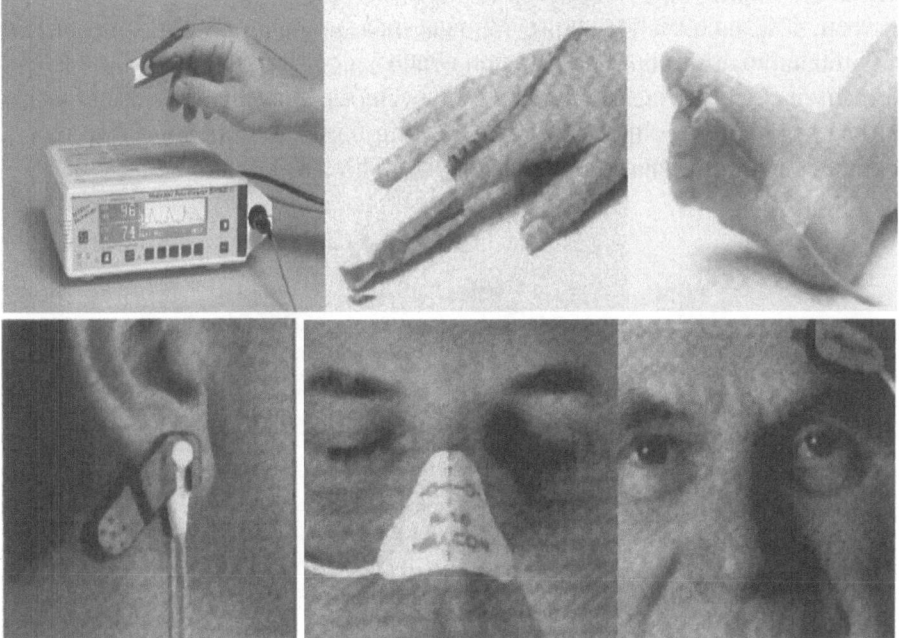

Fig. 6 Types of pulse oximeter

patients. As the brain is the organ most sensitive to oxygen depletion, the more obvious signs of hypoxaemia, such as visual and cognitive changes, will develop only when oxyhaemoglobin saturation falls to around 80-85%. Restlessness, agitation, confusion, cyanosis, hypotension and tachycardia are all delayed manifestations which may be missed or wrongly interpreted. As with all monitoring equipment, the reading should be interpreted in association with the patient's clinical condition. If the patient appears to be in perfect health and the saturation is reading 80%, this should alert you to the possibility of interference. Never ignore a reading which suggests the patient is becoming hypoxic. It is important to remember that pulse oximeters assess oxygen saturation, but give no indication of the level of CO_2, adequacy of ventilation or lung performance.

Limitations of pulse oximeter use

Precision, efficacy and application of the pulse oximeter have been investigated repeatedly; numerous studies have focused on the technical aspects of pulse oximeters and found that these instruments have a reasonable degree of accuracy [14, 15]. Most manufacturers claim that their instruments are accurate to within ±2% in the SaO_2 range between 70% and 100% and ±3% for saturations between 50% and 69% [16]. Pulse oximeter measurement of SaO_2 is physiologically related to arterial oxygen tension (PaO_2) according to the HbO_2 dissociation curve (Fig. 7). Because the HbO_2 dissociation curve has a sigmoid shape, oximetry is relatively insensitive in detecting the development of hypoxemia in patients with high baseline levels of PaO_2 [17, 18, 19].

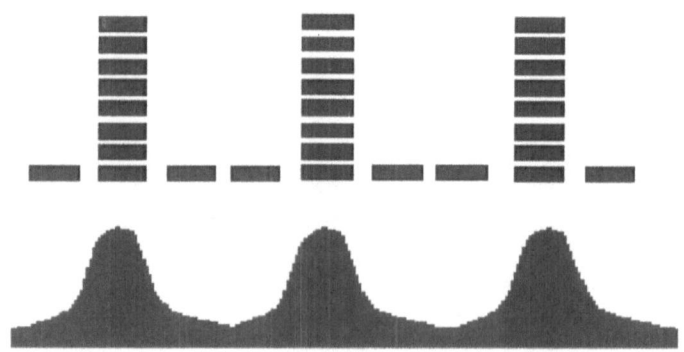

Fig. 7 HbO$_2$ dissociation curve

The limitations of the pulse oximeter in various clinical settings must be recognized in order to appropriately interpret results. The major limitations can be divided into two categories: technical and physiological (Table 4). The pulse oximeter utilizes a plethysmographic waveform to differentiate pulsatile arterial haemoglobin saturation from venous blood. The absence of a pulsatile waveform peripherally such as in hypothermia, hypovolaemia, peripheral vascular disease or vasopressors interferes with the oximeter's function. There must be adequate perfusion at the site of the probe. The pulse oximeter is not effective during cardiac arrest or with extreme heart rates (less than 30 or over 200). The patient's blood pressure generally needs to be at least 80 systolic. If plethysmography is not able to track the arterial pulse, the oximeter will be inaccurate or will not display oxygen saturation, a message will usually be displayed to alert the user to the inadequate pulse signal. The shape and stability of the photoplethysmographic waveform can be used as an indication of possible motion artefacts or low perfusion conditions. If the problem is limited to hand perfusion, it can be corrected by changing the location of the probe, warming the extremity, or applying a topical vasodilator. Problems may also be encountered in anaemic patients as the pulse oximeter reading depends on the light absorbed by haemoglobin, and the pulse oximeter will respond as if there is a state of low perfusion, giving erroneous results.

The presence of dysfunctional haemoglobin will cause the readings to be unreliable. The pulse oximeter is unable to detect other "types of haemoglobin" such as carboxyhaemoglobin (HbCO) or methaemoglobin (MetHb) (Table 3).

Table 3 Examples of dysfunctional haemoglobin

– Anaemia
– Carboxyhaemoglobin
– Foetal haemoglobin
– Methemoglobinaemia
– Sickle cell anaemia
– Thalassaemia

Therefore, if these are pathologically elevated, the pulse oximeter will give a falsely elevated reading. It will not be able to distinguish oxyhaemoglobin from carboxyhaemoglobin, and overestimate the true concentration of the latter in the blood (Fig. 1). The CO-Oximeter uses four different wavelengths and can measure total haemoglobin, HbO_2, HbCO and methaemoglobin. The value reported by a CO-Oximeter is commonly termed fractional HbO_2 and is equal to the amount of HbO_2 expressed as a fraction of the amount of total haemoglobin (the total of all active and inactive forms of haemoglobin with respect to the oxygen-binding capability). The pulse oximeters use only two wavelength and are not able to distinguish each type of haemoglobin derivative present in blood [10].

Functional $SaO_2 = HbO_2 / (HbO_2 + Hb)$
Fractional $SaO_2 = HbO_2 / (HbO_2 + Hb + HbCO + MetHb)$

Other compounds such as dyes, methaemoglobins and nail polish may affect readings. Skin pigmentation has also been found to affect the accuracy of pulse oximetry because the calibration curves for the initial machines were based on healthy white, rather than black, volunteers. However, manufacturers have addressed this problem in later models.

Table 4 Cause of physiological and technical limitations

– Improper positioning
– Motion artefact
– Venous congestion
– Electrocautery
– IV dyes (methylene blue, indigo carmine, indocyanine green)
– Nail polish
– Severe anaemia
– Dyshaemoglobinaemia
– Poor perfusion
– Shape of oxygen dissociation curve
– Ambient light
– Darkly pigmented skin

Conclusion

The use of the pulse oximeter for monitoring patients in the general surgical ward has become a standard procedure. The most important advantage of the pulse oximeter is its capability to provide continuous, safe, and noninvasive monitoring of blood oxygenation at the patient's bedside. Detection of hypoxia by clinical indicators alone is notoriously unreliable [20], whereas the pulse oximeter offers real-time assessment of oxygenation status on a moment-to-moment basis, reflecting efficacy of interventions as well as progression of disease processes.

The increasing cost of health care today makes the use of pulse oximetry even more attractive, because it allows effective oxygen monitoring without the time, risk, and costs associated with clinical laboratory analysis of blood samples.

References of images

Figures 2-3:
http://design.stanford.edu/Courses/me220/lectures/lect16/lect_16.html
Figures 4-7:
http:// gasbone.herston.uq.edu.au/teach/ su602/docs/d19_2pox.html
Figure 5: www.cheo.on.ca/english/ 2012d.html
Figure 6: http:// hsc.virginia.edu/medcntr/depts/ clinical-eng/po.html
Figure 6: www.bioengineering.swri.org/ pulseoximeter.htm
Equ 1, 2, 3: www.biomed.mtu.edu/osoykan/classes/ be304/week6/week6.htm

References

1. Stephen CR, Slater HM, Johnson AL, Sekelj P (1951) The oximeter - a technical aid for the anesthesiologist. Anesthesiology 12:541-545
2. Severinghaus JW, Astrup PB (1986) History of blood gas analysis. VI Oximetry. J Clin Monit; 2:270-288
3. Matthes K (1934) Uber den einfluss der atmung auf die sauerstoffsattingungen des arterienblutes. Arch Exp Pathol Pharmacol 176:683-696
4. Matthes K (1935) Untersuchungen uber die sauerstoffsattingungen des menschlichen arterien-blutes. Arch Exp Pathol Pharmacol 179:698-711
5. Millikan GA, Pappenheimer JR, Rawson AJ, Hervey JP (1941) Continuous measurement of oxygen saturation in man. Am J Physiol 133:390
6. Wood EH, Geraci JE (1949) Photoelectric determination of arterial oxygen saturation in man. J Lab Clin Med 34:387-401
7. Tremper KK (1989) Pulse oximetry. Chest 95:713-715
8. Aoyagi T, Kishi M, Yamaguchi K, Watanabe S (1974) Improvement of the earpiece oximeter. In: Abstracts of the Japanese Society of Medical Electronics and Biological Engineering:90-91
9. Cheney FW (1990) The ASA closed claims study after the pulse oximeter: a preliminary look. American Society of Anesthesiologists Newsletter 54:10-11
10. Mendelson Y (1992) Pulse oximetry: theory and applications for noninvasive monitoring. Cli Chem 38:1601-1607
11. Tremper Kk, Barker S (1989) Pulse oximetry. Anesthesiology 70:98-108
12. Sinex J (1999) Pulse oximetry: principles and limitations. Am J Emerg Med 17:59-66
13. Welch JP, DeCesara R, Hess D (1990) Pulse oximetry: instrumentation and clinical applications. Respir Care 35:584-601
14. Weeb RK, Ralston AC, Runciman WB (1991) Potential errors in pulse oximetry: II. Effects of changes in saturation and signal quality. Anaesthesia 46:207-212
15. Christensen, Lie C, Rosenberg J (1999) Continuous pulse oximetry in the general surgical ward:

Nellcor N-200 versus Nellcor N-3000. Anaesthesia 54:253-257

16. Hornberger C, Matz H, Konecny E, et al (2002) Design and validation of a pulse oximeter calibrator. Anesth Analg 94:S8-S12

17. Jubral A (1999) Pulse oximetry. Crit Care 3:R11-17

18. Ralston AC, Webb RK, Runciman WB (1991) Potential errors in pulse oximetry. I. Pulse oximeter evaluation. Anaesthesia 46:202-206

19. Jubran A, Tobin MJ (1996) Monitoring during mechanical ventilation. Clin Chest Med 17: 453-473

20. Mower WR, Sachs C, Nicklin EL, et al (1995) Effect of routine emergency department triage pulse oxymetry screening on medical management. Chest 108:1297-1302

Oximetry spectral analysis and sleep disordered breathing

P. V. Romero, C. Zamarrón

Pulse oximetry is one of the most widely used tools to determine a patient's cardiorespiratory stability. This technique has become a standard for obtaining valuable blood oxygenation data in a noninvasive and continuous way. Over the last 40 years, it has often replaced arterial blood gas analysis to obtain information about respiratory performance. Continuous pulse oximetry is also frequently used in a variety of settings, including preoperative evaluations, the operating room, post-anaesthesia recovery suites, intensive care units, hospitalisation units and sleep laboratories.

Utility of classical or time-based nocturnal oximetry analysis in the diagnosis of sleep apnea syndrome

Obstructive sleep apnoea (OSA) is a disorder in which repetitive apnoeas occur during sleep; these are associated with hypoxaemia, bradycardia, arousals, and fragmented sleep [1]. The prevalence of OSA in middle-aged populations is currently estimated to be 2% in women and 4% in men [2], and 7% among people 50-70 years of age [3].

Clinical diagnosis of OSA is inaccurate and, therefore, some form of monitoring procedure is generally required to make the diagnosis. Polysomnography (PSG) is the standard diagnostic test for OSA, however it is expensive and time consuming [4]. The morbidity and mortality in untreated patients [5-9] can be diminished with effective treatment [10-12], and thus early diagnosis is warranted.

The high prevalence of the disease and the inconvenience of PSG for the patient make simplified techniques desirable for diagnosing OSA [13]. It is known that pulse oximetry is an attractive candidate for the screening of OSA and that technological advances have made the pulse oximeter easier to use, cheaper, and more reliable. This device can receive and read both the oxygen saturation (SaO₂) and heart rate signals, at the same time. In fact, Bennet and Kinnear [14] called pulse oximetry "sleep on the cheap" in their 1999 editorial because it generates a lot of data at a very low cost.

To properly interpret overnight oximetry data, an understanding of the SaO₂ versus time waveform morphologies is essential. The oximetry signal can be studied by analysing oximetric tracing and oxygen desaturation indexes (ODI) from the oximeter recording in the time domain. The oxymetric recording has the advantage of providing quick and accessible visual information (Fig. 1a--d), which allows visual determination of quality of the respiratory disturbances. However, the variability of the tracing makes it difficult to interpret and a skilled reader is required, especially for some diagnostic applications. Another way of analysing SaO₂ tracing is by using the oximetry desaturation index (ODI). This parameter is obtained by dividing the number of desaturations (Fig. 2) by the

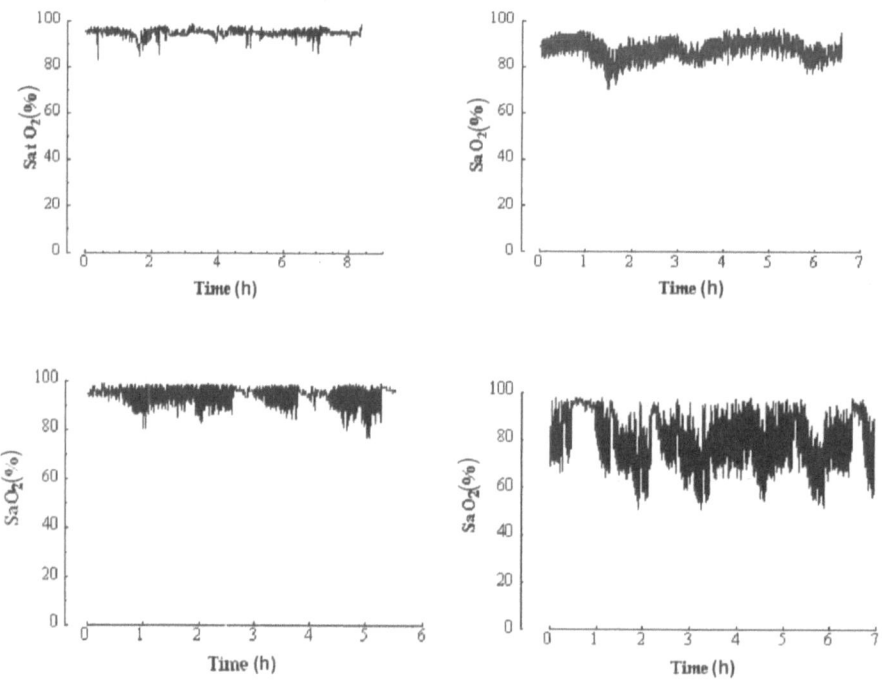

Fig. 1 Different types of pulse oximetry recordings in obstructive sleep apnoea (OSA) patients revealing different degrees of severity in sleep disordered breathing, ranging from a normal-shaped oximetry recording (**a**) to severe OSA high-amplitude oscillations (**d**). Intermediate recordings show middle-size oscillations with (**b**) or without keeping the baseline (**c**)

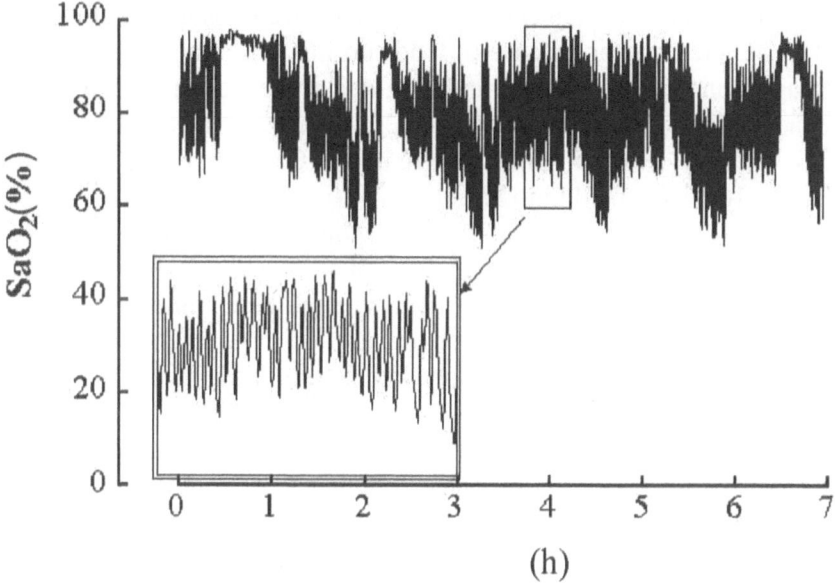

Fig. 2 Detailed view of the variations in a particular segment of oxygen saturation signal in OSA

total test time. There are generally three cutoff points indicating abnormality that are computer calculated. ODI4 indicates events with falls of $SaO_2 \geq 4\%$ per hour; ODI3 indicates events with falls of $SaO_2 \geq 3\%$ per hour and ODI2 for events with falls of $SaO_2 \geq 2\%$ per hour. The cumulative time spent with a SaO_2 below 90% (CT90) is also calculated, as an index of gravity.

The utility of oximetry tracing and ODI in the diagnosis of OSA has been the object of numerous studies. One of the first studies to use oximetric tracing in the diagnosis was carried out by Farney et al. [15]. In this study, the oximetry reading made it possible to differentiate REM from non-REM sleep stage. This technique has a sensitivity of 80% and a specificity of 71% in the diagnosis of OSA [15].

In 1991, Cooper et al. [16] studied a group of 41 patients with suspected OSA. They classified oximeter recordings according to "pattern recognition" of repetitive dips of SaO_2 and found that the sensitivity and specificity of this technique was dependent on the apnoea-hypopnoea index (AHI). When the AHI was greater than 5, sensitivity was 60% and specificity 95%. However, when AHI was greater than 25, sensitivity was 100% and specificity was 80%. The authors concluded that pulse oximetry is an effective tool for screening patients with moderate or severe OSA.

Williams et al. [17] evaluated the usefulness of pulse oximetry together with a clinical score in identifying OSA. Forty patients were assigned a clinical score based on the presence or absence of loud snoring, observations of interrupted breathing during sleep, hypersomnolence, obesity and essential hypertension. Each underwent a night of domiciliary pulse oximetry followed by PSG. They reported a sensitivity of 78% and specificity of 100% when screening patients with AHI $\geq$10 events per hour [17].

In a study by Gyulay et al. [18], 98 consecutive patients referred for assessment of snoring and/or daytime somnolence were assessed clinically and then underwent both unsupervised oximetries in their homes and PSG. The sensitivity of visual inspection of the oximetry tracing was 72%. The ODI4 had higher specificity and lower sensitivity. For desaturations of 4% or more from baseline, ODI4 > 15 per hour identified patients with AHI$\geq$ 15 with sensitivity 40% and specificity 98%. From the oximetry data, the percentage of time spent at SaO2 below 90% (CT90) was also calculated. A finding of CT90 > 1% identifies OSA patients with a 93% sensitivity and of 51% specificity.

In a sample consisting of 240 consecutive patients using a similar visual inspection, the oximetry test was classified as abnormal (suspicion of sleep-related breathing abnormalities) in the presence of repetitive, short-duration arterial oxyhaemoglobin saturation [19]. Series et al. [19] found a sensitivity of 98% for OSA, but specificity was only 48%.

Instead of studying desaturation, Rauscher et al. [20] investigated apnoeas and hypopnoeas by searching for rapid resaturations of $\geq 3\%$ SaO_2 within 10 s at the end of a respiratory event. They found the resaturation to be a more--accurate sign of respiratory events than the actual desaturation, and reported a sensitivity of 94% and a specificity of 45% for detecting OSA with an AHI $\geq$ 10 events per hour, and 95% sensitivity and 45% specificity with an AHI $\geq$ 20 events per hour, respectively.

Other researchers have used a saturation variability index (ΔIndex, the sum of differences between successive readings divided by the number of readings - 1). In a prospective study of 301 consecutive patients referred for suspected sleep disorders, they reported that ΔIndex of 0.8 yielded a sensitivity of 90% and a specificity of 75% for AHI $\geq$15 [21].

Olson et al. [22] studied 793 patients suspected of having OSA by unattended overnight oximetry in their homes followed by PSG. From the oximetry data we extracted cumulative percentage time at SaO2 < 90% (CT90) and a saturation variability index (ΔIndex). The sensitivity of ΔIndex cut-off of 0.4 for the detection of AHI $\geq$15 was 88%, for detection of AHI $\geq$20 it was 90%, and for the detection of AHI $\geq$25 it was 91%. The specificity of ΔIndex of 0.4 for AHI $\geq$15 was very low (40%). They concluded that oximetry using a saturation variability index is sensitive but nonspecific for the detection of OSA [22].

Vázquez et al. [23] studied 246 patients with suspected OSA by automated analysis of the oximetry signal. Using an AHI ≥ 15/h, the sensitivity and specificity were 98% and 88%, respectively.

Golpe et al. [24] assessed the value of home oximetry as a screening test in 116 patients with moderate to severe symptoms of OSA, in which both home oximetry and PSG were performed. A cutoff point for CT90% <0.79 had 84% sensitivity while ODI4 ≥ 31or ODI4 ≥ 40 diagnosed OSA with 97% specificity. Using these values, 38% of the patients would have been correctly classified by oximetry alone, 10% would have been incorrectly classified, and 50% could not have been classified. The greatest value of oximetry in this setting seems to be as a tool to rapidly recognize and treat more-severe OSA patients on the waiting list for PSG [24].

Roche et al. [25] carried out a prospective study to test the validity of two models for the prediction of OSA before PSG. Models were developed using a clinical index, pulmonary function tests, arterial blood gas pressure, and nocturnal pulse oximetry. Their results stress the need for systematic prospective testing of mathematical predictive models in OSA, because their diagnostic characteristics may differ markedly between populations.

Therefore, many authors advocate the use of pulse oximetry in the diagnosis of OSA, reserving more-complex, more-expensive, and less-convenient tests for patients whose oximetry studies are inconclusive.

The use of oximetry makes it possible to carry out fewer PSG tests. Deegan and McNicholas [26] studied 250 patients who underwent PSG. In one-third of these patients, patient history and pulse oximetry data would have been sufficient to make a diagnosis. In the other two-thirds, a final diagnosis was only possible with PSG. Chiner et al. [27], in another prospective study, which excluded COPD patients, used analysis of temporal oximetry recordings in suspected OSA and AHI ≥15. They concluded that with patients who have positive nocturnal oximetry and normal spirometric values it is possible to start treatment without PSG.

It is important to realize that not all desaturations are due to OSA and healthy individuals can experience this phenomenon as well as respiratory disease sufferers. The length of the desaturation waveform can also help to distinguish desaturations due to COPD from desaturations caused by OSA. Normally OSA patients present brief and cyclical desaturations and fast resaturations. The desaturations secondary to COPD tend to last much longer and have a much higher slope in the waveform, being cyclical. Furthermore, they are more intense during the REM stage [28].

Limitations of nocturnal oximetry

There are always some technical or physiological difficulties when using oximetry for recognizing OSA [29,30]. These difficulties increase false-positive results and decrease the specificity of any diagnostic technique.

Technical difficulties

It is important that the oximeter is set to the shortest time interval for measurement. Very short respiratory events may not be detected by the oximeter. However, the typical cyclical drop in SaO_2 in OSA patients lags 45-60 s behind a respiratory event, and should be accurately detected at this measurement speed. It is important to remember that some limitation in the value of **pulse oximetry** as a diagnostic tool may derive from the lack of consensus on oximetric interpretation.

Physiological difficulties

The body movements, vasoconstriction, and hypotension can cause artefacts through an interruption of the **pulse** signal [31, 32]. Changes in the haemoglobin structure and quantity will also cause artificially high (in cases of methemoglobinemia and carboxyhemoglobinemia) or low readings (in cases of anemia) that are not due to respiratory disturbances. Anemia would also lead to overestimating respiratory-caused desaturations.

Spectral analysis of pulse oximetry in the diagnosis of sleep disordered breathing

OSA is frequently accompanied by repetitive oxygen desaturation episodes that can be useful in its detection [33] (Fig. 2). Periodicities of ventilation have been found in subjects with and without OSA [34]. These ventilatory oscillations originate phase-lagged changes in arterial oxygen saturation with the same periodicity, and can therefore be detected by spectral analysis of oximetric signal. Basically, this process can be explained as follows: an apnoea is defined as a respiratory arrest lasting 10 s or more; including the awakening response after apnoea, the minimum cycle length of one apnoeic episode (during non-REM sleep) last about 25 s (0.04 Hz). On the other hand, the longest apnoea time usually observed in OSA during REM last about 2 min (0.008 Hz) [35]. Therefore, OSA-positive patients have a peak in the band of the oximetry spectrum between 0.008 and 0.04 Hz (or between 25 and 120 s if the oximetry periodogram is considered) as observed in Fig. 3. Throughout the night the amplitude of this peak is seen to vary in intensity, but its location on the periodogram remains fixed, as shown by continuous analysis of the variability of oximetry spectrum performed in patients (Fig. 4).

Furthermore, fluctuations in haemodynamic parameters during episodes of OSA, such as blood pressure and heart rate (Fig. 5), during sleep are well known phenomena [36-38]. In OSA, during apneas and the subsequent hyperventilation periods and arousals, a succession of bradycardia and tachycardia phases are seen in subjects with intact autonomic nervous system [39]. The physiological basis of abnormalities lies in the fight against upper airway obstruction, first by stimulation of the parasympathetic nervous system, then by a sudden sympathetic activation caused by the resultant hypoxia [40]. At night the changes of successive parasympathetic and sympathetic drives enhance heart rate variability, which can be characterized by power spectrum or periodogram analysis [41].

Spectral analysis of SaO$_2$ or heart rate variability has been suggested as a potential diagnostic tool for OSA. Using Holter-ECG recordings, Keyl et al.

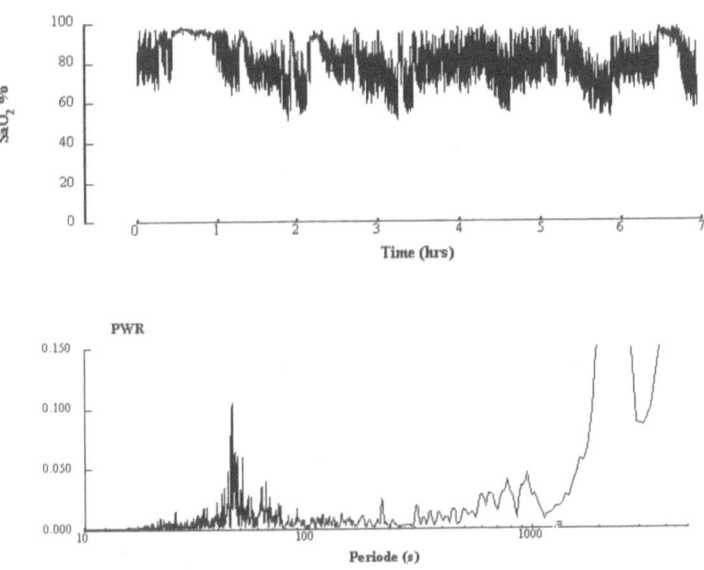

Fig. 3 The relationship between conventional oximetry recording (*top*) and subsequent spectral analysis

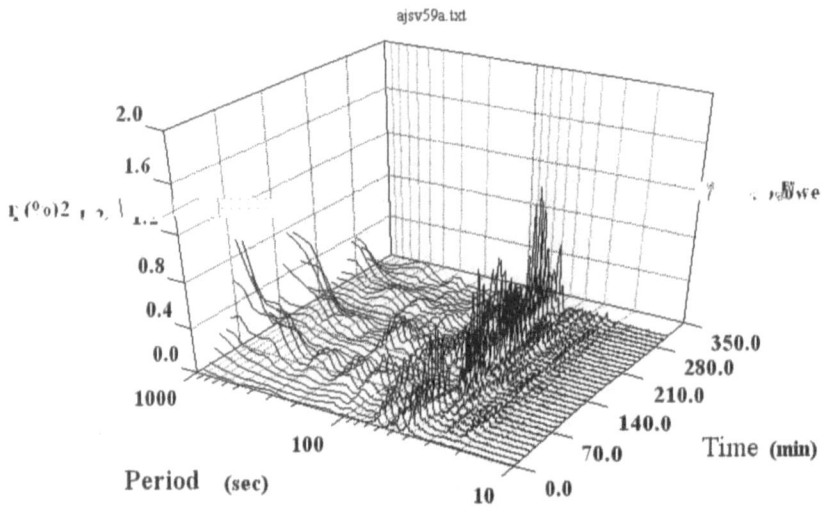

Fig. 4 Three-dimensional distribution of spectral analysis during the night recording. A peak in the periodogram is observe at about 50 s, and is constant throughout the night

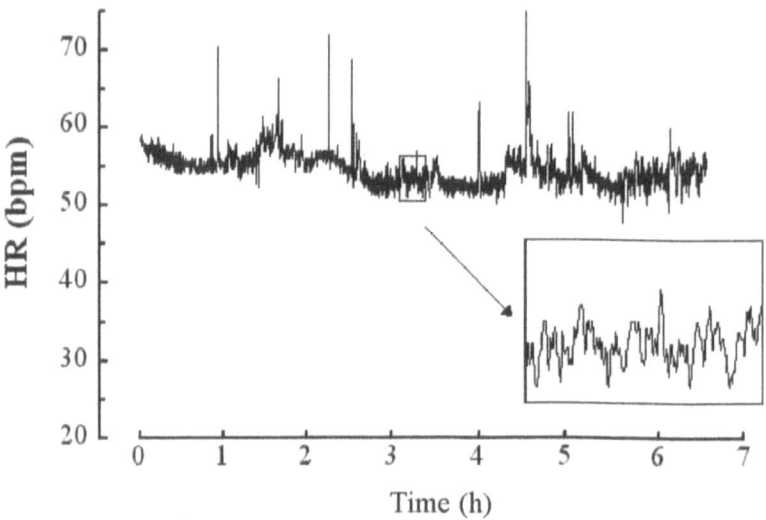

Fig. 5 Detail view of the variations in a particular segment of heart rate (*HR*) signal in OSA

[42] obtained a high accuracy of spectral analysis of heart rate variability, for discriminating between normal and periodic breathing, with a sensitivity of 90% and specificity of 77%. In another study, ROC curves and logistic regression analysis were applied to analyse parameters of heart rate variability in time domain associated with OSA status. The classification and regression methodology showed a sensitivity of 90%, and a specificity of 98% by using different thresholds for the same variable [43]. In a study by Hilton et al. [44], time domain analysis of heart rate variability showed a sensitivity of 90% in the diagnosis of OSA.

In previous studies we demonstrated that the spectral analysis and peak detection in the period 30-70 s of SaO_2 or heart rate signal obtained from nocturnal pulse oximetry could be useful as a first step in OSA diagnosis [45,46].

Methodology and clinical application of power spectral analysis of oxygen saturation and heart rate

SaO_2 and heart rate recording are performed with a finger probe, sampled at a frequency of 0.2 Hz (one sample every 5 s), and stored at internal memory buffer of the oximeter. In order to avoid aliasing, according to the Niqvist theorem [47], the system has to be tested to be sure that spectral power at frequencies near and over 0.1 Hz are negligible. Stored time-domain data are played back into a computer for Fast Fourier analysis. Fast Fourier Transform (FFT) of the signal inherently assumes that the data we have are a single period of a periodically repeating waveform with an infinite number of samples. However, we have a finite number of samples, of a signal that is randomly cut between two points in time. This can lead to an artefact known as spectral leakage, which is due to artefactual discontinuities that appear at the beginning and the end of the sampled signal. To avoid spectral leakage, signals are windowed. Applying a window to a signal is equivalent to multiplying the signal by the window function. A general-purpose window commonly used for analysing transients longer than the time duration of the window is the Hamming window:

$$w[n] = 0.54 - 0.46\cos(2?n/N) \text{ for } n=0,1,2,3,...,N-1$$

Then the power spectrum of SaO_2 and heart rate was analysed using the Fast Fourier Transformation of the Hamming-windowed signal [47]. Power spectra shows the power density or squared magnitude of the amplitude, in each of the frequency components of the signal, in the bandwidth defined by the interval:

$$f_{min} = Df = f_s/N$$
$$f_{max} = 1/f_s$$

where Df is the frequency resolution, f_s is the frequency of sampling (fs =

1/5 = 0.02 Hz), and N is the total number of points sampled. Periodogram is obtained by substituting frequency by period [T(s)=1/frequency(Hz)] in the power spectrum. Analysis was performed by using a Labview (National Instruments Corp. Austin, Tex., USA) based software.

The power contents of the signal are plotted against the logarithm of the period [45,46] for visual identifications of peaks. Furthermore, we measured the total area of the periodogram between 10 and 2,000 s (S_{TOT}), the area between the frequency boundaries of 30-70 s (S_{30-70}), the area between the frequency boundaries of the peak in percentage of the total area of the periodogram (S%), and the peak amplitude (PA) (Fig. 6).

A total of 240 patients (79.4% men, 20.6% women), clinically suspected of having OSA, were studied with this methodology. Subjects ranged in ages from 21 to 82 years, had a body mass index (BMI) of 30.4 ± 5.8 kg/m^2 and were prospectively evaluated using a single-night pulse oximetric recording (SaO$_2$ and heart rate) in conjunction with a simultaneous polysomnographic study analysed by segments of 8 h. The average of AHI was calculated in hourly

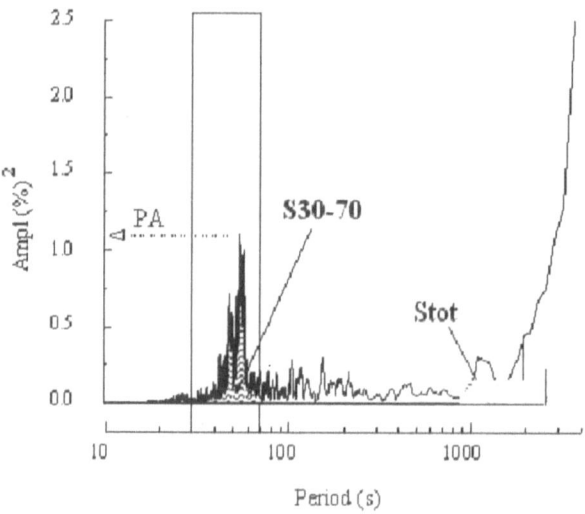

Fig. 6 Power contents of the signal plotted against the period: T(s)=1/frequency(Hz). We can observe a peak in the periodogram (30-70 s). S_{TOT} is total area of the periodogram between 10 and 2,000 s, S_{30-70} is the area between the frequency boundaries of the peak (30 -70 s), S% is ratio of the area enclosed in the periodogram between the frequency boundaries of the peak to the total area of the periodogram, and PA is the peak amplitude of the periodogram (30-70 s)

samples of sleep. In this study an AHI of 10 or more was considered as diagnostic of OSA.

As the differential frequency in the spectrum (df) depends on the total number of samples, which differs between subjects, the spectra were interpolated to obtain the spectral amplitude at equally distributed frequencies between 0 and 0.1 Hz, with a df = 4×10^{-5} Hz. Amplitudes were then averaged to obtain average SaO_2 spectra in OSA patients and in normal subjects. The average of the SaO_2 spectral signal shows the characteristic features (Fig. 7a). Average power amplitude and one standard deviation are shown. A peak is present in the range 0.014-0.028 Hz (corresponding to 35- to 70-s period), which is absent in normal subjects (Fig. 7b). Similar results are observed when heart rate is considered instead SaO_2 (Fig. 8), a peak in the spectrum is observed in the same range of frequencies.

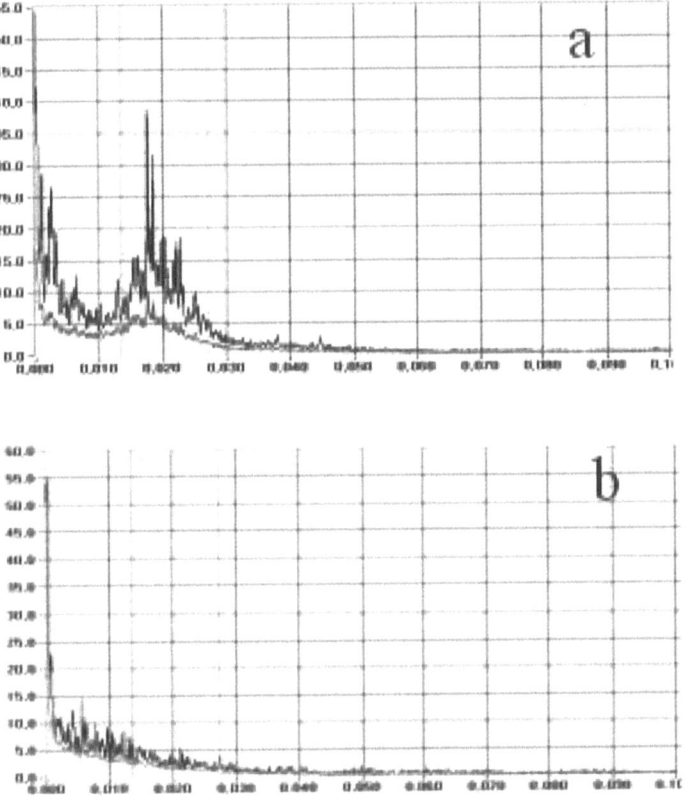

Fig. 7 The average periodogram of oxygen saturation for OSA patients (**a**) and non-OSA patients (**b**). Average and average+1 SD periodograms are shown

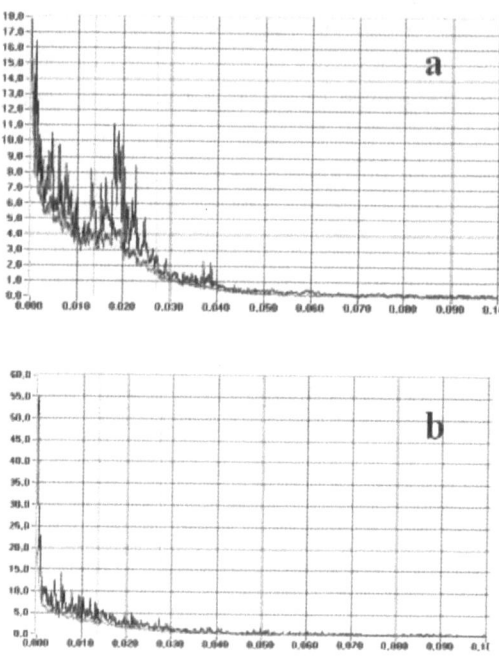

Fig. 8 The average periodogram of heart rate for OSA patients (**a**) and non-OSA patients (**b**). Average and average+1 SD periodograms are shown

Another interesting way to study low-frequency oscillations in cardio-respiratory signals is to decimate the signal in segments of the same length, and to determine the behaviour of the spectrum on the period-time plane, by applying the Short Fourier Transform without overlapping. Figure 4 shows the evolution of SaO_2 spectrum during the entire night in an OSA patient. Since the beginning of the sleeping time, a peak at about 50 s period appears, together with some secondary peaks between 40 and 60 s. Although some variations in the location of the peak can be occasionally detected, always in the range 30-100 s, in general the main peak seems to be relatively constant in the spectral location, but largely varying in amplitude (Fig. 9). In fact, when an OSA patient is treated with continuous positive airway pressure, this peak disappears (Fig. 10).

In our study, the diagnosis of OSA was confirmed in 124 patients using PSG. The presence of a peak in the periodogram (30-70 s) of SaO_2 and heart rate recordings was determined in each study, and we studied the utility of this peak in the diagnosis of OSA. The trace was classified as abnormal (suspicion of OSA) in the presence of a peak, regardless of the size of the peak in the

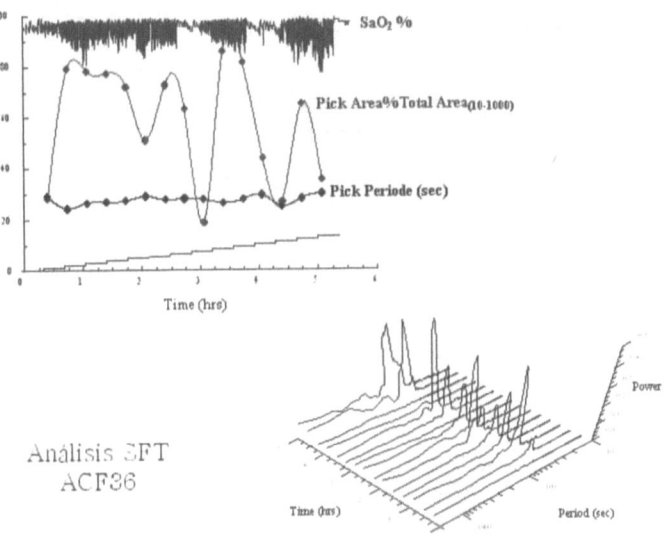

Fig. 9 Continuous periodogram analysis of nocturnal oximetry using Short Fourier Transform in segments of 20 min. At the *bottom* of the period-time plane, evolution of spectral characteristics of nocturnal oximetry during sleeping can be observed. A peak at about 60 s is nearly constant throughout the night. On the *top*, nocturnal variations of different spectral parameters (peak area as percentage of total area) show noticeable variations, while the peak period is nearly constant

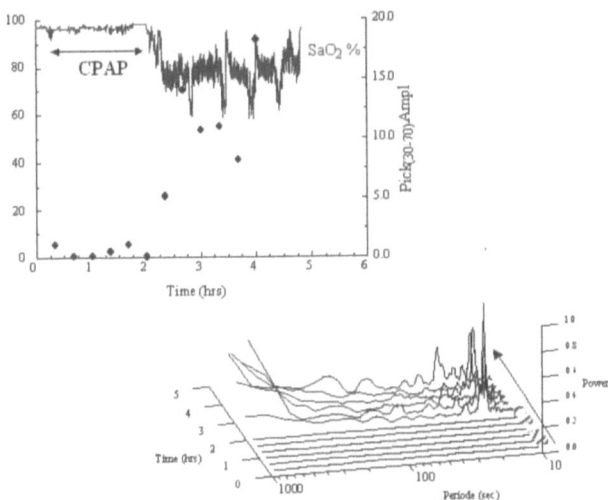

Fig. 10 The peak in the spectrum disappears with continuous positive airway pressure (CPAP) treatment. When CPAP is off during sleep, spectral disturbances appear again. At the *top*, linear evolution of oximetry and peak amplitude during sleeping are shown. *Bottom*, evolution of the spectrum in the period-time plane

periodogram (30-70 s), and normal in the absence of the same peak in the periodogram. Using this methodology, we determine the sensitivity, specificity in detecting OSA for each signal.

The presence of a peak in the SaO_2 spectrum of the pulse oximetric test had a sensitivity of 78.2% and a specificity of 89.0%, The presence of a peak in a heart rate spectrum had a sensitivity of 81.3% and a specificity of 91.5 %.

However, some patients may not present variations in SaO_2 or heart rate signals; consequently, the study of just one signal may not be sufficient to give a correct diagnosis. Since the pulse oximetric recording can display both signals, the study of the variations in one signal or another may improve the diagnosis of OSA patients at no additional cost. Using this methodology, the presence of a peak in the period within 30-70 s in the periodogram in either signal had a sensitivity of 94% a specificity of 82%.

In conclusion, pulse oximetry is inexpensive, can be performed either in hospital or at home, and is easily processed by computer to give reproducible and objective results. We think that spectral analysis of nocturnal pulse oximetric recording can become a supplementary method to the conventional indexes and could be incorporated into the same instruments at no additional costs. The presence of a peak within the period 30-70 s in the SaO_2 or in heart rate periodogram has a high sensitivity and specificity in the diagnosis of OSA. Furthermore, the combined spectral analysis that we use has a greater usefulness than conventional methods, utilizing only one signal (either SaO_2 or heart rate). From a clinical point of view, the inherent complexity of spectral analysis due to its mathematical component, is completely overcome when user-friendly software is used. Moreover, this software can be incorporated into the digitized oximeters already in use. Obviously, there is a lot of commercial software available for spectral analysis. We developed Labview-based software in order to improve the process of data intake from the oximeter and the screen presentation. In conclusion, the spectral characteristics of SaO_2 and heart rate signals obtained by nocturnal pulse oximetry in OSA patients are different from those in non-OSA subjects, and the presence of a peak in the periodogram of either signal allows us to distinguish OSA patients from non-OSA patients.

References

1. Guilleminault C, Van den Hoed J, Mitler MM (1978) Clinical overview of the sleep apnea syndromes. In: Guilleminault C, Dement WC (eds) Sleep apnea syndromes. Liss, New York
2. Young T, Platt M, Dempsey J, et al (1993) The occurrence of sleep-disordered breathing among middle-aged adults. N Engl J Med 328:1230-1235
3. Zamarrón C, Gude F, Otero Y, et al (1999) Prevalence of sleep disordered breathing and sleep apnea in 50 to 70 years old individuals. A survey. Respiration 66:317-322
4. Practice parameters for the indications for polysomnography and related procedures (1990) An American Sleep Disorders Association Report. Sleep 20:406-422
5. Mooe T, Rabben T, Wiklund U, et al (1996) Sleep disordered breathing in women: occurrence and association with coronary artery disease. Am J Med 101:251-256
6. Peppard PE, Young T, Palta M, et al (2000) Prospective study of the association between sleep disordered breathing and hypertension. N Engl J Med 342:1378-1384
7. Peker Y, Hedner J Kraiczi H, et al (2000) An independent predictor of mortality in coronary artery disease. Am J Respir Crit Care Med 162:81-86
8. Parra O, Arboix A, Bechich S, et al (2000) Time course of sleep related breathing disorders in first ever stroke or transient ischemic attack. Am J Respir Crit Care Med 161:375-380
9. Shahar E, Whitney CW, Redline S, et al (2001) Sleep-disordered breathing and cardiovascular disease: cross-sectional results of the Sleep Heart Health Study. Am J Respir Crit Care Med 163:19-25
10. Krieger J, Grucker D, Sforza E, et al (1991) Left ventricular ejection fraction in obstructive sleep apnea. Effects of long-term treatment with nasal continuous positive airway pressure. Chest 100: 917-921
11. Indications and standards for use of nasal continuous positive airway pressure (CPAP) in sleep apnea syndromes (1994) American Thoracic Society. Official statement adopted March 1944. Am J Respir Crit Care Med 150:1738-1745
12. Muñoz A, Mayoralas LR, Barbé F, et al (2000) Long-term effects of CPAP on daytime functioning in patients with sleep apnoea syndrome. Eur Respir J 15:676-681
13. Ryan PJ, Hilton MF, Boldy DAR, et al (1995) Validation of British Thoracic Society guidelines for the diagnosis of the sleep apnoea/hypopnoea syndrome. Can polysomnography be avoided? Thorax 50:972-975
14. Bennet JA, Kinnear WJ (1999) Sleep on the cheap: the role of overnight oximetry in the diagnosis of sleep apnea-hypopnea syndrome. Thorax 54:958-959
15. Farney RJ, Walker DE, Jensen RL, et al (1986) Ear oximetry to detect apnea and differentiate rapid eye movement (REM) and non-REM (NREM) sleep. Screening for the sleep apnea syndrome. Chest 89:533-539
16. Cooper BG, Veale D, Griffiths CJ, et al (1991) Value of nocturnal oxygen saturation as a screening test for sleep apnoea. Thorax 46:586-588
17. Williams AJ, Yu G, Santiago S, et al (1991) Screening for sleep apnea using pulse oximetry and a clinical score. Chest 100:631-635
18. Gyulay S, Olson LG, Hensley MJ, et al (1993) A comparison of clinical assessment and home oximetry in the diagnosis of obstructive sleep apnea. Am Rev Respir Dis 147:50-53
19. Series F, Marc I, Cormier I, et al (1993) Utility of nocturnal home oximetry for case finding in patients with suspected sleep apnea hypopnea syndrome. Ann Intern Med 119:449-453
20. Rauscher H, Popp W, Zwick H (1993) Model for investigating snorers with suspected sleep apnoea. Thorax 48:275-279
21. Levy P, Pépin JL, Deschaux-Blanc C, et al (1996) Accuracy of oximetry for detection of respiratory disturbances in sleep apnea syndrome. Chest 109:395-399
22. Olson LG, Ambrogetti A, Gyulay SG (1999) Prediction of sleep disordered breathing by unattended overnight oximetry. J Sleep Res 8:51-55
23. Vazquez JC, Tsai WII, Flemons WW, et al (2000) Automated analysis of digital oximetry in the diagnosis of obstructive sleep apnea. Thorax 55:302-307

24. Golpe R, Jimenz A, Carpizo, et al (1999) Utility of home oximetry as a screening test for patients with moderate to severe symptoms of obstructive sleep apnea. Sleep 22:932-937

25. Roche N, Herer B, Roig C, et al (2002) Prospective testing of two models based on clinical and oximetric variables for prediction of obstructive sleep apnea. Chest 121:747-752

26. Deegan PC, McNicholas WT (1996) Predictive value of clinical features for obstructive sleep apnea syndrome. Eur Respir J 9:117-124

27. Chiner E, Signes Costa J, Arrieiro JM, et al (1999)Nocturnal oximetry for the diagnosis of the sleep apnoea hypopnoea syndrome: a method to reduce the number of polysomnographies? Thorax 54: 968-971

28. Manni R, Cerveri I, Bruschi C, et al (1988) Sleep and oxyhemoglobin desaturation patterns in chronic obstructive pulmonary diseases. Eur Neurol 28:275-278

29. Jensen LA, Onyskiw JE, Prasad NGN (1998) Meta-analysis of arterial oxygen saturation monitoring by pulse oximetry in adults. Heart Lung 27:387-408

30. Sinex JE (1999) Pulse oximetry: principles and limitations. Am J Emerg Med 17:59-67

31. Boehlecke B (2001) Controversies in monitoring and testing for sleep-disordered breathing. Curr Opin Pulm Med 7:372-380

32. Barker SJ, Shah NK (1997) The effects of motion on the performance of pulse oximetry saturation. Eur J Pediatr 156:808-811

33. Netzer N, Eliasson AH, Netzer C, et al (2001) Overnight pulse oximetry for sleep disordered breathing in adults: a review. Chest 120:625-633

34. Pack AI, Silage DA, Millman RP, et al (1988) Spectral analysis of ventilation in elderly subjects awake and asleep. J Appl Physiol 64:1257-1267

35. Shiomi T, Guilleminault Ch, Sasanabe R, et al (1996) Augmented very low frequency component of heart rate variability during obstructive sleep apnea. Sleep 19:370-377

36. Guilleminault C, Connolly S, Winkle R, et al (1984) Cyclical variation of the heart rate in sleep apnoea syndrome. Lancet 21:126-131

37. Rüther E, Kreuzer H (1992) Changes in heart rate during obstructive sleep apnea. Eur Respir J 7:853-857

38. Leroy M, Van Surell C, Pilliere R, et al (1996) Short term variability of blood pressure during sleep in snorers with or without apnea. Hypertension 28:937- 943

39. Zwillich C, Devlin T, White D, et al (1982) Bradycardia during sleep apnea: characteristics and mechanism. J Clin Invest 69:1286-1292

40. Andreas S, Hajak G, Von Breska B, et al (1992) Changes in heart rate during obstructive sleep apnea. Eur Respir J 7:853-857

41. Pomeranz B, Macaulay JB, Caudill MA, et al (1985) Assessment of autonomic function in humans by heart rate spectral analysis. Am J Physiol 248:H151-H153

42. Keyl C, Lemberger P, Pfeifer M, et al (1997) Heart rate variability in patients with daytime sleepiness suspected of having sleep apnea syndrome: a receiver operating characteristics analysis. Clin Sci (Colch) 92:335-343

43. Roche F, Gaspoz JM, Court Fortune I, et al (1999) Screening of obstructive sleep apnea syndrome by heart rate variability analysis. Circulation 100:1411-1415

44. Hilton MF, Bates RA, Godfrey KR, et al (1999) Evaluation of frequency and time frequency spectral analysis of heart rate variability as a diagnostic marker of the sleep apnoea syndrome. Med Biol Eng Comput 37:760-769

45. Zamarrón C, Romero PV, Rodriguez JR, et al (1999) Oximetry spectral analysis in the diagnosis of obstructive sleep apnea. Clin Sci (Colch) 97:467-473

46. Zamarrón C, Romero PV, Gude F, et al (2001) Screening of obstructive sleep apnoea: heart rate spectral analysis of nocturnal pulse oximetric recording. Respir Med 95:759-765

47. Stearns SD, Hush DR (1990) Digital signal analysis, 2nd ed. Prentice Hall, Englewood Cliffs, N.J., pp 155-162

Post-occlusion rapid drop in pressure

W.A. ZIN

Since the post-occlusion rapid drop in pressure relates almost exclusively to respiratory resistance, the other sources of mechanical impediments to breathing (e.g., elastic, viscoelastic, plastoelastic forces) will be dealt with very briefly here. However, they will be discussed in depth in other chapters of this book.

Physical and physiological basis of respiratory resistance

Before dealing in detail with the rapid decay in pressure after end-inspiratory occlusion, some physiological mechanical concepts must be briefly revisited.

Friction always opposes the movement of an object. Thus, movement of gas (i.e., flow = V') through a tube requires a driving pressure to overcome frictional resistance. The magnitude of flow depends on the difference in pressures (ΔP) across the tube and the resistance (R) offered by the pipe itself:

$$V' = \Delta P / R \qquad (1)$$

and rearranging:

$$R = \Delta P / V' \qquad (2)$$

The same concept can be perfectly extended to thoracic tissue resistance. In other words, some pressure will be expended – and lost – to move pulmonary and chest wall tissues.

As a result, the pressure generated to overcome resistive forces dissipates when flow ceases. This is a fundamental concept that cannot be henceforth forgotten. As depicted in Fig. 1, the solid line that represents airway pressure shows a sudden rise at the beginning of inflation and a fast decay after airway occlusion at end-inspiration. The dashed line corresponds to the pressure used

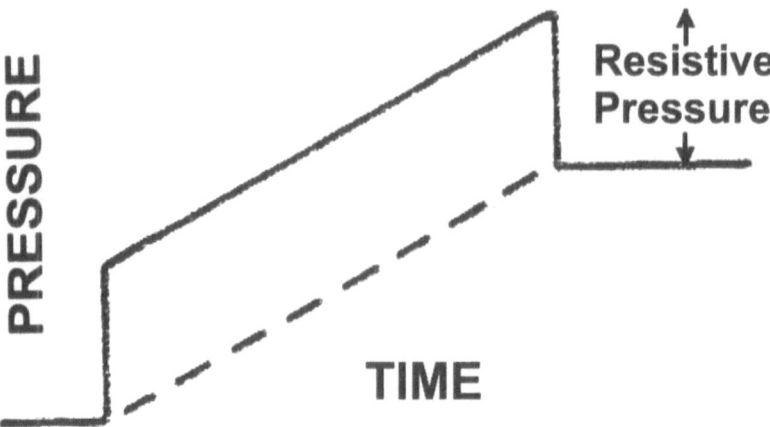

Fig. 1 Airway pressure plotted against inspiratory time. The *solid line* represents airway pressure and abruptly rises at the beginning of inflation and quickly decays after airway occlusion at end-inspiration. The *dashed line* corresponds to the pressure used to overcome elastic properties of the respiratory system

to overcome elastic properties of the respiratory system. Once again, resistive pressure is only present when there is flow.

Pulmonary resistance

Pulmonary resistance corresponds to the sum of airway resistance and the viscous resistance of lung tissues. Interestingly, it has been demonstrated in dogs [1] and rats [2] that the lung tissues do not contribute appreciably to pulmonary resistance.

Chest wall resistance

Chest wall resistance has been assessed in mechanically ventilated anaesthetized paralyzed cardiac patients during corrective heart surgery [3] and normal subjects [4]. Chest wall resistance represents a small fraction of total respiratory resistance. Together with the minute contribution of pulmonary tissue resistance, airway resistance is only slightly smaller than total respiratory resistance [5]. By means of the body plethysmographic method, respiratory system resistance was also found to be very similar to airway resistance [6].

Historical background of the interrupter technique

In 1915 Rohrer [7] described quantitatively for the first time the resistive and elastic pressures required to inflate the lung. His ideas were extended by his pupil Wirz [8], and later by von Neergaard and Wirz [9]. These authors were looking for means of alveolar pressure measurement to be able to determine airway resistance rather than pulmonary resistance. Their rationale was that the transient interruption of airflow would allow pressures to equilibrate all over the lung and airways (Pascal's principle). Under these circumstances mouth pressure during the short occlusion would represent the alveolar pressure responsible for generating the airflow immediately before and after the occlusion. Later Mead and Whittenberger [10] revived the sudden occlusion technique associated with the measurement of oesophageal pressure, but it was to be overshadowed by the whole-body plethysmography perfected by DuBois et al. [11]. In the mid-1980s the technique was revisited and applied to anaesthetized humans [12] and animals [13-15]. The physical and physiological aspects of the technique were established in a series of subsequent studies [16-18].

Technique of rapid airway occlusion during constant flow inflation

This technique essentially combines the elastic subtraction [19] and the interruption methods [9]. A similar approach was suggested in the mid-1960s[20, 21]. The airway can be occluded at different lung volumes and under diverse flows, but the results will vary accordingly.

The rapid airway occlusion during constant flow inflation is characterized by an immediate drop in pressure after the occlusion (resistive component). A slow decay in pressure follows (viscoelastic/inhomogeneous pressure) until an apparent plateau (Pel = elastic recoil pressure) is reached. In Fig. 2 representative tracings of tracheal (Ptr) and alveolar pressures (Pcap) can be seen. After airway occlusion, Ptr drops immediately to Pcap, being the pressure value represented by DP1. During the slow decay (DP2) both pressures are exactly superimposed.

Technical considerations

The end-inflation occlusion technique requires a rapidly closing valve, since the speed of closure influences the values of measured resistances [22]. Under ideal conditions the occlusion time would be nil, but a finite time always exists between the totally open and completely closed configurations of the valve. During that period, gas continues to flow through the valve, altering the

measured pressure signal [15, 17]. A simple correction for the proper determination of resistance otherwise biased by the flow of gas into the lungs during
valve closure has been broadly used [15]. A valve closing time of 10 ms or less
is long enough to yield an accurate measurement of resistance. In the clinical
situation, useful results can be gathered with a closing time of 20 ms or less [17].
Another crucial point is the precise identification of the inflexion point between
the fast and the slow pressure profiles after the airway occlusion. Oscillations
in the pressure signal subsequent to the occlusion can add extra noise on top of
the true value (Fig. 2). Additionally, the transition between both slopes may be
smoothed out by disease, as a result of the existence of inhomogeneity of time
constants in the system. To overcome this drawback the inflexion point can be
pinpointed by back-extrapolation of the pressure signal during the slow decay
in pressure to the point of zero flow [20]. The development of suitable
signal-processing techniques has made such measurement more rapid and
precise [22-24], as depicted in Fig. 3. Alternatively, ensemble averaging of
several consecutive inspirations can be used to get rid of the ripple and noise,
thus revealing the inflexion point [4].

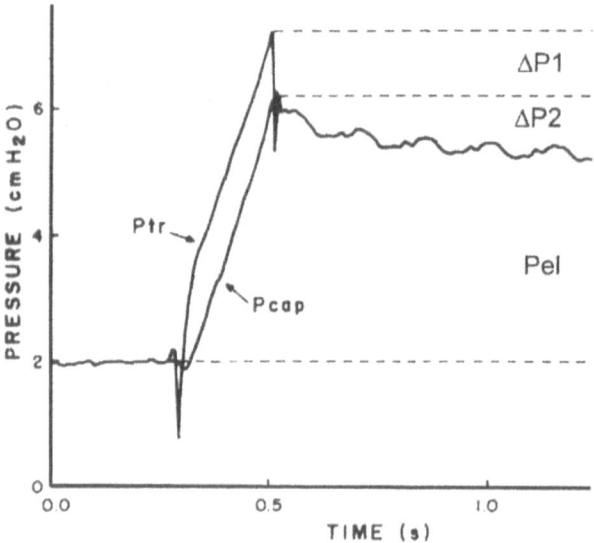

Fig. 2 Tracheal and alveolar pressures (Ptr and Pcap, respectively) plotted versus time in an
anaesthetized paralyzed mechanically ventilated rat. After end-inspiratory occlusion, Ptr drops
quickly toward Pcap, and this variation (DP1) represents the pressure required to overcome the
resistive properties of the lung. DP2 corresponds to the viscoelastic/inhomogeneous pressure
dissipation, and Pel is the elastic recoil pressure of the lung. (Modified from reference [2])

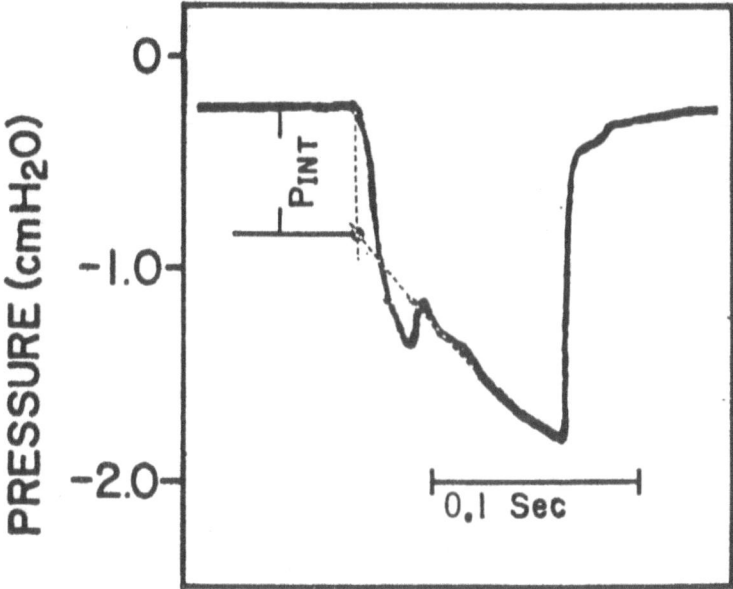

Fig. 3 Airway opening pressure plotted against time. *Dotted lines* illustrate the curvilinear back-extrapolation to the time of interruption and the predicted inflection point. *PINT* represents the resistive pressure. (Modified from reference [24])

Measurement of resistance

The difference between the maximal pressure at the beginning of the occlusion and the pressure value at the inflexion point divided by the flow immediately preceding the occlusion yields a resistance (Eq. 2). It has been termed minimum resistance (Rmin), interrupter resistance (Rint), and initial resistance (Rini). If airway opening, transpulmonary, and transthoracic pressures are used, respiratory system, pulmonary, and chest wall true resistances can be calculated, respectively. For clinical purposes, however, the initial rapid pressure drop in airway opening pressure corresponds to the pressure dissipation within the airways, especially in patients with chronic obstructive pulmonary disease (COPD) [25] and acute respiratory distress syndrome (ARDS) [26], in whom airway resistance is increased.

In Fig. 4 tracings of airflow, tracheal and transpulmonary pressures (Ptr and PL, respectively) obtained in an anaesthetized paralyzed human are shown. After end-inspiratory occlusion, peak Ptr and PL (Ptr,max and PL,max, respectively) fall suddenly, reaching the inflection points Ptr,i and PL,i, respectively. These pressure variations (ΔP1) divided by the flow immediately preceding the occlusion yield the respiratory system and pulmonary ($\approx$airway) resistances

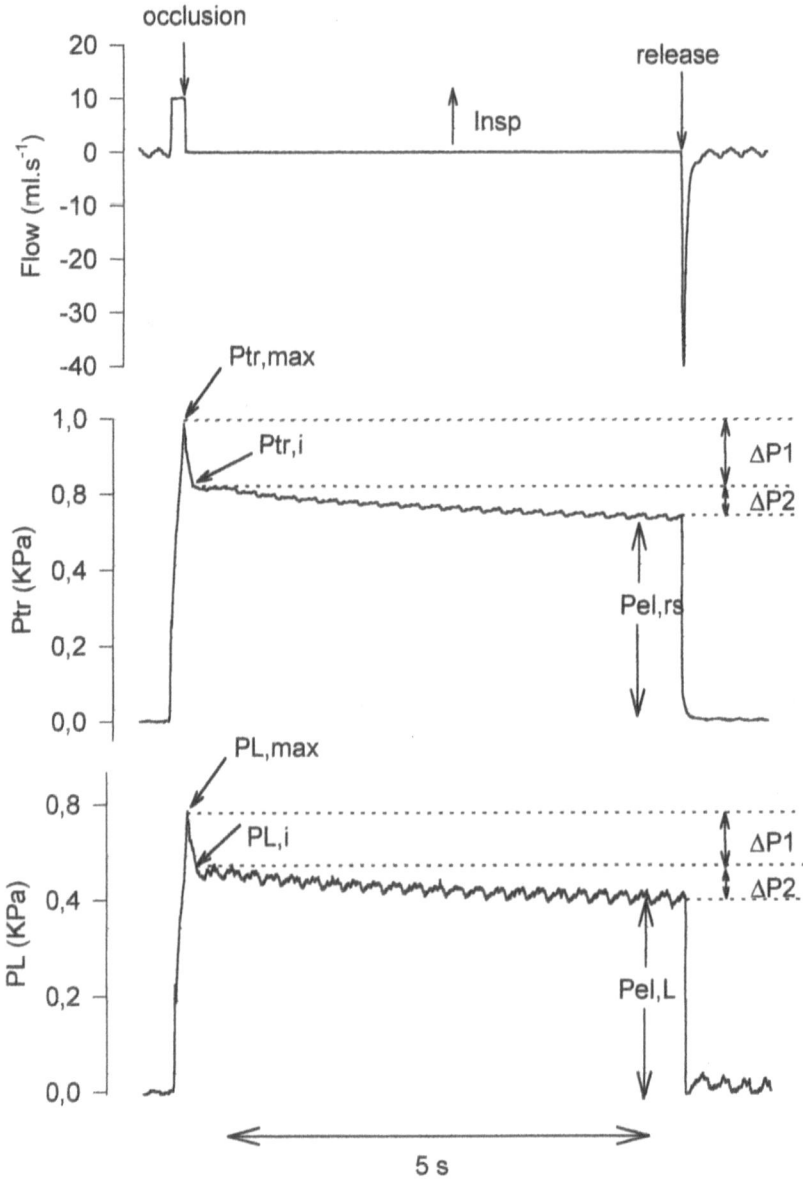

Fig. 4 Tracings of airflow, tracheal and transpulmonary pressures (Ptr and PL, respectively) obtained in an anaesthetized paralyzed human. After end-inspiratory occlusion, peak Ptr and PL (Ptr,max and PL,max, respectively) fall suddenly, reaching their respective inflection points, Ptr,i and PL,i. DP1 and DP2 correspond respectively to the pressures required to overcome resistive and viscoelastic properties of the respiratory system (Ptr tracing) and lung (PL tracing). Pel,rs and Pel,L are the elastic recoil pressures of the respiratory system and lung, respectively (*Insp* inspiration)

(Ptr and PL tracings, respectively). Chest wall information can be obtained by subtracting the pulmonary data from the corresponding respiratory system values.

For the precise measurement of $\Delta P1$, and, consequently, of resistance, the pressure required to overcome equipment resistance (tracheal tube, connectors, and so on) must be subtracted from raw $\Delta P1$. Conversely, the measurement of airway pressure can be performed by means of a catheter whose tip is placed distally to the tracheal tube tip.

Effects of flow and volume on resistance

Along with the traditional concepts about flow and volume dependences of resistance, the end-inflation occlusion method also indicates that pulmonary resistance should decrease with increasing lung volume and fall with decreasing flow in normal subjects [27, 28], and in patients with COPD [29, 30] and ARDS [26, 28, 31].

In the clinical setting the differences among patients, as well as in the same patient with time, may result from measurements performed under diverse ventilator settings, rather than reflect a true mechanical result of a medical manoeuvre or drug administration. Hence, the comparison of resistance values without standardized flow and volume is useless and may lead to erroneous (and dangerous) conclusions.

Conclusion

The fast drop in airway pressure after end-inspiratory occlusion may easily disclose the clinical evolution of a patient from the respiratory mechanical point of view. It suffices to perform the occlusion under the same ventilation settings (flow and volume), and to measure the change in pressure from peak value down to the inflexion point. If this variation is decreasing (i.e., resistance is falling) it means that the patient's condition is improving and vice-versa.

References

1. Bates JHT, Ludwig Ms, Sly PD, et al (1988) Interrupter resistance elucidated by alveolar pressure measurement in open-chest normal dogs. J Appl Physiol 6:808-814
2. Saldiva PHN, Zin WA, Santos RLB, et al (1992) Alveolar pressure measurement in open-chest rats. J Appl Physiol 72:302-306
3. Auler JOC Jr, Zin WA, Caldeira MPR, et al (1987) Pre- and postoperative inspiratory mechanics in ischemic and valvular heart disease. Chest 92:984-990
4. D'Angelo E, Prandi E, Tavola M, et al (1994) Chest wall interrupter resistance in anaesthetized paralysed humans. J Appl Physiol 77:883-887
5. Ingram RH Jr, Pedley TJ (1986) Pressure-flow relationships in the lungs. In: Macklem PT, Mead J (eds) Handbook of physiology. The respiratory system. Mechanics of breathing. American Physiology Society, Maryland, pp 277-293
6. Liistro GD, Stanescu D, Rodenstein D, et al (1989) Reassessment of the interruption technique for measuring flow resistance in humans. J Appl Physiol 67:933-937
7. Rohrer F (1915) Der Strömungswiderstand in den menschlichen Atemwegen und der Einfluss der unregelmässigen Verzweigung des Bronchialsystems auf den Atmungsverlauf verschiedenen Lungenbezirken. Pflügers Arch. Gesamte Physiol Menschen Tiere 162:225-229
8. Wirz K (1923) Das Verhalten des Druckes im Pleuraraum bei der Atmung und die Ursachen seiner Veränderlichkeit. Pflügers Arch. Gesamte Physiol Menschen Tiere 199:1-12
9. Von Neergaard K, Wirz K (1927) Die Messung der Strömungswiderstände in den Atemwegen des Menschen, insbesondere bei Asthma und Emphysem. Z Klin Med 105:51-82
10. Mead J, Whittenberger JL (1953) Physical properties of human lungs measured during spontaneous respiration. J Appl Physiol 5:779-796
11. DuBois AD, Botelho SY, Comroe JH Jr (1956) A new method for measuring airway resistance in man using a body plethysmograph; values in normal subjects and patients with respiratory disease. J Clin Invest 35:327-335
12. Rossi A, Gottfried SB, Higgs BD, et al (1985) Respiratory mechanics in mechanically ventilated patients with respiratory failure. J Appl Physiol 58:1849-1858
13. Gottfried SB, Rossi A, Calverley PMA, et al (1984) Interrupter technique for measurement of respiratory mechanics in anesthetized cats. J Appl Physiol 56:681-690
14. Bates JHT, Decramer M, Chartrand D, et al (1985) The volume-time profile during relaxed expiration in the normal dog. J Appl Physiol 59:732-737
15. Kochi T, Okubo S, Zin WA (1988) Flow and volume dependence of pulmonary mechanics in anesthetized cats. J Appl Physiol 64:441-450
16. Bates JHT, Baconnier P, Milic-Emili J (1988) A theoretical analysis of the interrupter technique for measuring respiratory mechanics. J Appl Physiol 64:2204-2214
17. Bates JHT, Milic-Emili J (1991) The flow interrupter technique for measuring respiratory resistance. J Crit Care 6:227-238
18. Milic-Emili J (1989) Pulmonary flow resistance. Lung 167:141-148
19. Neergaard K von, Wirz K (1927) Ueber eine Methode zur Messung der Lungen elastizität am lebenden Menschen insbesondere beim Emphysem. Z Klin Med 105:35-50
20. Don HF, Robson JC (1965) The mechanics of the respiratory system during anaesthesia: the effect of atropine and carbon dioxide. Anesthesiology 26:168-178
21. Rattenborg CC, Holaday DA (1966) Constant flow inflation of the lungs. Acta Anaesthesiol Scand [Suppl] 23:211-223
22. Bates JHT, Hunter I, Okubo S, et al (1987) Effect of valve closure time on the determination of respiratory resistance by flow interruption. Med Biol Eng Comput 25:136-140
23. Bates JHT, Sly PD, Okubo S (1987) General method for describing and extrapolating monotonic transients and its application to respiratory mechanics. Med Biol Eng Comput 25:131-135
24. Jackson AC, Milhorn HT, Norman JR (1974) A reevaluation of the interrupter technique for airway resistance measurement. J Appl Physiol 36:264-268

25. Guérin C, Coussa ML, Eissa NT, et al (1993) Lung and chest wall mechanics in mechanically ventilated COPD patients. J Appl Physiol 74:1570-1580
26. Eissa NT, Ranieri MV, Corbeil C, et al (1991) Analysis of behaviour of the respiratory system in ARDS patients: effects of flow, volume and time. J Appl Physiol 70:2719-2729
27. D'Angelo E, Calderini E, Torri G, et al (1989) Respiratory mechanics in anesthetized paralyzed humans: effects of flow, volume, and time. J Appl Physiol 67:2556-2564
28. Auler JOC Jr, Saldiva PHN, Carvalho CR, et al (1990) Flow and volume dependence of respiratory system mechanics during constant flow ventilation in normal subjects and in adult respiratory distress syndrome. Crit Care Med 18:1080-1086
29. Georgopoulos D, Mitrouska I, Markopoulou K, et al (1995) Effects of breathing pattern on mechanically ventilated patients with chronic obstructive pulmonary disease and dynamic hyperinflation. Intensive Care Med 21:880-886
30. Tantucci C, Corbeil C, Chassé M, et al (1991) Flow resistance in patients with chronic obstructive pulmonary disease in acute respiratory failure. Am Rev Respir Dis 144:384-389
31. Tantucci C, Corbeil C, Chassé M, et al (1992) Flow and volume dependence of respiratory system: flow resistance in patients with adult respiratory distress syndrome. Am Rev Respir Dis 145:355-360

Relaxed expiration

G.L. CHELUCCI

Passive deflation as exponential wash-out function

An exponential decay process is one in which the rate of change of the variable of interest is directly proportional to the variable itself. During passive exhalation, gas empties more or less exponentially after the end-inspiratory pause from the normal lung, driven by recoil pressure [1]. If respiratory system deflates as one compartment, the expression relating lung volume (V) at time "t" to the initial lung volume (V_0) is: $V(t) = V_0 e^{-kt}$. V_0 is the sum of tidal volume and any volume trapped above the relaxed equilibrium volume of the chest owing to dynamic hyperinflation. The constant "k" is equal to 1/(RC), in which R and C represent the resistance and pathway compliance of the respiratory system and "e" is the base of the natural (Napierian) logarithm system. The RC product is the time constant (τ), that is the time it takes to exhale 63% of the initial total lung volume contained above the equilibrium position of the respiratory system.

τ is a convenient expression for the *speed of response* of a system to external forcing (ΔP): C dictates, in a sense, *how far* the system has to go in response to a given ΔP, and R, *how fast it* can move while getting there. So, from the previous equation: $V(t) = V_0 e^{-t/\tau}$, when $t = \tau$: $V(t) = V_0 e^{-1}$ and, consequently: $V(t) = V_0 . 0.37$. Deflation is essentially complete 4 - 5 time constants after it begins. Increases in either R or C delay emptying. Briefly, lung emptying follows an exponential wash-out function [2, 3]. Thus, during expiration the rate of volume reduction changes at a rate, which decreases progressively with the reduction of aerated lung tissue. A wash-out function has the general form $y = y_0 . e^{-t/\tau}$, where the quantity of the variable "y" at time 0 is "y_0", the time constant is "τ", the elapsed time period is "t", and the base of the natural logarithm system is "e" [4]. After 1 time constant, "y" will have fallen to 1/e of its initial value or approximately 37 % of "y_0". After 2τ a change is 86.5 % complete, after 3τ it is 95 % and after 4τ it is 98.2 % complete. The *half-life*, which is the time required for "y" to change to half of its previous value, is 0.69τ. Time constant is ideally suited to compare the rate at which changes of lung volume occur during prolonged expiration, since τ is independent from the size of ventilated zones. Thus, it allows comparision of the dynamics of lung emptying in subjects with different levels of lung volumes.

Passive deflation in normal subjects

During passive expiration, the time-course of the fall in thoracic gas volume is determined by the mechanical properties of the respiratory system. The driven pressure is then provided entirely by the elastic recoil pressure of the total respiratory system, which is used to overcome the total expiratory flow resistance. Theoretical calculations, first proposed by Brody [1] in 1954 for a single-compartment model, indicate that if the compliance (Crs) and resistance (Rrs) of the respiratory system were fixed, the time-course of volume during passive expiration should follow a single exponential function:

$$V(t) = V_0 \cdot e^{-t/\tau rs} \quad (1)$$

where V is the volume of gas exhaled at any time "t", V_0 is the initial volume above the relaxation volume of the respiratory system, and τrs is time constant of the respiratory system, equal to the product of resistance and compliance ($\tau rs = Rrs.Crs$).

Bates et al. [5] have recently shown that in anaesthetized-paralyzed dogs the time-course of volume during passive expiration preceded by an end-inspiratory pause can better be described in terms of a double-exponential function:

$$V(t) = A_1 \cdot e^{-t/\tau_1 rs} + A_2 \cdot e^{-t/\tau_2 rs} \quad (2)$$

where A_1 and A_2 are the initial volumes of the fast and slow emptying compartment, $A_1 + A_2 = V_0$, τ_1 and τ_2 are the corresponding time constants, and where the relatively rapid first component reflects the pure resistive behaviour, while the second slower component is probably mainly due to the time constant inhomogeneities within the lung, i.e., "pendelluft", and to the viscoelastic properties of the pulmonary and chest wall tissues. In previous studies on humans, the time-course of volume during relaxed expirations has previously been studied in anaesthetized and paralyzed subjects, mechanically ventilated at zero end-expiratory airway pressure (ZEEP), but no mention has been made of a slow component during relaxed expiration [6-8]. Indeed, volume was obtained by electronic integration of the pneumotachograph signal and the late slow changes in volume during expiration were considered as integrator drift and, hence, were neglected. In normal humans [9,10], and dogs

[5], τ_2 is much longer than τ_1. This not only affects the time-course of lung emptying (Eq. 2) but also has profound implications in terms of dynamic work of breathing and frequency dependence (time dependency) of respiratory system resistance and compliance.

In the study of Chelucci et al. [9] on 11 comatose (self-poisoning) subjects with normal lungs, using the "*single-breath*" method, volume changes were measured by respiratory inductive plethysmography (RIP) placed around the rib cage. After a period of stable mechanical ventilation, end-inspiratory airway occlusions were performed with the manual tap. During the ensuing period of apnoea (5-6 s), relaxation of the respiratory muscles was shown by the rapid appearance of a plateau on the tracheal pressure tracing (Paw). The occlusion was then rapidly released, and the subjects allowed to expire freely at barometric pressure until full expiration was achieved, i.e., until the RIP signal was both steady for at least 1.5 s and indistinguishable from baseline (Fig. 1).

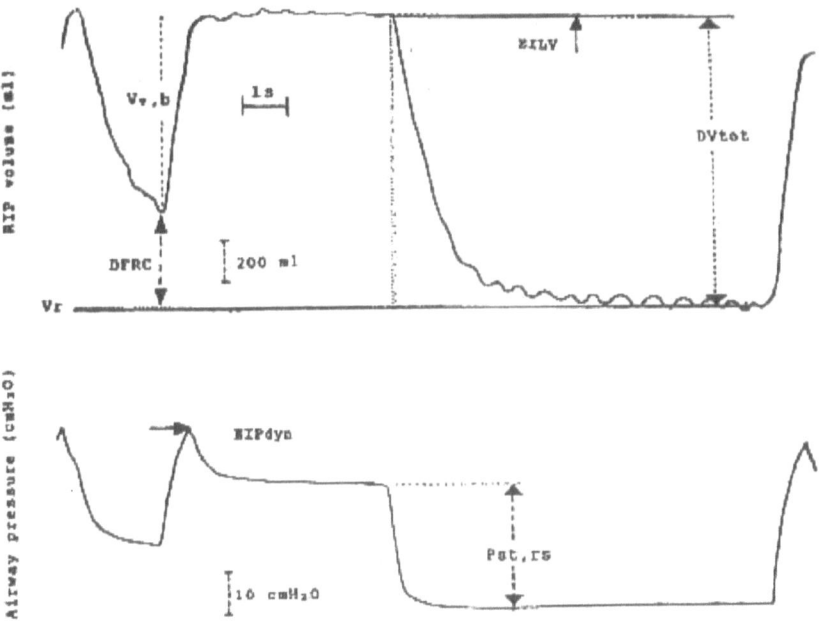

Fig. 1 *Top* example of changes in thoracic gas volume during passive expiration measured with a respiratory inductance plethysmograph (RIP) as a function of time. Passive lung deflation from baseline $V_T(V_T,b)$ starts from the end-inspiratory lung volume (EILV) and ends at relaxation volume (Vr). *DFRC* end-expiratory lung volume relative to Vr during baseline ventilation, *DVtot* total exhaled volume to Vr. *Bottom* changes in airway pressure measured at the airway opening as a function of time. *Pst,rs* represents the static elastic recoil pressure of the respiratory system. *EIPdyn* represents the end-inspiratory dynamic pressure

End-inspiratory occlusions were performed at baseline tidal volume (V_T) and at a lesser degree of lung inflation (partial inflation, V_Tp): about one-half of baseline V_T. RIP volume-time curves were digitized at 0.1 –s intervals (sampling frequency = 10 Hz) down to Vr and the data were analyzed for fitting in terms of a bi-exponential function.

The group average volume-time curves during passive expiration in the 11 normal subjects are shown in Fig. 2. These were clearly not mono- but rather bi-exponential. In all individuals, the bi-exponential model (Eq.2) better fitted the data than the mono-exponential one (Eq.1) for both V_T and V_Tp. The rapid component (Eq.2) represented 84±10% and 79±11 % of the total volume change at V_T and V_Tp, respectively. In line with previous reports [10-13] we assumed that the fast exponential compartment (corresponding to the rapid phase of passive expiration) of the volume-time decay reflects the time constant due to Cst,rs and the pure (Newtonian) resistance offered by the respiratory system plus that due to the endotracheal (ET) tube. Such behaviour, moreover, is in line with recent studies on anaesthetized paralyzed humans [10] and dogs [14], which showed that the respiratory system consists of two compartments: (1) a fast compartment, reflecting standard respiratory compliance (Cst,rs) and resistance; (2) a slow compartment, reflecting the viscoelastic properties of the thoracic tissues. These findings are consistent with a model of the respiratory system originally proposed by Mount [15].

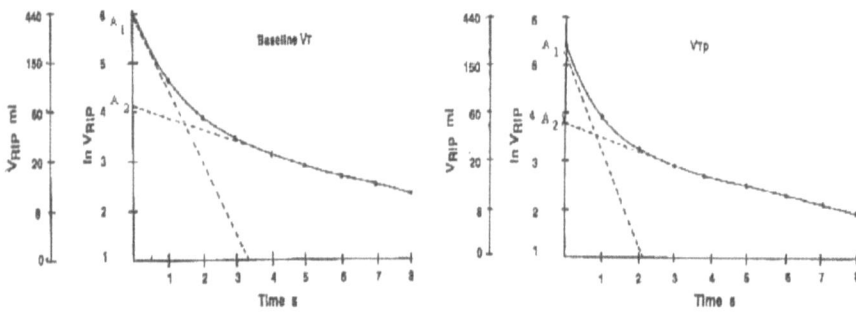

Fig. 2 Semilog plots of group-average volume-time curves for baseline tidal volume (V_T, *left panel*) and partial tidal volume (V_Tp, *right panel*). Curves were drawn through use of group-average parameters of the bi-exponential model. A_1 and A_2 are the coefficients of the equation, reflecting the volumes of the two compartments of lung emptying. *Dotted lines* represent the two exponential functions

In anaesthetized paralyzed dogs, Bates et al. [5] made computerized nume-
rical integration of the pneumotachograph flow signal, thus avoiding problems
due to drift. They were able to show that in dogs the volume-time profile
includes a slow compartment, as described by Eq.2. Moreover, Chelucci et al.
[9] indicated that in humans also the time-course of volume during relaxed
expiration is better described by a bi-exponential than by a mono-exponential
function. However, it is necessary to discuss the limitations of this analysis.
Both Eqs.1 and 2 are based on the assumption that the relevant time constants
are the product of a fixed compliance and expiratory resistance. The results of
Chelucci et al. [9], however, suggest that the system deviates from linearity.
Indeed, *firstly*, the lowering of Cst,rs with decreasing lung volume (V_{TP}) would
be expected to result in relatively faster lung emptying. Consequently, this
cannot explain the slow deflation compartment, which occurs late in expiration.
Secondly, when the resistance of the ET tube is taken into account, the flow
resistance of the respiratory system cannot be constant. Indeed, the ET tubes
offer a variable flow resistance that follows Rohrer's equation: $K_1 + K_2 V'$,
where K_1, K_2 are constants [8]. This should result in proportionately greater
diminution of expiratory flow rates during *early* passive expiration rather than
later on, and hence cannot explain the slow deflation component, which was
found in this study. *Moreover*, it is unlikely that changes in thoracic volume
due to continuing gas exchange in apnoea [16] would appreciably affect the
volume-time profile during the relatively short duration of expiration. *Thirdly*,
changes in thoracic blood volume could have an effect on the volume signals
of RIP. In fact, since positive end-expiratory pressure (PEEP) reduces both right
and left ventricular end-diastolic volumes [17], it is likely that intrathoracic
blood volume increased during passive expiration when intra-thoracic pressure
fell to barometric pressure. Therefore, changes in thoracic blood volume cannot
account for the slow compartment that we observed in these subjects during
passive expiration at barometric pressure. *Lastly*, small airway closure and gas
trapping or delayed gas emptying *via* collateral ventilation could have contributed to the slow expiratory compartment in these subjects. However, it is
highly likely that the slow compartment reflects the viscoelastic properties of
the pulmonary and chest wall tissues, as originally suggested by Bates et al.
[5]. In the subjects of Chelucci et al. [9], the rapid deflation component caused
emptying of 84±10% of the expired volume for inflation volume of 441±124
ml, whereas the slow component contributed only 16±7% of the expired
volume with a time constant about 6 times longer (3.27 s) than that of the fast
compartment (0.50 s). When the inflation volume was reduced to 249±91 ml,
the time constant of the slow compartment did not change significantly (2.95
s), while that of the rapid compartment decreased by 26% (0.37 s) ($P<0.05$).

This was probably due to both the concomitant decrease (-15%) in Cst,rs (46 ml/cmH$_2$O vs. 53 ml/cmH$_2$O) and the curvilinear pressure-flow relationships of the ET tubes [8]. As postulated by Bates et al. [5], the time constant of the fast compartment probably reflects the product of standard Rrs and Cst,rs, where Rrs is the pure (ohmic) component of total expiratory flow resistance (including the ET tube), whereas the time constant of the slow compartment reflects the viscoelastic properties of the pulmonary and chest wall tissues and time constants inequalities within the lung (*"pendelluft"*) [10,11]. In contrast, the values of time constant of the slow compartment should be less affected by the presence of the ET tubes. In fact, it is this slow compartment that may well explain the frequency dependence of compliance and flow resistance of the lung and chest wall found both in animals [14] and humans [10].

In conclusion, these results show that in intubated humans (as in anaesthetized paralyzed dogs), the time course of volume during passive expiration is characterized by a fast and a slow exponential compartment and suggest that the mono-exponential model is not suitable to determine the mechanical properties of the respiratory system in normal subjects.

Passive deflation in ARDS patients, mechanically ventilated on ZEEP

The first mechanical model of the respiratory system was introduced in 1950 by Otis et al. [18]. It consisted of a single compartment of constant elastance (Ers), served by a pathway of constant resistance (Rrs), and hence was characterized by a single energy storage time constant ($\tau rs = Rrs/Ers$). Based on this model, the time-course of volume (V), during the portion of passive deflation corresponding to decreasing flow, should be described by a single-exponential function [1]. However, recent studies on normal anaesthetized paralyzed dogs [5] and humans [9] have shown that passive expiration preceded by an end-inspiratory pause is better described by a double-exponential function.

In the study of Chelucci et al. [19], the authors determined the constants in Eq.2 in intubated paralyzed patients with acute respiratory distress syndrome (ARDS), together with static elastance of the respiratory system (Est,rs), showed their passive expiratory kinetics can be adequately described by a bi-exponential function (Eq.2), and interpreted the results in terms of a viscoelastic model of the respiratory system [11, 13] (Fig. 3). In its simplest form, this model consists of two compartments in parallel: a dashpot, which in humans represents airway resistance (Raw), and a Kelvin body. The latter consists of a spring representing the static elastance of the respiratory system (Est,rs) in parallel with a Maxwell body, i.e., a spring (E$_2$) and a dashpot (R$_2$) arranged serially. E$_2$ and R$_2$ represent the elastance and resistance of the viscoelastic

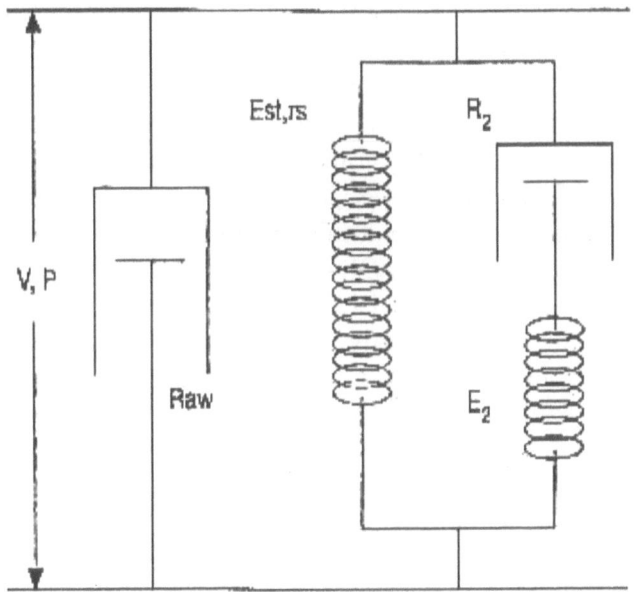

Fig. 3 Scheme of spring-and-dashpot model for interpretation of respiratory dynamics. Respiratory system consists of airway resistance (*Raw*), in parallel with standard elastance (*Est,rs*), and with a series spring-and-dashpot body (E_2, R_2, respectively) that represents stress adaptation units. Distance and tension between two *horizontal bars* are analogue of lung volume (*V*) and of pressure at airway opening (*P*), respectively, (modified from [13])

(stress adaptation) units within the pulmonary and chest wall tissues. The corresponding viscoelastic time constant (τ_2) is given by the ratio R_2/E_2. The distance between the two horizontal bars is analogue of lung volume (V), and the tension between these bars is analogue of Paw. Under elastic equilibrium condition (Paw = 0), the tension in both springs is nil, and V corresponds to the relaxation volume of the respiratory system (Vr).

When the model is elongated slowly (analogue to very low flow), the dashpot R_2 has time enough to move and dissipate the tension in spring E_2, the spring E_2 should remain at its elastic equilibrium length (l_0), at which its tension is nil, and Pel,rs = Pst,rs = Est,rs.ΔV.

In contrast, at higher elongation speeds (equivalent to higher inflation flows or when inflation time is very short in relation to τ_2), the dashpot R_2 will not move at all, there will be insufficient time for the tension in spring E_2 to be entirely dissipated through the dashpot R_2, so that Pel,rs will be necessarily > Pst,rs. With springs Est,rs and E_2 in parallel, the relationship between Pel,rs and ΔV will be: Pel,rs = (Est,rs+E_2).ΔV.

If a *"flow interruption"* manoeuvre (i.e., a pause) is performed by halting the relative movement of the two horizontal bars for a time $> 3\tau_2$, the spring E_2 will gradually return to l_0, i.e., spring E_2 will now exert zero tension. Under these conditions, the end-inspiratory Pel,rs will be given by Est,rs.ΔV, and passive expiration will necessarily include a slow compartment (A_2), representing the gradual relaxation of spring E_2 until it returns to l_0 at Vr.

In the study of Chelucci et al. [19], measurements were obtained following a 5- to 6-s end-inspiratory pause, a time long enough for spring E_2 to attain relaxation in both normal subjects [9] and ARDS patients. Accordingly, in these ARDS patients, A_1 amounted to 81±7% of V_T, while A_2 amounted to 19±6% of V_T and did not differ significantly from the values (16±7% of V_T) obtained using the same technique (*"single-breath"* method) in 11 comatose (self-poisoning) subjects with normal lungs [9]. The values of time constants were similar in both groups: $\tau_1 = 0.35\pm0.11$ s (ARDS) versus 0.50±0.22 s (normals); $\tau_2 = 4.67\pm2.38$ s (ARDS) versus 3.27±1.54 s (normals). The absence of a significant difference in $\tau2$ between ARDS patients and normal subjects suggests that in ARDS the tissues subtending the aerated and ventilated lung units exhibit relatively normal viscoelastic behaviour. This fits the notion that ARDS is characterized by a bi-modal distribution: (1) normal aerated and ventilated units; (2) abnormal non-aerated and non-ventilated units. Indeed, in such case, τ_2 of the remaining normal lung units should be the same as in normal subjects.

Figure 4 depicts the time-course of volume decay during passive lung

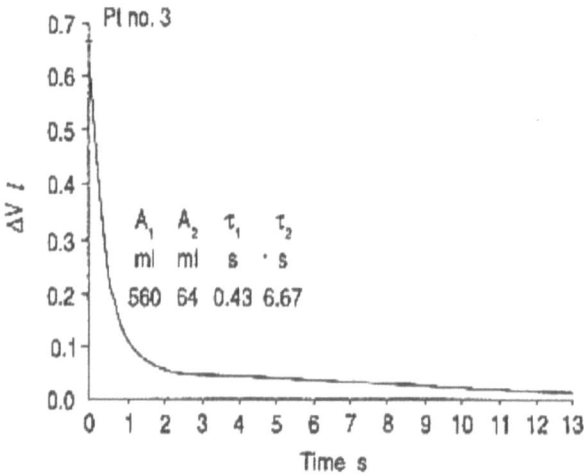

Fig. 4 Relationship between changes in volume (ΔV) and time during passive expiration in a representative acute respiratory distress syndrome (ARDS) patient. Experimental points closely fit Eq.2 ($r>0.99$). A_1 and A_2, τ_1 and τ_2: coefficients of bi-exponential model fit (Eq.2)

deflation in a representative patient. The change in volume as a function of time is well described by the bi-exponential model (Eq.2), as indicated by the high value of the correlation coefficient ($r>0.99$). Similar results were obtained in the other patients ($r>0.99$). On average, τ_2 was 13.3 times longer than τ_1..

Passive deflation in ARDS patients, mechanically ventilated on PEEP

Originally, ARDS was thought to be due to a generalized increase in *lung stiffness*, resulting in a decrease in lung volume [20]. In reality, the lungs of ARDS patients do not exhibit generalized stiffness but instead are functionally small (*baby lung*) [21]. Consequently, the common clinical practice of ventilating ARDS patients with a relatively large inflation volume may result in alveolar overdistension of "normally aerated" areas (*volutrauma*).

Moreover, recent reports indicate that with the respiratory system compliance decreasing, resistance increases markedly in ARDS [22], with expiratory resistance (strongly influenced by the mechanical properties of the airways and lung parenchyma) exceeding the inspiratory one. Moreover, measurement of resistance during expiration is problematic, because flow is continuously changing. However, previous studies in ARDS patients [19] and normal subjects [9], based on the *"single-breath"* method and the measurement of time constants of a passive expiration, have allowed computation of the respiratory system resistance (if compliance is known) and show that relaxed exhalation can be well characterized by a fast and a slow emptying compartment.

In mechanically ventilated ARDS patients, PEEP is generally assumed to cause a decrease in airway resistance due to the concomitant increase in lung volume. Indeed, PEEP is thought to augment lung volume by recruiting collapsed alveoli, thus improving pulmonary gas exchange. However, in ARDS patients the number of aerated lung units is markedly reduced and, as a result, the range of inflation volumes required to reach the flat portion of their static volume-pressure curve – corresponding to a deleterious zone from a mechanical point a view – is narrower [23]. Under these conditions it is not surprising that the use of high PEEP and relatively large tidal volumes can induce ventilator-induced lung injury. Moreover, there are no systematic studies in which the effect of the association of PEEP with different V_Ts on passive lung deflation has been quantified in ARDS patients, mechanically ventilated on PEEP. In the study of Chelucci et al. [24], the authors evaluated: (1) the presence of a two-compartment kinetic behaviour of the respiratory system during relaxed expiration; (2) how the constants describing these two compartments would be affected by different tidal volumes and PEEP; (3) the effect of the respiratory system resistance and elastance during mechanical ventilation on

PEEP and increasing tidal volume. Experimental procedure was not different from the previous experiments carried out on PEEP= 0 (ZEEP) conditions [19]. End-inspiratory occlusions were randomly performed on PEEP (13 ± 4 cmH$_2$O, on average) at baseline tidal volume (V_T,b = 8.5 ml/kg, on average) and at an inflation volume of about $0.5V_T$,b (4.3 ml/kg, on average) and compared with those on ZEEP at V_T,b. In each patient PEEP was adjusted as "*best*" PEEP [25]. This study shows two noteworthy observations: (1) the association of PEEP with two different tidal volumes does not modify the kinetic characteristics of the bi-exponential curve during passive expiration in ARDS patients. In other words, there is no significant difference among values characterizing passive lung deflation: this suggests that the mechanical properties of the recruited units are similar to those of the previously open lung; (2) airway resistance appears to increase as tidal volume increases (V_T,b vs. $0.5V_T$,b), in the presence of PEEP. In all patients the bi-exponential model fitted the data better than the mono-exponential one under PEEP. In all instances the V(t) curves closely fitted the bi-exponential function: $0.972 < r^2 < 6\,2.998$, and $0.978 < r^2 < 6\,2.998$ at $0.5V_T$,b and V_T,b, respectively. The group average curves obtained under the two experimental conditions are shown in Fig. 5. On PEEP the fast compartment (A_1) was responsible for $84\pm7\%$ ($0.5V_T$,b) and $86\pm5\%$ (V_T,b) versus $81\pm6\%$ on ZEEP (P=ns) of the total exhaled volume, with τ_1 of 0.50 ± 0.13 s and 0.58 ± 0.17 s versus 0.35 ± 0.11 s on ZEEP, respectively. There was a significant difference ($P<0.02$) in the mean τ_1 only between V_T,b on PEEP (0.58 s) and V_T,b on ZEEP (0.35 s). On PEEP the slow compartment (A_2) contributes $16\pm7\%$ ($0.5V_T$,b) and $14\pm5\%$ (V_T,b) versus $19\pm6\%$ on ZEEP (P=ns) of the total exhaled volume, with τ_2 of 6.46 ± 3.45 s ($0.5V_T$,b) and 6.44 ± 2.79 s (V_T,b) with PEEP versus 4.67 ± 2.38 s (V_T,b) on ZEEP, respectively (P=ns). Among the various conditions studied, Raw was significantly higher (46 %) ($P<0.05$) at V_T,b on PEEP that at V_T,b on ZEEP. These findings support the conclusion that the increase in τ_1 was due mainly to increased Raw. Indeed, the effects of PEEP on airway resistance may depend on the degree of lung distension. Possibly this behaviour is a consequence of longitudinal stretching of large airways by high lung volumes (V_T,b + PEEP), which results in a decrease in their calibre secondary to the mechanical interdependence of lung parenchyma and airways [26].

In conclusion, in ARDS patients: (1) the behaviour of airway resistance seems to depend on the degree of the prevailing lung distension; (2) PEEP changes the mechanical properties of the respiratory system fast-emptying compartment.

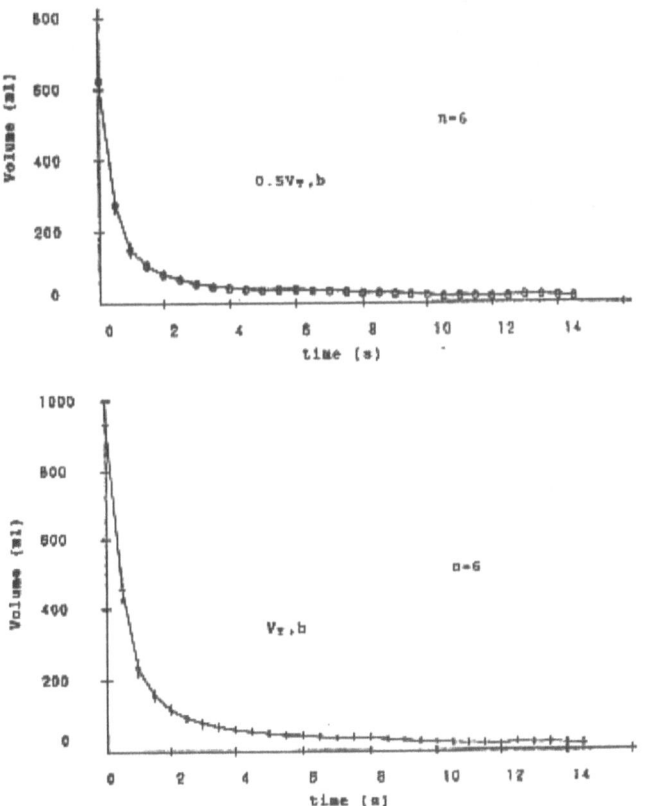

Fig. 5 Each data point corresponds to the group average changes of volume as a function of time during passive expiration after inspiration to half tidal volume (0.5V_T,b) *(top)* and to tidal volume (V_T,b) *(bottom)* of 6 ARDS patients on positive end-expiratory pressure. *Bars* represent ± 1 SD.

References

1. Brody AN (1954) Mechanical compliance and resistance of the lung-thorax calculated from the flow recorded during passive exhalation. Am J Physiol 178:189-196
2. Neumann P, Berglund JE, Mondejar EF, et al (1998) Dynamics of lung collapse and recruitment during prolonged breathing in porcine lung injury. J Appl Physiol 85:1533-1543
3. Rothen HU, Neumann P, Berglund JE, et al (1999) Dynamics of re-expansion of atelectasis during general anaesthesia. Br J Anaesth 82:551-556
4. Nunn JF (1993) Applied respiratory physiology, 2nd edn Butterworth-Heinemann, Oxford
5. Bates JHT, Decramer M, Chartrand D, et al (1985) Volume-time profile during relaxed expiration in the normal dog. J Appl Physiol 59:732-737
6. McIlroy MB, Tierney DF, Nadel JA (1963) A new method for measurement of compliance and resistance of lungs and thorax. J Appl Physiol 17:424-427
7. Bergman NA (1966) Measurement of respiratory resistance in anesthetized subjects. J Appl Physiol 21:1913-1917

8. Behrakis PK, Higgs BD, Baydur A, et al (1983) Respiratory mechanics during halothane anesthesia and anesthesia-paralysis in humans. J Appl Physiol 55:1085-1092
9. Chelucci GL, Brunet F, Dall'Ava-Santucci J, et al (1991) A single-compartment model cannot describe passive expiration in intubated, paralysed humans. Eur Respir J 4:458-464
10. D'Angelo E, Calderini E, Torri G, et al (1989) Respiratory mechanics in anesthetized paralyzed humans: effects of flow, volume, and time. J Appl Physiol 67:2556-2564
11. Bates JHT, Decramer M, Zin WA, et al (1986) Respiratory resistance with histamine challenge by single-breath and forced oscillation method. J Appl Physiol 61:873-880
12. Bates JHT, Baconnier P, Milic-Emili J (1988) A theoretical analysis of interrupter technique for measuring respiratory mechanics. J Appl Physiol 64:2204-2214
13. Bates JHT, Brown KA, Kochi T (1989) Respiratory mechanics in the normal dog determined by expiratory flow interruption. J Appl Physiol 67:2276-2285
14. Similowski T, Levy P, Corbeil C, et al (1989) Viscoelastic behaviour of lung and chest wall in dogs determined by flow interruption. J Appl Physiol 67:2219-2229
15. Mount LE (1955) The ventilation flow-resistance and compliance of rat lungs. J Physiol (Lond) 127:157-167
16. Dall'Ava-Santucci J, Armaganidis A, Brunet F, et al (1988) Causes of error of respiratory pressure-volume curves in paralyzed subjects. J Appl Physiol 64:42-49
17. Fewell JE, Abendschein DR, Carlson CJ, et al (1980) Mechanism of decreased right and left ventricular end-diastolic volumes during continuous positive-ventilation in dogs. Circ Res 47:467-472
18. Otis AB, Fenn WO, Rahn H (1950) Mechanics of breathing in man. J Appl Physiol 2:592-607
19. Chelucci GL, Dall'Ava-Santucci J, Dhainaut JF, et al (1993) Modelling of passive expiration in patients with adult respiratory distress syndrome. Eur Respir J 6:785-790
20. Bone RC (1993) A new therapy for the adult respiratory distress syndrome. N Engl J Med 328:431-432
21. Gattinoni L, Pesenti A, Avalli L, et al (1987) Pressure-volume curve of total respiratory system in acute respiratory failure: CT scan study. Am Rev Respir Dis 136:730-736
22. Pesenti A, Pelosi P, Rossi N, et al (1991) The effects of positive end-expiratory pressure on respiratory resistance in patients with adult respiratory distress syndrome and in normal anesthetized subjects. Am Rev Respir Dis 144:101-107
23. Amato M, Barbas C, Medeiros D, et al (1995) Beneficial effects of the "open lung" approach with low distending pressures in acute respiratory distress syndrome. A prospective randomized study on mechanical ventilation. Am J Respir Crit Care Med 152:1835-1846
24. Chelucci GL, Dall'Ava-Santucci J, Dhainaut JF, et al (2000) Association of PEEP with two different inflation volumes in ARDS patients: effects on passive lung deflation and alveolar recruitment. Intensive Care Med 26:870-877
25. Suter PM, Fairley B, Isenberg MD (1975) Optimum end-expiratory airway pressure in patients with acute pulmonary failure. N Engl J Med 292:284-289
26. Vincent NJ, Knudson R, Leith DE, et al (1970) Factors influencing pulmonary resistance. J Appl Physiol 29:236-243

Dynamic hyperinflation

W.A. ZIN

Although not difficult to accomplish, the precise identification of dynamic hyperinflation and the subsequent interpretation of the results demand awareness of exact theoretical and methodological concepts. The detection of dynamic hyperinflation is of paramount importance in critically ill patients because it may lead to increased work of breathing and respiratory muscle fatigue, cardiocirculatory collapse, interference with the triggering of the ventilator, and some other undesirable consequences.

Physiological basis

In normal subjects breathing at rest the end-expiratory lung volume (EELV) closely approximates the elastic equilibrium volume or relaxation volume (Vr) of the respiratory system [1]. When the rate of lung emptying is slowed down, there is a chance of EELV becoming higher than Vr, a condition termed dynamic hyperinflation [2-8]. Hence, dynamic hyperinflation is initiated when the tidal volume cannot be exhaled completely during the allotted expiratory duration [3]. The same process of incomplete emptying is repeated with subsequent tidal breaths. An equilibrium is quickly reached, allowing the entire tidal volume to be exhaled because the increased elastic recoil pressure and a wider airway caliber at the higher lung volume serve to enhance expiratory flow.

The existence of dynamic hyperinflation thus yields an increased static recoil pressure that is transmitted to the alveoli. Under these conditions, end-expiratory alveolar pressure is positive relative to airway opening pressure. This positive pressure is called auto-PEEP [9] or intrinsic PEEP (PEEPi) [2, 10]. Unfortunately, the increase in lung volume that allows the tidal volume to be exhaled may lead to alveolar hyperdistension, which in association with PEEPi may generate undesirable consequences.

In patients with airflow limitation [11-14], hyperinflation results from dynamic airway collapse. It can also arise in subjects without dynamic airway collapse if there is inadequate time available during expiration for the alveolar pressure to reach equilibrium with the airway opening pressure.

It is important to appreciate that dynamic hyperinflation with PEEPi and expiratory flow limitation need not always coexist. Patients who are not flow limited may develop significant PEEPi if expiratory duration is significantly shortened as a result of high ventilation or prolongation of inspiratory duration. Conversely, prolongation of expiration may allow some flow-limited patients to reach their Vr by the onset of the next inspiration.

Characteristics

Dynamic hyperinflation and the ensuing PEEPi can be characterized by:
-   alveolar pressure remaining greater than extrinsic PEEP throughout expiration, as depicted in Fig. 1;
-   detection of expiratory flow up to the beginning of the subsequent inspiration, unless airways collapse is present;
-   possible presence of high expiratory resistance or expiratory flow limitation;
-   dependence on respiratory system compliance, lung volume at the beginning of expiration, and expiratory duration;
-   being generated by any mode of artificial ventilation.

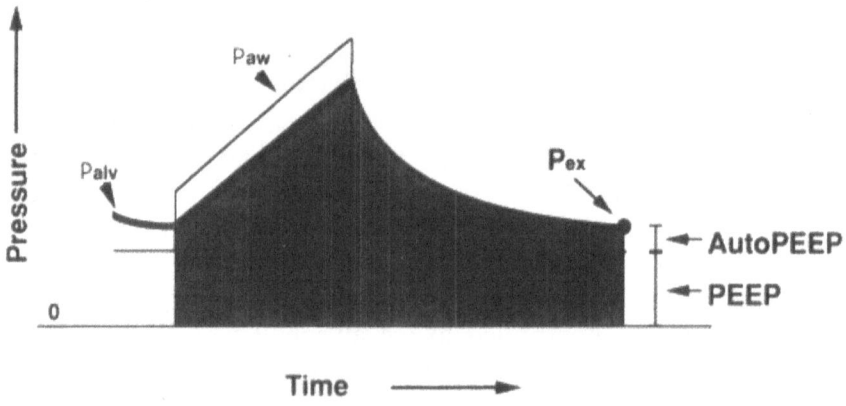

Fig. 1 Schematic diagram of the airway (Paw) and alveolar (Palv) pressures during a volume-cycled positive-pressure breath delivered to a passively ventilated patient with increased airway resistance. Positive end-expiratory alveolar pressure (Pex) equals the sum of applied positive end-expiratory pressure (PEEP) and the positive end-expiratory pressure resulting from dynamic hyperinflation (auto-PEEP)

Causes

Dynamic hyperinflation can be most frequently caused by either slow pulmonary emptying or inadequate ventilator setting. In intensive care unit patients, the main factors that may lead to dynamic hyperinflation are listed in Table 1.

Table 1 Factors that may lead to dynamic pulmonary hyperinflation in ICU patients (Ti inspiratory duration, $Ttot$ total duration of the breathing cycle)

Slow pulmonary emptying

  Patient's characteristics
    Increased compliance
    Increased expiratory resistance
    Airflow limitation

  Physical characteristics of the ventilation tubing
    Narrow tracheal tube
    Kinking of expiratory circuit
    Liquid accumulation in the tubing pathway
    Connectors, valves, humidifiers

Ventilator settings
    Large tidal volume
    High respiratory frequency
    High Ti/Ttot – inverse ration ventilation
    End-inspiratory pause

Patient's characteristics

Increased airway collapsibility has been recognized in patients with advanced chronic obstructive pulmonary disease [15]. This phenomenon has been attributed to destruction of lung parenchyma, with loss of lung elastic recoil, resulting in an increased compliance. In severe asthma, the structural changes within the airway wall itself (increases in airway smooth muscle, bronchomotor tone, and inflammatory infiltration) may stiffen it, and decrease collapsibility despite considerable reduction in airway calibre, yielding an increase in airflow resistance [16, 17].

Physical characteristics of the ventilation tubing

Tracheal tubes, exhalation valves, and PEEP devices play an important and frequently underestimated role in overall resistance, adding an expiratory delay [18-20]. One must always look for unnecessary pieces of tubing or valves and eliminate them off the circuit. Gay et al. [21] reported that the addition of a small resistive load, in the form of the expiratory circuit of the ventilator, reduced expiratory flow, thus facilitating the appearance of dynamic hyperinflation.

Ventilator settings

The ventilator setting can contribute to dynamic hyperinflation to the extent that a high respiratory frequency and the use of an elevated I:E ratio may yield too short an expiratory duration, thus impairing lung emptying. One should also consider that both pressure control and volume control ventilation can lead to dynamic hyperinflation, as shown in Fig. 2. Figure 2 shows that the introduction

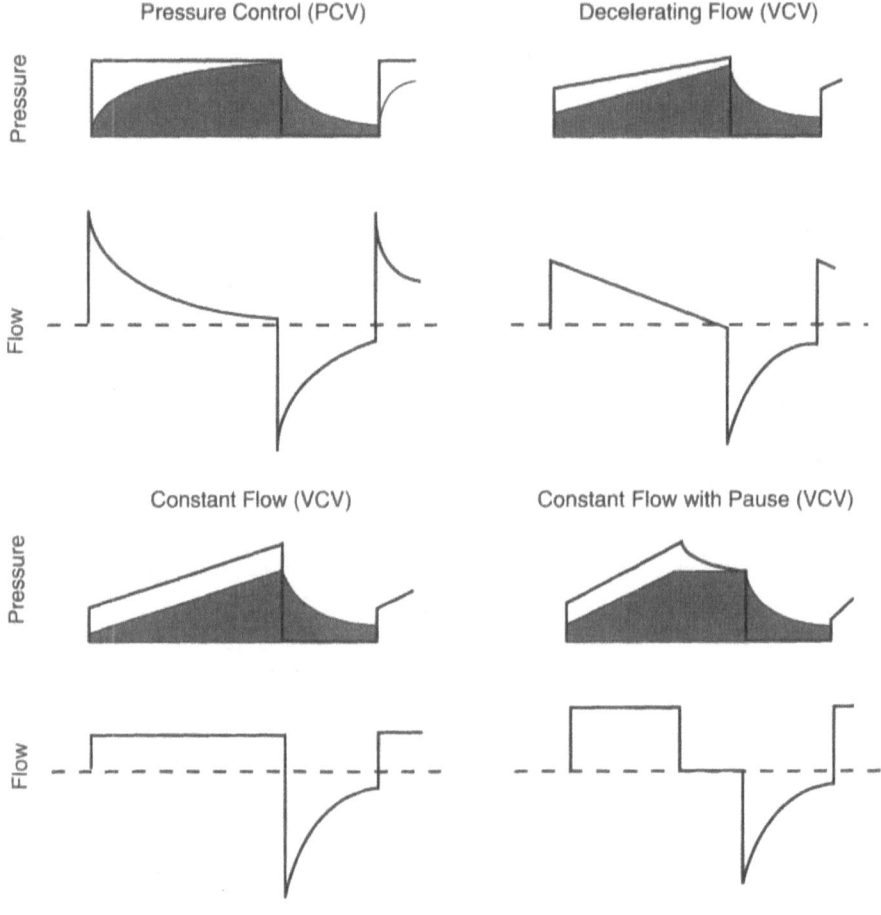

Fig. 2 Pressure and flow plotted against time of pressure control ventilation (PCV) and three variations of volume control ventilation (VCV): decelerating flow, slow constant flow, and constant flow with an end-inspiratory pause. The *shaded area* of the pressure-time tracing represents alveolar pressure, while the *solid line* depicts the airway pressure profile

of an end-inspiratory pause can also diminish expiratory duration. In this same context, if tidal volume is high, one should bear in mind the need to adjust expiratory duration accordingly [3, 22-25].

Consequences

Excessive pulmonary hyperinflation may yield serious pulmonary and cardio-vascular alterations (Table 2).

Table 2 Consequences of dynamic hyperinflation (*TLC* total lung capcity)

Barotrauma
The respiratory system will cycle at volumes closer to TLC, where compliance is decreased
Increased respiratory work during weaning attempts
Interference with ventilator triggering in assisted and pressure support modes
Respiratory muscle fatigue
Possible underestimation of respiratory system compliance
Cardiocirculatory collapse

Respiratory

As lung volumes become higher, barotrauma is the first obvious complication to be avoided. Pneumothorax, pneumomediastinum, subcutaneous emphyse-ma, and other forms of extra-alveolar air are collectively termed barotrauma. Alveolar rupture can lead to these different clinical manifestations, depending upon the amount of gas that enters the pulmonary interstitium and where the path of least resistante takes it. Although the term implies a lesion resulting from excessive pressure, under the present approach it is more likely that excessive alveolar distending volume, rather than high pressure per se, is the responsible agent [26, 27].

In the presence of dynamic hyperinflation the respiratory system will cycle at volumes closer to total lung capacity, where compliance is decreased [2, 28]. Both high lung volume and decreased compliance associated with elevated respiratory resistance will increase the work of breathing and the energy required for any level of minute ventilation. The work of breathing itself will increase CO_2 production, and thence the minute ventilation requirement. A further increase in energy expenditure because of increased anatomical and physiological dead space will occur.

Unfortunately, the respiratory muscles will be compromised too. The chest wall conformational changes resulting from the hyperinflation not only position the respiratory muscle fibres on a disadvantageous portion of their length-tension curve, but the altered orientation of the diaphragm to the rib cage reduces its mechanical efficiency [29-35]. Respiratory failure ensues when the respiratory muscles fail to compensate for the mechanical disadvantage and maintain sufficient minute ventilation to prevent abnormal values of blood gases and pH.

The concomitant PEEPi represents a threshold inspiratory load on the muscles of the respiratory system [36, 37], which will interfere with the ventilator triggering in assisted and pressure support modes [25, 28]. Respiratory work during weaning attempts will increase [38, 39].

Finally, during measurements the pressure gradient required to generate tidal breathing may be possibly overestimated, thus leading to underestimation of respiratory system compliance [2, 23]. PEEPi must be subtracted from the total static pressure to allow a correct determination of compliance.

Cardiocirculatory

The cardiovascular system is made up of several vascular compartments generally linked in series. In this context the abdominal and thoracic large veins, the right heart, alveolar and extra-alveolar pulmonary vascular beds, the left heart and the aorta (both thoracic and abdominal) represent diverse compartments subjected to the ever-changing extramural pressure during the breathing cycle. Thus, modifications of intrathoracic (pleural) pressure and volume significantly alter the haemodynamics of vascular beds within the thorax. On the other hand, the abdominal vasculature is affected by the movements of the diaphragm. Blood flow in each compartment is influenced by changes in the surrounding pressure, the compliance of the vessel, and the pre- and afterloads.

The predominant haemodynamic consequences of high lung volumes are the mechanical changes on the vasculature and cardiac chambers. Indeed, haemodynamics is jeopardized as if external PEEP were the causal agent [40, 41]. These effects are more prominent in volume-depleted patients and in those with pre-existing cardiac disease [42].

High intrathoracic pressure affects both the venous return to the right ventricle (RV) and the systemic left ventricle (LV) outflow [43]. There is a reduction of the venous gradient for right atrial filling (decreased RV preload), pulmonary vascular resistance may be elevated, thereby increasing RV afterload [40], which may compromise the forward output of that chamber. To overcome this effect, RV volume usually augments to maintain RV output. Intrapericardial pressure may increase, thwarting LV compliance [44]. Additionally, pulmonary hyperinflation can compress the heart, reducing the compliance of both ventricles [45].

Overzealous manual ventilation can rapidly worsen dynamic hyperinflation and drop cardiac output and blood pressure. Abrupt, severe hypotension caused by progressive dynamic hyperinflation ensues, with distended neck veins, severe dyspnea, agitation, cardiovascular collapse, and oxygen desaturation.

Measurement

The absolute functional residual capcity (FRC) can be measured during mechanical ventilation by an adaptation of the dilution method [46]. However, this method cannot determine total thoracic gas volume, but rather the gas contained in airspaces with open airways. On the other hand, the difference between EELV and Vr, defined as ΔFRC, can be easily obtained by prolonging the expiratory time and, hence, allowing the patient to exhale to Vr (Fig. 3) [47-49]. The monitoring of ΔFRC is recommended in patients with acute asthma to prevent excessive alveolar overdistension and barotraumas [48]. It has been

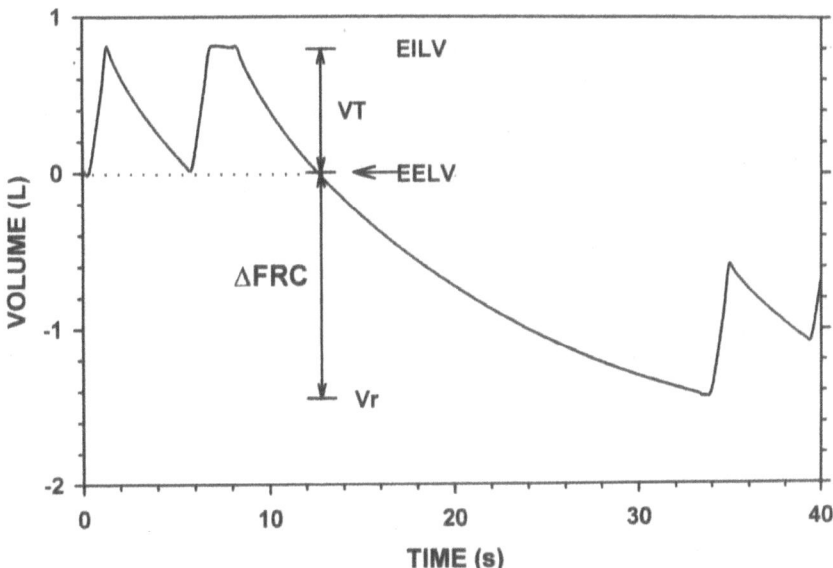

Fig. 3 Volume-time profile with a complete relaxed prolonged expiration following a short end-inspiratory pause in a ventilated patient. Lung volume above relaxation volume of the respiratory system (Vr), i.e., end-inspiratory lung volume (EILV) is composed of the tidal volume (VT) plus the amount of gas collected during the breathing pause from the end-expiratory lung volume (EELV) to Vr (=ΔFRC)

demonstrated that maintaining ΔFRC below 20 ml/kg can improve survival in asthma [48]. This manoeuvre is simple and adequate for bedside monitoring in relaxed patients. Its drawback rests on the fact that even 30 s may not suffice for patients with extreme airway obstruction to exhale to Vr.

The expired volume-flow loop could also be used to evaluate ΔFRC. For this purpose a complete relaxed expiration, allowing the patient to reach true Vr, would be superimposed on a control breath. ΔFRC is the difference between the apparent FRC level (control breath) and the volume when flow becomes nil on the relaxed expiration. Clearly, the same restriction pertaining to the prolongation of expiratory time applies to the volume-flow method.

References

1. Shee CD, Ploy-sang-song Y, Milic-Emili J (1985) Decay of inspiratory muscle pressure during expiration in conscious humans. J Appl Physiol 58:1859-1865
2. Rossi A, Gottfried SB, Zocchi L, et al (1985) Measurement of static compliance of the total respiratory system in patients with acute respiratory failure during mechanical ventilation. The effect of "intrinsic" PEEP. Am Rev Respir Dis 131:672-677
3. Marcy TW, Marini JJ (1994) Respiratory distress in the ventilated patient. Clin Chest Med 15:55-73
4. Kimball WR, Leith DE, Robins AG (1982) Dynamic hyperinflation and ventilator dependence in chronic obstructive pulmonary disease. Am Rev Respir Dis 126:991-995
5. Broseghini C, Brandolese R, Poggi R, et al (1988) Respiratory mechanics during the first day of mechanical ventilation in patients with pulmonary edema and chronic airway obstruction. Am Rev Respir Dis 138:355-361
6. Fleury B, Murciano D, Talamo C, et al (1985) Work of breathing in patients with obstructive pulmonary disease in acute respiratory failure. Am Rev Respir Dis 131:822-827
7. Gottfried SB, Rossi A, Higgs BD, et al (1985) Noninvasive determination of respiratory mechanics during mechanical ventilation for acute respiratory failure. Am Rev Respir Dis 131:414-420
8. Ranieri VM, Grasso S, Fiore T, Giuliani R (1996) Auto-positive end-expiratory pressure and dynamic hyperinflation. Clin Chest Med 17:379-394
9. Pepe PE, Marini JJ (1982) Occult positive end-expiratory pressure in mechanically ventilated patients with airflow obstruction: the auto-PEEP effect. Am Rev Respir Dis 126:166-170
10. Rossi A, Polese G, Brandi G, et al (1995) The intrinsic positive end expiratory pressure (PEEPi): physiology, implications, measurement, and treatment. Intensive Care Med 21:522-536
11. Fry DL, Ebert RV, Stead WW, et al (1954) The mechanics of pulmonary ventilation in normal subjects and in patients with emphysema. Am J Med 16:80-97
12. Fry DL, Hyatt RE (1960) Pulmonary mechanics: a unified analysis of the relationship between pressure, volume and gasflow in the lungs of normal and diseased human subjects. Am J Med 29:672-689
13. Dayman H (1951) Mechanics of airflow in health and in emphysema. J Clin Invest 30:1175-1190
14. Fry DL (1958) Theoretical considerations of the bronchial pressure-flow-volume relationships with particular reference to the maximum expiratory flow-volume curve. Phys Med Biol 3:174-194
15. Pride NB, Permutt S, Riley RL, et al (1967) Determinants of maximal expiratory flow from the lungs. J Appl Physiol 23:646-662

16. Djukanovic R, Roche WR, Wilson JW, et al (1990) Mucosal inflammation in asthma. Am Rev Respir Dis 142:434-457
17. Ebina M, Yaegashi H, Chiba R, et al (1990) Hyperreactive site in the airway tree of asthmatic patients revealed by thickening of bronchial muscles, Am Rev Respir Dis 141:1327-1332
18. Rocco PRM, Zin WA (1995) Modelling the mechanical effects of tracheal tubes on normal subjects. Eur Respir J 8:121-126
19. Marini JJ (1994) Airway resistance – an old friend revisited. Intensive Care Med 20:401-402
20. Wright PE, Marini JJ, Bernard GR (1989) In vitro versus in vivo comparison of endotracheal tube airflow resistance. Am Rev Respir Dis 140:10-16
21. Gay CC, Rodarte JR, Hubmayr RD (1989) The effects of positive expiratory pressures on isovolume flow and dynamic hyperinflation in patients receiving mechanical ventilation. Am Rev Respir Dis 139:621-626
22. Rossi A, Polese G, Milic-Emili J (1997) Monitoring respiratory mechanics in ventilator-dependent patients. In: Tobin MJ (ed) Principles and practice of intensive care monitoring. McGraw-Hill, New York, pp 553-596
23. Tobin MJ (1997) Monitoring respiratory mechanics in spontaneously breathing patients. In: Tobin MJ (ed) Principles and practice of intensive care monitoring. McGraw-Hill, New York, pp 617-654
24. Marini JJ (1988) Monitoring during mechanical ventilation. Clin Chest Med 9:73-100
25. Marcy TW, Marini JJ (1992) Modes of mechanical ventilation. Curr Pulmonol 13:43-90
26. Pierson DJ (1988) Alveolar rupture during mechanical ventilation: role of PEEP, peak airway pressure, and distending volume. Respir Care 33:472-484
27. Maunder RJ, Peirson DJ, Hudson LD (1984) Subcutaneous and mediastinal emphysema: Pathophysiology, diagnosis, and management. Arch Intern Med 144:1447-1453
28. Amato MBP, Barbas CSV, Bonassa J, et al (1992) Volume-assured pressure support ventilation (VAPSV). Chest 102:1225-1234
29. Roussos S, Macklem PT (1982) The respiratory muscles. N Engl J Med 307:786-797
30. Macklem PT (1980) Respiratory muscles: the vital pump. Chest 78:753-758
31. Rochester DF (1985) The diaphragm: contractile properties and fatigue. J Clin Invest 75:1397--1402
32. Grassino A, Macklem PT (1984) Respiratory muscle fatigue and ventilatory failure. Annu Rev Med 35:625-647
33. Macklem PT (1984) Hyperinflation. Am Rev Respir Dis 129:1-2
34. DeTroyer A, Kelly S, Zin WA (1983) Mechanical action of the intercostal muscles on the rib cage. Science 220 (4592):87-88
35. DeTroyer A, Kelly S, Macklem PT, Zin WA (1985) Mechanics of intercostal space and actions of external and internal intercostal muscles. J Clin Invest 75:850-857
36. Petrof BJ, Legaré M, Goldberg P, et al (1990) Continuous positive airway pressure reduces work of breathing and dyspnea during weaning from mechanical ventilation in severe chronic obstructive pulmonary disease. Am Rev Respir Dis 141:281-289
37. Smith TC, Marini JJ (1988) Impact of PEEP on lung mechanics and work of breathing in severe airflow obstruction. J Appl Physiol 65:1488-1499
38. Hubmayr RD, Abel MD, Rehder K (1990) Physiologic approach to mechanical ventilation. Crit Care Med 18:103-113
39. Eissa NT, Milic-Emili J (1991) Modern concepts in monitoring and management of respiratory failure. Respiratory mechanics. Anesthesiol Clin North Am 9:199-218
40. Harken AH, Brennan MF, Smith B, et al (1974) The hemodynamic response to positive end-expiratory pressure ventilation in hypovolemic patients. Surgery 76:786-793
41. Whittenberg JL, McGregor M, Berglund E, et al (1960) Influence of the state of inflation of the lung on pulmonary vascular resistance. J Appl Physiol 15:878-882
42. Hudson LD (1983) Cardiovascular complications in acute respiratory failure. Respir Care 28:627-631

43. Buda AJ, Pinsky MR, Ingels NB, et al (1979) Effects of intrathoracic pressure on left ventricular performance. N Engl J Med 301:453-459
44. Bove AA, Santamore WP (1981) Ventricular interdependence. Prog Cardiovasc Dis 23:356-388
45. Butler J (1983) The heart in good hands. Circulation 67:1163-1168
46. Suter PM, Scholobohm RM (1974) Determination of the functional residual capacity during mechanical ventilation. Anesthesiology 41:605-607
47. Tuxen DV, Lane S (1987) The effects of ventilatory pattern on hyperinflation airway pressures, and circulation in mechanical ventilation of patients with severe airflow obstruction. Am Rev Respir Dis 136:872-879
48. William TJ, Tuxen DV, Scheinkestel CD, et al (1992) Risk factors for morbidity in mechanically ventilated patients with acute severe asthma. Am Rev Respir Dis 146:607-615
49. Tuxen DV (1994) Permissive hypercapnic ventilation. Am J Respir Crit Care Med 150:870-875

Bronchodilation in chronic obstructive pulmonary disease

C. Tantucci

Bronchodilation and bronchoreversibility: two different concepts

In the management of patients with chronic obstructive pulmonary disease (COPD), the use of bronchodilators is recommended as central to prevent or reduce symptoms and to control bouts of bronchospasm during exacerbations. These drugs are given chronically on an as-needed basis and/or regularly, according to the severity of airflow obstruction, mostly to control exertional and resting dyspnea. Beta-2 agonists (short- and long-acting), anticholinergics, and theophilline (alone or in combination) are the bronchodilators most commonly used [1].

This could be seen as curious since, by definition, COPD sensu strictu is a disorder characterized by a chronic and progressive airflow obstruction that usually does not change significantly (not fully reversible..?) after bronchodilators [1]. Nevertheless, many COPD patients benefit from these drugs in terms of reduction in dyspnea, increased tolerance to effort, and better quality of life [2-4].

It is becoming increasingly clear, however, that the concept of bronchodilation should be kept distinct from that of reversibility of airway obstruction, especially in COPD patients.

Bronchoreversibility is an operational concept based usually on changes of forced expiratory volume in the 1st (FEV1) during a maneuver of maximal (full, forced) expiratory vital capacity, following the administration of a bronchodilating agent [5].

FEV1 has been chosen because it includes a large portion of the expiratory forced vital capacity (FVC) and thus is influenced by a decrease in large and small airway flow resistance. Moreover, FEV1 is a spirometric parameter that is remarkably reproducible within subjects when retested under the same circumstances. Since the intra-individual variability of FEV1 is less than 10%, any increase in FEV1 above this threshold after bronchodilators is considered as significant, reflecting the reversibility of the airway obstruction [6].

Many ways to assess the post-bronchodilator change in FEV1 have been suggested [7, 8], and even today there is no agreement among the different societies about the method for measuring the reversibility of airway obstruction [9, 10].

In any case, a given increase in FEV1 must be achieved after short-acting bronchodilators (usually nebulized beta-2 agonists, administered by a metered--dose inhaler at near-ceiling dosage), either immediately or after a period of anti-inflammatory therapy with steroids.

Therefore, bronchoreversibility is an "all or nothing" response and COPD patients are very often divided into *responders* (few) and *non-responders* (the vast majority).

Bronchodilation is a functional concept that is related to an enlargement of the narrowed airway lumen following the administration of bronchodilating agents. In COPD patients, this is obtained through different mechanisms of action of these drugs, may occur mainly on large or small airways, and actually represents a response that must be viewed as a *continuum*, from *nothing to something* [11,12].

Accordingly, bronchodilation may be also achieved in the absence of bronchoreversibility, i.e., without significant changes in FEV1 after bronchodilators.

Expiratory flow limitation, dynamic hyperinflation, and chronic dyspnea in COPD

Expiratory flow limitation (EFL) refers to a functional condition in which the expiratory flow cannot increase and, hence, is maximal at a given lung volume [13]. Many patients with moderate-to-severe COPD exhibit EFL during tidal breathing at rest [14, 15].

It has been increasingly recognized that in COPD patients the occurrence of tidal EFL at rest represents a critical functional step, because it promotes the development of dynamic pulmonary hyperinflation (DH) [16-18]. In fact, COPD patients who breathe using the maximal expiratory flow rates at rest (so--called flow limited), have an end-expiratory lung volume (EELV) greater than the relaxation volume of the respiratory system [Vr = static functional residual capacity (FRC)] at rest if the expiratory time is not long enough, and invariably in the presence of increased ventilatory requests (e.g., effort, fever, respiratory infections, etc.).

Under these circumstances, the inspiratory capacity (IC) is reduced, indicating the presence of DH and limiting the potential increment of tidal volume [18]. Hence, the baseline IC is almost always less than 80% of that predicted in stable COPD patients with EFL at rest, reflecting a specular increase in FRC [19].

DH implies the generation of some intrinsic positive end-expiratory pressure (PEEPi) [20] acting as a threshold elastic load on the inspiratory muscles, operationally weaker because of the lung volume-related shortening of their fibers [21].

Flow-limited COPD patients at rest have more chronic dyspnea, as evaluated by a modified MRC scale than non-flow-limited COPD at rest, even at a comparable degree of airway obstruction based on the FEV1 values [15,18]. In this respect, the chronic dyspnea, assessed by MRC scale, has been shown to correlate better with EFL than FEV1 in a large cohort of stable moderate-to--severe COPD patients [15].

In the last few years, the increase in DH, reflected by a progressive increase in both end-inspiratory and end-expiratory lung volume, and the ensuing neuro-ventilatory uncoupling, has been emphasized as the main mechanism determining the severity of the exertional dyspnea in COPD patients [22,23]. Recently, the presence of resting EFL has been indicated as a critical factor causing a significant increase in the EELV (i.e., rapid development of DH) during progressive exercise in patients with mild to severe COPD [24].

Therefore, there is evidence that COPD patients who are flow limited at rest exhibit a higher degree of dyspnea while performing their daily living activities and during incremental exercise.

Exertional dyspnea and bronchodilators in COPD

In a previous study, Belman et al. [25] have elegantly shown that the decrease in DH, through its favorable effect on dynamic lung volumes, inspiratory pressure reserve, and neuroventilatory coupling, was the main factor causing the reduction in breathlessness in a group of moderate-to-severe COPD patients at the end of a symptom-limited incremental exercise testing after administration of bronchodilator.

Under prevailing conditions, a decrease in DH induced by the bronchodilators implies a reduction in EELV (or dynamic FRC), which must be invariably associated with a concomitant increase in inspiratory capcity (IC), since total lung capacity (TLC) does not change acutely in COPD patients following bronchodilators [18].

This is expected to occur at baseline in COPD patients who are flow limited at rest and, probably, during effort in those COPD patients who rapidly develop EFL.

In fact, in a group of COPD patients divided according to the presence or absence of tidal EFL and with similar baseline FEV1 (% predicted), the acute administration of a bronchodilator induced a significant (greater than 10% of baseline) increase in IC only in the tidally flow limited COPD patients (about 75% of these patients) (Fig. 1). It should be remembered that only 6% (ERS criteria [10]) or 16% (ATS criteria [9]) of all COPD patients examined had reversibility of the airway obstruction after bronchodilator. Moreover, a significant post-bronchodilator decrease in EELV (or dynamic FRC) was observed only in the COPD subgroup with tidal EFL (Fig. 2). This suggests that the decrease in breathlessness found by Belman et al. [25] during incremental submaximal exercise after bronchodilator should be mostly due to the flow-limited COPD patients.

On the other hand, for moderate-to-severe COPD patients it could be more pleasant and useful to have their dyspnea reduced after bronchodilator during

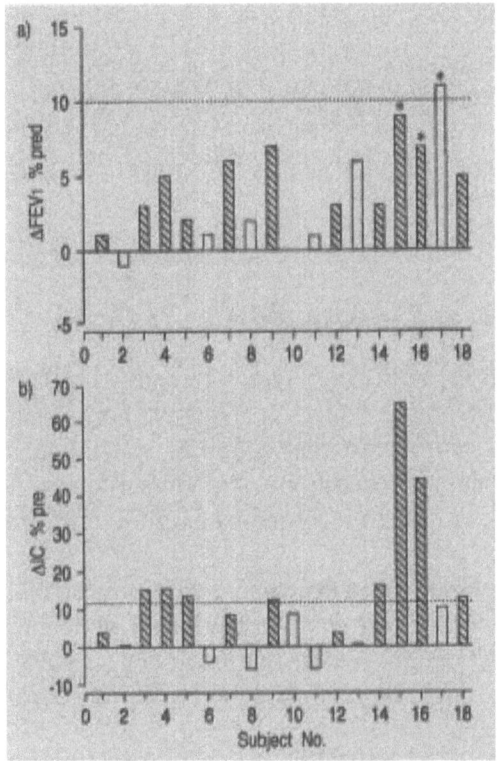

Fig. 1 a Changes in forced expiratory volume in the first second (DFEV1) and **b** inspiratory capacity (DIC) after salbutamol in 18 moderate-to-severe chronic obstructive pulmonary disease (COPD) patients, 11 with tidal expiratory flow limitation (EFL) at rest (*hatched columns*) and 7 without tidal EFL at rest (*blank columns*). The *dotted horizontal line* indicates in **a** an FEV1 increase of 10% relative to predicted value (% pred) and in **b** an IC increase of 12% relative to baseline (% pre).
* indicates the subjects with DFEV1 >12% of baseline and an absolute increase in FEV1 >200 ml

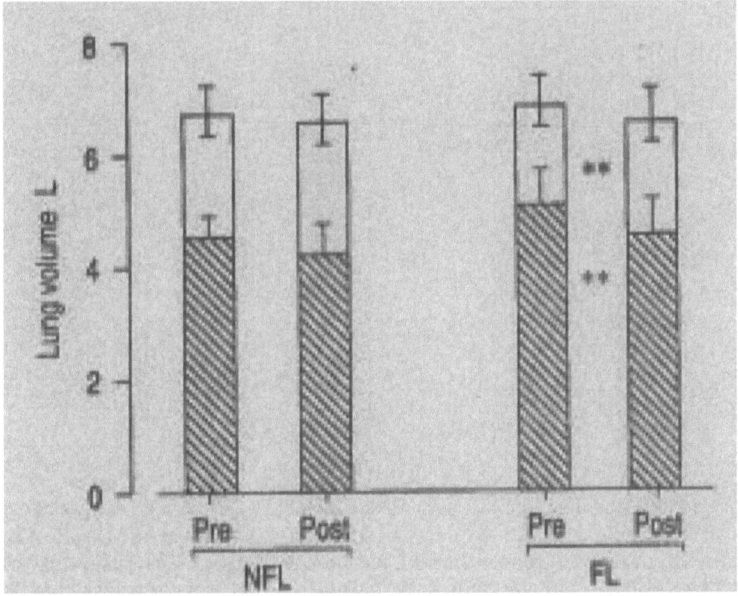

Fig. 2 Mean+SEM (*bars*) values of functional residual capacity (FRC) (*hatched columns*) and IC (*blank columns*) and total lung capacity (TLC) (*hatched plus blank columns*) in non-flow-limited (NFL, *n*=7) and flow-limited (FL, *n*=11) patients with COPD before (Pre) and after (Post) administration of the bronchodilator. While TLC remained essentially unchanged, the FRC decreased and IC increased significantly in the FL subgroup. ** P<0.01 Pre versus Post

daily living activities or even at rest, rather than at their maximal performance. This should occur, however, essentially in COPD patients with EFL at rest in whom the administration of bronchodilator may induce a reduction in DH either at rest or as soon as the ventilatory demand increases.

Indeed, in a recent study, changes in baseline IC (DIC %pre) and in both resting (DBorg,rest) and exertional dyspnea (DBorg,exercise) at the end of a low-intensity, steady-state exercise were measured in two groups of COPD patients, with and without tidal EFL at rest, but with comparable baseline FEV1 (% predicted), following administration of a short-acting bronchodilator.

A significant reduction in exertional dyspnea (DBorg,exercise) (Fig. 2) and a close relationship between DBorg,exercise (decrease) and DIC at rest (%pre) (increase) were found after salbutamol, regardless of the change in FEV1, in the group of COPD patients with tidal EFL at rest (Figs. 3 and 4). In contrast, no change in DIC at rest (%pre) and in DBorg,exercise was observed in the group of COPD patients without tidal EFL at rest (Figs. 3 and 4) [26]. Therefore,

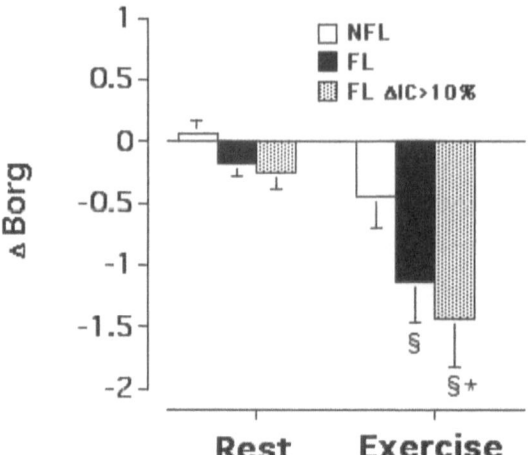

Fig. 3 Changes in dyspnea after administration of salbutamol (DBorg) before (Rest) and at the end of a steady-state light exercise (Exercise) in NFL and FL COPD patients at rest. DBorg,exercise was significantly greater than DBorg, rest only in FL patients (□= P<0.01). DBorg,rest was not significantly different between FL and NFL groups. Although DBorg,exercise was greater in FL than in NFL patients, this difference was significant only in FL patients with an increase in resting IC >10% (pre) after salbutamol (n= 8). *Columns* are means and bars represent SEM. * P<0.05 vs. DBorg,exercise in NFL

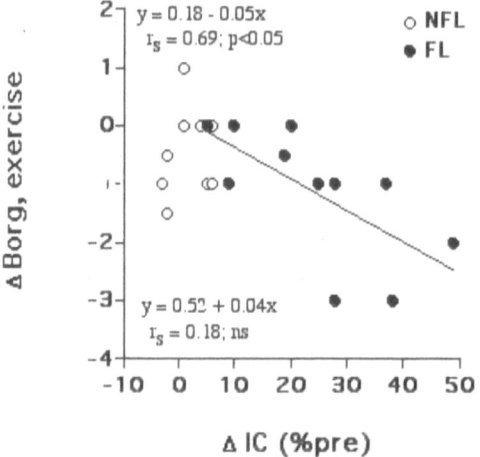

Fig. 4 Decrease in dyspnea during light exercise (DBorg,exercise) after bronchodilator was closely related to the increase in resting IC (DIC %pre) only in COPD patients with tidal EFL at rest (FL). The regression line is shown in this group. In contrast, no increase in IC and significant decrease in exertional dyspnea were observed in NFL COPD patients. Note that after administration of salbutamol in 3 FL patients, IC did not increase (DIC%pre) and the reduction in their dyspnea during exercise was also minimal in the presence of tidal EFL

in COPD patients the reduction in breathlessness during mild-to-moderate exercise following the administration of bronchodilator is heralded by an increase in IC at rest.

It has to be noted, however, that not all of the COPD patients with tidal EFL at rest exhibit a relevant increase in resting IC (10% compared with baseline) after bronchodilator (Fig. 4) [26]. This suggests that, in some COPD patients, either tidal EFL at rest may not be associated with some pulmonary dynamic hyperinflation or β_2-agonists have no appreciable bronchodilating effect.

Such a possibility should be borne in mind. In fact, only by removing the 3 flow-limited patients with DIC (%pre) less than 10% after salbutamol in a post-hoc analysis, did the difference of DBorg, exercise following bronchodilator become significant between the flow-limited and non-flow-limited COPD patients (Fig. 3) [26].

These results show the importance for COPD patients of being flow limited during tidal breathing at rest, to possibly achieve a prompt decrease in DH and PEEPi after bronchodilator [27] and, consequently, to have less dyspnea even during light effort.

Assessment of bronchodilation in COPD

In the past bronchodilation has been assessed exclusively in terms of FEV1 change in COPD patients, and, simply because we were looking at bronchoreversibility, often bronchodilators have been thought to be functionally ineffective and, thus, useless in these subjects.

On the other hand, despite no significant increase in FEV1, bronchodilators are frequently prescribed to COPD patients because many of them report symptomatic benefits from this treatment.

Comparisons between pre- and post-bronchodilator isovolume maximal expiratory flows, at fixed percentage (i.e., 25%,50%,75%) of the pre-bronchodilator FVC, have been made to detect an increase in the expiratory flow reserve at different lung volumes.

Although such a procedure is rational, in practice the natural large variability of these parameters in the same subjects and the complexity of calculations requiring specific software have reduced the utility of this method and its diffusion.

In keeping with these studies, the measurement of the IC variations after bronchodilator appears a very simple and valuable method to assess the so-called *volume effect* elicited by these drugs, at least in moderate-to-severe COPD patients with tidal EFL at rest. In fact, even a small increase in expiratory flow reserve at a lung volume corresponding to the tidal volume may be sufficient to cause a substantial decrement in the EELV in these patients. This is because whatever bronchodilation is provided, COPD patients with tidal EFL at rest choose to breathe (usually remaining flow limited) at a lower lung volume with less DH and PEEPi, rather than escape their chronic EFL without changing the EELV [18,26].

Therefore, in COPD patients with tidal EFL at rest, the measurement of the IC change after bronchodilators may represent an objective tool for prescribing these drugs, in order to attain symptomatic improvement and better quality of life, even in the absence of significant increase in FEV1.

How large the post-bronchodilator increment of IC should be, has yet to be determined. However, looking at the short-term reproducibility data of IC [28], an increase in IC above 10% of the baseline value, which has been found to be associated with a clinically significant decrease in dynamic FRC in moderate-to-severe COPD patients [18,26], can be currently recommended.

References

1. Global Initiative for Chronic Obstructive Lung Disease (2001) National Institutes of Health, Publication number 2701
2. Mahler DA, Matthay RA, Synder PE, et al (1985) Sustained release theophylline reduced dyspnoea in non-reversible obstructive airways disease. Am Rev Respir Dis131:22-25
3. Jones PW, Bosh TK, in association with an international study group (1997) Quality of life changes in COPD patients treated with salmeterol. Am J Respir Crit Care Med 155:1283-1289
4. Ramirez-Venegas A, Ward J, Lentine T, Mahler DA (1997) Salmeterol reduces dyspnea and improves lung function in patients with COPD. Chest 112:336-340
5. Weir DC, Burge PS (1991) Measures of reversibility in response to bronchodilators in chronic airflow obstruction: relation to airway caliber. Thorax 46:43-45
6. Dales RE, Spitzer WO, Tousignant P, et al (1988) Clinical interpretation of airway response to a bronchodilator. Epidemiologic considerations. Am Rev Respir Dis 138:317-320
7. Eliasson O, Degraff AC (1985) The use of criteria for reversibility and obstruction to define patient groups for bronchodilator trials. Am Rev Respir Dis 132: 858-864
8. Harf A (1992) How to express the reversibility of bronchial obstruction? Eur Respir J 5:919-920
9. ATS (1987) Standards for the diagnosis and care of patients with chronic obstructive pulmonary disease (COPD) and asthma. Am Rev Respir Dis 136:225-244
10. Siafakas NM, Vermeire P, Pride NB et al (1995) Optimal assessment and management of chronic obstructive pulmonary disease (COPD). Eur Respir J 8:1398-1420
11. Skorodin M (1993) Pharmacotherapy for asthma and chronic obstructive pulmonary disease: current thinking, practices and controversies. Arch Intern Med 153:814-828
12. Nisar M, Harris JE, Pearson MG, Calverley PMA (1992) Acute bronchodilator trials in chronic obstructive pulmonary disease. Am Rev Respir Dis 146:555-559
13. Fry DL, Hyatt RE (1960) Pulmonary mechanics: a unified analysis of the relationship between pressure, volume and gas flow in the lungs of normal and diseased subjects. Am J Med 29:672-689
14. Koulouris NG, Valta P, Lavoie A, et al (1995) A simple method to detect expiratory flow limitation during spontaneous breathing. Eur Respir J 8:306-313

15. Eltayara L, Becklake MR, Volta CA, Milic-Emili J (1996) Relationship between chronic dyspnea and expiratory flow limitation in patients with chronic obstructive pulmonary disease. Am J Respir Crit Care Med 154:1726-1734
16. Valta P, Corbeil C, Lavoie A, et al (1994) Detection of expiratory flow limitation during mechanical ventilation. Am J Respir Crit Care Med 150:1311-1317
17. Pellegrino R, Brusasco V (1997) Lung hyperinflation and flow limitation in chronic airway obstruction. Eur Respir J 10:543-549
18. Tantucci C, Duguet A, Similowski T, et al (1998) Effect of salbutamol on dynamic hyperinflation in chronic obstructive pulmonary disease patients. Eur Respir J 12:799-804
19. Diaz O, Villafranca C, Ghezzo H, et al (2000) Role of inspiratory capacity on exercise tolerance in COPD patients with and without tidal expiratory flow limitation at rest. Eur Respir J 16:269-275
20. Pepe AE, Marini JJ (1982) Occult positive end-expiratory pressure in mechanically ventilated patients with airflow obstruction: the auto-PEEP effect. Am Rev Respir Dis 26:166-170
21. Bellemare F, Grassino A (1983) Force reserve of the diaphragm in patients with chronic obstructive pulmonary disease. J Appl Physiol 55:8-15
22. O'Donnell DE (1994) Breathlessness in patients with chronic airflow limitation. Mechanisms and management. Chest 106:904-912
23. O'Donnell DE, Webb KA (1993) Exertional breathlessness in patients with chronic airflow limitation. The role of lung hyperinflation. Am J Respir Crit Care Med 148:1351-1357
24. Koulouris NG, Dimopoulou I, Valta P, et al (1997) Detection of expiratory flow limitation during exercise in COPD patients. J Appl Physiol 82:723-731
25. Belman MJ, Botnick WC, Shin JW (1996) Inhaled bronchodilators reduce dynamic hyperinflation during exercise in patients with chronic obstructive pulmonary disease. Am J Respir Crit Care Med 153:967-975
26 Boni E, Corda L, Franchini D, et al (2002) Volume effect and exertional dyspnoea after bronchodilator in patients with COPD with and without expiratory flow limitation at rest. Thorax 57:528-532
27. Dal Vecchio L, Polese G, Poggi R, Rossi A (1990) "Intrinsic" positive end-expiratory pressure in stable patients with chronic obstructive pulmonary disease. Eur Respir J 3:74-80
28. Hadcroft J, Calverley PMA (2001) Alternative methods for assessing bronchodilator reversibility in chronic obstructive pulmonary disease. Thorax 56:713-720

High-frequency oscillation in acute respiratory distress syndrome

R.M. KACMAREK

For over 40 years high-frequency ventilation (HFV) has been investigated for the management of acute respiratory failure [1-3]. A number of approaches to HFV have been developed over these years; high-frequency positive pressure ventilation (HFPPV), high-frequency jet ventilation (HFJV), and high-frequency oscillation (HFO). HFPPV has been defined as the application of conventional mechanical ventilation at rates of about 60-180 breaths / min or 1.0-3.0 Hz (1 Hz = 60/min) [3]. HFJV is established by the injection of a gas under high pressure into the airway at a rate of up to about 10 Hz while entraining a secondary gas [3]. HFO is the oscillation by use of a piston or diaphragm of a column of bias gas flow across the airway at frequencies up to about 20 Hz [3]. Currently, the high-frequency approach used in both neonatal respiratory failure and adult acute respiratory distress syndrome (ARDS) that has gained the most interest is HFO.

Rationale for the use of HFO

Over the last 10 years interest in HFO in the management of ARDS patients has markedly increased, because of the increased concern regarding ventilator--induced lung injury. HFO may be the ideal lung protective ventilatory approach, since theoretically it avoids both overdistension and repetitive recruitment and derecruitment of unstable lung units [4]. This is accomplished by the maintenance of a high mean airway pressure and the oscillation of a bias flow of gas around the mean airway pressure. Both a positive and negative pressure phase is applied with HFO, and at the high rates used, pressure fluctuations around the mean airway pressure at the alveolar level are assumed to be minimal [3]. In fact, with an 8-mm internal diameter endotracheal tube and a frequency of 8 Hz it is estimated that only 15% of the applied pressure amplitude is transmitted to the peripheral lung [5]. As a result, pressure maintained at the lung periphery fluctuates little about the mean airway pressure, particularly at high rates.

Mechanism of gas exchange

During HFO few variables are set (Table 1). A bias flow is maintained across the airway. Resistance to the free passage of the bias flow establishes the mean airway pressure. Frequency is maintained by the movement of a diaphragm or piston and the force of this movement establishes the pressure amplitude moving gas into and out of the airway. A pressure amplitude of 60 cmH_2O indicates that the pressure change around the mean airway pressure is 60 cmH_2O, plus 30 cmH_2O during inspiration and minus 30 cmH_2O during expiration. In addition, the inspiratory to expiratory (I:E) ratio can be adjusted between 1:1 and 1:2. As noted in Table 1, the applied ranges for these variables vary considerably, based on the size of the patient ventilated.

Table 1 Ventilatory setting during high-frequency ocillation (HFO) (*I* inspiratory, *E* expiratory)

	Neonates	Pediatric	Adults
Bias flow	Plain 15 l/min	15-30 l/min	30-40 l/min
Mean airway pressure	Plain 20 cmH_2O	20-30 cmH_2O	25-35 cmH_2O
Rate	8-15 Hz	6-12 Hz	3-8 Hz
Pressure amplitude	20-30 cmH_2O	30-60 cmH_2O	60-90 cmH_2O
I:E	1:1 to 1:2	1:1 to 1:2	1:1 to 1:2

Oxygenation and ventilation during HFO are considered uncoupled. Essentially, the mean airway pressure, and to a much lesser extent the I:E ratio, affect oxygenation, while the pressure amplitude, rate, and I:E ratio affect ventilation [1]. During HFO, especially at high rates, tidal volumes are less than anatomical dead space, and contrary to conventional ventilation tidal volume varies indirectly with rate [1, 3]. The higher the rate the lower the tidal volume [3]. This is essentially a result of pressure amplitude dissipation. Pressure is dissipated to a greater extent across the large airways at higher rates compared with lower rates, thus decreasing tidal volume as rates increase. However, pressure amplitude at a specific rate is directly related to tidal volume, but its effect on tidal volume is considerably less than the effect of rate on tidal volume [2]. Lengthening inspiratory time also increases tidal volume, but the effect is much less than that of rate or pressure amplitude.

A number of mechanisms have been proposed to account for carbon dioxide elimination during HFO when tidal volume is less than or equal to plain anatomical dead space (Table 2) [3]. Although mechanisms such as Taylor type dispersion, pendelluft, and enhanced molecular diffusion do improve ventilation during HFO, convection is still the predominant mechanism for carbon dioxide elimination, which is why increasing tidal volume (low rate) results in better ventilation [3].

Table 2 Factors responsible for gas exchange during HFO

• Convection (direct alveolar ventilation)
• Taylor type dispersion
• Pendaluf
• Convective dispersion
• Coaxial gas flow
• Cardiac oscillations
• Enhanced molecular diffusion

At a given HFO setting, impedance to gas exchange also has a large effect on tidal volume. The lower the lung compliance and the higher the airways resistance, the smaller the tidal volume at any specific ventilator setting. No data directly measuring tidal volume are available in patients, but in animal models (30 kg, sheep lavage lung injury) at low rates (4 Hz) and high pressure amplitudes (60 cmH$_2$O), tidal volumes approaching 5 ml/kg have been recorded [6]. As a result, it is difficult to be sure that tidal volumes during HFO in adult ARDS are not consistent with those now recommended during conventional ventilation (4-8 ml/kg).

Mean airway pressure during HFO is similar in its effects to positive end-expiratory pressure (PEEP) during conventional ventilation. With conventional ventilation, mean airway pressure is greatly affected by tidal volume and inspiratory time, as well as the PEEP level [3]. Whereas, during HFO mean airway pressure is set and essentially it is not affected by changes in rate or pressure amplitude. During neonatal, pediatric, and adult HFO, mean airway pressures are generally set above the mean airway pressure measured during conventional ventilation, and are much higher than the PEEP level [5, 7]. The use of these high mean airway pressures may in part be the reason why HFO appears in adult ARDS to improve oxygenation over conventional ventilation. During HFO, tidal recruitment is much less than during conventional ventilation. However, very few data are available to determine the best methodology for setting any variable during HFO. In one study it was demonstrated in an animal model that mean airway pressure equal to the point of maximum curvature on the deflation limb of the pressure-volume curve resulted in the best oxygenation without hemodynamic compromise [8].

Lung recruitment

Since the mid 1980s a lung recruitment maneuver has been recommended at the onset of HFO [2, 4]. This is usually accomplished by increasing the mean airway pressure above the level expected necessary, then reducing the mean pressure over time to the lowest level maintaining oxygenation. Generally recruitment mean airway pressures in adult ARDS are between 35 and 45 cmH_2O, and maintenance mean airway pressures between 25 and 35 cmH_2O [5, 7]. Although in some patients higher (up to 45 cmH_2O) maintenance mean airway pressures have been necessary [5, 7].

Fluid balance

Clearly there are differences regarding the use of fluids in ARDS. However, to accomplish HFO in adult ARDS, vascular volume to vascular space relationships need to be maximized [5, 7]. In general, pulmonary capillary wedge pressure needs to be maintained over 14 cmH_2O, or central venous pressures over 6 cmH_2O, to insure adequate cardiac output during HFO. Without adequate vascular volume, because of the high mean intrathoracic pressures, cardiac output can be markedly decreased during HFO.

Neonatal experience

To date nine randomized controlled trials of HFO in neonatal respiratory failure have been published [9-17]. The results of these trials are not overwhelmingly favourable to HFO. None of these nine trials demonstrated a significant decrease in mortality with HFO, and in some there was no difference whatsoever between conventional mechanical ventilation and HFO [12-14]. Some do demonstrate a decrease in chronic lung disease [9-11] (need for oxygen therapy at 30 days from onset of mechanical ventilation) with HFO, but in other trials patients managed with HFO had a higher incidence of severe intracranial hemorrhage and leukomalasia [15, 16]. Many have argued that the negative HFO trials were confounded because of a low lung volume strategy (lowest possible mean airway pressure). However, in all of these trials conventional ventilation was applied with low PEEP levels (plain 6 cmH$_2$O), synchronized intermittent mandatory ventilation, and modest mean airway pressures. It is difficult to determine whether results would have been different if conventional ventilation were applied with the same lung open strategy as HFO. However, in spite of these differences in approach to ventilation and the equivocal results of these trials, HFO has become the standard of care in neonatal respiratory failure with refractory hypoxemia.

Pediatric HFO

Only one pediatric randomized controlled trial has been published [18]. As with the neonatal trials, there was no difference in mortality between groups. However, similar to neonatal trials, the primary benefit attributed to HFO was a decrease in chronic lung disease. Less patients receiving HFO required oxygen therapy at 30 days post initiation of mechanical ventilation.

Adult HFO trials

Few clinical data have been published to date on the use of HFO in adult ARDS [5, 7, 19]. Fort et al. [5] reported 17 patients with severe ARDS managed with HFO. Before transition to HFO all patients were considered failing conventional ventilation and had a peak airway pressure (volume ventilation) of 54±13 cmH$_2$O, PEEP of 18±7 cmH$_2$O, mean airway pressure of 31±11 cmH$_2$O, and a PaO$_2$/F$_I$O$_2$ of 66±19 mmHg. As expected, mortality in this case series was high; 30-day survival was 46%. HFO was started at a mean airway pressure 2-3 cmH$_2$O higher than during conventional mechanical ventilation, and increased up to 45 cmH$_2$O to maintain an oxygen saturation ≥ 90%. Over time, the mean airway pressure was decreased as oxygenation improved. Frequency was set between 3 and 5 Hz, and pressure amplitude between 60 and 90 cmH$_2$O. If the PaCO$_2$ was 60 mmHg, the pressure amplitude was < 60 mmHg, if PaCO$_2$ was 60-70 mmHg the pressure amplitude was 75 cmH$_2$O, and if PaCO$_2$ was > 70 mmHg the pressure amplitude was set at 90 cmH$_2$O. Fluid was liberally administered to maintain cardiac output and inotropes were administered as needed. Thirteen patients demonstrated improved gas exchange by 24 h. However, in 3 patient oxygenation failed to improve and in 1 patient the oscillator failed to ventilate; 3 other patients demonstrated severe hypotension, in 1 patient the oscillator failed to operate properly, and 1 patient developed a pneumothorax during HFO. There was a relationship between the length of time conventional mechanical ventilation (CMV) was provided prior to HFO and mortality. The greater the number of days on conventional ventilation, the greater the mortality.

Similarly, Mehta et al. [7] reported the rescue use of HFO in 24 ARDS adults failing conventional ventilation. Prior to HFO, these patients had a PaO_2/F_IO_2 of 98 ± 39 mmHg, an oxygenation index of 32 ± 19, a plateau pressure of 36 ± 4 cmH_2O, a PEEP of 14.5 ± 2.4 cmH_2O, and a mean airway pressure set at 24 ± 3 cmH_2O. HFO was initiated at 5 Hz and mean airway pressure 5 cmH_2O above that during conventional ventilation. Pressure amplitude was adjusted to maintain $PaCO_2$ between 35 and 60 mmHg. If a maximum pressure amplitude (90 cmH_2O) could not maintain target $PaCO_2$, the rate was decreased to a minimum of 3 Hz. If oxygenation could not be maintained at the initial mean airway pressure, it was increased in 1 to 2 cmH_2O increments to a maximum of 45 cmH_2O. As with Fort et al. [5], liberal fluid and intotropes were administered to maintain cardiac output. Of the 24 patients rescued, 8 (33%) survived to intensive care discharge. There was also a strong relationship between survival and length of mechanical ventilation prior to HFO, survivors were ventilated 1.6 ± 1.2 days and non survivors 7.8 ± 5.8 days (P = 0.001).

Currently, there is one randomized controlled trial of HFO versus conventional mechanical ventilation in adult ARDS [19]. This was a multicenter (13 centers) study enrolling patients with a $PaO_2/F_IO_2 \leq 200$ mmHg while on 10 cmH_2O PEEP, with bilateral pulmonary infiltrates and no clinical evidence of heart failure. Patients were excluded if they had severe chronic obstructive pulmonary disease, asthma, intractable shock, severe airleak, an estimated survival < 6 months for non-pulmonary reasons, and having received an F_IO_2 > 0.80 for > 48 h. About 75 patients were randomized to each group. Table 3 list the approaches used to ventilate patients in each arm of the study. Conventional ventilation was provided with volume ventilation.

Table 3 Ventilatory strategies used in the randomized controlled trial of HFO versus conventional mechanical ventilation (CMV) (V_T tidal volume, *PEEP* positive end-expiratory pressure, *BW* body weight)[19]

	CMV	HFO
Initial V_T	6-10 ml/kg actual BW	-------
Initial rate	Maintain pH >7.15 (maximum 35/min)	5 Hz (3-5 hz)
Initial PEEP	10 cmH_2O (maximum 18 cmH_2O)	-------------
Initial mean airway pressure	------------	CMV + 5 (maximum 45 cmH_2O)
Initial pressure amplitude	------------	"Adequate chest wall vibration" (60-90 cmH_2O)

There were no significant differences at baseline between the two groups. Patients were about 50 years of age with an APACHE II of 22. About 50% of patients had sepsis syndrome, about 18% pulmonary infection, and 20% were trauma patients. At the time of enrollment, patients in the HFO group were ventilated 2.7±2.8 days and those in the CMV group 4.4±7.8 days.

Over the first 72 h of HFO, the mean airway pressure was about 28±6 cmH$_2$O, the pressure amplitude 65±13 cmH$_2$O and the rate 4.7±0.7 Hz. While in the CMV, group tidal volume was 10.2 ml/kg ideal body weight, PEEP 13±4 cmH$_2$O, and respiratory rate 20±6 breaths/minute. F$_1$O$_2$ was similar in both groups at about 0.55. There were no differences in any outcome variables between the two groups. The numbers of patients failing oxygenation or ventilation, those experiencing hypotension, or developing airleaks, or endo-tracheal tube obstruction were the same. Thirty-day mortality did favor HFO (37% vs. 52%, P = 0.102), but less difference existed at 6 months (47% vs. 56%).

One must conclude from the available data in adults that HFO is as safe and as effective as CMV. Although the randomized trial of Derdak et al. [19] indicates a trend toward better outcome with HFO, HFO must be prospectively compared with our best approach to CMV. Based on today's standards, a tidal volume of 10.2 ml/kg ideal body weight cannot be considered the most--appropriate approach. In addition, there was a trend toward a greater number of days ventilated prior to HFO in the CMV group, which has been shown to adversely affect mortality. Thus, although HFO is intriguing and theoretically an ideal lung protective strategy, the approach used to date (mean airway pressure up to 45 cmH$_2$O, pressure amplitude up to 90 cmH$_2$O, and slow rates of 3-5 Hz) in adults may not offer advantages over approaches recommended during CMV. Yes, HFO is equal to CMV, but there are no data to demonstrate it is better than CMV.

References

1. Mildner R, Cox P (2001) The preclinical history of HFV. Respir Clin North Am 7:523-534
2. Bohr D (2001) The history of high frequency ventilation. Respir Clin North Am 7:535-548
3. DosSantos CC, Slutsky AS (2001) Overview of high frequency ventilation modes clinical rationale and gas transport mechanisms. Respir Clin North Am 7:549-576
4. Froese AB (1997) High-frequency oscillatory ventilation for adult respiratory distress syndrome: let's get it right this time. Crit Care Med 25:906-908
5. Fort P, Farmer C, Westerman J, et al (1997) High-frequency oscillatory ventilation for adult respiratory distress syndrome: a pilot study. Crit Care Med 25:937-947
6. Sedeek KA, Takeuchi M, Suchodolski K, Kacmarek RM (2002) Determinants of tidal volume during high frequency oscillation. Crit Care Med (in press)

7. Mehta S, Lapinsky SE, Hallett DD, et al (2001) Prospective trial of high frequency oscillation in adults with acute respiratory distress syndrome. Crit Care Med 29:1360-1369
8. Goddon S, Fujino Y, Hromi JM, Kacmarek RM (2001) Optimal mean airway pressure during high-frequency oscillation. Anesthesiology 94:862-869
9. Gerstmann DR, Minton SD, Stoddard RA, et al (1996) The provo multicenter early high frequency oscillatory ventilation trial: improved pulmonary and clinical outcomes in respiratory distress syndrome. Pediatrics 98:1044-1051
10. Clark RH, Gerstmann DR, Null DN, deLemos RA (1992) Prospective randomized comparison of high-frequency oscillatory and conventional ventilation in respiratory distress syndrome. Pediatrics 89:5-12
11. Plavaka R, Kopecky P, Sebron V, et al (1999) A prospective randomized comparison of conventional mechanical ventilation and very early high frequency oscillatory ventilation in extremely premature newborns with respiratory distress syndrome. Intensive Care Med 25:68-74
12. Clark RH, Yoder BA, Sell MS (1994) Prospective, randomized comparison of high-frequency oscillation and conventional ventilation in candidates for extracorporeal membrane oxygenation. J Pediatr 124:447-454
13. Ogawa Y, Katsuyuki M, Kawano T, et al (1993) A multicenter randomized trial of high frequency oscillatory ventilation as compared with conventional mechanical ventilation in preterm infants with respiratory failure. Early Hum Dev 32:1-10
14. HIFO Study Group (1993) Randomized study of high-frequency oscillatory ventilation in infants with severe respiratory distress syndrome. J Pediatr 122:609-619
15. The HIFI Study Group (1989) High-frequency oscillatory ventilation compared with conventional mechanical ventilation in the treatment of respiratory failure in preterm infants. N Engl J Med 320:88-93
16. Moriette G, Paris-Llado J, Walti H, et al (2001) Prospective randomized multicenter comparison of high-frequency oscillatory ventilation and conventional ventilation in preterm infants of less than 30 weeks with respiratory distress syndrome. Pediatrics 107:363-372
17. Rettitz-Volk W, Veldman A, Roth B, et al (1998) A prospective, randomized, multicenter trial of high-frequency oscillatory ventilation compared with conventional ventilation in preterm infants with respiratory distress syndrome receiving surfactant. J Pediatr 132:249-254
18. Arnold JH, Hanson JA, Toro-Figuero LO, et al (1994) Prospective, randomized comparison of high-frequency oscillatory ventilation and conventional mechanical ventilation in pediatric respiratory failure. Crit Care Med 22:1530-1539
19. Derdak S, Mehta S, Stewart TE, et al (2002) High-frequency oscillatory ventilation for acute respiratory distress syndrome in adults: a randomized, controlled trial. Am J Respir Crit Care Med (in press)

Statics of normal lung

J. MILIC-EMILI, A. KOUTSOUKOU

Static behaviour of isolated lungs

Static volume-pressure curves of the excised lung were first obtained by Hutchinson [1] in 1949, who studied two human lungs immediately after death. Since then, many such studies on the lungs of different species have been reported, but adequate data pertaining to normal human lungs are still lacking. Accordingly, the lungs of other mammals will be used for purposes of illustration.

Pressure-volume relationships vary somewhat among species and are dependent on experimental parameters such as temperature and prior volume history. When these sources of variability are held constant, however, volume--pressure relationships are almost precisely reproducible. Typical pressure-volume behaviour is illustrated in Fig. 1.

In this example a rabbit lung was first degassed. Degassing the lungs can be accomplished by two methods. The first requires perfusion with blood to absorb all alveolar gas (after a period of O_2 breathing) until complete alveolar collapse (atelectasis) has occurred. The second, applicable to non-perfused lungs, requires placing the lung in a vacuum chamber containing some water or saline and reducing the pressure in and around the lung to the vapour pressure of the liquid. With only water vapour left in the alveolar spaces, the lung collapses gas free when atmospheric pressure is restored to the chamber.

When starting from the completely degassed (atelectatic) state, an initially high pressure is needed to begin inflation (Fig. 1, curve a). This peak indicates that the critical pressures for opening atelectatic units are in the range of 20-30 cmH_2O. With repeated cycling between 0 and 30 cmH_2O distending pressure, the pressure volume loops become consistent (curve b), undergoing about a fivefold volume change between minimal (Vo) and maximal (V30) inflation. This volume range is approximately that which a subject would achieve between a maximal expiratory effort [residual volume (RV)] and a maximal inspiratory effort [total lung capacity (TLC)]. At the high end the lung stiffens, presumably due to both connective tissue stiffness and increasing surface

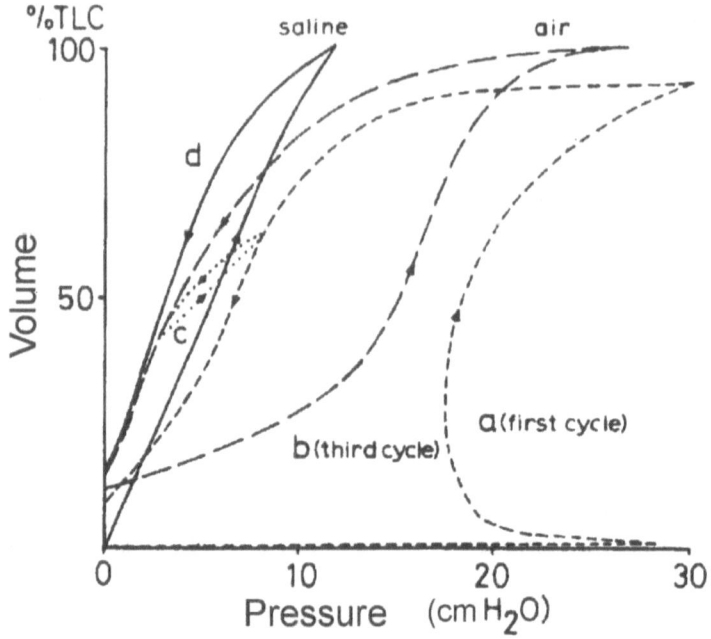

Fig. 1 Four inflation-deflation manoeuvres in excised rabbit lung generating characteristic volume-
-pressure loops. *a* Inflation from degassed state shows that transpulmonary pressures in excess of 20
cmH₂O are required before there is appreciable opening. On deflation to 0 cmH₂O emptying is
incomplete; *b* Repeated cycles between 0 and 30 cmH₂O show stable loops. Lung is now much more
easily opened than in *a*, but still becomes relatively stiff near 30 cmH₂O. *c* Small volume cycles (such
as in tidal breaths in vivo) run between 3 and 8 cmH₂O. *d* With air replaced by and saline, lung shows
much less recoil over same volume range (*TLC* total lung capacity) (from reference [2] with
permission)

tension. With inflation to pressures 30 cmH₂O, volume will continue to increase, although at a relatively low rate, until the lung ruptures and leaks develop.
A choice of an upper pressure limit (cmH₂O) could significantly underestimate
maximum physiological lung volume. This would be particularly likely in
studying lungs after collapse or degassing, because opening of atelectatic alveoli
might still be incomplete. When the lung is filled with saline (curve d), there is
much less recoil than with air filling because of absence of surface forces.

Figure 2 depicts static volume pressure curves of a freshly excised dog lung
with repeated cycling between -5 and 30 cmH₂O of transpulmonary pressure
(PL). The PL is the difference between the alveolar pressure (Palv) and the
pleural surface pressure (Ppl).

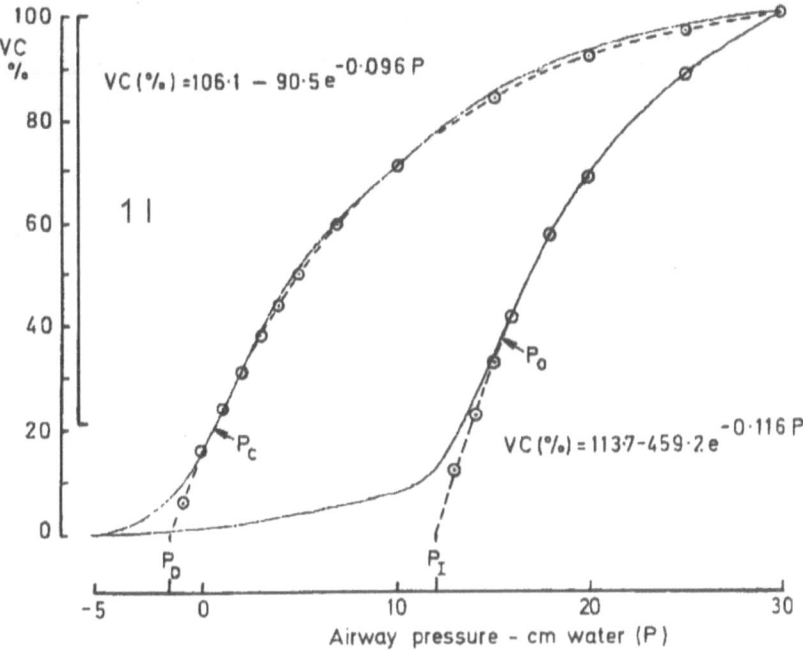

Fig. 2 Pulmonary static volume-pressure curves obtained on a freshly excised, exsanguinated dog lung. Lung gas volume is expressed as a percentage of the volume obtained at a transpulmonary pressure of 30 cmH₂O (%V30). *Filled and open circles:* exponential relations during lung deflation and inflation, respectively. *TGV* Trapped gas volume, *Pc* closing airway pressure, *Po* opening airway pressure (from reference [3] with permission)

Static volume-pressure hysteresis

The volume-pressure curve during lung deflation is not the same as during lung inflation. During deflation the lung exhibits a static hysteresis loop, and this may involve three main mechanisms [2-4]. The first is plastic behaviour of tissue elements and true tissue hysteresis. The second is surface hysteresis. The third is dependent on the difference in the number of lung units open at the beginning and at the end of lung inflation.

Resting lung volume

This is the pulmonary gas volume at zero PL and is commonly referred to as the 'minimal volume' or 'minimal air'. Clearly, these terms are misnomers, since by decreasing PL below zero we can decrease lung volume still further (Fig. 2). The magnitude of the 'minimal volume' (Vo) varies with the animal species. In the example in Fig. 2, Vo during deflation amounts to about 16% of V30. In exsanguinated dog and cat lungs, in general, the 'minimal air' appears to amount to about 10%-20% of V30, while in man higher values have been reported. For example, in the study by Stigol et al. [5] Vo ranged between 18% and 60% V30, which suggests that these results may not represent normal behaviour but have probably been influenced by the presence of stable foam in the airways. The variability of pulmonary blood content may also have affected Vo. In studies on excised cat lungs, Frank [6], repeating an earlier observation by von Basch [7], found that with pulmonary vascular engorgement the 'minimal air' increases by a small amount. Among other factors, the Vo depends on the previous volume history of the lung. As shown in Fig. 2, Vo is lower during inflation than deflation.

Trapped gas volume

In the older texts, where the term 'minimal air' is used to define the volume of gas in the freely collapsed lung, it is stated that this gas is trapped by closure of non-cartilaginous airways, the assumption being that at zero PL the airways leading to all pulmonary alveoli are closed. Kleinman et al. [8] were probably the first to point out that in the freely collapsed lung at least some airways must remain patent throughout their length. In fact, when PL is decreased below zero (Fig. 2), there is a further decrease in lung volume. On the other hand, when a critical PL of about -3 to -5 cm H_2O is reached, expulsion of gas from the lung ceases abruptly, suggesting that all pulmonary pathways are now closed. The volume of gas trapped behind the closed airways is generally referred to as the *trapped gas volume* (TGV). Hughes et al. [9] demonstrated that it was the terminal bronchioles that closed.

Airway closing pressure

The critical PL at which lung emptying ceases reflects the pressure at which the terminal airways are closed throughout the lung. Since some of the airways may begin to close at higher PL, it seems appropriate to term the PL at which TGV is reached as the *minimum airway closing pressure*, while *maximum airway closing pressure* should refer to the PL at which airway closure begins. The available data concerning the minimum airway closing pressure in excised lungs are scanty. In excised dog lungs it averages about -2.5 cm H_2O of PL, while in some excised 'normal' human lungs complete airway closure appears to occur close to zero PL [5]. In open-chest cats and dogs the corresponding values range between −1 and −2 cm H₂O [10]. Little is known with regard to the maximum airway closing pressures. Some inferences can, however, be drawn from analysis of the shape of the static deflation volume-pressure relations of the lung.

In the volume range between V30 and about 20% V30, the relationship between volume and pressure during deflation can be described with good approximation by the following exponential function [3]

$$V = V_{max} - b.e^{-KP} \quad (1)$$

where V_{max} is the *predicted* volume at infinite PL, K is constant, and b is the difference between Vmax and the predicted lung volume at zero PL. Thus, in the volume range above 20% V30, the static deflation volume-pressure curve is of exponential character, as defined by Eq. 1. Such a function has been shown also to fit volume-pressure relationships in man [11]. At lung volumes lower than 20% V30, the experimental relationship deviates to the left of the exponential function as a result of progressive airway closure (inflection point on deflation in Fig. 2). Clearly, when the airways leading to parts of the lung close, a greater PL change will be required to produce a given volume change, and hence the overall lung compliance will be reduced, resulting in a shift to the left of the volume-pressure curve. If this interpretation is correct, the PL at the inflection point should represent the maximum airway closing pressure (max. Pc in Fig. 2), while the pressure at which TGV is reached reflects the minimum value (min. Pc). In view of the complexities of the multitudinous pathways within the lung, it seems likely that there is a range of airway closing pressures rather than a unique value pertinent to all of the airways.

The finding of negative Pc min indicates that at low lung volumes at least some of the peripheral airways offer resistance to collapse. A full discussion of the factors stabilizing the peripheral airways can be found elsewhere [12]. Although the small airways do offer some resistance to collapse, relatively small negative pressures are normally required to close them (Pc min ∼ -3 cmH₂O). The closing pressures for airways, however, appear to be less negative than those for alveoli. Indeed, in experiments on rabbits, cats and dogs, Cavagna et al. [10] demonstrated that the closing pressure for the airways amounts to −1 to −2 cmH₂O, while for the alveoli it ranges between −2 and −6 cmH₂O. As a result, during lung deflation, TGV is reached before there is alveolar collapse. This is a functionally useful feature because smaller PLs are required to reopen closed airways than closed alveoli.

Airway opening pressure

The PL necessary to reopen a closed airway would be expected to be greater than that required to close it, because surface forces would be different under the two circumstances [12]. Indeed, as shown in Fig. 2, during lung inflation from TGV there is very little volume change until a critical P_L of about 10 cmH$_2$O is reached. This pressure probably represents the *minimum* airway opening pressure (min *Po*). As for airway closing pressure, different airways probably have different opening pressures. An evaluation of the *maximum* airway opening pressure (max *Po*) may be possible by analysis of the shape of the inflation volume-pressure curve of the lung in Fig. 2.

In the volume range between the lung volume corresponding to the minimum opening pressure (about 10 cmH$_2$O of PL) and about 36% of V30, the slope of the inflation curve increases progressively (Fig. 2). This phenomenon probably reflects, at least in part, progressive opening of closed airways and therefore progressive recruitment of lung units that were initially at their TGV. At lung volumes higher than about 36% of V30, the relationship between volume and pressure again fits with good approximation an exponential function of the type described by Eq. 1. The point where the experimental curve joins the exponential function (inflection point on inflation in Fig. 2) probably reflects max Po, the latter being about 5 cmH$_2$O higher than the min Po.

"Knee" on static inflation volume-pressure curve

As shown in Fig. 2, up to PL of 10 cmH$_2$O there is little increase in volume, the latter mainly reflecting expansion of the central airways with increasing applied positive pressure. At PL of about 10 cmH$_2$O, which corresponds to Po min, there is a rapid increase in volume, as reflected by a rapid change in the slope dV/dPL. As a result, the inflation V-P curve at this point is characterized by an apparent "knee", which is commonly termed "lower inflection point". This, however, is a misnomer because an inflection point is actually said to occur when the slope of a curve changes direction (from increasing to decreasing or vice versa). The "knee", on the other hand, corresponds to the region where the rate of change in slope dV/dPL is highest.

Isotropic behaviour of lungs

Isotropic behaviour implies that all parts of the lungs fill or empty proportionately [13]. In studies on excised exsanguinated dog lobes, Frank [14] has shown that there is a small difference in the static volume-pressure relationships between the upper and lower lobes but not between the right and left upper lobes or the right and left lower lobes. This has been confirmed in a large series of dog lobes [15] and has also been demonstrated in rabbits [16], but not in humans [17]. However, some indirect evidence suggests that in man there may also be differences similar to those observed in dogs and rabbits [18], although other indirect estimates [19] support the notion of equal static volume-pressure relationships among the various human lobes. At the sublobar level, the available evidence suggests that the static mechanical properties are relatively uniform. In radioactive xenon studies on excised dogs lobes, Faridy et al. [15] demonstrated that, at least at the gross regional lobar level, the static mechanical properties within each lobe are substantially uniform. Morphometric studies in isolated lungs of dogs [20] have also shown that the alveoli expand uniformly, both in the sense that all undergo a proportional increase in size and that this increase is equal in all directions. In experiments on excised dog lungs, Hughes et al. [21] demonstrated that during lung inflation and deflation the percentage changes of bronchial length and diameter for airways of different sizes are approximately the same, and changes in length and in many cases of diameter were reasonably well correlated with changes in the cube root of absolute lung volume. All of these findings are consistent with the notion that in the absence of airspace or airway closure, the isolated lungs or lobes expand virtually uniformly.

Static behaviour of lungs in situ

While in the absence of airspace or airway closure the isolated lungs or lobes expand virtually uniformly, this is not the case when the lungs are inside the thorax. This different behaviour can probably be accounted for almost entirely by the fact that, whereas in excised preparations the pleural surface pressure is uniform, this is not so in the intact thorax. Indeed, it is now recognized that in situ the pleural surface pressure is not uniform, but that there is normally a vertical 'gradient' in pleural surface pressure, with the more-negative values at the upper parts. As a result of the vertical gradient of pleural surface pressure, the static PL is greater in upper lung zones and consequently the upper lung units are normally more expanded than those in the lower zones.

The effects of the vertical gradient of PL on regional ventilation distribution and on regional gas exchange have been fully described in the literature [11, 18, 22-26]. Here we will consider the implications to the conventional measurements of the elastic properties of the lung.

Figure 3 shows the static volume-pressure curves of a normal subject

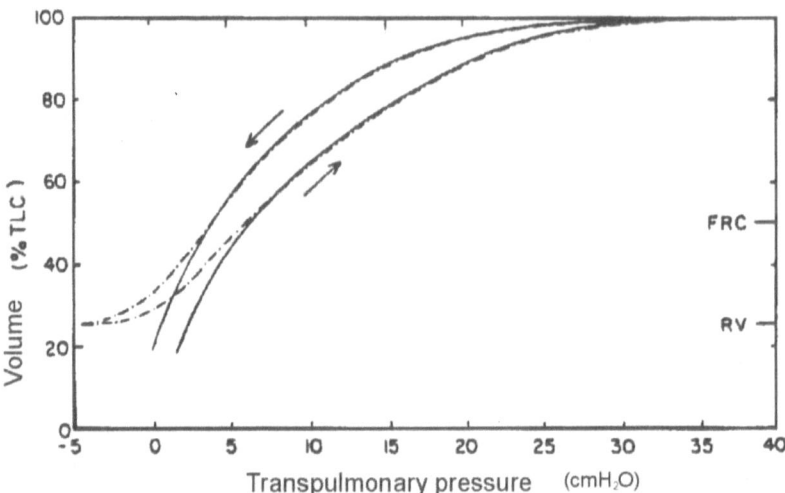

Fig. 3 Pulmonary static volume-pressure curves obtained in a normal subject in situ. Lung gas volume is expressed as a percentage of the total lung capacity (*% TLC*). *Broken lines* experimental relationships, *solid lines* exponential relationships. *FRC* functional residual capacity, *RV* residual volume. The point at which the experimental relationship during deflation deviates from the corresponding exponential curve indicates the maximal critical closing pressure (Pc max), while the same point during inflation reflects the maximal critical opening pressure (Po max) (from reference [19] with permission)

measured in situ using the oesophageal balloon technique [19]. Similar to Fig. 2 the exponential volume-pressure relationships during lung deflation and inflation are also shown. In situ, maximal Pc (reflecting onset of peripheral airway closure) occurs at a much higher lung volume (~ 50% TLC) than in the isolated lung (~ 20% V30), because of the vertical gradient in pleural surface pressure. Furthermore, with intact thorax, some of the airways remain patent even at full expiration. Thus, in situ the morphology of the static volume-pressure curves of the lung is profoundly altered by the pleural pressure gradient. It should be noted, however, that artefacts in oesophageal pressure measurements probably also affect the volume-pressure curve of the lungs particularly in the supine position [26].

Conclusions

Based on the present review it can be concluded that (1) lower static PL values are required to close the alveoli than peripheral airways; (2) much higher static

PL values are required to reopen atelectatic alveoli than closed peripheral airways; (3) in isolated lungs peripheral airway closure during lung deflation and opening during inflation occur over a smaller volume range than in situ; and (4) the "knee" on the static inflation volume-pressure curve of the lungs reflects reopening of peripheral airways and not alveoli. Further studies are, however, required for better definition of the elastic properties of the normal human lungs.

References

1. Hutchinson J (1949-52) Thorax. In: Todd RB (ed) Cyclopaedia of anatomy and physiology 4. Longmans, London, V1016
2. Hoppin FG Jr, Stothert JC Jr, Greaves IA, et al (1986) In: Macklem P, Mead J (eds) Lung recoil: elastic and rheological properties. In: Handbook of physiology, section 3. The respiratory system, vol. III. Mechanics. I. American Physiology Society, Bethesda, Maryland, pp 195-215
3. Glaister DH, Schroter RC, Sudlow MF, et al (1973) Bulk elastic properties of excised lungs and the effect of transpulmonary pressure gradient. Respir Physiol 17:347-364
4. Hoppin FG Jr (1999) Sources of lung recoil. In: Milic-Emili J (ed) Respiratory mechanics. Eur Respir Monogr 12:33-53
5. Stigol LC, Vawter GF, Mead J (1972) Studies on the elastic recoil of the lung in pediatric population. Am Rev Respir Dis 105:552-563
6. Frank NR (1959) Influence of acute pulmonary congestion on recolling force of excised cat's lung. J Appl Physiol 14:905-908
7. Basch S von (1887) Ueber eine Function des Capillardruckes in den Lungen-alveol. Wien Med Blatter 10:465-467
8. Kleinman LE, Poulos DA, Siebens AA (1964) Minimal air in dogs. J Appl Physiol 19:204-206
9. Hughes JMB, Rosenzweig DY, Kivitz PB (1970) Site of airway closure in excised dog lungs: histologic demonstration J Appl Physiol 29:340-344
10. Cavagna GA, Stemmler EJ, DuBois AB (1967) Alveolar resistance to atelectasis. J Appl Physiol 22:441-452
11. Milic-Emili J, Henderson JAM, Dolovich MB, et al (1966) Regional distribution of inspired gas in the lung. J Appl Physiol 21:749-759
12. Macklem PT, Proctor DF, Hogg JC (1969-70) The stability of peripheral airways. Respir Physiol 8:191-203
13. Radford EPJ (1964) Static mechanical properties of mammalian lungs. In: Fenn WO, Rahn H (eds) Handbook of physiology. Respiration 1. Am Physiol Soc, Washington DC, pp 429-449
14. Frank NR (1963) A comparison of static volume-pressure relations of excised pulmonary lobes of dogs. J Appl Physiol 18:274-278
15. Faridy EE, Kidd R, Milic-Emili J (1967) Topographical distribution of inspired gas in excised lobes of dogs. J Appl Physiol 22:760-766
16. D'Angelo E (1972) Local alveolar size and transpulmonary pressure in situ and in isolated lungs. Respir Physiol 14:251-266
17. Berend N, Shoog C, Thrulbeck WM (1981) Exponential analysis of lobar pressure-volume characteristics. Thorax 36:452-455
18. Bake B, Bjure J, Grimby G, et al (1967) Regional distribution of inspired gas in supine man. Scand J Respir Dis 48:189-196
19. Sutherland PW, Katsura T, Milic-Emili J (1968) Previous volume history of the lung and regional distribution of gas. J Appl Physiol 25:566-574

20. Glazier JB, Hughes JMB, Maloney JE, et al (1967) Vertical gradient of alveolar size in lungs of dogs frozen intact. J Appl Physiol 23: 694-705
21. Hughes JMB, Hoppin FG, Mead J (1972) Effect of lung inflation on bronchial length and diameter in excised lungs. J Appl Physiol 32: 25-35
22. Milic-Emili J (1974) Pulmonary statics. In: Widdicombe JG (ed) Respiratory physiology I, vol 2. International Review of Physiology Series, Butterworth, Baltimore, pp105-137
23. Milic-Emili J (1977) Ventilation. In: West J (ed) Regional differences in lung. Academic Press, New York, pp167-199
24. Milic-Emili J (1986) Static distribution of lung volumes. In: Macklem P, Mead J (eds) Handbook of physiology: mechanics of breathing, vol 2. American Physiology Society, Bethesda, Maryland, pp 561-574
25. Milic-Emili J, Mead J, Turner JM (1964) Topography of esophageal pressure as a function of posture in man. J Appl Physiol 19: 212-216
26. Milic-Emili J (1997) Topographical inequality of ventilation. In: Crystal RG, West J (eds) The Lung: scientific foundations, 2nd edn. Lippinson-Raven, Philadelphia, pp 1415-1423

Definition of spectrum of acute lung injury

C.S. VALENTE BARBAS, C. HOELZ, V.L. CAPELOZZI

Acute lung injury (ALI) and acute respiratory distress syndrome (ARDS) are part of a spectrum of the same syndrome that reflect the clinical expression of the alveolar-capillary membrane permeability alterations leading to a protein--rich pulmonary edema and consequent acute respiratory failure after a genetically predisposed human organism is exposed to a trigger [1-3].

The pathogenic pathway or underlying disease responsible for the inflammatory injury in ARDS may occur either directly in lung cells, as with aspiration pneumonia, pulmonary infection (bacterial pneumonia, viral pneumonia, and protozoa pneumonia), inhalation injury, pulmonary contusion, near drowning, or indirectly via the bloodstream, as with sepsis, severe trauma with prolonged hypotension and or multiple fractures, multiple transfusions of blood products, acute pancreatitis, fat emboli, cardiopulmonary bypass, endovenous drug overdose, disseminated intravascular coagulation, reperfusion injury burns and head injury [3-5].

It is important to analyze the pulmonary and extrapulmonary origin of ALI/ARDS because, in the case of direct insult, lung injury is characterized by a lesion of the pulmonary epithelium due to the activation of alveolar macrophages, and the prevalent damage is intra-alveolar, with the occupation of pulmonary units by biological material. Physiological experiments indicate that it is the alveolar epithelium, rather than the capillary endothelium, that determines the permeability of the alveolar-capillary barrier to large molecules. Hence, considering the extensive damage to the alveolar epithelium in pulmonary ARDS, the escape of fluid and macromolecules from capillaries and the interstitial space into the alveoli would no longer be impeded. Morphological experiments with ALI induced by the subcutaneous administration of *N*-nitroso-*N*-methyurethane in dogs (causing extensive necrosis of the alveolar epithelium, while the capillary endothelium remains essentially intact) described diffuse perivascular and interstitial edema and alveolar collapse when epithelial cell necrosis became more widespread. The direct injury to the surfactant-producing system leads to a decrease in the amount of surfactant, followed by increases in surface tension and alveolar collapse. This increased surface tension, transmitted to the alveolar wall, might alter intravascular hydrostatic pressure gradients across the capillaries, causing interstitial and perivascular edema. Important clinical studies designed to assess the function of the alveolar epithelial barrier in early ARDS have demonstrated that the alveolar epithelium is more resistant than the lung endothelium, particularly after extrapulmonary ARDS, and alveolar epithelial barrier function may be clinically useful as a prognostic index [3, 4]. Hoelz et al. [4] found histological quantitative morphometric differences between pulmonary and extrapulmonary ARDS. In pulmonary ARDS there is a predominance of alveolar collapse, fibrinous exudate, and alveolar wall edema compared with extrapulmonry ARDS. In addition, Negri et al. [5], based on extracellular matrix remodeling analysis, demonstrated that pulmonary ARDS shows a greater content of collagen compared with extrapulmonary ARDS. Gattinoni et al. [6] suggested that patients suffering direct pulmonary insults show lower compliance and have alveolar units that are less susceptible to recruitment by mechanical ventilation than do those with an extrapulmonary initiating process. In 1999, Goodman et al. [7], studying the computed tomography patterns of pulmonary and extrapulmonary ARDS, described more-extensive consolidations in patients with pulmonary ARDS and correlated their findings with higher shunt fraction, higher mean pulmonary arterial pressure, and less recruitment with positive pressure ventilation. They hypothesized that these findings may represent a combination of edema, atelectasis, or early hyaline membrane formation, and may be the area most responsible for improved gas exchange with mechanical ventilation. The authors still noticed that more consolidation was associated with increased mortality [7].

Identifying risk factors for the development of ALI/ARDS is particularly important in evaluating treatments that may prevent progression to lung injury in high-risk populations [8]. Three prospectives studies from the early 1980s evaluated the incidence of ARDS in patients with known risk factors [9-11]. The data from these prospective studies identified sepsis as the most-common risk factor for developing ALI/ARDS, followed by aspiration pneumonia, pneumonia, trauma (lung contusion), and multiple transfusions [9-11]; overall approximately 20-40% of patients with well-established risk factors and respiratory failure develop ARDS and the more risk factors in any individual, the greater the likelihood of developing the syndrome. Of the patients that developed ARDS, 76% had done so within 2-24 h of the inciting event and 93% by 72 h [9].

In addition to the risk factors discussed, recent reports have identified additional conditions that influence the susceptibility of individuals to develop lung injury. In a prospective study of 351 patients, the incidence of ARDS with one of the seven known at-risk diagnoses was compared in patients with and without a history of chronic alcohol abuse. The incidence of ARDS was 43% in patients with a history of chronic alcohol abuse compared with 22% in the control group [12]. Patients with higher APACHE II scores at the time of the at-risk diagnosis also had a significantly higher incidence of ARDS. Both the history of chronic alcohol abuse and the APACHE II score remain significant with multivariate analysis. The same investigators hypothesized that patients with diabetes mellitus may be protected from an ARDS due to the impaired neutrophil function associated with hyperglycemia. In a study of 113 patients with septic shock , the incidence of ARDS was 25% in diabetic and 47% in non-diabetic patients [13]. Mortality was not significantly different between the two groups.

Several prospective studies identified risk factors that are independent predictors of mortality [14-17]. Although identification of independent predictors of mortality using multivariate analysis in any single study depends on which risk factors are evaluated, cumulative data convincingly show that patients with ALI/ARDS and sepsis, liver disease, non-pulmonary organ dysfunction , or advanced age have higher mortality rates. Equal distribution of these risk factors among experimental and control groups is essential when enrolling patients in clinical trials [14-17].

Histologically, lungs were characterized by diffuse alveolar damage (DAD), with a subdivision of the temporal course into early and late lesions, designated as acute and chronic or fibroproliferative diffuse alveolar damage. The acute stage of DAD is characterized by interstitial and intra-alveolar edema and hyaline membranes, described as important diagnostic features of early DAD. This stage is followed by a consecutive proliferation of fibroblastic cells, characterizing chronic or fibroproliferative DAD [3-5]. It is important to differentiate between the acute and chronic phases of the ARDS because it was recently shown in a prospective and randomized clinical trial that methylprednisolone (2 mg/kg per day) can improve the gas exchange and patient survival in the chronic phase compared with placebo.

According to the last North American-European Consensus conference (NAECC) a revised definition for acute lung injury and ARDS includes [18]:

Onset:	Acute and persistent
Oxygenation criteria	PaO_2/FIO_2 300 for ALI
	PaO_2/FIO_2 200 for ARDS
Haemodynamic criteria	PAOP 18mmHg
	No clinical evidence of left atrial hypertension
Radiographic criteria	Bilateral opacities consistent with pulmonary edema

The consensus conference recognized that accurate estimates of the inciden-ce and outcomes of ARDS were hindered by the lack of a simple uniform definition , especially one that could be used to enrol patients in clinical studies. However, as a group that participate in clinical trials of ARDS we have some concerns about this definition.

1. Onset: acute and persistent. Clinicians have to try to detect the exact moment that the patient was exposed to the cause of ARDS, as well as the time that the deterioration of gas exchange started (room air without PEEP). Clinicians have to try to classify the syndrome into the early or exudative or late fibroproliferative stage (radiological, pressure-volume curve meas-urement, tomographic findings) as the response to mechanical ventilation and PEEP and pharmacological agents (corticosteroids) may be different.

2. Oxygenation criteria. We all know that the PaO_2/FIO_2 depends on the ventilator settings. For example, a patient with the diagnosis of ARDS has a PaO_2/FIO_2 ratio of 100. After a recruitment maneuver and with a PEEP level of 19 cmH_2O the same patient has PaO_2/FIO_2 ratio of 350 (no longer an ARDS according to the definition).

Then it is very important to compare the PaO_2/FIO_2 ratio with the ventilator settings at which it was calculated. This allows us to standardize the PaO_2/FIO_2 calculation.

3. Hemodynamic criteria: POAP18 mmHg or no clinical evidence of left atrial hypertension. We all know PAOP pressure depends on volemic status, left cardiac function, and level of airway (alveolar) pressurization. Hence, it is important to refer to the ventilator settings while measuring the PAOP pressure, as well as to know the volemic status of the patient (Hidric balance or daily weight comparisons). It is important also that while measuring the PAOP with the Swan-Ganz catheter we also measure the cardiac output or a better profile index, such as left ventricular work/ PAOP pressure [19].

4. Radiographic criteria: bilateral opacities consistent with pulmonary ede-ma. We all know that pulmonary bilateral infiltrates can reflect more than the alveoli capillary membrane permeability alterations. For example, these two thoracic scans show bilateral pulmonary infiltrates without signals of left ventricular failure (PAOP < 18 mmHg) (Fig. 1). However, the computerized thoracic tomography shown in the first case is typical of ALI/ARDS: gravitational dependent lungs densities (lung biopsy ARDS). In the second case, the computerized thoracic tomography showed bilateral pulmonary condensation with airway bronchograms (lung biopsy bron-chiolitis obliterative organizing pneumonia).

Computerized thoracic tomography is a very important tool in the diagnosis of ALI/ARDS, showing bilateral infiltrates (edema) and gravitational depend-

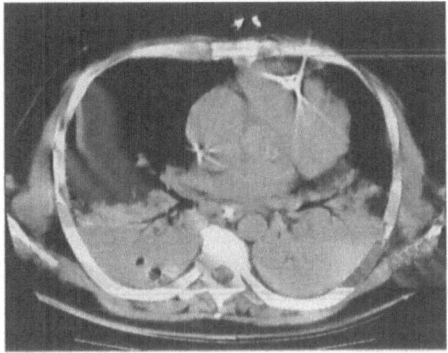 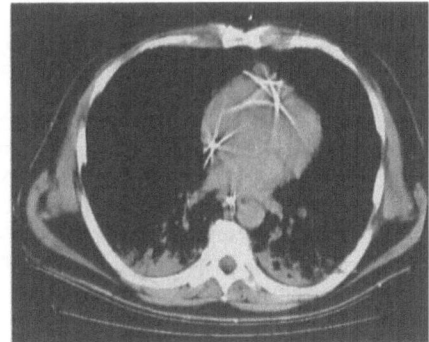

Fig. 1 Thoracic computerized tomography in a patient with acute respiratory distress syndrome (*left*) with gravitational dependent lung densities, and in a patient with bronchiolitis obliterative organizing pneumonia (*right*) showing bilateral pulmonary condensation

ent alveolar densities (edema and collapse) that can be graded at the time of tomography as a histogram or percentage of collapse. Thoracic tomography can show other concomitant infiltrates, associated pulmonary infections, and/or inflammation that can alert the physician to an associated diagnosis. Thoracic tomography can show the redistribution of the infiltrates when turning the patient to the prone position and can detect the response to mechanical ventilation, different PEEP levels, and recruitment maneuvers [20].

In patients with clinical and functional deterioration despite the standard treatment and in patients with atypical tomographic findings, a pulmonary biopsy can help in establishing the diagnosis. We evaluated 12 patients with open lung biopsy after clinical deterioration, after optimizing the medical treatment and mechanical ventilation and we found DAD associated with viral infections in 6 of the patients (cytomegalovirus, herpes and influenza virus) and unsuspected diseases (such as leukemic infiltrates and malaria) [21].

As well as taking in account the pulmonary infiltrates in the chest scan, the gas exchange, and the PAOP pressures, the physicians have to understand the spectrum of alveolar-capillary membrane permeability dysfunction and the associated conditions to try to correct the precipitating and causes avoid increasing the injury using appropriate ventilatory protective strategies [22, 23], while recovery of the integrity of the alveolar capillary membrane is taking place.

References

1. Marshall RP (2002) Genetic polymorphisms associated with susceptibility and outcome in ARDS. Chest 121 [Suppl]: 68S-69S
2. Wong HR (2002) ARDS: the future. Crit Care Clin 18:177
3. Albertine KH (1998) Histopathology of pulmonary oedema and the acute respiratory distress syndrome in pulmonary oedema. Dekker, New York, vol 116, pp 37-83
4. Hoelz C, Negri EM, Lichtenfels AJFC, et al (2001) Morphometric differences in pulmonary lesions in primary and secondary ARDS. Pathol Res Pract 197:521-530
5. Negri EM, Hoelz C, Barbas CSV, et al (2002) Acute remodeling of parenchyma in pulmonary and extrapulmonary ARDS. An autopsy study of collagen-elastic system fibers. Pathol Res Pract 198:355-361
6. Gattinoni L, Pelosi P, Suter P, et al (1998). Acute respiratory distress syndrome caused by pulmonary and extrapulmonary disease. Different syndromes? Am J Respir Crit Care Med 158:3-11
7. Goodman L, Fumagalli R, Tagliabue P, et al (1999) Adult respiratory distress syndrome due to pulmonary and extrapulmonary causes: CT, clinical and functional correlations. Radiology 213:545-552
8. Atabai K, Matthay MA (2002) The pulmonary physician in critical care: acute lung injury and the respiratory distress syndrome: definitions and epidemiology. Thorax 57:452-458
9. Fowler AA, Hamman RF, Good JT, et al (1983) Adult respiratory distress syndrome: risk with common predisposition. Ann Intern Med 98: 593-597
10. Hudson LD, Milberg JA, Anardi D, et al (1995) Clinical risks for development of the acute respiratory distress syndrome. Am J Respir Crit Care Med 151:293-301
11. Pepe PE, Potkin RT, Reus DH, et al (1982) Clinical predictors of the adult respiratory distress syndrome . Am J Surg 144:124-30
12. Moss M, Bucher B, Moore FA, et al (1996) The role of chronic alcohol abuse in the development of acute respiratory distress syndrome. JAMA 275:50-54
13. Moss M, Guidot DM, Steiberg KP, et al (2000) Diabetic patients have a decreased incidence of acute respiratory distress syndrome. Crit Care Med 28:2187-2192
14. Doyle RL, Szaflarski N, Modin GW, et al (1995) Identification of patients with acute lung injury. Predictors of mortality. Am J Respir Crit Care Med 152:1818-1824
15. Monchi M, Bellenfant F, Cariou A, et al (1998) Early predictive factors of survival in the acute respiratory distress syndrome. A multivariate analysis. Am Respir Crit Care Med 158:1076-1081
16. Zilberberg MD, Epstein SK (1998) Acute lung injury in the medical ICU: comorbid conditions, age, etiology, and hospital outcome. Am J Respir Crit Care Med 157:1159-1164
17. Lurh OR, Antonsen K, Karlsson M, et al (1999) Incidence and mortality after acute respiratory failure and acute respiratory distress syndrome in Sweden, Denmark and Iceland. The ARF Study Group. Am J Respir Crit Care Med 159:1849-1861
18. Artigas A (1998) The American-European Consensus Conference on ARDS, II. Ventilatory, pharmacologic, supportive therapy, study design strategies and issues related to recovery and remodeling. Intensive Care Med 24:378-398
19. Taylor AE, Cope DK, Allison RC, et al (1991) Capillary pressure measurement in human lungs in adult respiratory distress syndrome. Dekker, New York, vol 50, pp 353-366
20. Gattinoni L (2001) What has computed tomography taught us about the acute respiratory distress syndrome? Am J Respir Crit Care Med 164:1701-1711
21. Barbas CSV, Capelozzi VL, Hoelz C, et al (2002) Impact of lung biopsy in acute respiratory failure. Am J Respir Crit Care Med 165:A218
22. Amato MBP, Barbas CSV, Medeiros DM, et al (1998) Effect of a protective ventilatory strategy on mortality in the acute respiratory distress syndrome. N Engl J Med 338:347-354
23. ARDS Network (2000) Ventilation with lower tidal volumes as compared with traditional tidal volumes for acute lung injury and the acute distress syndrome. The Acute Respiratory Distress Syndrome Network. N Engl J Med 342:1301-1308

Primary and secondary ARDS

P.R.M. Rocco

The first descriptions of acute respiratory distress syndrome appeared in 1967, when Ashbaugh and colleagues [1] described 12 patients with acute respiratory distress, cyanosis refractory to oxygen therapy, decreased lung compliance, and diffuse infiltrates evident on the chest radiograph. It is not defined by a specific pathogenesis, but reflects the lung's non-selective response to numerous insults and precipitating factors. Based on these observations, the term "syndrome" defined as "group of symptoms and signs of disordered function related to one another by means of some anatomic, physiologic, or biochemical peculiarity" was used. Although the term acute respiratory distress syndrome (ARDS) is often used interchangeably with acute lung injury (ALI), by strict criteria ARDS should be reserved for the most severe end of the spectrum (Table 1) [2].

Table 1. Recommended criteria for acute lung injury (ALI) and acute respiratory distress syndrome (ARDS) [2]

	Timing	Oxygenation	Chest radiograph	Pulmonary artery wedge pressure
ALI criteria	Acute onset	PaO_2/FIO_2_300 (regardless of PEEP level)	Bilateral infiltrates seen on frontal chest radiograph	≤18 mmHg when measured or no clinical evidence of left atrial hypertension
ARDS criteria	Acute onset	PaO_2/FIO_2_200 (regardless of PEEP level)	Bilateral infiltrates seen on frontal chest radiograph	≤18 mmHg when measured or no clinical evidence of left atrial hypertension

Despite recent advances in intensive care, mortality rates persist at between 40-60%. The acute respiratory distress syndrome is thought to be a uniform expression of a diffuse and overwhelming inflammatory reaction of the pulmonary parenchyma to a variety of serious underlying diseases. In 1994, the American-European Consensus Conference [2] defined two pathogenetic pathways leading to ARDS: a direct ("primary" or "pulmonary") insult, that directly affects lung parenchyma, and an indirect ("secondary" or "extrapulmonary') insult, that results from an acute systemic inflammatory response (Table 2) [3]. Sepsis, usually from gram-negative infections, is the most prevalent and lethal cause of ARDS (50%). Much of the scientific research in ALI has centred on sepsis and lung injury [4]. Pulmonary aspiration and trauma account for a further 25%. Drug overdose, pancreatitis, smoke inhalation, lung contusion, and other causes comprise the remaining risk factors.

Table 2. Major categories of acute lung injury risk

Direct lung injury	Indirect lung injury
Common causes	Common causes
Pneumonia (bacterial, fungal, viral, atypical)	Sepsis syndrome
Aspiration of gastric contents	Severe non-thoracic trauma with shock and multiple transfusions (multiple long bone fractures, hypovolemic shock)
Less common causes	Less common causes
Severe thoracic trauma (pulmonary contusion)	Cardiopulmonary bypass
Fat emboli	Hypertransfusion of blood products for emergency resuscitation
Near-drowning	Drug overdose (opiates, paraldehyde, thiazides, paraquat)
Inhalation injury (smoke, oxygen, chorine, phosgene)	Acute pancreatitis
Reperfusion pulmonary edema after lung transplantation or pulmonary embolectomy	Disseminated intravascular coagulation

There are many causes that trigger ALI, but the determination of its precise pathophysiology needs to be clarified. Extensive animal studies have examined the inflammatory cascades initiated by infection, trauma, burns, and haemorrhage [5]. These studies have demonstrated the complexity and multiplicity of pathways involved in these pathophysiologic processes, and they indicate that differences in the initial insult, combined with underlying conditions, can result in the activation of different inflammatory mechanisms. Understanding the range of pathways that lead to pulmonary dysfunction, it may be possible to assess several novel treatments to specific areas of the pathologic cascade in an attempt to modify lung injury. Although various causes of ARDS result in a uniform pathology in the late stage [6-9], evidence indicates that the pathophysiology of early ARDS may differ according to the type of the primary insult [8, 10-12].

This chapter presents a brief overview of primary and secondary ARDS, especially its functional, histological and inflammatory differences. In addition, we will describe the effects of different ventilatory therapies and pharmacological agents in primary and secondary ARDS.

Pathogenesis

The alveolar-capillary barrier is formed by two separate histological entities, the microvascular endothelium and the alveolar epithelium. It has been thought that, whatever the insult applied to the lung, through the airways or the circulation, the final result is diffuse alveolar damage [13].

In experimental models of ALI/ARDS, different response and morphological alterations of lung parenchyma have been reported as a consequence of direct insult (intratracheal instillation of endotoxin, complement, tumour necrosis factor, or bacteria) or indirect insult to the alveoli (endotoxin injected intravenously or intraperitoneally). This distinction is important, as the pathway may govern the expression of the pulmonary abnormalities.

After a direct insult, the primary structure injured is the pulmonary epithelium. The normal alveolar epithelium is composed of two types of cells: flat type I cells (which make up 90% of the alveolar surface area and are easily injured) and cuboidal type II cells (which make up 10% of the alveolar surface area and are more resistant to injury). Type II cells have many functions: surfactant production, ion transport, and proliferation and differentiation to type I cell after injury. The lesion of alveolar epithelium leads to activation of alveolar macrophages and of inflammatory network, determining the onset of pulmonary inflammation. The epithelial damage determines: a) alveolar flooding (the epithelial barrier is much less permeable than the endothelial barrier) [10], b) reduction in the removal of oedema fluid from the alveolar space (loss of epithelial integrity and injury of type II cells disrupt normal epithelial fluid transport) [14], c) lessening the production and turnover of surfactant (lesion of type II cells)[15], and d) fibrosis (severe and disorganised alveolar epithelium injury leads to fibrosis) [16]. Thus, the prevalent damage following the direct insult is intra-alveolar with alveolar filling by oedema, fibrin, collagen, neutrophilic aggregates, and/or blood.

When the insult is indirect, pulmonary lesions are originated by the mediators released from extrapulmonary foci into the blood (e.g., peritonitis, pancreatitis). The main target damage is the pulmonary endothelial cell. The activation of the inflammatory network results in increased permeability of the endothelial barrier and recruitment of monocytes, neutrophils, platelets, and other cells [17]. Thus, the pathologic alteration due to an indirect insult is mainly represented by microvessels congestion and interstitial oedema, with a relatively sparing of the intra-alveolar spaces.

It is probable that direct and indirect insults can coexist. This may be observed in patients with pneumonia when one lung is initially directly affected, and the other is indirectly injured hours or days later as the inflammation spreads by means of loss of compartmentalization (indirect insult).

It is important to differentiate between direct and indirect pathophysiologic pathways, as the underlying pathology seems to be different in the two conditions (consolidation versus interstitial oedema and collapse), at least during the early phase, and this may influence the approach to treatment [18].

Histopathology

There is a general belief that ARDS is the extreme form of a spectrum of lung injury caused by a uniform inflammatory mechanism that is independent of the precipitating disease. This assumption mainly originates from pathology studies, which have consistently indicated that the lung response to injury is stereotyped, with transition from acute alveolar capillary damage to a late proliferative phase, quite independently of the initial cause [19]. Unfortunately, most of the studies report late or terminal events, and pathologic features of early phases of ARDS such as interstitial oedema and alveolar collapse are not easily recognised.

Hoelz and colleagues described the morphological differences between pulmonary lesions in acute respiratory distress syndrome originating from primary and secondary ARDS [20]. They observed a predominance of alveolar collapse, fibrinous exudate and alveolar wall oedema in primary ARDS. The morphological difference between primary and secondary ARDS was mainly quantitative in extent and distribution according to the underlying disease.

We studied lungs morphometrically with primary and secondary ARDS induced by intratracheal and intraperitoneal injection of lipopolysaccharide (LPS) of *Escherichia coli* [21]. Interestingly, light microscopy analyses showed similar increment in alveolar collapse and tissue cellularity 24 hours after the induction of the lesion (Figure 1). However, analysing the electron microscopy in primary ARDS, we observed extensive injury of alveolar epithelium, swollen and fragmented type I and II cells (lamellar bodies in the alveolar space), intact capillary endothelium, ductal hyperdistension, neutrophil recruitment into the alveolar space, proliferation of fibroblasts into the alveolar septa, the presence of collagen fibre type III and hyaline membranes. Secondary ARDS showed interstitial oedema and intact types I and II cells. The amount of apoptotic neutrophils was higher in primary than in secondary ARDS (Figure 2).

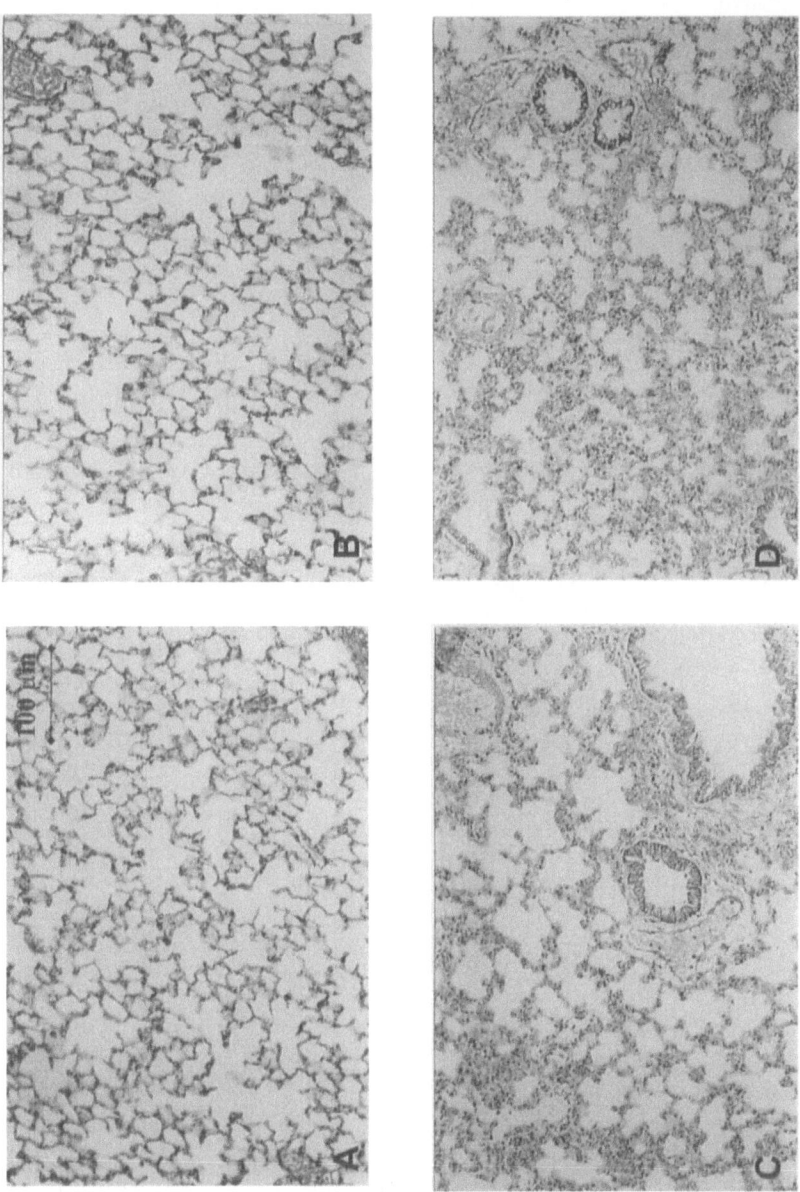

Fig. 1. Lung histology from the lungs of the control (A and C) and primary and secondary acute lung injury groups (B and D). Photographs were taken at an original magnification of x100 from slides stained by HE.

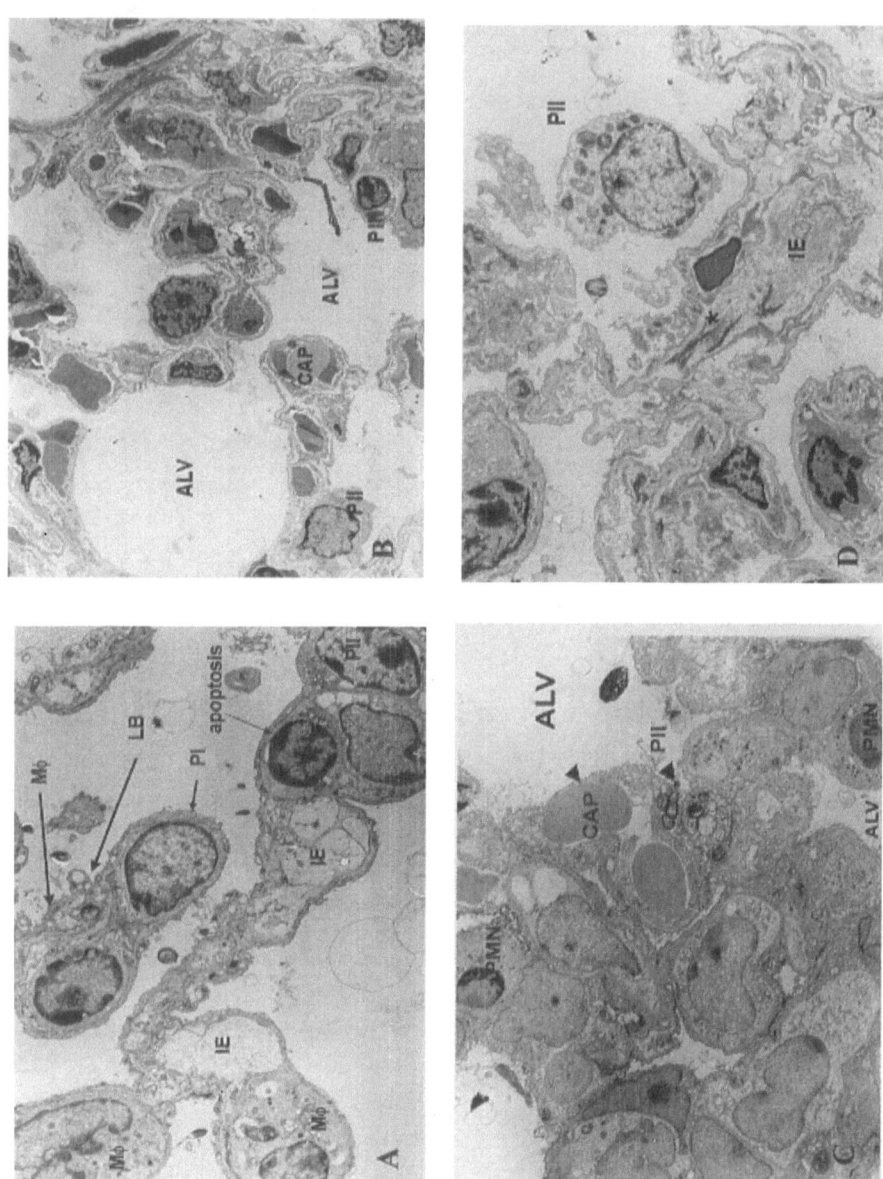

Fig. 2. Electron micrographs of rat lungs obtained 24 hours after intratracheal instillation (A and D) or intraperitoneal (B and D) injection of *Escherichia coli* LPS (x5000). ALV = alveolus, LB = lamellar bodies, PI = pneumocyte type I, PII = pneumocyte type II, IE = interstitial edema, MΦ = macrophages, PMN = polymorphonuclear. In C the alveolar epithelium is destroyed (arrowhead) while the capillary endothelium (CAP) is intact. Asterisk = collagen fibre.

Morphological analysis

Over the past 15 years, many experimental and clinical reports have described the different morphological patterns found in ALI/ARDS by means of computed tomography (CT). Unfortunately, most of the series were limited in size, used different methodological approaches, different generations of CT equipment, and varied greatly in terminology for describing morphological changes [23]. CT scan has conclusively shown that ALI/ARDS is !n inhomogeneous process, ALI/ARDS morphology varies with aetiology, and ALI/ARDS morphology changes with time, mechanical ventilation, and patient position. Since anatomic descriptors varied so broadly, it is worthwhile to define the CT terminology on the basis of the Fleischner Society Nomenclature Committee: a) ground-glass opacification: a hazy increase in lung attenuation, with preservation of bronchial and vascular margins; b) consolidation: a homogeneous increase in lung attenuation that obscures bronchovascular margins in which an air-bronchogram may be present; and c) reticular pattern: innumerable interlacing line shadows that may be fine, intermediate or coarse [24]. In ALI/ARDS the ground glass opacification is thought to reflect an active inflammatory process involving both the lung interstitium, with abnormal thickening of the alveolar wall, and incomplete filling of the alveolar space with inflammatory cells, cellular debris, and oedema. Consolidation, otherwise referred to as a dense parenchymal opacification, whether patchy or diffuse, usually refers to pulmonary parenchyma, which is completely or almost completely airless. This may be due to either a complete filling of the alveolar spaces with liquid and cells or to total collapse of potentially recruitable pulmonary units (atelectasis), or to a combination of both. Reticular pattern usually refers to discrete, recognisable linear thickening of the interstitium. This may be acute (oedema or interstitial inflammation) or chronic (fibrosis) [24, 25].

In ALI/ARDS due to the direct insult via the airway (aspiration, pneumonia), one should expect multifocal involvement of the lung parenchyma, whereas with indirect insult, one should expect a more diffuse and uniform parenchymal alteration due to hematogenously distributed mediators. It has been experimentally shown that with indirect insult, the alteration is primarily interstitial [26]. In addition, as the indirect pulmonary insult is commonly due to abdominal diseases, basilar atelectasis increases due to the augmented abdominal pressure from the cephalad shift of the diaphragm. Indeed, the morphological CT patterns in primary and secondary ALI/ARDS should be somewhat different [23, 27].

Goodman and coworkers compared 22 patients with early primary ARDS with 11 patients with secondary ARDS [28]. They observed that secondary ARDS depicted predominantly symmetric ground glass opacification and dorsal consolidation (atelectasis), whereas primary ARDS tended to be asymmetric, with a mix of dense parenchymal opacification and ground grass opacification. Rouby et al [12], Desai et al [29], and Winer-Muram et al [30] reached similar but not identical results. Unfortunately, these studies presented some limitations: a) all reported a small number of patients, b) secondary ARDS group included patients with abdominal disease and patients after cardiac surgery, in which the left lower lobe collapse is a frequent finding, c) direct and indirect insults may coexist, making the morphological pattern difficult to interpret. Recently, Desai and coworkers showed that seven of 25 patients with secondary ARDS, and five of 16 patients with primary ARDS had typical CT features [31]. Thus, the differentiation of primary from secondary ARDS, is not assured on the basis of CT alone; no single CT feature can be shown in isolation to accurately predict whether ARDS is of the primary or secondary type. These findings highlight a fundamental limitation of the aforementioned studies [12, 27-30].

Respiratory mechanics

Gattinoni and colleagues observed different responses of respiratory mechanics in ARDS of primary versus secondary origin [27]. This may correspond to different underlying processes resulting from two different pathogenetic pathways. It is traditionally thought that in ARDS the high respiratory system elastance is mainly attributed to the lung, with little changes in chest wall mechanics. However, Gattinoni noticed that in primary ARDS chest wall elastance was nearly normal, while during secondary ARDS it was increased because of the augmentation in intra-abdominal pressure. The changes in respiratory mechanics parameters in primary ARDS could be attributed to alveolar and interstitial oedema, and atelectasis. On the other hand, patients with primary abdominal alteration determined an increase in intra-abdominal pressure that caused the augmentation in chest wall elastance.

However, the authors described only direct insult including primarily diffuse pneumonia or indirect insult related to abdominal causes. In other situations such as cardiac surgery, trauma, near drowning, aspiration, or meningitis the precise identification of the pathogenetic pathway is somewhat questionable. In addition, it is difficult to be confident of the onset of ARDS, the phase and the severity of the lesion in all patients.

In order to bypass these drawbacks, we have recently developed a model of primary and secondary ARDS induced by intratracheal or intraperitoneal injection of LPS of *E. coli* with similar degrees of lung injury; as indicated by lung mechanics. We wished to correlate the mechanical changes (resistive, elastic and viscoelastic pressures) in ARDS originating from either primary or secondary aetiologies with the levels of inflammatory cytokines (IL-6, IL-8, and IL-10) in the bronchoalveolar lavage fluid (BALF) and lung histology (light and electron microscopy). Although pulmonary mechanical and morphological changes were similar independently of the aetiology of ARDS, direct insult yielded more pronounced inflammatory responses, e.g., primary ARDS group presented a threefold increase of IL-8 and IL-10 in relation to secondary ARDS, whereas IL-6 was two times larger in primary ARDS group [21]. Furthermore, tissue resistance (R), elastance (E), and hysteresivity (h), the amount of collagen and elastic fibers (oxytalan + elaunin + fully developed elastic fiber), and tissue cellularity were determined in these models of primary and secondary ARDS. R, E, h increased similarly in primary and secondary ARDS, which are accompanied by collagen fiber content and tissue cellularity augment. Elastic fiber content remained unchanged in all groups [22].

Responses to therapeutic intervention

Ventilation strategies can affect outcome, but there are several other potential therapeutic strategies for ARDS [32, 33]. These include, but are not limited to, the use of high levels of PEEP, sigh, prone position, inhaled agents including nitric oxide and nebulized prostaglandin I2 (PGI2). It seems likely that the success will be determined by the stage of ARDS/ALI at which they are applied (early or late) and on the basis of the aetiology of ARDS [34].

Different respiratory mechanics in primary and secondary ARDS can affect transpulmonary pressure considering a given applied airway pressure, i.e., the distending pressure of the lungs, is higher in primary than in secondary ARDS. Distinct underlying pathology (prevalent consolidation versus prevalent collapse) and different transpulmonary pressures for the same applied airway pressure lead to diverse ventilatory strategy [35]. In fact the potential for recruitment is higher in case of collapse and lower in case of consolidation. On the other hand the applied opening pressures for lung recruitment may lead to different transpulmonary pressures according to chest wall elastance. In this line, Gattinoni and coworkers have provided evidence of different responses of respiratory mechanics in ARDS of primary versus secondary origin. Increasing PEEP to 15 cmH_2O induced mainly overstretching, increasing respiratory system static elastance in primary ARDS, whilst in secondary ARDS, PEEP induced recruitment, thus decreasing elastance [27]. Pelosi and coworkers observed the effects of three sighs per minute at 45 cmH_2O plateau pressure on oxygenation and recruitment in primary and secondary ARDS [36]. In primary ARDS the amount of atelectasis is scarce, and the predominant damage is the consolidation of alveolar units. Consequently, for a given applied plateau pressure the average change of transpulmonary pressure (the difference between the plateau pressure and PEEP minus the difference between oesophageal pressure at end-inspiration and end-expiration) is relatively high. Thus, in primary ARDS the lung is stiffer, with low potential for recruitment, and a transpulmonary pressure sufficient for lung opening cannot be achieved. On the other hand, in secondary ARDS the amount of atelectasis is greater, transpulmonary pressure is low, and the lung appears more amenable generally to recruitment strategies [36]. These clinical findings are in line with animal experiments. Van der Kloot and coworkers compared the effect of baseline ventilatory strategy and recruitment manoeuvres on end-expiratory lung volume and oxygenation in three models of acute lung injury (saline lavage, oleic acid, and intratracheal instillation of *Escherichia coli*) [37]. They observed that each model of ALI behaved differently in response to a recruitment manoeuvre superimposed on a chosen mechanical ventilatory strategy. The model of intratracheal instillation of bacterial pneumonia (more similar to primary ARDS) was less responsive to PEEP than was the oleic acid model (more similar to secondary ARDS). However, recently Grasso and coworkers examined the hypothesis that the effectiveness of a recruiting manoeuvre to improve oxygenation in patients with ARDS would be influenced by the elastic properties of the lung and chest wall independently of the aetiology of ARDS [38]. They observed that application of recruiting manoeuvres improves oxygenation only in patients with early ARDS who do not have impairment of chest wall mechanics and with a large potential for recruitment, as indicated by low values of lung static elastance. Thus, the underlying disease responsible for ARDS did not influence the amount of improvement in arterial oxygenation after application of the recruiting manoeuvre. In addition, it is true that a significant part of the alteration in chest wall mechanics can be explained by abdominal distension in patients with abdominal surgery and in patients in whom ARDS is caused by extrapulmonary causes, but chest wall mechanics can be significantly altered also by the presence of pleural effusions [39-42]. Consequently, the potential for alveolar recruitment is probably related to the changes in lung and chest wall mechanics, independently of the underlying disease.

On the other hand, Puybasset and colleagues observed in patients with ARDS that the effects of PEEP were affected by lung morphology rather than by the cause of the lung injury (primary versus secondary ARDS) [43]. The regional distribution of the loss of aeration and the type of atelectasis [mechanical (massive loss of lung volume) x inflammatory (preservation of lung volume)] were the main determinants of the respiratory effects of PEEP. The differences between Puybasset and Gattinoni's studies [27, 43] could be attributed to the population studied and/or to the ventilatory and clinical management at the moment of the study. In the study of Puybasset and colleagues most of the patients included in secondary ARDS had extra-abdominal sepsis and only 1 presented intra-abdominal sepsis [43], while in the study of Gattinoni and coworkers most of them presented intra-abdominal sepsis [27]. Thus, probably we should describe another group of ARDS, the extra-abdominal ARDS. In addition, I think it is important to understand the mechanisms of each aetiology of ARDS, not the syndromes.

A recent National Heart, Lung, and Blood Institute ARDS Network randomised controlled trial demonstrated that a low tidal volume mechanical ventilation strategy (6 ml/kg) reduced mortality by 22% compared with traditional mechanical ventilation (12 ml/kg) in patients with ALI/ARDS [33]. Using data from patients enrolled in ARDS Network randomised controlled trials, Eisner and colleagues retrospectively examined whether the efficacy of low tidal volume ventilation varied by clinical risk factors for ALI/ARDS [44]. They found that patients with sepsis had the largest risk of death, whereas those with trauma had the lowest risk. Despite these differences in disease severity, they observed no evidence that the efficacy of low tidal volume ventilation strategy differed among clinical risk factor subgroups for ALI/ARDS. Consequently the low tidal volume strategy should be broadly applied to patients with ALI/ARDS.

The response to prone position is also different in primary and secondary ARDS. Lim and coworkers showed that the response of prone positioning on respiratory function appears to be different in patients with early primary and secondary ARDS [45]. They found that in prone position the response in oxygenation (defined as an increase of PaO_2/FiO_2 greater than 40% from the baseline) was more marked in secondary than in primary ARDS, the kinetic of the increase in oxygenation was slower in primary ARDS, the decrease of respiratory system compliance was greater in secondary ARDS, and the densities determined on the chest radiography decreased to a greater degree in secondary ARDS.

Observational clinical studies have suggested that inhaled nitric oxide (NO) may be beneficial in patients with ARDS [46, 47]. The potential therapeutic value was based on reports of improved oxygenation from a decrease in intrapulmonary shunt, lowered pulmonary arterial pressure, and a potential reduction in morbidity or mortality. Many experimental studies have been done with inhaled NO in a large number of animal models of acute lung injury. Some animal studies have reported improvement in the severity of lung injury with inhaled NO, while an equal number have reported no benefit, or occasionally a worsening of lung injury [48, 49]. Dellinger and colleagues reported the results of randomised, double-blinded phase II study of different doses of inhaled NO for patients with ARDS. The primary objective was to evaluate safety and the physiologic responses of different doses of inhaled NO with the hope that the results would demonstrate enough benefit to warrant a phase III trial [50]. However, patients were excluded from the trial if they had ARDS from non-pulmonary sepsis and hypotension, or if they were immunocompromised. Thus, they could not analyse the effects of NO in primary and secondary ARDS. In addition, the results of this phase II trial were not encouraging. Brett and coworkers have tried to determine whether responses to inhaled nitric oxide can be related to aetiology of ARDS [51]. They examined the relationship between responsiveness to inhaled NO and features of underlying disease: the authors were unable to identify aspects (morphology, inflammatory response, and pathophysiology) of the disease likely to be associated with a clinical response to inhaled NO. In this study, the analysis was done without considering a clinical assignment to the two forms (primary and secondary) of the disease. Recently, Rialp and coworkers compared the gas exchange and haemodynamic effects induced by the combination of NO inhalation and prone position in patients with ARDS and analysed whether or not primary and secondary ARDS patients behave differently [52]. They observed that prone position was associated with a marked improvement in oxygenation, irrespective of the causes of ARDS, and additive effects of NO inhalation were mainly seen in patients with primary ARDS. These findings were attributed to the fact that there was a redistribution of ventilation toward dorsal (nondependent) zones in prone position, and thus, it is conceivable that NO may reach lung regions with low V'/Q' ratios.

Domenighetti and colleagues examined the hypothesis that the response to inhaled prostacyclin (PGI2) on oxygenation and pulmonary haemodynamics may be related to different morphologic features that are supposed to be present in acute respiratory distress syndrome originating from primary and secondary ARDS [53]. Unlike NO, PGI2 and its stable degradation products do not have toxic side effects requiring special monitoring; both NO and PGI2 have nearly identical profiles of efficacy on oxygenation and pulmonary haemodynamics, but PGI2 is easier to administer in the critical care setting [54]. Fifteen consecutive, mechanically ventilated patients with ARDS received nebulised PGI2. Blood gas, gas exchange, and haemodynamic measurements were performed at the following time points: a) baseline; b) during the optimal or maximum dose of PGI2; and c) 1 hr after withdrawal of the drug. Patients underwent a computed tomographic scan. Patients were considered responders to PGI2 if an increase in PaO_2 of 7.5 torr or an increase in PaO_2 /FiO_2 ratio of

10% occurred. For the group as a whole, mean pulmonary artery pressure decreased during PGI2 nebulisation, whereas pulmonary vascular resistance decreased 1 hour after withdrawal of nebulisation; oxygenation did not change significantly. Eight patients responded to PGI2 on oxygenation (53%), whereas seven (47%) did not. All responders were secondary ARDS patients, whereas all primary ARDS patients (plus one secondary ARDS patient) were nonresponders. In primary ARDS, the nebulised PGI2 was distributed to a higher extent into predominantly non-functionally active alveolar areas, whereas in secondary ARDS, PGI2 reached more alveolar-accessible areas because the consolidations were less distributed (mainly gravity-dependent): this last interpretation in secondary ARDS patients seems again to be reinforced by the CT number frequency distribution analysis, which showed a characteristic bimodal pattern corresponding to thresholds defined as aerated and consolidated (gravity-dependent) areas. In patients presenting with primary ARDS, PGI2 induced a reduction in PaO_2/FiO_2 (from 146 ± 16 to 135 ± 17) and PaO_2 (from 87 ± 2 to 79 ± 2 torr), whereas in patients with secondary ARDS there was an increase in PaO_2/FiO_2 (from 161 ± 23 to 171 ± 22) and in PaO_2 (from 76 ± 4 to 84 ± 4 torr) with a decrease in mean pulmonary artery pressure. They concluded that the clinical recognition of the two types of the syndrome together with the CT number frequency distribution analysis might be associated with a prediction of the PGI2 nebulisation response on oxygenation.

No pharmacological treatment has been found effective in the reduction of mortality in ARDS. The control of the complex network of pro-inflammatory pathways and mediators at the early phase of ARDS with anti-inflammatory drugs has been a tempting idea. In this line, corticosteroid was used to prevent this inflammatory process with disappointing results. The most likely reason for the failure of corticosteroid trials has been speculated to be the short duration of treatment in patients with persistent exaggerated inflammation. Varpula and colleagues retrospectively analysed the effects of late steroid therapy on the severity of respiratory failure, multiorgan dysfunction and the degree of acute phase reaction, and on the outcome of patients with primary ALI, with special attention to ALI caused by *Streptococcus pneumonia* [55]. They concluded that in direct ALI, corticosteroid therapy might be beneficial, if signs of systemic inflammation persist.

Recently, we compared the effects of corticosteroid in experimental model of primary and secondary ALI induced by LPS of *Escherichia coli*. These models exhibited similar degrees of lung injury. Contrary to what have been observed, the response of corticosteroid on respiratory mechanics, lung morphometry and cytokines was more intense in primary in comparison to secondary ARDS [22].

Although these ventilatory strategies and pharmacological therapies did better in secondary ARDS in comparison to primary ARDS none yielded a better outcome. Suntharalingam and coworkers showed no differences between primary and secondary ARDS groups with respect to the primary outcome measures [56]. However, there was a trend toward increased mortality in the direct aetiology group, which after *post-hoc* analysis also indicated a require-ment for a significantly longer duration of pressure-controlled inverse-ration ventilation. Angus and colleagues measured quality-adjusted survival in the first year only in patients with primary ARDS. They demonstrated that patients who appear in good health until presenting with primary ARDS are at signifi-cant risk of death for several months beyond the traditional end point of 28 days [57]. Furthermore, the quality of life in those that do survive is markedly impaired.

Conclusions

Since its description, the acute respiratory distress syndrome has been consi-dered a morphological and functional expression of a similar underlying lung injury caused by a variety of insults. Two distinct forms of ARDS/ALI are described, since there are differences between primary ARDS (direct lung injury) and secondary ARDS (reflecting lung involvement in a more distant systemic inflammatory response). These differences could be detectable radio-graphically, functionally, and analysing the responses to therapeutic interven-tion (PEEP, prone position, drugs). However, the distinction between primary and secondary ARDS is not always clear and simple, and the observation of some overlapping in pathogenetic mechanisms and morphological alterations may be frequent. Thus, we need to strongly reconsider ARDS as a consistent response to its diverse aetiology. We think that if we consider each pathogenetic mechanism, clinical management would be more precise.

References

1. Ashbaugh DG, Bigelow DB, Petty TL et al (1967) Acute respiratory distress syndrome. Lancet 2: 319-323
2. Bernard GR, Artigas A, Bringham KL et al (1994) The American-European consensus conference on ARDS: definitions, mechanisms, relevant outcomes, and clinical trial coordination. Am J Respir Crit Care Med 149:818-824
3. Pepe PE, Potkin RT, Resus DR et al (1982) Clinical predictors of the adult respiratory distress syndrome. Am J Surg 144:124-130
4. Fein AM, Lippmann M, Hotzman H et al (1983) The risk factors, incidence, and prognosis of ARDS following septicemia. Chest 83:40-42
5. Bone RC, Grodzin CJ, Balk RA (1997) Sepsis: A new hypothesis for pathogenesis of the disease process. Chest 112: 235-243
6. Blaisdell FW (1974) Pathophysiology of the respiratory distress syndrome. Arch Surg 108: 44-49
7. Nash G, Foley FD, Langlinais PD (1974) Pulmonary interstitial edema and hyaline membranes in adult burn patients. Electron microscopic observations. Hum Pathol 5: 149-160
8. Lamy M, Fallat RJ, Koeniger E et al (1976) Pathologic features and mechanisms of hypoxemia in adult respiratory distress syndrome. Am Rev Respir Dis 114: 267-284
9. Bachofen M, Weibel ER (1977) Alterations of the gas exchange apparatus in adult respiratory insufficiency associated with septicemia. Am Rev Respir Dis 116: 589-615
10. Wiener-Knonish JP, Albertine KH, Mattahay MA (1991) Differential response of the endothelial and epithelial barriers of the lung in sheep to *Escherichia coli* endotoxin. J Clin Invest 88: 864-875
11. Terashima T, Marsubara H, Nakamura M (1996) Local pseudomonas instillation induces contralateral lung injury and plasma cytokines. Am J Respir Crit Care Med 153: 1600-1605
12. Rouby JJ, Puybasset L, Cluzel P et al (2000) Regional distribution of gas and tissue in acute respiratory distress syndrome. II Physiological correlation and definition of an ARDS Severity Score. CT Scan ARDS Study Group. Intensive Care Med 26: 1046-1056
13. Ware LB, Matthay MA (2000) The acute respiratory distress syndrome. New Engl J Med 342: 1334-1349
14. Modelska K, Pittet JF, Folkesson HB et al (1999) Acid-induced lung injury: protective effect of anti-interleukin-8 pretreatment on alveolar epithelial barrier function in rabbits. Am J Respir Crit Care Med 160: 1450-1456
15. Greene KE, Wright JR, Steinberg KP et al (1999) Serial changes in surfactant-associated proteins in lung and serum before and after onset of ARDS. Am J Respir Crit Care Med 160: 1843-1850
16. Bitterman PB (1992) Pathogenesis of fibrosis in acute lung injury. Am J Med 92: 39S-43S
17. Pelosi P (2000) What about primary and secondary ARDS? Minerva Anestesiol 66: 779-785
18. Gattinoni L, Pelosi P, Brazzi L et al (1999) Acute Respiratory Distress Syndrome, In: Albert RK (ed) Comprehensive Respiratory Medicine. Mosby, New York, pp 69.1-69.16
19. Tomashefski JF Jr (2000) Pulmonary pathology of acute respiratory distress syndrome. Clin Chest Med 21: 435-466
20. Hoelz C, Negri EM, Lichtenfels AJ et al (2001) Morphometric differences in pulmonary lesions in primary and secondary ARDS. A preliminary study in autopsies. Pathol Res Pract 197: 521-530
21. Menezes SLS, Laranjeira AP, Castro-Faria Neto HC et al (2001) Inflammatory responses in pulmonary and extrapulmonary acute lung injury. Am J Respir Crit Care Med 163: A460
22. Rocco PRM, Leite-Junior JH, Souza AB et al (2001) Effects of corticosteroid in acute lung injury caused by pulmonary and extrapulmonary disease. Proceedings of the 8th World Congress of Intensive Care Medicine 1: 191
23. Gattinoni L, Caironi P, Pelosi P et al (2001) What has computed tomography taught us about the acute respiratory distress syndrome? Am J Respir Crit Care Med 164: 1701-1711
24. Austin JHM, Müller NL, Friedman PJ et al (1996) Glossary of terms for CT of the lungs:

recommendations of the nomenclature committee of the Fleichner Society. Radiology 200: 327-331

25. Remy-Jardin M, Remy J, Giraud F et al (1993) Computed tomography assessment of ground-glass opacity: semiology and significance. J Thorac Imag 8: 249-264

26. Müller-Leisse C, Klosterhalfen B, Hauptmann S et al (1993) Computed tomography and histologic results in the early stages of endotoxin-injured pig lungs as a model for adult respiratory distress syndrome. Invest Radiol 28: 39-45

27. Gattinoni L, Pelosi P, Suter PM et al (1998) Acute respiratory distress syndrome caused by pulmonary and extrapulmonary disease. Different syndromes? Am J Respir Crit Care Med 158: 3-11

28. Goodman LR, Fumagalli R, Tagliabue P et al (1999) Adult respiratory distress syndrome due to pulmonary and extrapulmonary causes: CT, clinical, and functional correlation. Radiology 213: 545-552

29. Desai SR, Wells AU, Rubens MB et al (1999). Acute respiratory distress syndrome: CT abnormalities at long-term follow up. Radiology 210: 29-35

30. Winer-Muram HT, Steiner RM, Gurney JW et al (1998) Ventilator-associated pneumonia in patients with adult respiratory distress syndrome: CT evaluation. Radiology 208: 193-199

31. Desai SR, Wells AU, Suntharalingam G et al (2001) Acute respiratory distress syndrome caused by pulmonary and extrapulmonary injury: a comparative CT study. Radiology 218: 689-693

32. Amato MB, Barbas CS, Medeiros DM et al (1998) Effect of a protective-ventilation strategy on mortality in the acute respiratory distress syndrome. N Engl J Med 338: 347-354

33. The Acute Respiratory Distress Syndrome Network (2000) Ventilation with lower tidal volumes as compared with traditional tidal volumes for acute lung injury and the acute respiratory distress syndrome. N Engl J Med 342: 1301-1308

34. Rocker GM (2001) Acute respiratory distress syndrome. Different syndromes, different therapies? Crit Care Med 29: 210-211

35. Pelosi P, Gattinoni L (2001) Acute respiratory distress syndrome of pulmonary and extrapulmonary origin: fancy or reality? Intensive Care Med 58:503-509

36. Pelosi P, Cardringher P, Bottino N et al (1999) Sigh in acute respiratory distress syndrome. Am J Respir Crit Care Med 159: 872-880

37. Van der Kloot T, Blanch L, Yougblood M et al (2000) Recruitment maneuvres in three experimental models of acute lung injury. Am J Respir Crit Care Med 161: 1485-1494

38. Grasso S, Mascia L, Del Turco M et al (2002) Effects of recruiting maneuvers in patients with acute respiratory distress syndrome ventilated with protective ventilatory strategy. Anesthesiology 96:795-802

39. Aberle DR, Wiener-Kronish JP, Webb WR et al (1988) Hydrostatic vs increased permeability pulmonary edema: diagnosis based on radiologic criteria in critically ill patients. Radiology 168: 73-79

40. Katz JA, Zinn SE, Ozanne GM et al (1981) Pulmonary, chest wall and lung-thorax elastances in acute respiratory failure. Chest 80: 304-311

41. Mattison LE, _oppage L, Alderman DF et al (1997) Pleural effusions in the medical ICU: Prevalence, causes and clinical implications. Chest 111: 1018-1023

42. Mutoh T, Lamm WJE, Emdree LJ et al (1992) Volume infusion produces abdominal distension, lung compression, and chest wall stiffening in pigs. J Appl Physiol 72: 575-582

43. Puybasset L, Gusman P, Muller JC et al (2000) Regional distribution of gas and tissue in acute respiratory distress syndrome. III Consequences for the effects of positive end-expiratory pressure. Intensive Care Med 26: 1215-1227

44. Eisner MD, Thompson T, Hudson LD et al (2001) Efficacy of low tidal volume ventilation in patients with different clinical risk factors for acute lung injury and the acute respiratory distress syndrome. Am J Respir Crit Care Med 164: 231-236

45. Lim C, Kim EK, Lee LS et al (2001) Comparison of the response to the prone position between pulmonary and extrapulmonary acute respiratory distress syndrome. Intensive Care Med 27: 477-485

46. Rossaint R, Falke KJ, Lopez F et al (1993) Inhaled nitric oxide for the adult respiratory distress syndrome. N Engl J Med 328: 399-405
47. Zapol W, Rimar S, Gillis N et al (1994) Nitric oxide and the lung. Am J Respir Crit Care Med 149: 1375-1380
48. Garat C, Jayr C, Eddahibi S et al (1997) Effects of inhaled nitric oxide or inhibition of endogenous nitric oxide formation on hyperoxia in rats. Am J Physiol 272: L631-L638
49. Kavanagh BP, Mouchawar A, Goldsmith J et al (1994) Effects of inhaled NO and inhibition of endogenous NO synthesis in oxidant-induced acute lung injury. J Appl Physiol 76: 1324-1329
50. Dellinger RP, Zimmerman JL, Taylor RW et al (1998). Effects of inhaled nitric oxide in patients with acute respiratory distress syndrome: results of randomized phase II trial. Crit Care Med 26: 15-23
51. Brett SJ, Hansell DM, Evans TW (1998). Clinical correlates in acute lung injury: Response to inhaled nitric oxide. Chest 114: 1397-1404
52. Rialp G, Betbesé AJ, Pérez-Márquez M et al (2001) Short term effects of inhaled nitric oxide and prone position in pulmonary and extrapulmonary acute respiratory distress syndrome. Am J Respir Crit Care Med 164: 243-249
53. Domenighetti G, Stricker H, Waldispuehl B (2001) Nebulized prostacyclin (PGI2) in acute respiratory distress syndrome: impact of primary (pulmonary injury) and secondary (extrapulmonary injury) disease on gas exchange response. Crit Care Med 29:57-62
54. Walmrath D, Schneider T, Schermuly R et al (1996) Direct comparison of inhaled nitric oxide and aerosolized prostacyclin in acute respiratory distress syndrome. Am J Respir Crit Care Med 153: 991-996
55. Varpula T, Pettilä V, Rintala E et al (2000) Late steroid therapy in primary acute lung injury. Intensive Care Med 26: 526-531
56. Suntharalingan G, Regan K, Keogh BF et al (2001) Influence of direct and indirect etiology on acute outcome and 6-month functional recovery in acute respiratory distress syndrome. Crit Care Med 29: 562-566
57. Angus DC, Musthafa AA, Clermont G et al (2001) Quality-adjusted survival in the first year after the acute respiratory distress syndrome. Am J Respir Crit Care Med 163: 1389-1394

Effect of positive end-expiratory pressure on gas exchange in acute respiratory distress syndrome

A. Koutsoukou, C. Roussos, J. Milic-Emili

Since the first description of the adult respiratory distress syndrome (ARDS) in 1967 [1], there has been a large number of publications encompassing many aspects of the syndrome. This is because ARDS is still a significant source of morbidity, mortality and expenditure among critically ill patients. By definition, patients with ARDS are severely hypoxic and require supplemental oxygen and mechanical ventilation.

Physiological basis of hypoxaemia

The severe hypoxaemia that is both the hallmark and a diagnostic criterion for ARDS is caused mainly by markedly increased intrapulmonary shunt (commonly accounting for more than 20% of cardiac output) due to alveolar atelectasis. Originally this gas exchange abnormality was considered to reflect a bimodal phenomenon, i.e., pulmonary blood flow supplying two areas, one with ventilation that is normal and proportional to blood flow and the other that is not ventilated because of atelectasis [2]. In most ARDS patients, however, there are also areas with low V/Q ratio, which may be caused by maldistribution of ventilation due to cyclic reopening and closure of the peripheral airways, time constant inhomogeneity, or partial obstruction of the peripheral airways as a result of interstitial oedema. A few ARDS patients also exhibit lung units with high V/Q ratios together with increased dead space. The last findings may reflect areas with reduced blood flow due to effects of mechanical ventilation, although the additional influence of pulmonary vascular derangement cannot be ruled out [3]. Using computed tomographic scans, Gattinoni et al. [4] demonstrated lung densities primarily in the dependent regions. The average lung density and the absolute weight of non-inflated tissue were positively related to venous admixture ratio and negatively to PaO_2.

According to Dantzker et al. [2], there is no limitation to O_2 diffusion in

ARDS. Mixed venous oxygen desaturation plays an important role in hypoxemia in ARDS. If mixed venous saturation is decreased in the presence of a high shunt, the desaturated venous blood mixing with oxygenated blood from the functioning lung units, can substantially decrease the arterial PO_2.

Effects of supplemental O_2

Increased fractional concentration of inspired O_2 (FiO_2) can partially improve the refractory hypoxemia of ARDS. Oxygen toxicity, however, occurs when clinicians are forced to use high concentrations of FiO_2 (0.7) [5]. Fibrin membranes, interstitial oedema and fibrosis, and alveolar cell hyperplasia have all been found after prolonged ventilation on FiO_2 of 0.9-1.0 [6]. In addition, such high values of FiO_2 promote absorption atelectasis and increased cardiac output. In ARDS patients breathing 100% O_2, there is in general a modest increase in intrapulmonary shunt with a parallel increase in dead space along with a small increases of $PaCO_2$ [7-10].

In general, the increase in FiO_2 is not sufficient to correct hypoxia in ARDS. Accordingly, the use of positive end-expiratory pressure (PEEP) to recruit atelectatic alveoli [1] and, more recently, to reduce PEEPi inequality within the lung [11], has been advocated.

Effects of PEEP

Since its introduction 35 years ago [1], PEEP continues to be a cornerstone in the management of patients with ARDS. Many papers on the effects of PEEP in ARDS have been published and "prophylactic", "super", or "minimal" PEEP have all been proposed as the "most"-suitable strategy [12, 13]. Although there is no dispute that PEEP is a powerful means of improving oxygenation in these patients, a reasonable approach to determine the appropriate level of PEEP requires a comprehensive understanding of the mechanism(s) by which this improvement occurs.

It was originally postulated that PEEP increases the functional residual çapacity, lung compliance, and PaO_2 by decreasing pulmonary oedema consequent to an increase in the interstitial hydrostatic pressure, and thus decreasing fluid flux into the lungs [14]. However, studies in animals with normal lungs or with oleic acid-induced pulmonary oedema showed that PEEP had no effect on any measurable index of pulmonary oedema [15-17]. Next, it has been postulated that PEEP improves lung mechanics and gas exchange because it redistributes water from flooded alveoli into the compliant interstitial space of the perivascular cuffs without altering the total amount of lung water [18,19]. A reduction in intrapulmonary shunt, caused by decreased cardiac output, has also been advocated to explain the PEEP-induced improvement in oxygenation [20]. Dantzker et al. [2,21] found that in ARDS patients PEEP produced a uniform decrease in cardiac output associated with a proportional reduction in flow to shunt areas, without altering the overall V/Q distribution, and concluded that the decrease in cardiac output was responsible for the decrease in shunt, and that this was the major mechanism of improved PaO_2 with PEEP.

Alveolar recruitment

Matamis et al. [22] used dopamine to prevent the drop in cardiac output with PEEP, and still found an improvement in V/Q relationships with a redistribution of blood flow from regions of shunt to normal V/Q regions. Based on this and other studies, Matamis et al. [22] concluded that the improvement in V/Q distribution and PaO_2 with PEEP was mainly due to recruitment of previously unventilated but perfused airspaces, rather than a to a decrease in total blood flow per se. Likewise, Ralph et al. [23] found that improvement in PaO_2 with PEEP was associated with a redistribution of blood flow from shunt regions to either low or normal V/Q regions, while the moderate decrease in cardiac output was unrelated to the changes in PaO_2.

PLIP

Lemaire's group [24] described a lower inflection point (PLIP, knee) on the static inflation pressure-volume (P-V) curve of the respiratory system, which should reflect the critical pressure required to open previously closed peripheral airways and/or alveoli. On this basis the investigators proposed that the therapeutic level of PEEP ("ideal PEEP", PEEPIDEAL) should correspond to PLIP plus one or 2 cmH_2O. Since then many investigators have suggested that PEEP settings based on PLIP should essentially abolish atelectasis within the lung. This notion implies that recruitment is an "all or none" phenomenon, i.e., that there is a critical pressure at which all closed units reopen. As a corollary, there should be a sudden increase in PaO_2 and alveolar recruited volume (Vrec) when PEEP exceeds PLIP. However, Ranieri et al. [25] showed that alveolar recruitment usually continues as PEEP is raised well beyond PLIP, i.e., there is not a single critical pressure at which all closed alveoli reopen. Ranieri et al. [25] also stressed that in terms of alveolar recruitment it is the end-inspiratory plateau pressure (Pplat) that counts rather than PEEP. This is because the pressure required to reopen atelectatic alveoli is much higher than the PEEP levels usually applied in ARDS (< 15 cmH$_2$O). In fact, Ranieri et al. [25] suggested that Pplat levels of about 30 cmH$_2$O are required to significantly recruit most atelectatic alveoli. In line with this notion, Crotti et al. [26] have recently shown that in ARDS patients a Pplat of at least 25 cmH$_2$O is required to reverse most atelectasis. The recognition that high end-inspiratory pressures are required to fully reverse atelectasis has recently led to the adoption of high--pressure recruitment manoeuvres [27]. Based on these developments, the physiological nature of PLIP and its clinical relevance needs to be reassessed.

In experiments on excised dog and monkey lungs, it has been shown that the inflation PLIP reflects reopening of peripheral airways rather than alveoli [28, 29]. Furthermore, these studies have shown that the critical closing pressure of the peripheral airways is much smaller than the critical opening pressure. Accordingly, in terms of maintaining the peripheral airways open, it is the PLIP measured on static deflation rather than inflation V-P curves that counts. In other words, in order to avoid peripheral airway closure, PLIP should be obtained from the static deflation V-P curve rather than inflation one, and the PEEP set accordingly. In this connection it should be stressed that PLIP should be actually assessed from static V-P curves of the lung and not of the total respiratory system, as is commonly done in intensive care unit patients. This is because PLIP assessed from V-P curves of the total respiratory system may be contaminated by curvilinearities in the static V-P curve of the chest wall [25, 30]. It should be noted, however, that measurement of the static V-P curve of the lung is problematic in humans in decubitus position because of artefacts in the oesophageal pressure measurements [31].

The shape of the static [30] and dynamic [25] inflation V-P curve of the respiratory system has been found useful to predict the effects of PEEP on alveolar recruitment, gas exchange, and haemodynamics in ARDS patients.

Regional inequality of dynamic PEEPi

The improvement of PaO_2 as a result of PEEP-induced recruitment of previously atelectatic alveoli or reopening of peripheral airways of trapped gas units [12, 22, 24, 25] is a well-recognized mechanism. Recently, however, it has been shown that in ARDS patients $PaO2$ may also increase as a result of PEEP-induced reduction of regional inequality of dynamic PEEPi (PEE-Pi,dyn).

In a study of patients with chronic airway obstruction (CAO) in acute respiratory failure, Rossi et al. [32] have proposed another mechanism for PEEP-induced improvement of arterial oxygenation, namely reduction of regional inequality of intrinsic PEEP (PEEPi). To mechanically ventilated CAO patients who exhibited dynamic hyperinflation due to expiratory flow limitation with high concurrent values of static PEEPi (PEEPi,st) on zero PEEP (ZEEP), they administered external PEEP amounting to 50% and 100% of PEEPi,st, respectively. In spite of the fact that in CAO patients there is no atelectasis and hence no alveolar recruitment [33], the PaO_2 improved significantly at both levels of PEEP. Since in these studies there was no change in cardiac output with PEEP, Rossi et al. attributed the improvement in PaO_2 to a reduction in regional inequality of dynamic PEEPi (PEEPi,dyn), leading to more-homogeneous distribution of inspired gas and improved gas exchange.

As a result of regional time constant inhomogeneity within the lung of CAO patients, there are regional differences in PEEPi during ventilation, as reflected by the observation that dynamic PEEPi is lower than static PEEPi [34]. The dynamic PEEPi (PEEPi,dyn) corresponds to the minimal change in airway pressure required to initiate lung inflation [30], and reflects the lowest intrapulmonary value of PEEPi. In contrast, PEEPi,st is thought to represent the average PEEPi within the non-homogeneous lung, because it is measured after gas re-distribution between lung units with different regional pressures during airway occlusion at end-expiration, a phenomenon referred to as *pendelluft* [35, 36]. Maltais et al. [37] measured the ratio PEEPi dyn/PEEPi,st an index of the extent of regional PEEPi inequality within the lung, in a variety of mechanically ventilated patients on ZEEP, and found that the ratio was almost invariably less than unity. According to Rossi et al. [32], the PEEPi inequality index should have increased with PEEP (i.e., less inequality) to explain the observed improvement in PaO_2 in their CAO patients, but they did not actually measure this index.

Administration of PEEP to ARDS patients should also contribute to the improvement of arterial oxygenation by reducing the regional differences in PEEPi. In fact, tidal expiratory flow limitation (FL), which is commonly present on ZEEP in ARDS patients [11], promotes regional inequality of PEEPi within the lung, because tidal FL implies sequential dynamic compression of peripheral airways during expiration [38], with concurrent non-homogeneous regional lung, emptying (the dependent lung zones achieving FL earlier because of the vertical pleural pressure gradient). Presence of tidal FL, which can be assessed using the negative expiratory pressure (NEP) method [39], entails cyclic dynamic compression and re-expansion of the peripheral airways with maldistribution of ventilation and presence of PEEPi inequality [40,41].

In a recent study on 13 mechanically ventilated ARDS patients [11], we assessed at different PEEP levels (1) presence of tidal FL; (2) regional PEEPi inhomogeneity based on measurement of the PEEPi inequality index; (3) alveolar recruitment; and (4) arterial blood gases. On ZEEP, 7 of 13 ARDS patients exhibited FL. They had higher PEEPi,st ($P<0.001$) and lower PEEPi inequality index ($P<0.001$) than the 6 non-flow-limited (NFL) patients. Two FL patients became NFL with PEEP of 5 cmH$_2$O and the other 5 with PEEP of 10 cmH$_2$O. In both FL and NFL patients, PaO_2 increased progressively with PEEP. A significant correlation was found between PaO_2 and PEEPi inequality index in the FL patients (Fig.1), but not in the NFL group. For any given level of applied PEEP, total PEEP (PEEPt=PEEPi,st+PEEP) increased more markedly in the NFL patients, because in the FL group external PEEP replaced PEEPi, and hence PEEPt increased less. As a result of the latter, over the experimental range of PEEP used (up to 15 cmH$_2$O), the increase in alveolar recruited volume was much smaller in the FL than NFL patients. This explains the lack of significant correlation of PaO_2 and PaO_2/FiO_2 to Vrec in the FL patients. In contrast, in the NFL patients such correlation was significant (Fig. 2).

Thus, a PEEP-induced reduction of PEEPi,dyn inequality may also explain the improvement in PaO_2 in ARDS patients. In this connection, it should be stressed that such improvement may occur in the absence of any increase in end-expiratory lung volume and hence of alveolar recruitment.

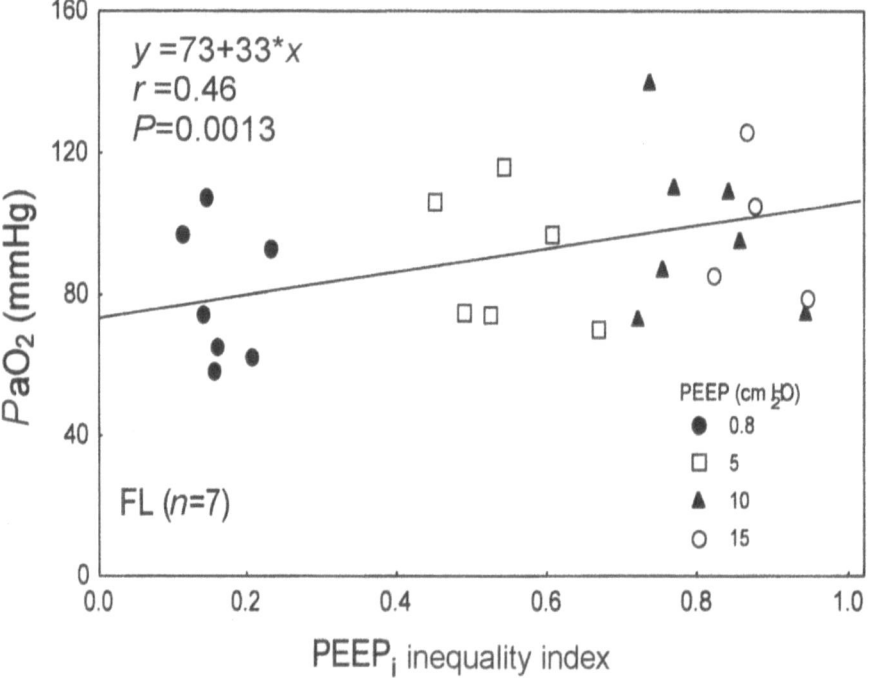

Fig. 1 Relationship of PaO_2 to PEEPi inequality index of 7 flow-limited (*FL*) ARDS patients

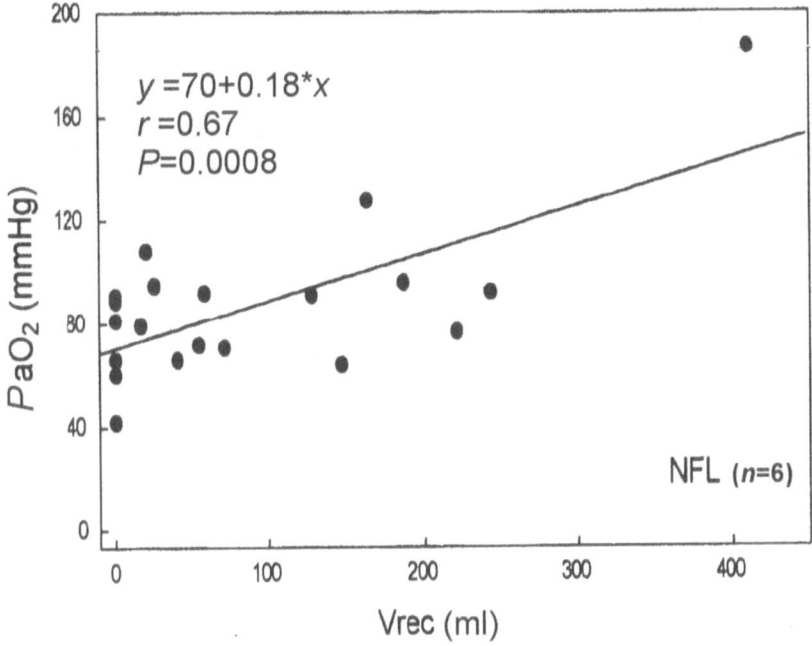

Fig. 2 Relationship of PaO_2 to Vrec in 6 non-flow-limited (*NFL*) ARDS patients

Koutsoukou et al. [11] also assessed the role of PLIP on alveolar recruitment and arterial PaO_2. When total static PEEP exceeded PEEPIDEAL, there was no abrupt increase in PaO_2 and Vrec in any of the 13 ARDS patients studied. In contrast, the changes in PEEPt,st were associated with a monotonic increase in both PaO_2 (Fig. 3) and Vrec. If PLIP should represent the critical pressure beyond which there is "massive" alveolar recruitment, there should be a sudden increase in PaO_2 and Vrec when the values of PEEPt,st-PEEPIDEAL exceed zero.

Risk of lung injury

In order to avoid large inflation pressures and volumes, and thus "high lung volume" injury, the current recommendation is to keep Pplat below 35 cmH$_2$O [42]. Several studies, however, have shown that mechanical ventilation with physiological tidal volumes from ZEEP may result in a significant increase of the histological injury scores in the respiratory and membranous bronchioles relative to ventilation with PEEP, in both an ex vivo model of lavaged rat lung [40] and normal, open-chest rabbit [43].

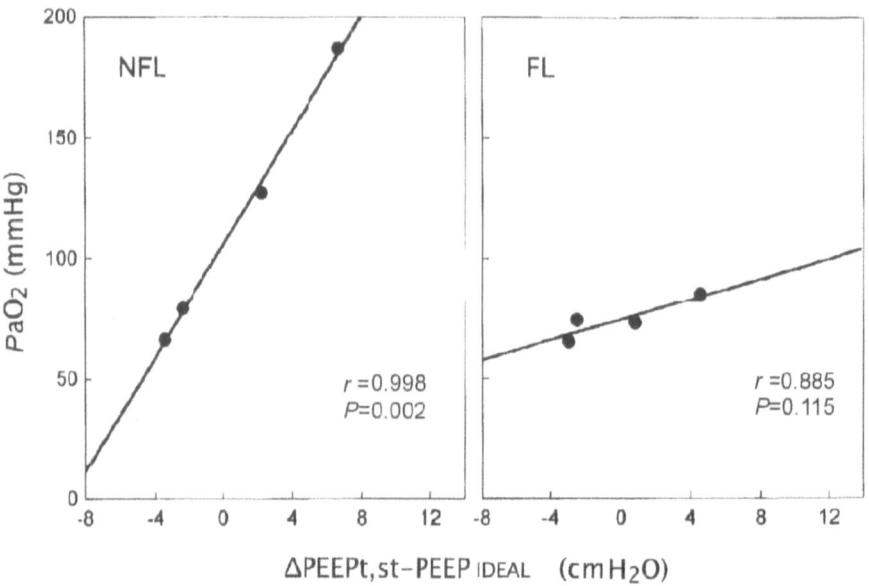

Fig. 3 Relationship of PaO_2 to PEEPt-PEEPIDEAL in two representative ARDS patients (PEEPI-DEAL exceeds PLIP by 1 cm H_2O)

Using the negative expiratory pressure (NEP) technique, it has been recently shown that on ZEEP many ARDS patients exhibit tidal expiratory FL with concurrent PEEPi up to 12 cmH$_2$O [39]. Presence of FL implies cyclic dynamic compression and re-expansion of the peripheral airways with concurrent inhomogeneous filling of airspaces. In non-homogeneous ARDS lungs, this should entail development of high shear forces with risk of "low lung volume" injury [40,43]. To avoid this, external PEEP has to be applied in order to increase the end-expiratory lung volume above the "FL" volume. Such therapeutic levels of PEEP can be readily determined by on-line inspection of the effect of NEP on the expiratory flow-volume loops: PEEP should be increased until tidal FL disappears. In general, when PEEP of 10 cmH$_2$O is applied, FL is abolished in most ARDS patients. It should be stressed that assessment of FL in ARDS patients provides the first objective assessment of cyclic compression and re-expansion of peripheral airways that has been advocated as a potential cause for "low lung volume" injury [40].

Thus, in FL patients application of PEEP is beneficial because it abolishes tidal FL with concurrent risk of "low lung volume" injury, and improves PaO_2 through reduction of PEEPi inhomogeneity within the lung. In contrast, in NFL patients, PEEP improves gas exchange mainly through alveolar recruitment.

Conclusion

Ensuring adequate ogygenation and avoidance of ventilator-induced lung injury are the main goals for the management of mechanically ventilated ARDS patients.

Improvement of PaO_2 can be achieved with PEEP by alveolar recruitment, which implies increased lung volume, and/or reduced PEEPi inequality within the lung, which can occur in the absence of changes in lung volume. Applying external PEEP based on inflation PLIP does not result in "massive" alveolar recruitment nor improvement in PaO_2. Significant alveolar recruitment requires relatively high pressures, and hence should be monitored in terms of Pplat rather than PEEP or PEEPt. The values of Pplat required to reverse atelectasis are close to those eliciting "high lung volume" injury, and hence should be closely monitored. Detection of tidal FL with the NEP technique is a potentially useful bed-side approach to avoid development of high shear forces within the peripheral airways and risk of "low lung volume" injury.

References

1. Ashbaugh DG, Bigelow DB, Petty TL (1967) Acute respiratory disease in adults. Lancet II:319-23
2. Dantzker DR, Brook CJ, Dehart P, et al (1979) Ventilation-perfusion distributions in the adult respiratory distress syndrome. Am Rev Respir Dis 120:1039-1052
3. Rodriguez-Roisin R (1993) Ventilation-perfusion relationships. In : Pinsky MR, Dhainaut JF A (eds) Pathophysiologic foundations of critical care. Williams and Wilkins, Baltimore, pp 389-413
4. Gattinoni L, Pesenti A, Bombino M, et al (1988) Relationship between lung computed tomographic density, gas exchange, and PEEP in acute respiratory failure. Anesthesiology 69: 824-832
5. Binger CAL, Faulkner JM, Moore RL (1927) Oxygen poisoning in mammals. J Exp Med 45: 849-864
6. Nash G, Blennershassett JB, Pontoppidan H (1967) Pulmonary lesions associated with oxygen therapy and artificial ventilation. N Engl J Med 276:368-374
7. Santos Ch, Ferrer M, Roca J, et al (2000) Pulmonary gas exchange response to oxygen breathing in acute lung injury. Am J Respir Crit Care Med 161:26-31
8. West JB (1971) Causes of carbon dioxide retention in lung disease. N Engl J Med 284:1232--1236
9. Suter PM, Fairley HB, Schlobohm RM (1975) Shunt, lung volume and perfusion during short periods of ventilation with oxygen. Anesthesiology 43:617-627
10. Dantzker DR, Wagner PD, West JB (1975) Instability of lung units with low /Q ratios during O2 breathing. J Appl Physiol 38:886-895

11. Koutsoukou A, Bekos V, Sotiropoulou, et al (2002) Effects of PEEP on gas exchange and expiratory flow limitation in ARDS. Crit Care Med (in press)
12. Falke KJ, Pontoppidan H, Kumar A, et al (1972) Ventilation with end-expiratory pressure in acute lung disease. J Clin Invest 51:2315-2323
13. Suter PM, Fairley HB, Isenberg MD (1975) Optimum end-expiratory pressure in patients with acute pulmonary failure. N Engl J Med 292:284-289
14. Dunegan LJ, Knight DC, Harken A, et al (1975) Lung thermal volume in pulmonary edema: effect of positive end-expiratory pressure. Ann Surg 190:809-812
15. Woolverton WC, Brigham KL, Staub NC (1978) Effect of positive pressure breathing on lung lymph flow and water content in sheep. Circ Res 42:550-557
16. Laver MB, Strauss W, Pohost GM (1979) Right and left ventricular geometry: adjustments during acute respiratory failure. Crit Care Med 7: 509-519
17. Luce JM, Robertson HT, Huang T, et al (1982) The effects of expiratory positive airway pressure on the resolution of oleic acid-induced lung injury in dogs. Am Rev Respir Dis 125:716-722
18. Malo J, Ali J, Wood LDH (1984) How does PEEP reduce intrapulmonary shunt in canine pulmonary edema?. J Appl Physiol 57:1002-1010
19. Puybasset L, Muller JC, Cluzel P, et al (2000) Regional distribution of gas and tissue in acute respiratory distress syndrome. 3. Consequences on the effects of positive end-expiratory pressure. Intensive Care Med 26:1215-1227
20. Dueck R, Wagner PD, West JB (1977) Effects of positive end-expiratory pressure on gas exchange in dogs with normal and edematous lungs. Anesthesiology 57:359-366
21. Dantzker DR, Lynch JP, Weg JG (1977) Depression of cardiac output is a mechanism of shunt reduction in the therapy of acute respiratory failure. Chest 65:636-642
22. Matamis D, Lemaire F, Harf A, et al (1984) Redistribution of pulmonary blood flow induced by positive end-expiratory pressure and dopamine infusion in acute respiratory failure. Am Rev Respir Dis 129:39-44
23. Ralph DD, Robertson TH, Weaver LJ, et al (1985) Distribution of ventilation and perfusion during positive end-expiratory pressure in the adult respiratory distress syndrome. Am Rev Respir Dis 131:54-60
24. Matamis D, Lemaire F Hart A, et al (1984) Total respiratory pressure-volume curves in the adult respiratory distress syndrome. Chest 86:58-66
25. Ranieri VM, Eissa NT, Corbeil C, et al (1991) Effects of positive end-expiratory pressure on alveolar recruitment and gas exchange in patients with the adult respiratory distress syndrome. Am Rev Respir Dis 144:544-551
26. Crotti S, Mascheroni D, Caironi P, et al (2001) Recruitment and derecruitment during acute respiratory failure. Am J Respir Crit Care Med 164:131-140
27. Marini JJ, Amato MB (1998) Lung recruitment during ARDS. In: Marini JJ, Amato MB (eds) Acute lung injury. Springer-Verlag, Berlin Heidelberg New York, pp 236-257
28. Glaister DH, Schroter RC, Sudlow MF, et al (1973) Bulk elastic properties of excised lung and the effect of transpulmonary pressure gradient. Respir Physiol 17:347-364
29. Glaister DH, Schroter RC, Sudlow MF, et al (1973) Transpulmonary pressure gradient and ventilation distribution in excised lungs. Respir Physiol 17:365-385
30. Rossi A, Gottfried SB, Zocchi L, et al (1985) Measurement of static compliance of the total respiratory system in patients with acute respiratory failure during mechanical ventilation. Am J Respir Dis 131:672-677
31. Milic-Emili J, Mead J, Turner M (1964) Topography of esophageal pressure as a function of posture in man. J Appl 19:212-216
32. Rossi A, Santos C, Roca J, et al (1994) Effects of PEEP on V/Q mismatching in ventilated patients with chronic airflow obstruction, Am J Respir Crit Care Med 149:1077-1084
33. Guerin C, LeMasson S, Varax R de, et al (1997) Small airway closure and positive end-expiratory pressure in mechanically ventilated patients with chronic obstructive pulmonary disease. Am J Respir Crit Care Med 155:1949-1956

34. Petrof BJ, Legare M, Golberg P, et al (1990) Continuous positive airway pressure reduces work of breathing and dyspnea during weaning from mechanical ventilation in severe chronic obstructive pulmonary disease. Am Rev Respir Dis 141:281-289
35. Otis AB, McKerrow CB, Bartlett RA, et al (1956) Mechanical factors in distribution of pulmonary ventilation. J Appl Physiol 8:427-443
36. Bates JTM, Rossi A, Milic-Emili J (1985) Analysis of the behavior of the respiratory system with constant inspiratory flow. J Appl Physiol 58:1840-1848
37. Maltais F, Reissman H, Navalesi P, et al (1985) Comparison of static and dynamic measurements of intrinsic PEEP in mechanically ventilated patients. Am J Respir Crit Care Med 150:1318-1324
38. Rodarte JR, Hyatt RE, Cortese DA (1975) Influence of expiratory flow on closing capacity at low expiratory flow rates. J Appl Physiol 39:60-65
39. Koutsoukou A, Armaganidis A, Stavrakaki-Kallergi K, et al (2000) Expiratory flow limitation and intrinsic positive end-expiratory pressure at zero positive end-expiratory pressure in patients with adult respiratory distress syndrome, Am J Respir Crit Care Med 161:1590-1596
40. Muscedere JM, Mullen JB, Gun K, et al (1994) Tidal ventilation at low airway pressures can augment lung injury. Am J Respir Crit Care Med 149:1327-1334
41. Ranieri VM, Giunto F, Suter PM, et al (2000) Mechanical ventilation as a mediator of multisystem organ failure in acute respiratory distress syndrome. JAMA 284:43-44
42. International consensus conference in intensive care medicine (1999) Ventilatory-associated lung injury in ARDS. Am J Respir Crit Care Med 160:2118-2124
43. D'Angelo E, Pecchiari M, Baraggia P, et al (2002) Low volume ventilation induces peripheral airways injury and increased airway resistance in normal open-chest rabbits. J Appl Physiol 92: 949-956

Experimental evidence for the use of corticosteroids in acute respiratory distress syndrome

P.R.M. Rocco

Effective management of acute respiratory distress syndrome (ARDS) has remained problematic since this syndrome was first described in 1967. Ashbaugh et al. [1] described 12 adult patients with severe respiratory distress, severe dyspnea, reduced lung compliance, diffuse chest radiographic infiltrates, and hypoxemia that was refractory to supplemental oxygen but was responsive to mechanical ventilation with positive end-expiratory pressure (PEEP). In 1994, a Consensus Conference of American and European investigators [2] agreed that ARDS should be regarded as the most-severe end of the spectrum of acute lung injury (ALI). The American-European Consensus Conference members also agreed that the diagnostic criteria for ALI and ARDS should include: (1) acute onset; (2) bilateral chest radiographic infiltrates; (3) a pulmonary artery occlusion pressure of 18 mmHg or no evidence of left atrial hypertension; and (4) impaired oxygenation regardless of the PEEP concentration, with a PaO_2 ratio of 300 torr (40 kPa) for ALI and 200 torr (27 kPa) for ARDS. Despite recent advances in understanding the pathophysiology of ARDS and improved life support of patients with ARDS, the mortality rates persist at between 40% and 60% [3].

The causes for development of ARDS are varied, and although some authors believe that the syndrome is a heterogeneous collection of diseases, the pulmonary pathological findings are consistent and uniform. The pathological features of the lung in ARDS derive from severe injury to the alveolocapillary unit. The morphological picture of the lung in ARDS has been labelled diffuse alveolar damage, and extravasations of intravascular fluid dominate the onset of the disease [4]. Microscopic findings are dependent on the stage of the illness. Traditionally, ARDS has been divided into three stages in which an initial inflammatory phase (exudative) is followed by fibroproliferation, which can lead to established interstitial and intra-alveolar fibrosis, the final phase. The histological features of the exudative phase are: (1) hyaline membranes, (2) alveolar collapse, and (3) swollen type I pneumocytes with cytoplasmic vacuoles. The endothelial cells swell, the intercellular junctions widen, and pinocytic vesicles increase, causing disruption in the capillary membrane and resulting in a capillary leak and oedema formation [4, 5] The proliferative phase was described to begin as early as the 3rd day and was most prominent in the 2nd and 3rd week after symptom onset. However, recently, some authors described that fibroproliferation is an early response to lung injury [6-9]. Thus, inflammatory and repair mechanisms occur in parallel rather than in series. Fibroproliferation is a stereotypical reparative reaction to tissue injury and is characterized by the replacement of damaged epithelial cell by accumulation of mesenchymal cells, in particular interstitial fibroblasts, which migrate, replicate, and secrete extracellular matrix proteins such as collagen; type II cells begin to proliferate and reline the denuded basement membrane; epithelial cells migrate over the surface of the organizing granulation tissue and transform the intra-alveolar exudate into the interstitial tissue. In the fibrotic phase, extensive remodelling of the lung by sparsely cellular collagenous tissue occurs, air spaces are irregularly enlarged, and there is alveolar duct fibrosis. Type III collagen is replaced by type I collagen, leading to a stiff lung over time [4].

A wide variety of animal models have been developed to explore the effects of corticosteroids in ARDS. Both direct (e.g., pneumonia, aspiration) and indirect (e.g., sepsis, drug overdose) insults to the alveolocapillary membrane have been used in various animal species to model ARDS [10]. Common to a majority of these models has been the description of a diffuse inflammatory reaction in the lung's microvasculature. The recognition that neutrophils, macrophages, and other components of the inflammatory cascade participate in the progression of ARDS has resulted in the use of anti-inflammatory agents particularly glucocorticoids [3, 11-13], as pharmacological probes to further define the pathophysiology of this syndrome.

Corticosteroids were administered to 9 of the 12 patients with ARDS in the original series [1]; 2 of these patients were thought to have benefited from corticosteroid therapy. In a subsequent publication from Petty and Ashbaugh [10], the authors indicated that corticosteroid is highly beneficial in patients with ARDS. Because of this enthusiastic support of clinical responses and the good experimental evidence for the use of corticosteroid in ARDS, corticosteroids have been administered to thousands of patients, and their use has been studied and reviewed extensively. Corticosteroid therapy in ARDS has been studied in three main situations: (1) prevention in high-risk patients [14-20], (2) early treatment with high-dose, short course therapy [21], and (3) prolonged therapy in unresolving cases [22-32]. It is clear that there is no evidence to support the use of corticosteroids for the prevention of ARDS in all patients at high risk. In addition, although there is intense inflammatory activity in the early stages of ARDS, early corticosteroid therapy similarly does not appear to be justified. In unresolving ARDS, corticosteroid effects have been investigated. The failure of the benefit effect of corticosteroid during the early phase of ARDS could be due to the population studied, in particular to the fact that those studies were multicentric, and were very heterogeneous in terms of the case mix and of management of the patients. In addition, negative effects due to the profound immunodepression or other side effects induced by high doses of steroids could counterbalance positive effects, so that the overall effect could be neutral or even deleterious. Corticosteroid therapy should be ineffective if many of the patients, who were considered to have ARDS based on clinical definitions, did not develop activation of inflammatory cascades in their lungs. When comparing the corticosteroid trials of the past with recent ones, three major differences are seen: (1) timing of administration (in the recent trials treatment was initiated 2-10 days after disease onset in patients that failed to improve, thus selecting a sicker patient population), (2) dosage (in the past trials the daily corticosteroid doses employed were 5-140 times greater than those used in the recent trials), and (3) in the past trials treatment consisted of administering one to four doses every 6 h versus aiming to achieve disease resolution and prolonging treatment as long as necessary (5-32 days) in the new trials. The recent randomized studies achieved statistical significance using a small number of patients [16, 30-32] compared with the large number of subjects collectively evaluated in past trials [21]. Such significant results most likely reflect a strong beneficial effect of therapy, although there is some concern that the small sample may be insufficient to confidently evaluate an outcome benefit. The National Institutes of Health (NIH) is conducting a large prospective, randomized, double-blind trial to further assess the efficacy of corticosteroid therapy for fibroproliferative ARDS.

Because of the great difficulties in designing and interpreting studies in humans, much of our knowledge about the pathophysiology of ARDS comes from animal experimentation. The results of animal studies have greatly increased our knowledge of lung injury.

This chapter reviews the results of experimental studies for the use of corticosteroids in ARDS. Firstly, in the following section it is important to discuss the mechanisms of action of corticosteroids.

Mechanisms of action of corticosteroids

Corticosteroids modulate the host defence response at virtually all levels, protecting the host from immune system over-reaction. Corticosteroids are mainly transported in the blood complexed to transcortin (corticosteroid-binding globulin) and albumin, although a small portion is in a free, metabolically active state. The free corticosteroid molecules cross the plasma membrane into the cytoplasm, where they bind to a specific receptor, the glucocorticoid receptor (GR). The GR is located in the cytoplasm of nearly all human cells [33]. After hormone binding, the GR complex migrates to the cell nucleus and inhibits inflammatory gene transcription, including nuclear factor (NF)-κB and activator protein (AP)-1, which are activated by extracellular inflammatory signals received by cell surface receptors.

NF-κB consists of two subunits arranged as homodimers (e.g., *p50/p50*) or heterodimers (e.g., *p65/p50*). The most-common form of activated NF-κB consists of a *p65* and *p50* heterodimer. Under basal conditions, NF-κB is retained in the cytoplasm in an inactive state by a related inhibitory protein known as IκB. Currently the most commonly accepted mechanism leading to the activation of NF-κB involves the activation of recently described IκBkinase, which rapidly phosphorylates IkB in response to various pro-inflammatory signals, such as endotoxin, tumor necrosis factor (TNF)-α, interleukin (IL)-1β, oxidants, bacteria, viruses, and phorbol esters. The liberated NF-κB then translocates into the nucleus and binds to promoter regions of target genes to initiate the transcription of multiple cytokines, cell adhesion molecules, and growth factors [34]. Products of the genes that are stimulated by NF-κB activate this transcription factor. Thus, TNF-α and IL-1β both activate and are activated by NF-κB by forming a positive regulatory loop that amplifies and perpetuates inflammation.

Activated GRs mediate transcriptional interference via the following mechanisms: (1) by physically interacting with the *p65* subunit and formation of an inactive (GRα-NF-κB) complex, (2) by inducing the transcription of inhibitory protein IκBαgene, which traps NF-κB in inactive cytoplasmic complexes catabolized by the ubiquitin-proteasome pathway, (3) by blocking degradation of IκBα via enhanced synthesis of IL-10, (4) by impairing TNF-α-induced degradation of IκBα, and (5) by competing for limited amounts of GRα coactivators such as CREB-binding protein and steroid receptor coactivator-1 [35-39]. GRs may also interact directly with protein transcription factors in the cytoplasm and nucleus and thereby influence the synthesis of certain proteins independently of an interaction with DNA in the cell nucleus.

Although it is not certain what the most-critical aspects of corticosteroid action are, it is likely that their inhibitory effects on cytokine synthesis are particularly important (Table 1) [35]. Corticosteroids inhibit NΦ-κB and consequently NΦ-κB-dependent pro-inflammatory gene expression [39, 40]. Thus, they inhibit the transcription of several cytokines that are relevant to ARDS, including IL-1, IL-3, IL-4, IL-5, IL-6, IL-8, TNF-α, and granulocyte-macrophage colony stimulating factor (GM-CSF). Furthermore, corticosteroids suppress the synthesis of nitric oxide synthase genes, decreasing the production of prostanoids and nitric oxide – key molecules in the inflammatory pathway – but increasing the synthesis of lipocortin-1, which has an inhibitory effect on phospholipase A_2, and therefore may inhibit the production of lipid mediators such as leukotrienes, prostaglandins, and platelet-activating factor (PAF) in leukocytes and airway epithelial cells [41, 42]. Corticosteroids also have an inhibitory effect on fibrogenesis [43], and act in synergy with IL-1 receptor antagonist [44] and the anti-inflammatory cytokines IL-4, IL-10, and IL-13 [45] to control the host defence response.

Table 1 Effects of corticosteroids on gene transcription (*IL* interleukin, *TNF* tumor necrosis factor)

Increased transcription	Decreased transcription
Lipocortin-1	Cytokines (IL-1β,2,3,4,5,6,11,13,TNF-α), granulocyte-macrophage colony stimulating factor (GM-CSF), stem cell factor
β2-Adrenoceptor	Chemokines (IL-8, RANTES, macrophage inhibitory protein 1 (MIP-1 α), macrophage chemotactic protein (MCP)-1, MCP-3, MCP-4, eotaxin)
Secretory leukocyte protease inhibitor	Enzymes [inducible nitric oxide synthase (iNOS), inducible cyclooxygenase (COX-2), cytoplasmic phospholipase A_2 (cPLA$_2$)]
Clara cell protein	Receptors [neurokinin receptor (NK)1, NK2], IL-2R
IL-1 receptor antagonist	Adhesion molecules [intercellular adhesion molecule 1 (ICAM-1), E-selectin)
IL-1R2	Endothelin-1
I-κBα	

Corticosteroid inhibits the synthesis of endothelin-1, a peptide with potent bronchoconstrictor properties in lung and airway epithelial cells. In addition, corticosteroid has effects on adhesion molecules, inhibiting the gene transcription of intercellular adhesion molecule-1 (ICAM-1) and E-selectin. Lastly, corticosteroids increase the synthesis of secretory leukocyte protease inhibitor (SLPI) by airway epithelial cells [33].

The response of a single cell exposed to corticosteroid is the result of the interplay between the following: (1) the concentration of the free hormone, (2) the relative potency of the hormone (influenced by biological activity, affinity for the GR in the nucleus), and (3) the ability of the cell to receive and transduce the hormonal signal [46]. Since it is the receptor that ultimately controls the expression of pertinent genes, anything that affects its concentration or binding affinity, translocation to the nucleus, and/or final transactivating or transrepressing conformation can also influence the response of the cells to corticosteroids. Thus, to be responsive to corticosteroids, a system must fulfil the following criteria: (1) sufficient amounts of corticosteroid must be made available, (2) corticosteroid must be present and responsive, and (3) target genes of interest must be active and regulated by corticosteroid. If one of these factors is defective, the system does not respond properly.

Animal research

Corticosteroid reduced pulmonary arterial and venous resistances and decreased the net transudation of fluid from pulmonary vasculature in a model of ALI induced by endotoxin in dogs [47]. In contrast, Demling et al. [48] observed in pre-treatment studies using an *Escherichia coli* endotoxin-induced ALI that the increase in pulmonary artery pressure was generally unaffected by methylprednisolone (MP) in the treated sheep, and a consistent benefit of steroids on oxygenation was not reported. On the other hand, corticosteroid in large doses given before or shortly after endotoxin in sheep prevented the subsequent increased lung vascular permeability, but did not reverse the abnormality once it occurred [49].

Several studies in animal models of sepsis and lung injury showed that corticosteroids decreased morbidity and mortality if given at the same as or before the experimental insult [50-52]. Pre-treatment with corticosteroid also increased the survival rate in ALI induced by aspiration pneumonitis [53] and oleic acid-induced pulmonary oedema [51, 54]. Thomas and Brockman [50] reported that steroid administration before induction of endotoxin shock in dogs improved the survival rate, but treatment after the development of shock had no influence on the animals' survival.

The beneficial effects of corticosteroid on oxygenation in animal models of ARDS have also been contradictory: the mean PaO_2 was increased over the control group in two studies [55, 56], but was not different from that found in untreated animals in the two other studies [48, 57].

Both endotoxin-induced leukopenia and increased pulmonary neutrophil migration were unaffected by MP treatment [48, 55]. Conversely, Lutch et al. [58] observed that endotoxin caused the release of substances into lung lymph-

-activating neutrophils. Pre-treatment by MP did not prevent early activity (1 h), but did significantly reduce such activity 3-4 h after *E. coli* endotoxin administration, when the permeability defects caused by it are most pronounced.

The effects of post-insult treatment with corticosteroid in an animal model of ARDS induced by endotoxaemia also presented contradictory results. In some studies [56, 59], MP treatment was associated with an improved PaO_2 and prevented the increase in extravascular lung water, while in the investigation of Harvey et al. [60], MP had no effect on the mean pulmonary arterial pressure or extravascular lung water and demonstrated only a slight inhibitory effect on the generation of cyclooxygenase metabolites.

In experimental ALI, corticosteroid administration was effective in decreasing lung collagen and oedema formation as long as treatment was prolonged, whereas steroid withdrawal rapidly negated this positive effect [61-63]. Limiting corticosteroid therapy to the first 6 days after ALI was also shown to enhance accumulation of collagen after discontinuing treatment in an experimental model [62]. These observations, together with the appreciation of the role of an exaggerated and protracted host defence response in producing non-resolving ARDS, may explain the difference between initial studies using a short course of corticosteroids early in ARDS versus the results of later studies reporting benefit with prolonged corticosteroid administration in the late or fibroproliferative phase of ARDS. In addition, the use of corticosteroids after a certain period may not be effective in changing the outcome of ARDS. On the other hand, recently we observed that fibroelastogenesis occurred at an early phase of ARDS, and even in a mild abnormal lung parenchyma [64]. In line with this, corticosteroid was used during the early phase of ALI, modifying the structural remodelling of lung parenchyma. After 24 h, tissue mechanics, collagen, and elastic fibres (elaunin, oxytalan, and fully developed elastic fibres) contents were measured in two different degrees of paraquat-induced ALI. Corticosteroid (MP) was injected 1 and 6 h after the induction of ALI. We concluded that corticosteroid acted differently depending on the degree of ALI, leading to a complete maintenance of tissue mechanics and collagen content in a mild lesion, whereas it minimized the changes in tissue impedance and extracellular matrix components in a severe lesion (Figs. 1 and 2) [65]. Interestingly enough the early (24 h after ALI induction) beneficial effects of corticosteroid in extracellular matrix remained unaltered 30 days after paraquat-induced ALI.

Corticosteroids also inhibited both the vascular and cellular aspects of acute inflammation induced by intratracheal instillation of endotoxin (LPS) by dowregulation of a broad spectrum of inflammatory cytokines and chemokines. Corticosteroid inhibited: (1) the LPS-initiated vascular leak of plasma proteins

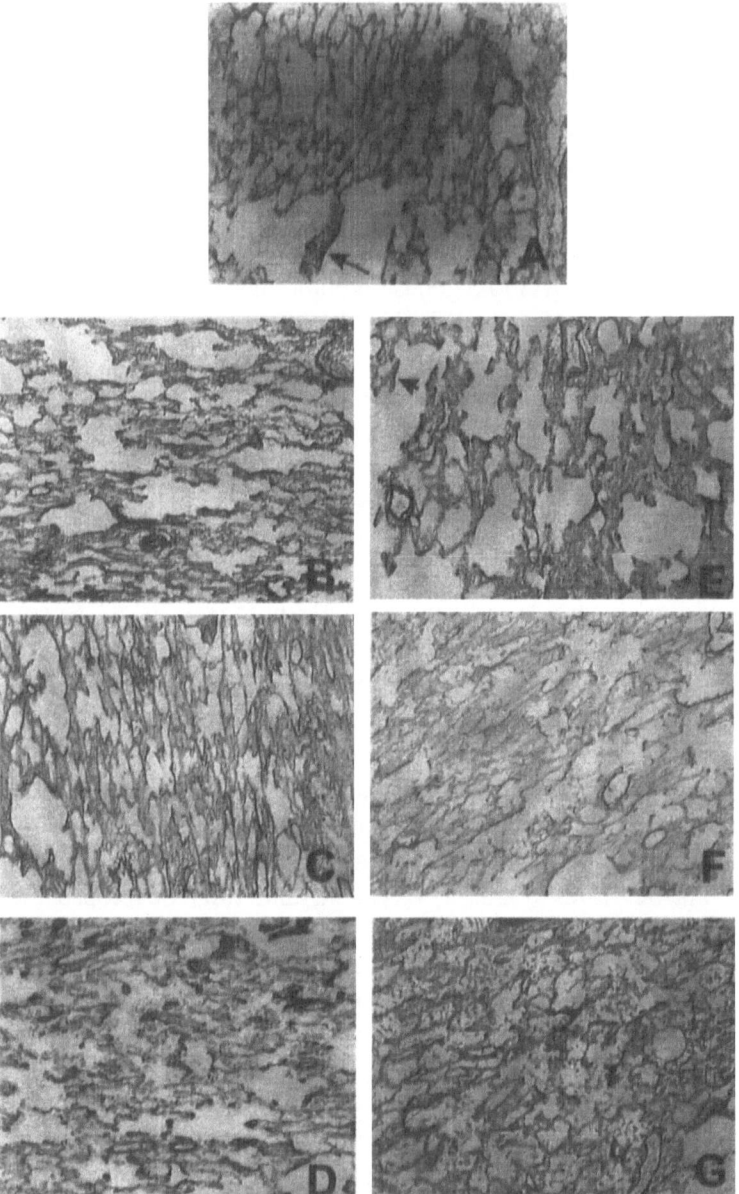

Fig. 1 Photomicrographs of parenchymal strips stained with Sirius red with polarization for collagen in control (**A**) and paraquat-treated lung [10 mg/kg (P10-**B**) and 25 mg/kg (P25-**E**)]. Panels **C**, **D**, **F**, and **G** correspond to M1P10, M6P10, M1P25, and M6P25, respectively, i.e., groups that received methylprednisolone (2 mg/kg, i.v.) 1 and 6 h after the induction of acute lung injury. All brightly birefringent structures, which shine against a dark background, contain orientated collagen molecules. Photographs were taken at an original magnification of x200

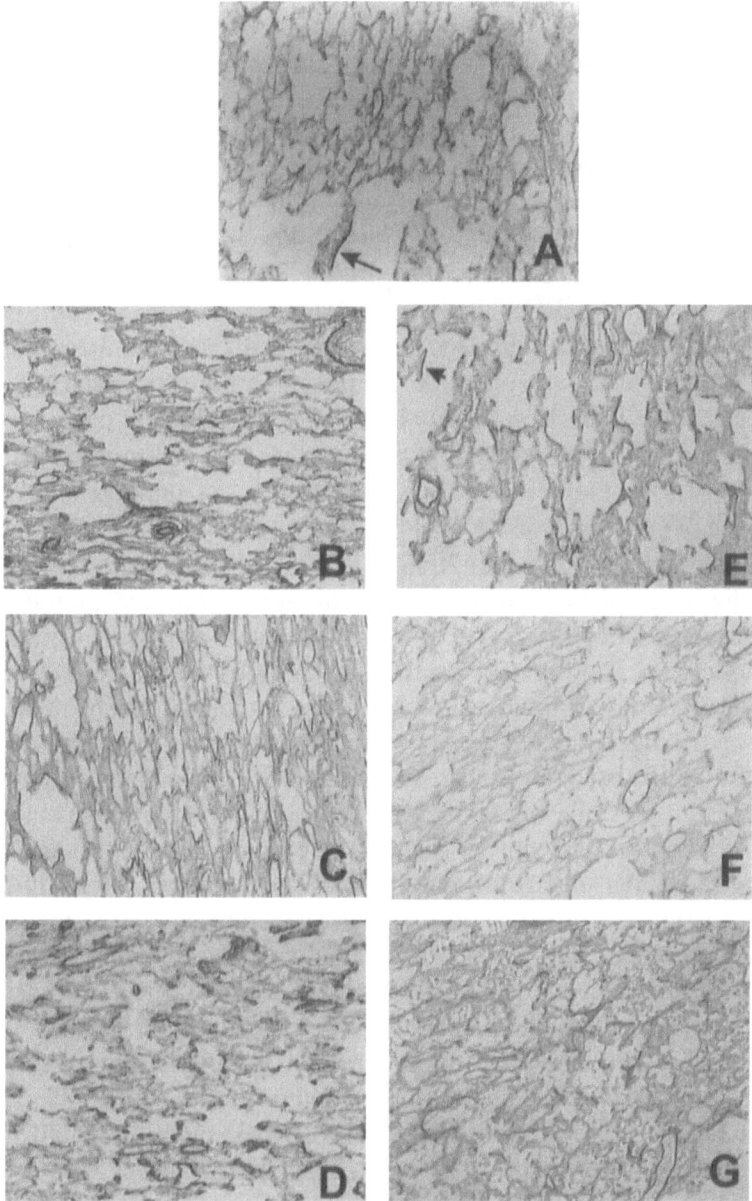

Fig. 2 Photomicrographs of parenchymal strips stained with Weigert's resorcin-fuchsin with oxidation, illustrating elastic system fibre distribution in control (**A**) and paraquat-treated lung [10 mg/kg (P10-**B**) and 25 mg/kg (P25-**E**)]. Panels **C**, **D**, **F** and **G** correspond to M1P10, M6P10, M1P25, and M6P25, respectively, i.e., groups that received methylprednisolone (2 mg/kg, i.v.) 1 and 6 h after the induction of acute lung injury. Elastic fibres are stained in black within alveolar walls (*arrow*). Photographs were taken at an original magnification of x200

into the airspace, (2) the LPS-initiated emigration of neutrophils and lymphocytes into the airspace in a dose-dependent fashion, and (3) the LPS-initiated mRNA and/or bronchoalveolar lavage protein expression of cytokines (TNF, IL-1, and IL-6) and chemokines [macrophage inflammatory protein (MIP)-1 α, MIP-2, and MCP-1] [66].

Reactive oxygen species (ROS) may have both beneficial and deleterious effects in the setting of critical illness. For example, ROS play a positive role in aiding neutrophils to kill bacteria. Thus, if the production of ROS by neutrophils is suppressed, increased susceptibility to bacterial infection is present. On the other hand, excessive generation of ROS appears to contribute to the development of ARDS, and may potentiate multiple organ system dysfunction associated with sepsis [67]. Dandona et al. [68] demonstrated that the administration of relatively modest doses of hydrocortisone (100 mg) produces prolonged depression in the ability of neutrophils to generate ROS. Because similar or larger doses of corticosteroids are commonly given to critically ill patients, these results may have important implications in the intensive care unit. Corticosteroid administration has long been known to increase susceptibility to infection, and it is likely that suppression of ROS generation by neutrophils contributes to corticosteroid-induced immunosuppression. Conversely, because production of ROS by activated neutrophils in the lung appears to play an important contributory role in ARDS, Dandona et al. [68] suggested a mechanism through which corticosteroids might be beneficial in this setting. However, there are some limitations that need to be mentioned before indicating the use of corticosteroid in ARDS: (1) Dandona's study was performed in normal subjects and the effects of corticosteroids on neutrophil function in critically ill patients are different, (2) neutrophils that infiltrate the lungs in ARDS demonstrate substantially greater pro-inflammatory properties than those of peripheral blood neutrophils, and generate excessive amounts of ROS, and (3) the release of ROS by peripheral blood neutrophils was examined in an in vitro system, in which the neutrophils were stimulated in culture [69].

One of the main arguments against intravenous corticosteroid therapy is its deleterious effects on the cellular immune response, which results in lowered host defence against infection. In 1990, Forsgren et al. [70] studied the effects of prophylactic treatment with an aerosolized corticosteroid liposome (CSL) in high dose in a porcine model of ARDS induced by endotoxaemia. They observed that CSL might be valuable as a modulator, modifying and partially counteracting the endotoxin impairment in resistance, compliance, and mean pulmonary artery pressure, without systemic side effects. In addition, Walther et al. [71] observed that nebulized corticosteroid protected pulmonary function in sepsis, indicating a therapeutic role in the treatment of ARDS. Probably, corticosteroids given directly to the lung via the inhaled/nebulized route might provide an opportunity for clinicians to administer appropriate dosages of corticosteroids to the lung in late ARDS without exposing the critically ill patient to the potentially harmful systemic steroid effect.

A variety of animal studies suggest a pivotal role of NF-κB during the development of ARDS [72]. In a clinically relevant model of sepsis, cecal ligation and puncture in the mouse, early activation of NF-κB could be detected after 3 h in the liver and the lung, associated with activated NF-IL-6 [73]. In rats, induction of NF-κB and AP-1 was observed in pulmonary tissue 2 h after trauma [74]. The pulmonary inflammatory response on systemic administration of pancreatic enzymes in the mouse was linked to the increased activity of NF-κB in the lung, providing an explanation for the systemic inflammation during acute pancreatitis [75]. Held et al. [76] showed that overinflation triggers activation of NF-κB and elicits the release of α-chemokines (MIP-2, KC), β-chemokines (MIP-1α), and cytokines (TNF-α, IL-6) from perfused lungs in a qualitatively and quantitatively similar manner to that of LPS. Since in the case of LPS these mediators were known to contribute to LPS-induced inflammation, comparable consequences might be assumed in the case of overinflation. Because steroids interfered with this process by blocking NΦ-κB activation, steroids might be considered as a subsidiary treatment during artificial mechanical ventilation [76].

Corticosteroid was also used combined with surfactant in rats with paraquat--induced lung injury. In view of the fact that corticosteroid: (1) selectively increased lamellar body and alveolar saturated phosphatidylcholine and surfactant protein A pools in adult rats [77, 78], (2) reduced the recruitment of inflammatory cells in the bronchoalveolar cavity and limited TNF-α [79], and (3) decreased inflammatory cells and protein levels in the bronchoalveolar lavage fluid in oleic acid-induced ALI [80], Chen et al. [81] hypothesized that exogenous surfactant instillation might improve gas exchange and facilitate distribution of corticosteroid to collapsed alveoli, and the combined use of surfactant and corticosteroid might enhance the effects of exogenous surfactant in paraquat-induced ALI. They observed that the intratracheal combined administration of high doses of surfactant and dexamethasone improved gas exchange, ameliorated lung inflammation, and alleviated lung damage after paraquat-induced lung injury.

Recently, London et al. [82] showed that corticosteroid treatment did not attenuate the infiltration of inflammatory leukocytes, did not suppress cytokine/chemokine expression, and did not inhibit the development of fibrotic changes in the lungs caused by reovirus 1/L infection, suggesting that as with ARDS in human patients, corticosteroids are ineffective in the early treatment of reovirus 1/L-induced ARDS. Similarly, Kuwabara et al. [83] observed that MP did not attenuate oleic acid-induced ALI, and this could be explained partly by its failure to reduce the increase of phospholipase A_2 activity and the surfactant degradation in the lung, which might also account for clinical ineffectiveness against early ARDS. However, corticosteroid treatment presented different effects in endotoxin-induced ARDS. Corticosteroid attenuated some features of endotoxin-induced ARDS in sheep, including the late-phase increase in lung lymph flow, late-phase leukopenia and hypoxia, and accumulation of granulocytes [55, 58]. Steroids also reduced both neutrophil infiltration and cytokine/chemokine expression in LPS-induced ARDS in rats [66, 84]. Conversely, the beneficial effect of corticosteroid treatment on non-ARDS--related pulmonary fibrosis in animal models has also been variable [85-88].

Two distinct forms of ARDS/ALI are described, since there are differences between primary ARDS (direct lung injury) and secondary ARDS (reflecting lung involvement in a more-distant systemic inflammatory response). These differences could be detected radiographically, functionally, and by analyzing the responses to therapeutic intervention. In line with this, we compared the effects of corticosteroid in an experimental model of primary and secondary ALI induced by intratracheal or intraperitoneal injection of LPS of E. coli [89]. MP (2 mg/kg) was intravenously injected 1 and 6 h after the induction of ALI. Primary and secondary ALI exhibited similar degrees of lung injury as indicated by in vivo (resistive, elastic, and viscoelastic pressures) and in vitro (tissue resistance, elastance, and hysteresivity) lung mechanics, pulmonary histology, the amount of collagen fibre in the alveolar septa, and tissue cellularity, but corticosteroid attenuated these changes only in primary ALI [90]. Bronchoalveolar lavage (BAL) levels of IL-8, IL-6, and neutrophils increased more in primary than in secondary ALI. Corticosteroid reduced IL-8, IL-6, and neutrophils in the BAL only in primary ALI. Thus, corticosteroid acted differently depending on the aetiology of ALI, leading to a complete maintenance of in vivo and in vitro mechanics and lung morphometry in ALI caused by pulmonary disease. The variable response of ARDS to corticosteroid treatment could be attributed to the heterogeneous biochemical and molecular mechanisms to different initial insults. Furthermore, numerous important factors need to be taken into account when corticosteroid was used as a strategy to treat ARDS (the specificity of inhibition, the duration and degree of inhibition, and the timing of inhibition).

Conclusions

Improving the course and outcome of patients with ARDS presents a considerable challenge. An important component of meeting this challenge is a more--comprehensive understanding of the heterogeneous pathophysiology of ARDS and the biological response of the individual patient. By understanding the immune status of a given patient at a given point in the disease process, the physician can consider manipulating pro-inflammatory systems more rationally. In this context, corticosteroid could be a therapeutic tool in the armamentarium against ARDS. Results obtained from corticosteroid therapy on animal models of ARDS have been controversial. On the basis of animal research, corticosteroid was subjected to clinical trials as adjunctive therapy for patients with ARDS.

References

1. Ashbaugh DG, Bigelow DB, Petty TL, et al (1967) Acute respiratory distress syndrome. Lancet II:319-323
2. Bernard GR, Artigas A, Bringham KL, et al (1994) The American-European consensus conference on ARDS: definitions, mechanisms, relevant outcomes, and clinical trial coordination. Am J Respir Crit Care Med 149:818-824
3. Ware LB, Matthay MA (2000) The acute respiratory distress syndrome. N Engl J Med 342: 1334-1349
4. Tomashefski JF Jr (2000) Pulmonary pathology of acute respiratory distress syndrome. Clin Chest Med 21:435-466
5. Fein AM, Calalang-Colucci MG (2000) Acute lung injury and acute respiratory distress syndrome in sepsis and septic shock. Crit Care Clin 16:289-317
6. Chesnutt AN, Matthay MA, Tibayan FA, et al (1997) Early detection of type III procollagen peptide in acute lung injury. Pathogenic and prognostic significance. Am J Respir Crit Care Med 156:840-845
7. Liebler JM, Qu Z, Buckner B, et al (1998) Fibroproliferation and mast cells in the acute respiratory distress syndrome. Thorax 53:823-829
8. Pugin J, Verghese G, Widmer MC, et al (1999) The alveolar space is the site of intense inflammatory and profibrotic reactions in the early phase of acute respiratory distress syndrome. Crit Care Med 27:304-312
9. Marshall RP, Bellingan G, Webb S, et al (2000) Fibroproliferation occurs early in the acute respiratory distress syndrome and impacts on outcome. Am J Respir Crit Care Med 162: 1783-1788
10. Petty TL, Ashbaugh DG (1971) The adult respiratory distress syndrome: clinical features, factors influencing prognosis and principles of management. Chest 60:233-239
11. Luce JM (2002) Corticosteroids in ARDS. An evidence-based review. Crit Care Clin 18:79-89
12. Brower RG, Ware LB, Berthiaume Y, et al (2001) Treatment of ARDS. Chest 120:1347-1367
13. McIntyre Jr RC, Pulido EJ, Bensard DD, et al (2000) Thirty years of clinical trials in acute respiratory distress syndrome. Crit Care Med 28:3314-3331
14. Sibbald WJ, Driedger AA, Finley RJ, et al (1982) High dose corticosteroids in the treatment of pulmonary microvascular injury. Ann NY Acad Sci 384:496-516
15. VanDerMerwe CJ, Louw AF, Welthagen D, et al (1985) Adult respiratory distress syndrome in

cases of severe trauma: the prophylactic value of methylprednisolone sodium succinate. S Afr
Med J 57:279-284

16. Weigelt JA, Norcross JR, Borman KR, et al (1985) Early steroid therapy for respiratory failure.
Arch Surg 120:536-540

17. Luce JM, Montgomery AB, Marks JD, et al (1988) Ineffectiveness of high-dose methylprednisolone in preventing parenchymal lung injury and improving mortality in patients with septic
shock. Am Rev Respir Dis 138:62-68

18. Bone RC, Fisher CJ Jr, Clemmer TP, et al (1987) Early methylprednisolone treatment for septic
syndrome and the adult respiratory distress syndrome. Chest 92:1032-1036

19. VA (1987) Effects of high dose glucocorticoid therapy on mortality in patients with clinical signs
of systemic sepsis. The Veterans Administration Systemic Sepsis Cooperative Study Group. N
Engl J Med 317:659-665

20. Sprung CL, Caralis PV, Marcial EH, et al (1984) The effects of high-dose corticosteroids in
patients with septic shock. A prospective, controlled study. N Engl J Med 311:1137-1143

21. Bernard GR, Luce JM, Sprung CL, et al (1987) High dose corticosteroids in patients with the
adult respiratory distress syndrome. N Engl J Med 317:1365-1370

22. Ashbaugh DG, Maier RV (1985) Idiopathic pulmonary fibrosis in adult respiratory distress
syndrome. Diagnosis and treatment. Arch Surg 120:530-535

23. Hooper RG, Kearl RA (1990) Established ARDS treated with a sustained course of adrenocortical steroids. Chest 97:138-143

24. Biffl WL, Moore FA, Moore EE, et al (1995) Are corticosteroids salvage therapy for refractory
acute respiratory distress syndrome? Am J Surg 170:591-596

25. Meduri GU, Chinn AJ, Leeper KV, et al (1994) Corticosteroid rescue treatment of progressive
fibroproliferation in late ARDS: patterns of response and predictors of outcome. Chest 105:1516-
-1527

26. Meduri GU, Headley S, Golden E, et al (1998) Effect of prolonged methylprednisolone therapy
in unresolving acute respiratory distress syndrome: a randomised controlled trial. JAMA
280:159-165

27. Meduri GU (1996) The role of the host defence response in the progression and outcome of
ARDS: pathophysiologic correlations and response to glucocorticoid treatment. Eur Respir J
9:2650-2670

28. Meduri GU, Headly S, Kohler G, et al (1995) Persistent elevation of inflammatory cytokines
predicts a poor outcome in ARDS: plasma IL-1β and IL-6 are consistent and efficient predictors
of outcome over time. Chest 107:1062-1073

29. Meduri GU, Kohler G, Headley S, et al (1995) Inflammatory cytokines in the BAL of patients
with ARDS: persistent elevation over time predicts poor outcome. Chest 108:1303-1314

30. Meduri GU, Headley S, Tolley E, et al (1995) Plasma and BAL cytokine response to corticosteroid rescue treatment in late ARDS. Chest 108:1315-1325

31. Meduri G U, Tolley EA, Chinn A, et al (1998) Procollagen types I and III aminoterminal
propeptide levels during acute respiratory distress syndrome and in response to methylprednisolone treatment. Am J Respir Crit Care Med 158:1432-1441

32. Meduri GU, Tolley EA, Chrousos GP, et al (2002) Prolonged methylprednisolone treatment
suppresses systemic inflammation in patients with unresolving acute respiratory distress syndrome. Evidence for inadequate endogenous glucocorticoid secretion and inflammation-induced
immune cell resistance to glucocorticoids. Am J Respir Crit Care Med 165:983-991

33. Jantz MA, Sahn AS (1999) Corticosteroids in acute respiratory failure. Am J Respir Crit Care
Med 160:1079-1100

34. Bauerle PA, Baltimore D (1996) NF-kappa B: ten years after. Cell 87:13-20

35. Payne DNR, Adcock IM (2001) Molecular mechanisms of corticosteroid actions. Pediatr Respir
Rev 2:145-150

36. Senftleben U, Karin M (2002) The IKK/NF-κB pathway. Crit Care Med 30:S18-S26

37. Wang P, Wu P, Siegel MI, et al (1995) Interleukin (IL)-10 inhibits nuclear factor kappa B

(NF-kappa B) activation in human monocytes: IL-10 and IL-4 suppress cytokine synthesis by different mechanisms. J Biol Chem 270: 9558-9563

38. Sheppard KA, Phelps KM, Williams AJ, et al (1998) Nuclear integration of glucocorticoid receptor an nuclear factor-κB signalling by CREB-binding protein and steroid receptor coactivator-1. J Biol Chem 273:29291-29294

39. Wissink S, Heerde EC van, Burg B van der, et al (1998) A dual mechanism mediates repression of NF-kappa B activity by glucocorticoids. Mol Endocrinol 12:355-363

40. Scheinman RI, Cogswell PC, Lofquist AK, et al (1995) Role of transcriptional activation of Ikappa B alpha in mediation of immunosuppression by glucocortioids. Science 270:283-286

41. Albina JE, Reichner JS (1995) Nitric oxide in inflammation and immunity. New Horiz 3: 46-64

42. Pruzanski W, Vadas P (1991) Phospholipase A2 – a mediator between proximal and distal effectors of inflammation. Immunol Today 12:143-146

43. Meduri GU, Belenchia JM, Estes RJ, et al (1991) Fibroproliferative phase of ARDS: clinical findings and effects of corticosteroids. Chest 100:943-952

44. Santos AA, Scheltinga MR, Lynch E, et al (1993) Elaboration of interleukin 1-receptor antagonist is not attenuated by glucocorticoids after endotoxemia. Arch Surg 128:138-144

45. Hart PH, Whitty GA, Burgess DR, et al (1990) Augmentation of glucocorticoid action on human monocytes by interkeukin-4. Lymphokine Res 9:147-153

46. Bamberger CM, Shulte HM, Chrousos GP (1996) Molecular determinants of glucocorticoids function and tissue sensitivity to glucocorticoids. Endocr Rev 17:245-261

47. Motsay GJ. Alho AV, Romero LH, et al (1973) The pulmonary microcirculation of endotoxin shocked dogs: effect of phenoxybenzamine and methylprednisolone on the precapillary and post-capillary resistances. J Surg Res 14:406-411

48. Demling RJ, Proctor R, Grossman J, et al (1980) Comparison of the systemic and pulmonary vascular response to endotoxin with plasma and lung lymph lysosomal enzyme release: effect of steroid pretreatment. Circ Shock 7:317-331

49. Brigham KL, Bowers RE, McKeen CR (1981) Methylprednisolone prevention of increased lung vascular permeability following endotoxemia in sheep. J Clin Invest 67:1103-1110

50. Thomas CS, Brockman SK (1968) The role of adrenal corticosteroid therapy in Escherichia coli endotoxin shock. Surg Gynecol Obstet 126:61-69

51. Wertzberger JJ, Peltier LF (1968) Fat embolism: the effect of corticosteroids on experimental fat embolism in the rat. Surgery 64:143-147

52. White GI, Archer LJ, Beller BK, et al (1978) Increased survival with methylprednisolone treatment in canine endotoxin shock. J Surg Res 25:357-364

53. Lawson DW, Defalco AJ, Phelps JA, et al (1966) Corticosteroids as treatment for aspiration of gastric contents: an experimental study. Surgery 59:845-852

54. Jones RL, King AG (1975) The effects of methylprednisolone on oxygenation in experimental hypoxemic respiratory failure. J Trauma 15:297-303

55. Begley CJ, Ogletree ML, Meyrick BO, et al (1984) Modification of pulmonary responses to endotoxemia in awake sheep by steroidal and nonsteroidal anti-inflammatory agents. Am Rev Respir Dis 130:1140-1146

56. Modig J, Borg T (1985) High dose methylprednisolone in a porcine model of ARDS induced by endotoxemia. Acta Chir Scand 526:94-103

57. Cefalo RC, Lewis PE, O'Brien WF, et al (1980) The role of prostaglandins in endotoxemia: comparisons in response in the nonpregnant, maternal, and fetal models. Am J Obstet Gynecol 137:53-57

58. Lutch WD, Bernard GR, Butka B, et al (1988) Corticosteroids inhibit endotoxin-induced lung lymph neutrophil stimulating activity in sheep. Am J Med Sci 296:98-102

59. Borg T, Gerdin B, Modig J (1985) Prophylactic and delayed treatment with high-dose methylprednisolone in a porcine model of early ARDS induced by endotoxaemia. Acta Anaesthesiol Scand 29:831-845

60. Harvey CR, Sugerman JH, Tatum JL, et al (1987) Ibuprofen and methylprednisolone in a pig *Pseudomonas* ARDS model. Circ Shock 21:175-183
61. Hesterberg TW, Last JA (1981) Ozone-induced acute pulmonary fibrosis in rats. Prevention of increased rates of collagen synthesis by methylprednisolone. Am Rev Respir Dis 123:47-52
62. Hakkinen PJ, Schmoyer RL, Witschi HP (1983) Potentiation of butylated-hydroxytoluene-induced acute lung damage by oxygen: effects of prednisolone and indomethacin. Am Rev Respir Dis 128:648-651
63. Kehrer JP, Klein-Szanto AJP, Sorensen EMB, et al (1984) Enhanced acute lung damage following corticosteroid treatment. Am Rev Respir Dis 130:256-261
64. Rocco PRM, Negri EM, Kurtz PM, et al (2001) Lung tissue mechanics and extracellular matrix remodeling in acute lung injury Am J Respir Crit Care Med 164:1067-1071
65. Rocco PRM, Lima JGM, Barros AS, et al (2001) Effects of corticosteroid on lung parenchyma remodeling at an early phase of acute lung injury. Am J Respir Crit Care Med 164:A451
66. Yi ES, Remick DG, Lim Y, et al (1996) The intratracheal administration of endotoxin: dexamethasone downregulates neutrophil emigration and cytokine expression in vivo. Inflammation 20: 165-175
67. Chabot F, Mitchell JA, Gutteridge JM, et al (1998) Reactive oxygen species in acute lung injury. Eur Respir J 11:745-757
68. Dandona P, Suri M, Hamouda W, et al (1999) Hydrocortisone-induced inhibition of reactive oxygen species by polymorphonuclear neutrophils. Crit Care Med 27:2442-2444
69. Abraham E (1999) Corticosteroid and the neutrophil: cutting both ways. Crit Care Med 27: 2583-2584
70. Forsgren PE, Modig JA, Dahlbäck CMO, et al (1990) Prophylactic treatment with an aerosolized corticosteroid liposome in a porcine model of early ARDS induced by endotoxaemia. Acta Chir Scand 156:423-431
71. Walther S, Jansson I, Berg S, et al (1993) Corticosteroid by aerosol in septic pigs-effects on pulmonary function and oxygen transport. Intensive Care Med 19:155-160
72. Blackwell TS, Yull FE, Chen CL, et al (1999) Use of genetically altered mice to investigate the role of nuclear factor-kappa B activation and cytokine gene expression in sepsis-induced ARDS. Chest 116:73S-74S
73. Browder W, Ha T, Chuantu L, et al (1999) Early activation of pulmonary nuclear factor kappa B and nuclear factor interleukin-6 in polymicrobial sepsis. J Trauma 46:590-596
74. Armstead VE, Opentanova IL, Minchenko AG, et al (1999) Tissue factor expression in vital organs during murine traumatic shock: role of transcription factors AP-1 and NF-kappaB. Anesthesiology 91:1844-1852
75. Jaffray C, Yang J, Carter G, et al (2000) Pancreatic elastase activates pulmonary nuclear factor kappa B and inhibitory kappa B, mimicking pancreatitis-associated adult respiratory distress syndrome. Surgery 128:225-231
76. Held HD, Boettcher S, Hamann L, et al (2000) Ventilation-induced chemokine and cytokine release is associated with activation of nuclear factor-kB and is blocked by steroids. Am J Respir Crit Care Med 163:711-716
77. Young SL, Silbajoris R (1986) Dexamethasone increased adult rat lung surfactant lipids. J Appl Physiol 60:1665-1672
78. Young SL, Ho YS, Silbajoris R (1991) Surfactant apoprotein in adult rat lung compartments is increased by dexamethasone. Am J Physiol 260:161-167
79. Williams CM, Smith L, Flanagan BF, et al (1997) Tumour necrosis factor-alpha expression and cell recruitment in Sephadex particle-induced lung inflammation. Effects of dexamethasone and cyclosporin A. Br J Pharmacol 122:1127-1134
80. Volpe BT, Lin W, Thrall RS (1994) Effect of intratracheal dexamethasone on oleic acid induced lung injury in the rat. Chest 106:583-587
81. Chen CM, Fang CL, Chang CH (2001) Surfactant and corticosteroid effects on lung function in a rat model of acute lung injury. Crit Care Med 11:2169-2175

82. London L, Majeski E, Altman-Hamamdzic S, et al (2002) Respiratory reovirus 1/L induction of diffuse alveolar damage: pulmonary fibrosis is not modulated by corticosteroids in acute respiratory distress syndrome in rats. Clin Immunol 103:284-295

83. Kuwabara K, Furue S, Tomita Y, et al (2001) Effect of methylprednisolone on phospholipase A2 activity and lung surfactant degradation in acute lung injury in rats. Eur J Pharmacol 433: 209-216

84. O'Leary EC, Marder P, Zuckerman SH (1996) Glucocorticoid effects in an endotoxin-induced rat pulmonary inflammation model: differential effects on neutrophil influx, integrin expression, and inflammatory mediators. Am J Respir Cell Mol Biol 15:97-106

85. Mapel DW, Samet JM, Coultas DB (1996) Corticosteroids and the treatment of idiopathic pulmonary fibrosis: past, present, and future. Chest 110:1058-1067

86. Khalil N, Whitman C, Zuo L, et al (1993) Regulation of alveolar macrophage transforming growth factor beta secretion by corticosteroids in bleomycin induced pulmonary inflammation in the rat. J Clin Invest 92:1812-1818

87. Phan SH, Thrall RS, Williams C (1981) Bleocycin-induced pulmonary fibrosis: effect of steroid on lung collagen metabolism. Am Rev Respir Dis 124:428-434

88. Sterling KM, DiPetrillo T, Cutroneo K, et al (1982) Inhibition of collagen accumulation by glucocorticoids in rat lung after intratracheal bleomycin instillation. Cancer Res 42:405-408

89. Menezes SLS, Laranjeira AP, Castro-Faria Neto HC, et al (2001) Inflammatory responses in pulmonary and extrapulmonary acute lung injury. Am J Respir Crit Care Med 163:A460

90. Rocco PRM, Leite-Junior JH, Souza AB, et al (2001) Effects of corticosteroid in acute lung injury caused by pulmonary and extrapulmonary disease. Proceedings of the 8th World Congress of Intensive Care Medicine 1:191

Evidence of biological efficacy for prolonged corticosteroid treatment in unresolving acute respiratory distress syndrome

G.U. MEDURI, E. GOLDEN, S. RATNAKANT

Acute respiratory distress syndrome (ARDS) is a disease of multi-factorial etiology characterized by rapid development of severe diffuse and non-homogenous inflammation of the pulmonary lobules, causing life-threatening hypoxemic respiratory failure. We have tested a therapeutic intervention on a previously defined pathophysiological model of ARDS [1]. The model was defined by investigating during the longitudinal course of ARDS, the relationship among the three fundamental elements of a disease process *pathogenesis*, *structural alterations*, and *functional consequences* [2]. In these studies, we provided biological and morphological evidence indicating that ARDS patients failing to improve after 1 week of mechanical ventilation (unresolving ARDS) have intense and protracted pulmonary and systemic inflammatory and neo-fibrogenetic activity.

Nuclear factor-κB (NF-κB) and the glucocorticoid receptor (GR) have diametrically opposed functions in regulating inflammation. In this chapter, we will review recent data indicating that poor outcome in ARDS is associated with failure of the activated GRs to downregulate the transcription of inflammatory cytokines, despite elevated levels of circulating cortisol. In a randomized study of patients with unresolving ARDS, we have shown that prolonged glucocorticoid (GC) supplementation improved all aspects of GR function and enhanced GC-mediated anti-inflammatory action by interfering with NF-κB activation.

Acute respiratory distress syndrome

ARDS is a term applied to a relatively specific morphological lesion of multi-factorial etiology termed "diffuse alveolar damage" (DAD) [3]. ARDS develops rapidly, in most patients within 12-48 h of exposure to infectious or non-infectious insults that can affect the lung directly (via the alveolar compartment) or indirectly (via the vascular compartment) [4]. At presentation (early), ARDS manifests with severe, diffuse, and non-homogenous acute host inflammatory response (HIR) of the pulmonary lobules, leading to a breakdown in the barrier and gas exchange function of the lung. Injury to the alveolo-capillary membrane (ACM) causes flooding of the airspaces with protein-rich neutrophilic oedema fluid, resulting in severe gas exchange and lung compliance abnormalities [5].

Overall mortality in ARDS is 40%-60% [5, 6], with most non-survivors dying within 2 weeks of disease development [7]. While a regulated inflammatory response is critical to survival [8], a major predictor of poor outcome in ARDS patients is persistence of pulmonary and systemic inflammation after 1 week of lung injury [9, 10]. Failure to downregulate the production of inflammatory mediators (dysregulated HIR) is associated with maladaptive lung repair and inability to improve ACM permeability, gas exchange, and lung mechanics over time.

The lung injury score (LIS) quantifies the physiological respiratory impairment in ARDS through the use of a four-point score, based on the levels of positive end-expiratory pressure (PEEP), PaO_2:FiO_2, the static lung compliance (Cst), and the degree of infiltration present on chest radiograph [11]. Patients failing to improve the LIS or its components by day 7 of ARDS (non-improvers) have a poor outcome [12-14]. We have previously reported that patients meeting predefined criteria for unresolving ARDS (LIS on day 7 of ARDS $\geq$ 2.5 and < 1-point reduction from day 1 of ARDS) have a mortality rate in excess of 80% (Table 1) [15].

Table 1 Definitions of resolving and unresolving acute respiratory distress syndrome (ARDS) (*LIS* lung injury score

Findings on day 7 of ARDS	Resolving	Unresolving
LIS from day 1 to day 7 of ARDS	$\geq$1 point reduction	< 1 point reduction
Clinical definition	Improver	Non-improver
Host inflammatory response	Regulated	Dysregulated
Progression of lung histology	Adaptive	Maladaptive
Observed mortality[a]	14%	83%

[a] Data obtained from reference [15]

Model of translational research

Because there is no animal model to study the progression of ARDS, translational clinical research has an important role to play for advancing understanding in this field. The University of Tennessee's research model has followed a "holistic" level of inquiry in constructing a pathophysiological model of ARDS attempting to fit pathogenesis (biology) with morphological (pathology) and clinical (physiology) findings observed during the longitudinal course of the disease (Fig. 1) [2]. Most importantly, we have attempted to define the differences over time between patients with an adaptive (resolving ARDS) versus maladaptive (unresolving ARDS) reparative response, and the time span of disease reversibility (prior to reaching end-stage disease) that is potentially amenable to anti-inflammatory treatment. In patients failing to improve after 1 week of ARDS onset (unresolving ARDS), we also have investigated the effect

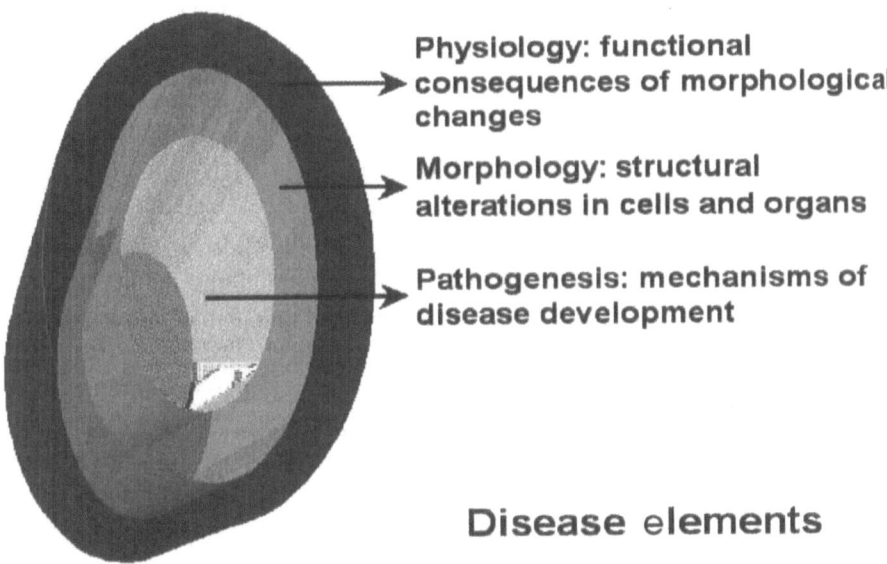

Physiology: functional consequences of morphological changes

Morphology: structural alterations in cells and organs

Pathogenesis: mechanisms of disease development

Disease elements

Fig. 1 Disease elements

of prolonged anti-inflammatory (GC) treatment. In relation to the treatment investigation, we assumed that the closer our treatment intervention was to the core pathogenetic mechanisms of disease development, the more likely treatment would affect all "layers" of the disease process (Fig. 1). In this context, a positive or negative biological and physiological response to treatment was used to prove or disprove the pathogenetic relevance (central vs. peripheral) of the factor or pathway affected by treatment.

Controversy continues on the use of GC treatment in ARDS [16] and sepsis [17, 18]. Meduri [19] provided a historical review of GC treatment in sepsis and ARDS in relation to the evolving pathophysiological understanding of systemic inflammation. Similar to the original reports from Ashbaugh and Maier [20] and Hooper and Kearl [21], we investigated the use of prolonged methylprednisolone (MP) administration in patients with unresolving ARDS. The differences between GC dosage and duration of administration of older (1980s) versus newer trials are outlined in the Table 2.

Table 2 Comparison of old and new trials investigating methylprednisolone use in ARDS (*HIR* host inflammatory response, *GCT* glucocorticoid treatment)

	1980s trials	1990s trials
Timing of ARDS	< 2 days	7-14 days (unresolved)
Dosage	120 mg/kg per day	2 mg/kg per day
Duration	1 day	Average 30 days
Understanding of the HIR in ARDS	Massive, short-lived	Prolonged, initial intensity affects duration
Understanding of GCT in ARDS	Reversibility lost early	Reversibility lost with end-stage fibrosis
Glucocorticoid treatment	Massive, short-course	Lower dose, prolonged until resolution

Over the last decade our understanding of the intermediary events that occur between the reception of a biological signal at the cell membrane and the eventual conversion of that signal to a change in gene expression at the nuclear level (i.e., signal transduction) has grown immensely [22]. It is now recognized that two cellular signalling pathways are central to the regulation of inflammation, the *stimulatory* nuclear factor-κB (NF-κB) and the *inhibitory* GRα-mediated signal transduction cascades. In unstimulated cells, both NF-κB and GR are predominantly sequestered in the cytoplasm.

Nuclear factor-kB

NF-κB is recognized as the central transcription factor that drives the inflammatory response to insults. NF-kB activation is an essential step in the experimental development of neutrophilic lung inflammation [23-25]. NF-κB is found in essentially all cell types and is involved in activation of an exceptionally large number of target genes (over 100) [26]. NF-κB is a heterogenous collection of dimers, composed of various combinations of the NF-κB/Rel family. The p65:p50 heterodimer was the first form of NF-κB to be identified and is the most abundant in most cell types [26]. NF-κB is maintained in an inactive form by sequestration in the cytoplasm through interaction with inhibitory proteins IkBs (most important being IκBα) (Fig. 2) [27]. Activation of NF-κB is a rapid, immediate early event that occurs within minutes after exposure to a relevant inducer, including innate immunity stimulating molecules (e.g., lipopolysaccharide and hsp60), double-stranded DNA, physical and chemical stresses, and inflammatory cytokines [e.g., tumour necrosis factor (TNF)-α and interleukin (IL)-1β]. In response to these various stimuli, the latent NF-κB/IκB complex is activated by phosphorylation and proteolytic degradation of IκB, with exposure of the NF-κB nuclear localization sequence (NSL) [26]. Proteolytic degradation of IκB is an irreversible step in the signaling pathway that constitutes a commitment to transcriptional activation [26].

The liberated NF-κB then translocates into the nucleus and binds to promoter regions of target genes to initiate the transcription of multiple cytokines including TNF-α, and IL-1β, IL-2, IL-6, chemokines such as IL-8, cell adhesion molecules (e.g., intercellular adhesion molecule-1, E-selectin), interferon, receptors involved in immune recognition such as members of the MHC, proteins involved in antigen presentation, receptors required for neutrophil adhesion and migration, and inflammation-associated enzymes [cyclooxygenase (COX), phospholipase A2 (PLA$_2$), inducible nitric oxide (iNOS)] [27, 28]. Products of the genes that are stimulated by NF-κB activate this transcription factor. Thus, TNF-α and IL-1β both activate and are activated by NF-κB, by forming a positive regulatory loop that amplifies and perpetuates inflammation [29]. NF-κB also operates in conjunction with other transcription factors, including activator protein-1 (AP-1) [30].

Glucocorticoid receptor

Peripherally generated TNF-α, IL-1β, and IL-6 activate the hypothalamic-pituitary-adrenal (HPA) axis independently at some or all of its levels [31, 32]. The HPA axis responds in a graded manner to greater intensities of stress with

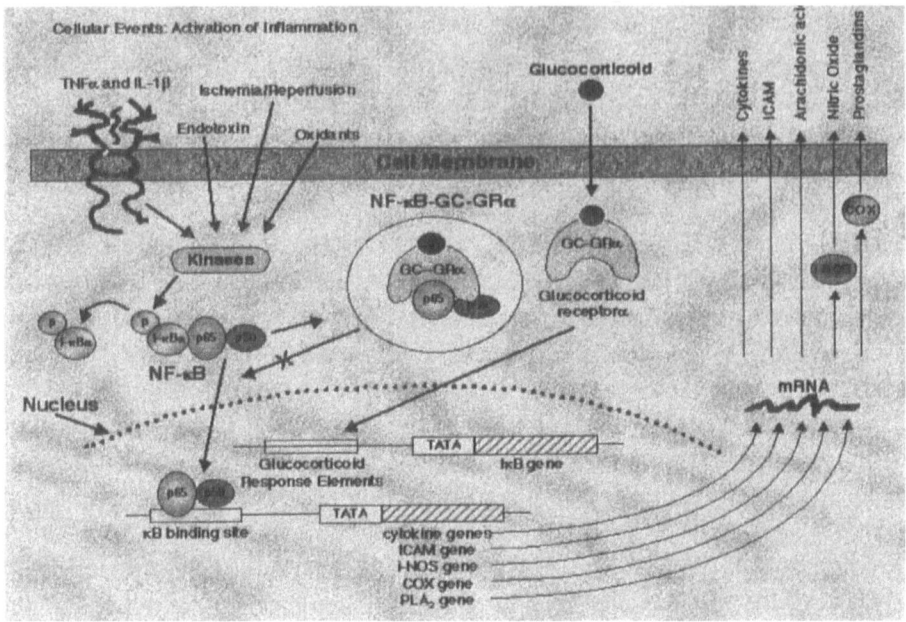

Fig. 2 Interaction between NF-κB and the activated glucocorticoid receptor. When cells are stimulated by inflammatory signals, specific kinases phosphorylate the inhibitory protein IkB and cause its rapid degradation. The activated form of NF-κB then moves to the nucleus, initiating the transcription of mRNA of inflammatory cytokines, chemokines, cell adhesion molecules, and inflammation-associated enzymes (cyclooxygenase, phospholipase A2, inducible nitric oxide). Cortisol or exogenous glucocorticoids freely cross into the cytoplasm and bind to their specific glucocorticoid receptors (GRα) to form the activated receptor (GC-GRα). GC-GRα complexes may influence NF-κB activity in five major ways: (1) physically interacting with the p65 subunit with formation of an inactive (GC-GRα/NF-κB) complex (2), inducing the synthesis of the inhibitory protein IκBα via interaction with glucocorticoid-responsive element DNA in the promoter of the IκB gene (3), blocking degradation of IκBα via enhanced synthesis of IL-10 (4), impairing TNF-α-induced degradation of IκBα, and (5) competing for limited amounts of GR co-activators such as CREB-binding protein (CBP) and steroid receptor coactivator-1 (SRC-1). GC-GRα may also decrease the stability of mRNA of several proinflammatory cytokines and other molecules. Products of the genes that are stimulated by NF-κB activate this transcription factor. Thus, TNF-α and IL-1β both activate and are activated by NF-κB, by forming a positive regulatory loop that amplifies and perpetuates inflammation.

increased production of adrenocorticotropic hormone (ACTH) and GCs. Due to their hormonal and lipophilic nature, GCs pass freely through the cell membrane. GCs exert most of their effects by activating ubiquitously distributed (2,000-30,000 per cell) cytoplasmic heat shock protein-complexed GR with formation of GC-GR complexes [33]. It is now appreciated that the GC-GR complexes modulate transcription in a *hormone-dependent manner* by binding as a dimer to GC-responsive elements (GREs) located in the promoter regions of GC-responsive genes and by interfering with the activity of other transcription factors such as NF-κB on genes regulated by these factors [34]. As a dimer and/or a monomer, GR-mediated transcriptional interference is achieved by five important mechanisms (Fig. 2): (1) physically interacting with the p65 subunit and formation of an inactive (GR-NF-κB) complex [33], (2) by inducing the transcription of the inhibitory protein IκBα gene [33, 35, 36], (3) by blocking degradation of IkBa via enhanced synthesis of IL-10 [37-39], (4) by impairing TNF-α-induced degradation of IκBα [40, 41], and (5) by competing for limited amounts of GR co-activators such as CREB-binding protein (CBP) and steroid receptor coactivator-1 (SRC-1) [42]. In addition to transcriptional modulation GCs also influence the processing of mRNA and translation of proteins, probably through transactivation or transrepression of genes that regulate mRNA stability and translation [43].

Inflammation-associated GC inadequacy/resistance

GCs as end-effectors of the hypothalamic-pituitary-adrenal axis are the most--important natural inhibitors of inflammation [44]. However, endogenous GCs are not always effective in suppressing life-threatening systemic inflammation, even though the degree of cortisolemia frequently correlates with severity of illness and mortality rate [45-48]. Unquestionably, the elevation of GC secretion in non-survivors is inadequate to meet the needs of the concurrent inflammatory response and its adverse systemic effects. Failure to suppress inflammation could be due to tissue resistance to GCs, inadequacy of the level and duration of endogenous GC elevation, or both [49].

The concept of acquired GC resistance was first introduced by Kass and Finland [50] in 1957. These investigators suggested that increased blood cortisol levels in patients with sepsis may reflect a block to steroidal activity or transport, as a consequence of the infection. In this situation, a small increase in blood levels with a low (equal or less than physiological) dose of exogenous GCs was believed to be sufficient for facilitating the passage of steroids into host cells [50]. GR-mediated resistance was originally described as a *primary* inherited familial syndrome [51, 52], and was recently recognized as an *acquired* condition. Among others, *acquired* immune tissue-specific GR resistance has been described in patients with asthma [53-56], acquired immunodeficiency syndrome (AIDS) [57], and severe sepsis [58].

Recent in vitro studies have shown that cytokines may induce resistance to GCs by reducing GR binding affinity to cortisol and/or GREs [59-61]. Such abnormalities of GR function were demonstrated in T cells incubated with a combination of IL-2 and IL-4 [60], IL-1, IL-6, and interferon (IFN)-γ [59], or IL 13 [61]. GC resistance was induced in a cytokine concentration-dependent fashion and was reversed by the removal of cytokines [60]. GR-mediated resistance in the presence of systemic inflammation was also studied in experimental models of sepsis and sepsis-induced ARDS [58, 62, 63]. In a sheep model of sepsis-induced ARDS, maximal binding capacity of GR decreased continuously after endotoxin infusion, while there was a marked elevation of cortisol levels [62]. The reduced GR binding correlated negatively ($r = -0.87$, $P <0.01$) with PLA_2 activity, a gene that is stimulated by NF-κB. In a rat model of septic shock, GR blockade by mifepristone (RU 486) exacerbated the physiological and pathological changes induced by endotoxemia [63]. PLA2 activity in rats with 80% GR blockade was more marked than in those with 50% GR blockade [63]. Monocytes of patients with sepsis developed near total glucocorticoid resistance in vitro, when cytokines, especially IL-2, were added [58].

Several inflammatory cytokines, including TNF-α, IL-1β, and IL-6 activate NF-kB [64]. It has been proposed that when cytokine-activated NF-κB forms protein-protein complexes with activated GR, the availability and activity of effective GR molecules are reduced [33, 56]. This functional reduction in GR availability is associated with decreased GR-GRE DNA binding and GC-mediated anti-inflammatory activity [33, 56].

Longitudinal studies of biomarkers of HIR in ARDS

We previously reported data to support a single "hit" model for ARDS progression, where degree and duration of the HIR determined the *adaptive* versus *maladaptive* evolution of the reparative process and final outcome. In a series of studies [65-68], we have shown that patients with ARDS failing to improve in the 1st week of mechanical ventilation (unresolving ARDS) had biological and morphological evidence of intense and protracted pulmonary and systemic inflammatory and neo-fibrogenetic activity. Over time, patients with unresolving ARDS had persistent and exaggerated elevation in plasma and bronchoalveolar lavage (BAL) levels of TNF-α, IL-1β, IL-6, IL-8 [65-68], soluble intercellular adhesion molecule-1 (sICAM-1) [67], and procollagen aminoterminal propeptide type I (PINP) and type III (PIIINP) [69]. During the 1st week of ARDS, pro-inflammatory cytokine levels declined in all survivors, while levels remained persistently elevated in all non-survivors. Recent data from our group indicate that cytokine levels reflected true biological activity [70]. Furthermore, histological findings of open lung biopsies obtained in patients with unresolving ARDS (day 15±7 of mechanical ventilation) provided morphological evidence of persistent activation of the HIR. Histological findings in previously spared pulmonary lobules included new injury to the endothelial and epithelial surfaces, with associated intravascular coagulation and extravascular fibrin deposition [9, 10]. Histological findings in previously involved pulmonary lobules included progressive fibroproliferative obliteration with transformation of the initially fibrinous exudate into myxoid connective tissue matrix and eventually into dense acellular fibrous tissue [9, 10]. Histological differences between survivors and non-survivors placed advanced pulmonary fibrosis with acellular fibrosis and loss of alveolar architecture at the upper boundary of disease reversibility [9].

GC treatment of unresolving ARDS

In a prospective, randomized, double-blind, placebo-controlled trial we evaluate the efficacy of prolonged MP treatment in patients with unresolving ARDS [71]. MP or placebo was given daily as intravenous push every 6 h (one-quarter of the daily dose) and changed to a single per os dose when oral intake was restored. The MP dosage regimen is shown in Table 3. If the patient was

Table 3 Methylprednisolone treatment in unresolving ARDS

Loading dose	2 mg/kg IV bolus followed by:		
Days 1-14	2 mg/kg/day as	0.5 mg/kg	IV push every 6 h
Days 15-21	1 mg/kg/day as	0.25 mg/kg	IV push every 6 h
Days 22-28[a]	0.5 mg/kg/day as	0.125 mg/kg	IV push every 6 h

[a] From days 29 to 32, methylprednisolone was given in a single per os dose of 0.25 mg/kg per day for 2 days and 0.125 mg/kg per day for 2 days

extubated prior to day 14, treatment was advanced to day 15 of drug therapy and tapered according to schedule [71]. The protocol contained (1) a provision for blindly crossing over patients who did not improve LIS by at least 1 point after 10 days of treatment and (2) procedures for infection surveillance, including weekly bronchoscopy with bilateral BAL [71]. Because MP blunts the febrile response to an infection, this latter intervention was essential for minimizing the random variation generated by the potential morbidity and mortality of untreated nosocomial infections. The study was designed as a sequential phase III clinical trial and projected to recruit 100 patients. The decision to end the trial was made when the test statistic exceeded the upper boundary of the triangular test of Whitehead, and the null hypothesis was rejected at a significance less than 0.05 and a power greater than 0.95.

The two groups were similar at study entry. By study day 10, all patients in the MP group improved (> 1 point reduction in LIS) versus 2 of 8 (25%) in the placebo group. Intensive care unit and hospital-associated mortality were significantly reduced: 0% versus 62% ($P=0.002$) and 12% versus 62% ($P=0.03$), respectively. The small number of patients may have biased the estimate of the treatment effect. The rate of complications between the two groups was similar. During MP treatment, pneumonia frequently developed in patients without fever (44%). Therefore, infection surveillance, including weekly bilateral bronchoscopic BAL, was useful for early detection of pneumonia and other serious infections. None of the recognized and appropriately treated infections developing during MP therapy affected resolution of ARDS or clinical outcome.

The therapeutic anti-inflammatory and anti-fibrotic efficacy of prolonged MP was assessed with serial measurements of HIR biomarkers. MP was associated with a rapid and sustained reduction in mean plasma and BAL TNF-α, IL-1β, IL-6, IL-8, sICAM-1, IL-1 receptor antagonist (IL-1ra), soluble TNF receptor 1 and 2 (sTNFR1 and sTNFR2), procollagen aminoterminal propeptide type I and III (PINP, and PIIINP), and with increases in IL-10 and in anti-inflammatory to pro-inflammatory cytokines ratios (IL-1ra/IL-1β, IL-10/TNF-α, IL-10/IL-1β) [68, 69, 72]. Placebo administration was not associated with reductions in HIR biomarkers. We believe that failure of older trials investigating massive doses of MP in early ARDS (Table 2) was attributable to the short duration of administration and not to timing of administration.

Evidence of inflammation-associated GC inadequacy/resistance in unresolving ARDS

Using an ex vivo model of systemic inflammation in ARDS we investigated intracellular upstream and downstream events associated with DNA binding of NF-κB and GRa in the paripheral blood lymphocytes (PBLs) (naïve cells) obtained from a healthy volunteer (laboratory work conducted by Dr. Frankie Stentz) [73]. PBLs were incubated for 3 h with 98 plasma samples obtained longitudinally from 17 patients with ARDS before and after randomization to either placebo ($n=6$) or MP ($n=11$). The cells were processed for fractionation into cytosolic and nuclear components, RNA extraction, and intracellular labelling. The primary objectives of these studies were to quantify the relationships among circulating levels of inflammatory cytokines TNF-α and IL-1β

and HPA axis hormones (ACTH and cortisol), and intracellular activities mediated by NF-κB (NF-κB κb-binding and transcription of TNF-α and IL-1β) and GRα (GRα binding to NF-kB, GRa binding to GRE DNA, stimulation of inhibitory protein IκBα, and stimulation of IL-10 transcription).

In the observation period prior to randomization, the biological and physiological characteristics of the MP and placebo groups were similar. Patients had persistent elevations in plasma levels of inflammatory (TNF-α, IL-1β, and IL-6) cytokines and HPA-axis (ACTH and cortisol) hormones, and similar severity of organ dysfunction scores. In PBLs exposed to patients' plasma, GRa-mediated activities were essentially unchanged over time, while NF-κB κb binding and transcription of TNF-α and IL-1β progressively increased. We hypothesized that inadequate secretion of cortisol and/or immune tissue resistance to endogenous GCs might explain the observed failure of activated GR to suppress inflammation (progressive increase in NF-kB-mediated activities) in the presence of persistently elevated ACTH and cortisol levels.

Patients treated with MP had rapid, progressive and sustained reductions in plasma TNF-α, IL-1β, IL-6, ACTH and cortisol levels over time. These were associated with parallel improvements in pulmonary and extrapulmonary organ dysfunction scores (previously reported in reference [71]). Normal PBLs exposed to plasma samples collected during MP versus placebo treatment also exhibited rapid, progressive significant increases in GRα-mediated activities (GRα binding to NF-κB, GRα binding to GRE DNA, stimulation of inhibitory protein IκBα, and stimulation of IL-10 transcription), and significant reductions in NF-κB κb binding and transcription of TNF-α and IL-1β. With MP, the intracellular relationships between the NF-kB and GRa signalling pathways changed from an initial NF-κB-driven and GR-resistant state to a GR-driven and GR-sensitive one.

We interpret the responses observed during MP treatment to support the concept of inflammation-dependent *acquired* GC resistance in patients with unresolving ARDS. Our findings also underscore the central role played by activated GRα in regulating inflammation and provide strong mechanistic evidence for the efficacy of prolonged MP treatment in unresolving ARDS

Acknowledgments

The authors recognize the assistance of Gail Spake in the preparation of the manuscript. This work was supported by the Baptist Memorial Health Care Foundation and the Assisi Foundation of Memphis.

References

1. Meduri GU (1996) The role of the host defence response in the progression and outcome of ARDS: pathophysiological correlations and response to glucocorticoid treatment. Eur Respir J 9:2650-2670

2. Cotran RS, Kumar V, Robbins SL (1994) Cellular injury and cellular death. In: Cotran RS, Kumar V, Robbins SL (eds) Pathologic basis of disease, 5 edn. Saunders, Philadelphia, pp 1-34

3. Katzenstein AL, Bloor CM, Leibow AA (1976) Diffuse alveolar damage – the role of oxygen, shock, and related factors. A review. Am J Pathol 85:209-228

4. Hudson LD, Milberg JA, Anardi D, et al (1995) Clinical risks for development of the acute respiratory distress syndrome. Am J Respir Crit Care Med 151:293-301

5. Steinberg KP, Hudson LD (2000) Acute lung injury and acute respiratory distress syndrome. The clinical syndrome. Clin Chest Med 21:401-417

6. Krafft P, Fridrich P, Pernerstorfer T, et al (1996) The acute respiratory distress syndrome: definitions, severity and clinical outcome. An analysis of 101 clinical investigations. Intensive Care Med 22:519-529

7. Sloane PJ, Gee MH, Gottlieb JE, et al (1992) A multicenter registry of patients with acute respiratory distress syndrome. Physiology and outcome. Am Rev Respir Dis 146:419-426

8. McKay LI, Cidlowski JA (1999) Molecular control of immune/inflammatory responses: interactions between nuclear factor-kappa B and steroid receptor-signaling pathways. Endocr Rev 20:435-459

9. Meduri GU, Chinn AJ, Leeper KV, et al (1994) Corticosteroid rescue treatment of progressive fibroproliferation in late ARDS. Patterns of response and predictors of outcome. Chest 105:1516--1527

10. Meduri GU, Eltorky M, Winer-Muram HT (1995) The fibroproliferative phase of late adult respiratory distress syndrome. Semin Respir Infect 10:154-175

11. Murray JF, Matthay MA, Luce JM, et al (1988) An expanded definition of the adult respiratory distress syndrome. Am Rev Respir Dis 138:720-723

12. Bone RC, Maunder R, Slotman G, et al (1989) An early test of survival in patients with the adult respiratory distress syndrome. The PaO2/FIo2 ratio and its differential response to conventional therapy. Prostaglandin E1 Study Group. Chest 96:849-851

13. Bernard GR, Luce JM, Sprung CL, et al (1987) High-dose corticosteroids in patients with the adult respiratory distress syndrome. N Engl J Med 317:1565-1570

14. Meduri GU (1997) Host defense response and outcome in ARDS. Chest 112:1154-1158

15. Headley AS, Tolley E, Meduri GU (1997) Infections and the inflammatory response in acute respiratory distress syndrome. Chest 111:1306-1321

16. Brower RG, Ware LB, Berthiaume Y, et al (2001) Treatment of ards. Chest 120:1347-1367

17. Lefering R, Neugebauer EA (1995) Steroid controversy in sepsis and septic shock: a meta-analysis. Crit Care Med 23:1294-1303

18. Cronin L, Cook DJ, Carlet J, et al (1995) Corticosteroid treatment for sepsis: a critical appraisal and meta- analysis of the literature. Crit Care Med 23:1430-1439

19. Meduri GU (1999) An historical review of glucocorticoid treatment in Sepsis. Disease pathophysiology and the design of treatment investigation. Sepsis 3:21-38

20. Ashbaugh DG, Maier RV (1985) Idiopathic pulmonary fibrosis in adult respiratory distress syndrome. Diagnosis and treatment. Arch Surg 120:530-535

21. Hooper RG, Kearl RA (1990) Established ARDS treated with a sustained course of adrenocortical steroids. Chest 97:138-143

22. Shanley TP, Wong HR (2001) Signal transduction pathways in acute lung injury: NF-kB and AP-1. In: Wong HR, Shanley TP (eds) Molecular biology of acute lung injury Kluwer, Boston, pp 1-16

23. Ross SD, Kron IL, Gangemi JJ, et al (2000) Attenuation of lung reperfusion injury after transplantation using an inhibitor of nuclear factor-kappaB. Am J Physiol Lung Cell Mol Physiol 279:L528-L536

24. Lentsch AB, Czermak BJ, Bless NM, et al (1999) Essential role of alveolar macrophages in intrapulmonary activation of NF-kappaB. Am J Respir Cell Mol Biol 20:692-698
25. Christman JW, Sadikot RT, Blackwell TS (2000) The role of nuclear factor-kappa B in pulmonary diseases. Chest 117:1482-1487
26. Karin M, Ben-Neriah Y (2000) Phosphorylation meets ubiquitination: the control of NF-[kappa]B activity. Annu Rev Immunol 18:621-663
27. Baeuerle PA, Baltimore D (1996) NF-kappa B: ten years after. Cell 87:13-20
28. Yamamoto Y, Gaynor RB (2001) Therapeutic potential of inhibition of the NF-kappaB pathway in the treatment of inflammation and cancer. J Clin Invest 107:135-142
29. Barnes PJ, Karin M (1997) Nuclear factor-kappa B: a pivotal transcription factor in chronic inflammatory diseases. N Engl J Med 336:1066-1071
30. Stein B, Baldwin AS Jr, Ballard DW, et al (1993) Cross-coupling of the NF-kappa B p65 and Fos/Jun transcription factors produces potentiated biological function. EMBO J 12:3879-3891
31. Perlstein RS, Whitnall MH, Abrams JS, et al (1993) Synergistic roles of interleukin-6, interleukin-1, and tumor necrosis factor in the adrenocorticotropin response to bacterial lipopolysaccharide in vivo. Endocrinology 132:946-952
32. Hermus AR, Sweep CG (1990) Cytokines and the hypothalamic-pituitary-adrenal axis. J Steroid Biochem Mol Biol 37:867-871
33. Bamberger CM, Schulte HM, Chrousos GP (1996) Molecular determinants of glucocorticoid receptor function and tissue sensitivity to glucocorticoids. Endocr Rev 17:245-261
34. Didonato JA, Saatcioglu F, Karin M (1996) Molecular mechanisms of immunosuppression and anti-inflammatory activities by glucocorticoids. Am J Respir Crit Care Med 154:S11-S15
35. Scheinman RI, Cogswell PC, Lofquist AK, et al (1995) Role of transcriptional activation of I kappa B alpha in mediation of immunosuppression by glucocorticoids. Science 270:283-286
36. Wissink S, Heerde EC van, Burg B van der, et al (1998) A dual mechanism mediates repression of NF-kappa B activity by glucocorticoids. Mol Endocrinol 12:355-363
37. Wang P, Wu P, Siegel MI, et al (1995) Interleukin (IL)-10 inhibits nuclear factor kappa B (NF kappa B) activation in human monocytes. IL-10 and IL-4 suppress cytokine synthesis by different mechanisms. J Biol Chem 270:9558-9563
38. Lentsch AB, Shanley TP, Sarma V, et al (1997) In vivo suppression of NF-kappa B and preservation of I kappa B alpha by interleukin-10 and interleukin-13. J Clin Invest 100:2443-2448
39. Shames BD, Selzman CH, Meldrum DR, et al (1998) Interleukin-10 stabilizes inhibitory kappaB-alpha in human monocytes. Shock 10:389-394
40. Hoffman SL, Punjabi NH, Kumala S, et al (1984) Reduction of mortality in chloramphenicol-treated severe typhoid fever by high-dose dexamethasone. N Engl J Med 310:82-88
41. Poppers DM, Schwenger P, Vilcek J (2000) Persistent tumor necrosis factor signaling in normal human fibroblasts prevents the complete resynthesis of I kappa B-alpha. J Biol Chem 275:29587--29593
42. Sheppard KA, Phelps KM, Williams AJ, et al (1998) Nuclear integration of glucocorticoid receptor and nuclear factor- kappaB signaling by CREB-binding protein and steroid receptor coactivator-1. J Biol Chem 273:29291-29294
43. Bamberger CM, Bamberger AM, Castro M de, et al (1995) Glucocorticoid receptor beta, a potential endogenous inhibitor of glucocorticoid action in humans. J Clin Invest 95:2435-2441
44. Chrousos GP (1995) The hypothalamic-pituitary-adrenal axis and immune-mediated inflammation. N Engl J Med 332:1351-1362
45. Melby JC, Spink WW (1958) Comparative studies on adrenalcortical function and cortisol metabolism in healthy adults and in patients with shock due to infection. J Clin Invest 37:1791--1798
46. Reincke M, Allolio B, Wurth G, et al (1993) The hypothalamic-pituitary-adrenal axis in critical illness: response to dexamethasone and corticotropin-releasing hormone. J Clin Endocrinol Metab 77:151-156

47. Briegel J, Forst H, Hellinger H, et al (1991) Contribution of cortisol deficiency to septic shock. Lancet 338:507-508

48. Annane D, Sebille V, Troche G, et al (2000) A 3-level prognostic classification in septic shock based on cortisol levels and cortisol response to corticotropin. JAMA 283:1038-1045

49. Meduri GU, Chrousos GP (1998) Duration of glucocorticoid treatment and outcome in sepsis: is the right drug used the wrong way? Chest 114:355-360

50. Kass EH, Finland M (1957) Adrenocortical hormones and the management of infection. Annu Rev Med 8:1-18

51. Chrousos GP, Detera-Wadleigh SD, Karl M (1993) Syndromes of glucocorticoid resistance. Ann Intern Med 119:1113-1124

52. Lamberts SW, Koper JW, Biemond P, et al (1992) Cortisol receptor resistance: the variability of its clinical presentation and response to treatment. J Clin Endocrinol Metab 74:313-321

53. Lane SJ, Lee TH (1991) Glucocorticoid receptor characteristics in monocytes of patients with corticosteroid-resistant bronchial asthma. Am Rev Respir Dis 143:1020-1024

54. Sher ER, Leung DY, Surs W, et al (1994) Steroid-resistant asthma. Cellular mechanisms contributing to inadequate response to glucocorticoid therapy. J Clin Invest 93:33-39

55. Adcock IM, Lane SJ, Brown CR, et al (1995) Differences in binding of glucocorticoid receptor to DNA in steroid-resistant asthma. J Immunol 154:3500-3505

56. Barnes PJ, Greening AP, Crompton GK (1995) Glucocorticoid resistance in asthma. Am J Respir Crit Care Med 152:S125-140

57. Norbiato G, Bevilacqua M, Vago T, et al (1992) Cortisol resistance in acquired immunodeficiency syndrome. J Clin Endocrinol Metab 74:608-613

58. Molijn GJ, Spek JJ, Uffelen JC van, et al (1995) Differential adaptation of glucocorticoid sensitivity of peripheral blood mononuclear leukocytes in patients with sepsis or septic shock. J Clin Endocrinol Metab 80:1799-1803

59. Almawi WY, Lipman ML, Stevens AC, et al (1991) Abrogation of glucocorticoid-mediated inhibition of T cell proliferation by the synergistic action of IL-1, IL-6, and IFN-gamma. J Immunol 146:3523-3527

60. Kam JC, Szefler SJ, Surs W, et al (1993) Combination IL-2 and IL-4 reduces glucocorticoid receptor-binding affinity and T cell response to glucocorticoids. J Immunol 151:3460-3466

61. Spahn JD, Szefler SJ, Surs W, et al (1996) A novel action of IL-13: induction of diminished monocyte glucocorticoid receptor-binding affinity. J Immunol 157:2654-2659

62. Liu LY, Sun B, Tian Y, et al (1993) Changes of pulmonary glucocorticoid receptor and phospholipase A_2 in sheep with acute lung injury after high dose endotoxin infusion. Am Rev Respir Dis 148:878-881

63. Fan J, Gong XQ, Wu J, et al (1994) Effect of glucocorticoid receptor (GR) blockade on endotoxemia in rats. Circ Shock 42:76-82

64. Baeuerle PA, Baichwal VR (1997) NF-kappa B as a frequent target for immunosuppressive and anti- inflammatory molecules. Adv Immunol 65:111-137

65. Meduri GU, Headley S, Kohler G, et al (1995) Persistent elevation of inflammatory cytokines predicts a poor outcome in ARDS. Plasma IL-1 beta and IL-6 levels are consistent and efficient predictors of outcome over time. Chest 107:1062-1073

66. Meduri GU, Kohler G, Headley S, et al (1995) Inflammatory cytokines in the BAL of patients with ARDS. Persistent elevation over time predicts poor outcome. Chest 108:1303-1314

67. Golden E, John B, Stentz F, et al (2000) Interleukin-8 and soluble intercellular adhesion molecule-1 during acute respiratory distress syndrome and in response to prolonged methylprednisolone treatment (abstract). Shock 13:42S

68. Headley AS, Meduri GU, Tolley E, et al (2000) Infections, SIRS, and CARS during ARDS and in response to prolonged glucocorticoid treatment (Abstract). Am J Respir Crit Care Med 161:A378

69. Meduri GU, Tolley EA, Chinn A, et al (1998) Procollagen types I and III aminoterminal propeptide levels during acute respiratory distress syndrome and in response to methylprednisolone treatment. Am J Respir Crit Care Med 158:1432-1441

70. Carratu P, Quasney MW, Stentz FB, et al (2002) TNF-a and LT-a gene polymorphism in acute respiratory distress syndrome (ARDS) (abstract). Am J Respir Crit Care Med 165: A474
71. Meduri GU, Headley S, Carson S, et al (1998) Prolonged methylprednisolone treatment improves lung function and outcome of unresolving ARDS. A randomized, double-blind, placebo-controlled trial. JAMA 280:159-165
72. Meduri GU, Tolley EA, Chrousos GP, et al (2002) Prolonged methylprednisolone treatment suppresses systemic inflammation in patients with unresolving acute respiratory distress syndrome. Evidence for inadequate endogenous glucocorticoid secretion and inflammation-induced immune cell resistance to glucocorticoids. Am J Respir Crit Care Med 165:983-991
73. Stentz F, Tolley EA, Headley AS, et al (2001) Mechanisms of NF-kB and glucocorticoid receptor (GRa) in activation and regulation of systemic inflammation (SI) in ARDS (abstract). Am J Respir Crit Care Med 163:A450

Effects of nitric oxide on haemodynamics and gas exchange in acute respiratory distress syndrome

K. Lewandowski, M. Lewandowski, K.J. Falke

Acute respiratory distress syndrome (ARDS) is characterized by an insult to the alveolar-capillary membrane that results in increased permeability and subsequent interstitial and – to a lesser degree – alveolar oedema. The hallmarks of the diagnosis of the syndrome include (1) a risk factor for the development of ARDS (pneumonia, sepsis, trauma, pancreatitis or a variety of other insults and illnesses), (2) severe hypoxaemia, even if the lungs are ventilated with a high fraction of inspired oxygen, (3) markedly elevated pulmonary artery pressure, (4) decreased pulmonary compliance, (5) bilateral pulmonary infiltrates on chest radiograph, and (6) all these features appear in a setting in which cardiogenic pulmonary oedema has been excluded.

Since its first description in 1968, no causal therapy of ARDS has been found, medical treatment has been limited to symptomatic therapeutic measures, mainly aimed at the restoration of a sufficient gas exchange to tide the patient over the acute phase of the syndrome. This, however, is a real challenge in severe ARDS, where partial pressure of arterial oxygen (PaO_2) levels below 50 mmHg during mechanical ventilation with positive end-expiratory pressure (PEEP) and a fraction of inspired oxygen (FiO_2) of 1.0 are no rarity. For years, there was no alternative to the extracorporeal membrane oxygenation (ECMO) to improve the severely impaired gas exchange in this situation.

In 1987 Ignarro et al. [1] discovered that nitric oxide (NO) was an important endothelium-derived relaxing factor of vascular smooth muscle. The vasodilating features of NO prompted researchers to study this gaseous agent in diseases where pulmonary vasodilation was impaired. In an animal model, inhaled NO had impressive effects on gas exchange and pulmonary hypertension [2]. Inhaled NO reduced the mean pulmonary artery pressure significantly and improved gas exchange markedly. With no further delay, these beneficial effects of inhaled NO where studied in patients with ARDS.

This essay seeks to outline the role of NO in combating pulmonary hypertension, hypoxaemia, and right ventricular dysfunction, and to give a concise overview of the current state of the art.

Systemic vasodilators

ARDS is characterized by a sudden, mostly generalized, inflammation of the lung, which, as it proceeds, induces noncardiogenic pulmonary oedema, pulmonary artery hypertension, reduction of total compliance of the lung, and progressive systemic hypoxaemia due to pulmonary ventilation/perfusion mismatching associated with increased intrapulmonary right-to-left shunt areas [3]. Pulmonary arterial hypertension is the result of a combination of three major factors: vascular obstruction, obliteration, and vasoconstriction. The vasoconstrictive element in ARDS may represent a basic alteration of pulmonary vasoreactivity. Treatment of the pulmonary arterial hypertension as a main contributor to the impaired gas exchange was tried for quite a while. Inhalational anaesthetics, intravenous nitrates, nitroprusside, calcium-channel blockers, or bronchodilators are able to impact on hypoxic vasodilation; however, they act nonselectively upon the pulmonary and systemic circulation. Simultaneous dilatation of pulmonary and systemic vessels increases cardiac output and intrapulmonary right-to-left shunt, hence, restricting hypoxic pulmonary vasoconstriction may produce a maldistribution of ventilation relative to perfusion and a further deterioration in oxygenation. Therefore, none of these agents has gained major clinical importance.

In search of a selective pulmonary vasodilator

The shortcomings of the intravenously applied, nonselectively effective vasodilators made the researchers look for a selective vasodilator acting exclusively upon the pulmonary circulation. The gas NO, administered by inhalation, turned out to be an "ideal", selectively acting, pulmonary vasodilatator. NO is able to reverse an acute pulmonary vasoconstriction in a moment, without affecting systemic vascular resistance, cardiac output, left atrial pressure, or central venous pressure.

The characterization of NO synthesis and its physiological pathways has been elucidated, and this was recently honoured by the Nobel prize. Endogenous NO is synthesized in endothelial cells by the enzyme NO synthase. NO diffuses into the vascular smooth muscle cells and convert the inactive soluble enzyme guanylate cyclase into its active form, inducing synthesis of cyclic guanosine monophosphate from guanosine triphosphate. Cyclic guanosine monophosphate finally initiates vasodilation (Fig.1).

Inhaled NO, directly diffuses from the ventilated alveoli into the vascular smooth muscle cell and there exerts the vasodilative effect. The gas NO, applied by inhalation, exclusively reaches ventilated pulmonary areas and achieves an increase of perfusion in these areas only. It can also be assumed that blood flow is being redistributed from non-aerated, atelectatic areas to ventilated lung regions. A systemic vasodilation is excluded, because NO binds to haemoglobin within seconds after diffusion into the intravascular lumen, and is inactivated by this mechanism. Hence, NO acts selectively in a twin sense: (1) it acts selectively in the pulmonary circulation and (2) it is active only in aerated lung areas, where it increases perfusion. The overall effect is an improvement of the ventilation/perfusion mismatching. It should, however, be mentioned that an overdose of NO may cause a "spill over" phenomenon, i.e., the gas may diffuse into the vasculature of unventilated lung regions. Pulmonary vasodilation in these regions may further lower pulmonary artery pressure but induce an unwanted decrease in PaO_2.

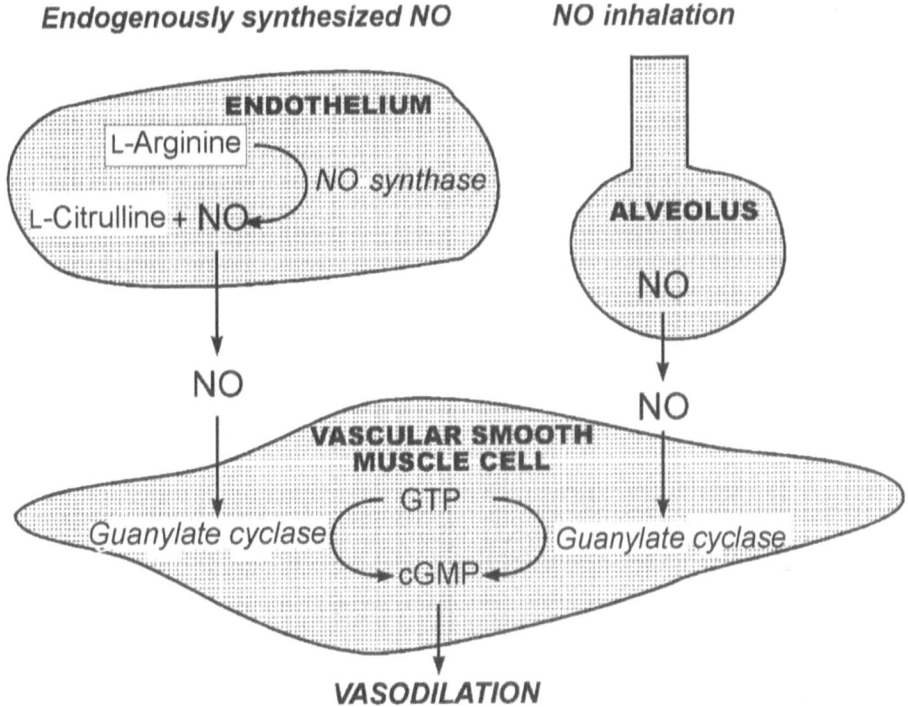

Fig. 1 Physiological pathway of nitric oxide (NO)

Inhalation of NO improves gas exchange

Inhalation of NO was first studied in animal models. Frostell et al. [2] have shown in awake, spontaneously breathing lambs that inhalation of NO in doses of more than 40 parts per million (ppm) reversed acute pulmonary vasoconstriction within 3 min. The pulmonary vascular resistance, the systemic vascular resistance, cardiac output, left atrial and central venous pressures were unaltered by NO inhalation. No significant adverse effects were reported.

Falke et al. [4] were the first who tried NO inhalation in a patient with severe ARDS. They compared the short-term effects of inhaled NO with intravenous prostacyclin (PGI_2). The inhaled selective pulmonary vasodilator lowered pulmonary hypertension and improved right ventricular ejection fraction, as did intravenous PGI_2. But, in contrast to intravenous PGI_2, NO increased PaO_2 and decreased intrapulmonary right-to-left shunt (Fig. 2).

The impressive results of this experiment prompted Rossaint et al. [5] to investigate a series of nine consecutive patients with severe ARDS who inhaled NO at two concentrations for 40 min each. Inhalation of NO in a concentration of 18 ppm significantly reduced the mean pulmonary artery pressure from 37 mmHg to 30 mmHg and decreased Q_S/Q_T from 36% to 31%. The PaO_2/FiO_2

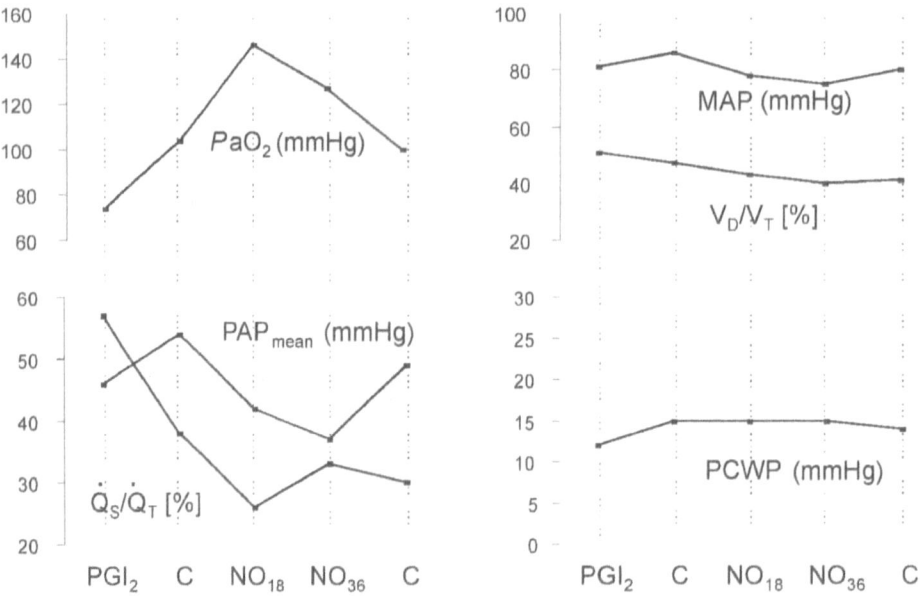

Fig. 2 First inhalation of NO in an ARDS patient (*PGI2* IV prostacyclin, *NO18* 18 ppm NO, *NO36* 36 ppm NO, *C* control, *PAPmean* mean pulmonary artery pressure, *MAP* mean arterial pressure, *VD/VT* deadspace, *PCWP* pulmonary occlusion pressure, *Qs/QT* intrapulmonary right-to-left shunt)

ratio increased during NO administration from 152 mmHg to 199 mmHg. Mean arterial pressure and cardiac output remained unchanged. The results demonstrated the potential of inhaled NO to enable a selectively improved perfusion of ventilated pulmonary areas, making it possible to significantly improve oxygenation, thus lowering ventilatory pressure and oxygen concentrations to less dangerous levels. This report initiated the clinical use of inhaled NO in ARDS, and, subsequently, there were numerous observational studies revealing beneficial effects in ARDS patients.

Bigatello et al. [6] published results of short-term and long-term application of inhaled NO in 13 ARDS patients. Inhalation of NO in concentrations of 2-40 ppm reduced mean pulmonary artery pressure markedly and improved oxygenation. The systemic circulation remained unaffected. Long-term use of inhaled NO (up to 27 days) did not exert tachyphylactic effects. Benzing et al. [7] studied the effects of inhaled NO and transvascular albumin flux in nine patients with acute lung injury using a double-radioisotope technique. The authors reported that short-term inhalation of NO induced a decrease in pulmonary artery pressure and reduced transvascular albumin flux. Further investigations showed that NO inhalation reduced pulmonary artery hypertension, unloaded the right ventricle, and improved right ventricular ejection fraction in ARDS patients [8].

Finding the correct dosage

As there remains concern about toxic effects of NO, it is crucial to apply the lowest possible dose to achieve the desired effect. Gerlach et al. [9] have shown that in ARDS patients effective doses for improvement of oxygenation can be low, i.e., ED_{50} was about 100 parts per billion (ppb). The median effective dose (ED_{50}) for reduction of mean pulmonary artery pressure was 2-3 ppm. Oxygenation improved at a much lower concentration than needed to decrease mean pulmonary artery pressure. These data also suggest that individual dose response curves are helpful to determine the dose for either improvement in oxygenation and/or decrease in mean pulmonary artery pressure in a given patient. In another study in three consecutive ARDS patients [10], the authors found that the lowest effective NO dose, i.e., the dose that increased PaO_2/FiO_2 ratio by 30%, was 60, 100, and 230 ppb. Changes in mean pulmonary artery pressure were not observed. The authors concluded that improvement in oxygenation by NO inhalation in ARDS does not necessarily require reduction of pulmonary vascular resistance (Fig. 3).

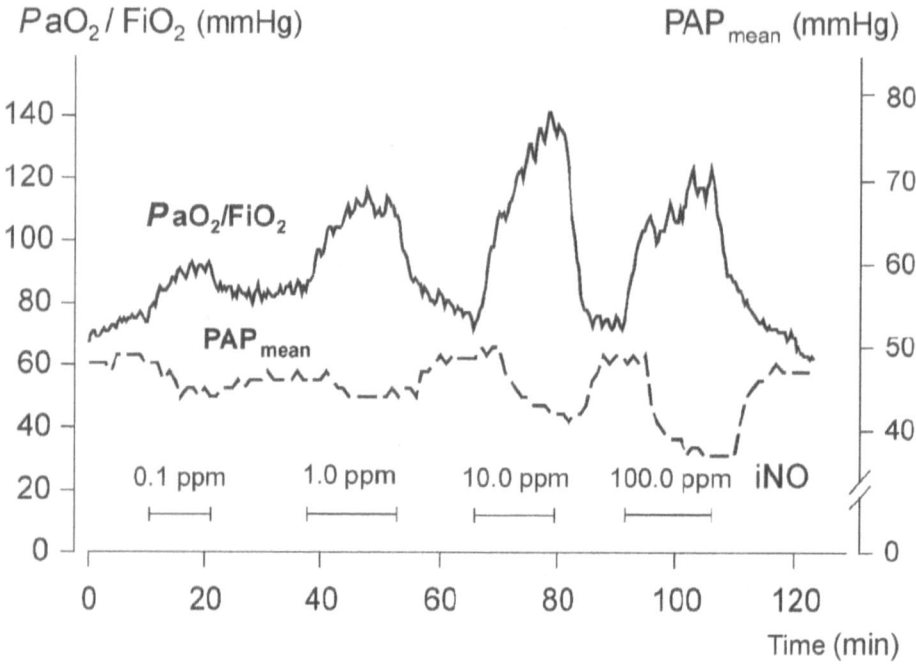

Fig. 3 Dose-response registration of NO inhalation (iNO). (Figure reprinted from [9] with permission)

Inhalation of NO does not improve outcome

Many studies have impressively shown that in a critical situation of ARDS inhaled NO has the potential to markedly improve oxygenation and lower high pulmonary arterial pressures. The question arises whether this potential effects the mortality rates of severe ARDS.

Two unblinded pilot randomized controlled studies of single ARDS treatment centres compared NO inhalation therapy with standard treatment. Both studies reported only temporary improvements in arterial oxygenation. Inhaled NO did not affect the mortality rates [11, 12]. Two large-scale randomized controlled trials followed the pilot studies and, disappointingly, confirmed the results.

Dellinger et al. [13] presented the results of the United States randomized double-blind placebo-controlled phase II trial. The aim of this study was to assess safety issues and physiological effects of various inhaled NO doses; it was not primarily designed to detect a statistical difference in outcome parameters. A total number of 177 patients, fulfilling criteria of early ARDS in accordance with the American European Consensus Conference criteria [14] for less than 72 h prior to randomization, were enrolled in 30 hospitals. Patients with sepsis, severe burns of larger surface area, persistent hypotension, and multi-system organ dysfunction were excluded, because these are conditions in which mortality and duration of mechanical ventilation are unlikely to be altered by an improvement in lung function alone. Patients were randomized to either receive inhaled NO at concentrations of 1.25, 5, 20, 40, or 80 ppm (n=120), or to receive placebo gas (n=57). In the treatment group, 60% of the patients responded with a marked improvement of PaO_2/FiO_2, which, however, only lasted during the first 24 h of treatment. The same accounted for changes in pulmonary artery pressure. Overall, the patients treated with inhaled NO, when compared with controls, did not show differences in the days alive and off mechanical ventilation.

Lundin et al. [15] presented the results of the prospective unblinded randomized European multicentre trial on inhaled NO in acute lung injury. The authors studied 286 patients with acute lung injury, who initially received NO in doses of 2,10, and 40 ppm for 10 min. Only the 66% responders to NO were randomized to either inhale NO or to be treated conventionally for 30 days. Reversal of acute lung injury was reported in 61% of patients receiving NO and in 54% of controls, the difference being not significant. Inhaled NO, however, significantly reduced the frequency of severe respiratory failure (2.2% NO, 10.3% control). Additionally, renal failure was found to be a possible adverse effect of NO inhalation. Thirty-day mortality rate was not different between groups.

Enhancement of NO effects

Some studies evaluated possible additive beneficial effects of NO. The question whether a combination of inhaled NO with PEEP is of advantage was addressed by Puybasset et al. [16]. The authors studied 21 ARDS patients who received moderate PEEP levels. Only the patients in whom PEEP induced alveolar recruitment showed an improvement in PaO_2 when exposed to inhaled NO. A study by Okamoto et al. [17] also reported synergistic effects of inhaled NO and PEEP. Papazian et al. [18] found an additive effect of inhaled NO and prone positioning on PaO_2 and right-to-left shunt. This finding was confirmed by other studies. Recruitment of lung tissue by application of surfactant or partial liquid ventilation and inhalation of NO has also been studied in animal models of acute lung injury. The results suggested that recruiting lung tissue might augment the effect of inhaled NO.

In 1993 Payen et al. [19] were the first to combine inhalation of NO with intravenous almitrine, a substance initially developed to improve pulmonary gas exchange in chronic obstructive pulmonary disease by an increase of ventilatory drive. Furthermore, almitrine is a selective pulmonary vasoconstrictor that reduces intrapulmonary right-to-left-shunt by enhancing the hypoxic pulmonary vasoconstriction. Co-administration of inhaled NO and intravenous almitrine induced an additive improvement of gas exchange while pulmonary artery pressure was reduced. There are also hints that the effects of inhaled NO plus almitrine can be further intensified by addition of prone positioning [20].

Toxicology and side effects

The first studies on inhaled NO did not report any side effects; however, further studies on larger patient collectives noted quite a number of unwanted effects. Inhaled NO inhibits the thrombocyte aggregation and prolongs the bleeding time. In ARDS patients treated with inhaled NO in concentrations of 3 - 100 ppm, a prolongation of the in vitro ivy bleeding time was observed, but the in vivo bleeding time was unchanged. The effects of inhaled NO on the bleeding time are not dose dependent for 0-40 ppm [21]. In ARDS patients, effects on thrombocyte aggregation are always detectable with NO. We do not have enough data yet to give a recommendation on the avoidance of bleeding complications, nevertheless the present data emphasize caution.

The other side effects of NO are strongly linked to the toxicity of the substance. NO easily binds to haemoglobin, which may result in a methaemoglobinaemia, which can reach clinical relevance. Consequently, it is necessary, to control the methaemoglobin levels during a long-term application of inhaled NO. Methaemoglobinaemia, however, is rare; in a meta-analysis Steudel et al. [22] reported 3 cases in 471 patients, only.

Other side effects of NO relate to its toxic by-products. Nitric oxide is a radical, freely diffusible gas, soluble in water and lipid. NO easily reacts with oxygen forming nitrogen dioxide (NO_2), a toxic gas. Inhalation of NO_2 in concentrations higher than 10 ppm may result in lung oedema, alveolar bleeding, and severe damage of the lung tissue. Such high NO_2 concentrations are not observed in usual NO therapies. A strict monitoring of NO_2, however, is mandatory during every NO treatment.

Even after termination of a NO inhalation, the physician should be prepared for side effects. After discontinuation of NO, the pulmonary artery pressure may rise markedly, intrapulmonary right-to-left shunt may increase, and PaO_2 may fall [5]. These rebound effects might be explained by suppression of the endogenous NO synthesis; however, animal experiments did not confirm the theory. Nevertheless, to avoid such rebound phenomena, a cautious reduction of the inhaled NO dose over a longer period is recommended.

Long-term damages to the lung were not reported in connection with NO therapy. Lung function tests, 8 months after NO treatment, showed similar results in the NO group and conventionally treated group. The European multicentre study on inhaled NO [15], however, noted a higher morbidity of renal failure in the NO group. There is still a lot of discussion of this finding and further investigation is needed.

Alternatives to NO

The selectivity of the NO effect is partly based on its inhalatory application. The inhalation of the pulmonary vasodilator affects only aerated lung tissue by improving perfusion in these areas. The idea that other vasodilators might be as effective as NO when given by inhalation prompted Walmrath et al. [23] to investigate the effect of aerosolized PGI_2 applied by inhalation. Similar to inhaled NO, PGI_2 significantly reduced pulmonary artery pressure and increased PaO_2. During inhalation, however, the selectivity of vasodilation is greatly dependent on the dose applied. High doses of PGI_2 seem to be absorbed into the blood where they exert systemic vasodilation that neutralizes the selective pulmonary effect. An advantage of NO is that its concentration can easily be controlled during therapy by chemiluminescence, the nebulized dose of PGI_2 has thus to be calculated. Doses as low as 10 ng/kg per min were reported to be effective in improving gas exchange in ARDS. However, we do not know enough about inhalation of PGI_2 in ARDS to give a general recommendation.

Conclusion

The introduction of NO into the therapy of ARDS has made it possible to treat one of the most-important pathophysiological features of the syndrome, the ventilation-perfusion mismatch of the diseased lung. NO, when applied via inhalation, selectively improves perfusion in aerated lung areas and recruits blood flow from the non-ventilated areas. Hereby it significantly improves gas exchange, lowers the high intrapulmonary right-to-left shunt and decreases the elevated pulmonary artery pressure. The effect of NO can be enhanced by application of PEEP, prone positioning, or other manoeuvres recruiting lung tissue. Disappointingly, NO has not shown its potential to affect the high mortality rate of ARDS. Important side effects of NO inhalation are the prolonged bleeding time and the methaemoglobinaemia. NO concentrations and NO_2, the toxic by-product of NO, have to be monitored during therapy. A promising alternative might be the aerosolized vasodilators; however, they are currently under evaluation. The future perspective of these innovative therapies will hinge upon cost and efficacy issues.

References

1. Ignarro LJ, Buga GM, Wood JS, et al (1987) Endothelium-derived relaxing factor produced and released from artery and vein is nitric oxide. Proc Natl Acad Sci U S A 84:9265-9269
2. Frostell C, Fratacci MD, Wain JC, et al (1991) Inhaled nitric oxide. A selective pulmonary vasodilator reversing hypoxic pulmonary vasoconstriction. Circulation 83:2038-2047
3. Zapol WJ, Snider MT (1977) Pulmonary hypertension in severe acute respiratory failure. N Engl J Med 296:476-480
4. Falke K, Rossaint R, Pison U, et al (1991) Inhaled nitric oxide selectively reduces pulmonary hypertension in severe ARDS and improves gas exchanges as well as right heart ejection fraction - a case report. Am Rev Respir Dis 143 [Suppl]:A248
5. Rossaint R, Falke KJ, Lopez F, et al (1993) Inhaled nitric oxide for the adult respiratory distress syndrome. N Engl J Med 328:399-405
6. Bigatello LM, Hurford WE, Kacmarek RM, et al (1994) Prolonged inhalation of low concentrations of nitric oxide in patients with severe adult respiratory distress syndrome. Effects on pulmonary hemodynamics and oxygenation. Anesthesiology 80:761-770
7. Benzing A, Brautigam P, Geiger K, et al (1995) Inhaled nitric oxide reduces pulmonary transvascular albumin flux in patients with acute lung injury. Anesthesiology 83:1153-1161
8. Putensen C, Hörmann C, Kleinsasser A, et al (1998) Cardiopulmonary effects of aerosolized prostaglandin E1 and nitric oxide inhalation in patients with acute respiratory distress syndrome. An J Respir Crit Care Med 157:1743-1747
9. Gerlach H, Rossaint R, Pappert D, et al (1993) Time-course and dose-response of nitric oxide inhalation for systemic oxygenation and pulmonary hypertension in patients with adult respiratory distress syndrome. Eur J Clin Invest 23:499-502
10. Gerlach H, Pappert D, Lewandowski K, et al (1993) Long-term inhalation with evaluated low doses of nitric oxide for selective improvement of oxygenation in patients with adult respiratory distress syndrome. Intensive Care Med 19:443-449
11. Troncy E, Collet JP, Shapiro S, et al (1998) Inhaled nitric oxide in acute respiratory distress syndrome: a pilot randomized controlled study. Am J Respir Crit Care Med 157:1483-1488
12. Michael JR, Barton RG, Saffle JR, et al (1998) Inhaled nitric oxide versus conventional therapy: effect on oxygenation in ARDS. Am J Respir Crit Care Med 157:1372-1380
13. Dellinger RP, Zimmerman JL, Taylor RW, et al (1998) Effects of inhaled nitric oxide in patients with acute respiratory distress syndrome: results of a randomized phase II trial. Crit Care Med 26:15-23
14. Bernard GR, Artigas A, Brigham KL, et al (1994) The American-European consensus conference on ARDS. Definitions, mechanisms, elevant outcomes, and clinical trial coordination. Am J Respir Crit Care Med 149:818-824
15. Lundin S, Mang H, Smithies M, et al (1999) Inhalation of nitric oxide in acute lung injury: results of a European multicentre study. Intensive Care Med 25:911-919
16. Puybasset L, Rouby JJ, Mourgeon E, et al (1995) Factors influencing cardiopulmonary effects of inhaled nitric oxide in acute respiratory failure. Am J Respir Crit Care Med 152:318-328
17. Okamoto K, Kukita I, Hamaguchi M, et al (2000) Combination of inhaled nitric oxide therapy and inverse ratio ventilation in patients with sepsis-associated acute respiratory distress syndrome. Artif Organs 24:902-908

18. Papazian L, Bregenon F, Gaillat F, et al (1998) Respective and combined effects of prone position and inhaled nitric oxide in patients with acute respiratory distress syndrome. Am J Respir Crit Care Med 157: 580-585
19. Payen DM, Gatecel C, Plaisance P (1993) Almitrine effect on nitric oxide inhalation in adult respiratory distress syndrome. Lancet 341:1664
20. Jolliet P, Bulpa P, Ritz M, et al (1997) Additive beneficial effects of the prone position, nitric oxide, and almitrine bismesylate on gas exchange and oxygen transport in acute respiratory distress syndrome. Crit Care Med 25:786-794
21. Gries A, Herr A, Motsch J, Holzmann A, et al (2000) Randomized, placebo-controlled, blinded and cross-matched study on the anti-platelet effect of inhaled nitric oxide in healthy volunteers. Thromb Haemost 83:309-315
22. Steudel W, Hurford WE, Zapol WM (1999) Inhaled nitric oxide. Basic biology and clinical applications. Anesthesiology 91:1090-1121
23. Walmrath D, Schneider T, Pilch J, et al (1993) Aerosolized prostacyclin in adult respiratory distress syndrome. Lancet 342:961-962

Lung function, dyspnoea, and exercise tolerance in stable chronic obstructive pulmonary disease patients

J. Milic-Emili, C. Tantucci

During the last 50 years, the correlation of exercise tolerance with routine pulmonary function testing in patients with chronic obstructive pulmonary disease (COPD) has been investigated in many studies. In almost all instances, the degree of airway obstruction was assessed in terms of FEV_1. Since, a weak correlation was found between exercise tolerance and FEV_1 (% predicted), it has been concluded that other factors than lung function impairment (e.g., deconditioning and peripheral muscle dysfunction) play a predominant role in limiting exercise capacity in COPD patients. Recent studies, however, have shown that in moderate to very severe COPD patients the inspiratory capacity, a marker of hyperinflation, is a better predictor of exercise tolerance than FEV_1 and forced vital capacity (FVC), suggesting that the main cause of exercise intolerance in these patients is dynamic pulmonary hyperinflation due to concurrent expiratory flow limitation (FL).

Dynamic hyperinflation

In normal individuals at rest, the end-expiratory lung volume (functional residual capacity, FRC), corresponds to the relaxation volume (Vr) of the respiratory system, i.e., the lung volume at which the elastic recoil pressure of the respiratory system is zero [1]. Pulmonary hyperinflation is defined as an increase in FRC above the predictable normal range, which may be due to increased Vr as a result of loss of lung recoil (e.g., emphysema) and/or to dynamic pulmonary hyperinflation, which is said to be present when the FRC exceeds Vr. Dynamic hyperinflation exists whenever the duration of expiration is insufficient to allow the lungs to deflate to Vr prior to the next inspiration. This may occur when expiratory flow is impeded (e.g., increased airway resistance) and/or expiratory time shortened (e.g., increased breathing frequency). Expiratory flow may also be reduced by other mechanisms, such as persistent contraction of the inspiratory muscles during expiration and expiratory narrowing of the glottal aperture. In COPD patients, dynamic hyperinflation is common and is due mainly to expiratory FL [2, 3].

Expiratory FL

FL should be used only for describing a condition in which flow cannot augment at a given lung volume. Thus, expiratory FL reflects the incapacity to increase expiratory flow by further increasing pleural and, therefore, alveolar pressure at that lung volume. It is exhibited by both normal subjects and patients with respiratory disorders during correctly performed maximal forced expiratory manoeuvres, in which, after peak expiratory flow, isovolumic expiratory flow rates cannot be increased by increasing expiratory effort and, thus, are maximal. In contrast, FL does not occur during tidal breathing in normal subjects in either the supine or sitting position. In respiratory disease, however, FL may be present during tidal breathing. Tidal FL is said to occur when expiratory flow rates are maximal under the prevailing conditions, either at rest or during exercise [2,3].

Pathophysiological factors

Several factors may contribute to the occurrence of tidal FL: airway obstruction, lung volume, expiratory flow rate, and body posture. Airway obstruction limits maximal expiratory flow rates, reducing expiratory flow reserve. Reduced FRC, as in gross obesity, restrictive disorders, congestive heart failure, etc., is usually associated with decreased expiratory flow reserve in the tidal breathing volume range. Increased ventilatory requirements augment the expiratory flows because of greater tidal volume and faster respiratory frequency, predisposing to tidal FL [3].

In the supine position, the Vr is lower than upright as a result of gravitational forces, and hence the end-expiratory lung volume (EELV) tends to decrease in recumbency. Since the maximal flow-volume curve shows little postural [4] variation, recumbency promotes FL because tidal breathing occurs at a lower lung volume at which the expiratory flow reserve is necessarily smaller [2].

Methods for assessing FL

Comparison between full (or partial) maximal and tidal flow-volume loops has been widely used in the past to detect FL, which is assumed to be present when tidal expiratory flow impinges on or exceeds the maximal expiratory flows at the same lung volume [5]. This method, however, is not reliable because of the different volume and time history of the lung and airways prior to the maximal and tidal expirations [3, 6].

Recently, the negative expiratory pressure (NEP) method has been introduced to detect FL [2, 7]. It consists of applying a small negative pressure during tidal expiration (usually between -3 and -5 cmH$_2$O), thus widening the pressure gradient between the alveoli and the airway opening. In the absence of FL, with NEP there is an increase in expiratory flow compared with the preceding control breath. In contrast, in the presence of FL the expiratory flow does not increase throughout the whole or part of the tidal expiration over that of the preceding control expiration. The NEP method, which has been validated using iso-volume flow-pressure curves [7], does not require cooperation from the subjects nor use of a plethysmograph, and is axiomatically devoid of problems caused by the different previous time and volume history of the lung between tidal and maximal expiration.

Dyspnoea and exercise limitation

Dyspnoea and exercise limitation are the predominant complaints of COPD patients, and are commonly the reason for seeking medical attention. However, routine assessment of lung function is in general focused almost entirely on FEV$_1$ and FVC, although there is ample evidence that in COPD patients these parameters correlate poorly with *both* dyspnoea and exercise tolerance [2]. In fact, in COPD it is hyperinflation that plays a central role in eliciting dyspnoea, exercise intolerance, and ventilatory failure [2, 3, 8]. Hyperinflation is commonly assessed through measurement of the FRC with body plethysmography, which is complex, expensive, and, in patients with severe airway obstruction, may lead to overestimation of the actual FRC because the transmission of alveolar pressure to the mouth during the panting manoeuvre is delayed by increased airway resistance [9]. However, in patients with airway obstruction, the increase of FRC is necessarily accompanied by a reduction in inspiratory capacity (IC). In contrast to FRC, measurement of IC is simple, cheap, and reliable. Thus, IC testing provides a useful marker for the indirect assessment of pulmonary hyperinflation. Indeed, in such patients a reduction of IC implies hyperinflation, with concurrent increase of dyspnoea [10, 11] and decreased exercise tolerance [3, 8, 12].

IC and exercise tolerance

Most normal subjects and endurance athletes do not exhibit tidal expiratory FL even during maximal exercise [13]. In contrast, in COPD patients tidal expiratory FL is frequently present at rest [2, 3, 8], as first suggested by Hyatt [5]. Tidal FL promotes dynamic hyperinflation with a concomitant decrease in IC, as shown in Fig. 1 (right). In fact, Diaz et al. [8] have recently shown that in most COPD patients who are FL at rest, the IC is lower than normal, while in the patients who are non-FL at rest the IC is within normal limits (Fig. 2).

In normal subjects there is a large expiratory flow reserve both above and below the FRC, as evidenced by the fact that the maximal expiratory flow rates available are much higher than the flow rates used during resting breathing (Fig. 1, left). As a result, in normal subjects the tidal volume during exercise can increase both at the expense of the inspiratory and expiratory reserve volumes [3]. In contrast, in COPD patients who exhibit FL at rest, the flows available

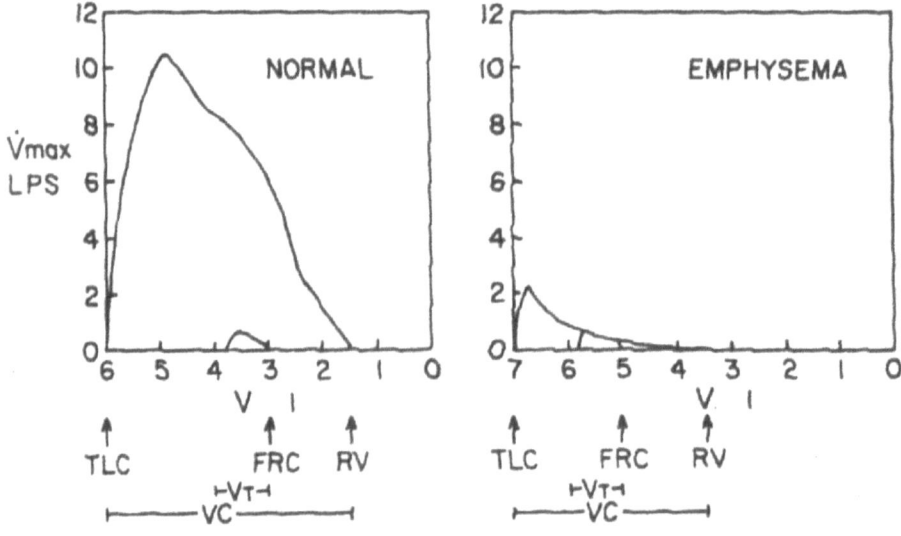

Fig. 1 Flow-volume curves during quiet and forced expiration in a normal subject *(left)* and a patient with severe emphysema *(right)* (*TLC* total lung capacity, *FRC* functional residual capacity, *RV* residual volume, *VC* vital capacity, *VT* tidal volume during quiet breathing). While in the normal subject there is considerable flow reserve in the resting tidal volume range, in the patient the tidal expiratory flow is maximal, i.e. expiratory flow limitation is present. The latter promotes an increase in FRC with concomitant reduction of inspiratory capacity (IC = TLC-FRC) (modified from reference [14], with permission)

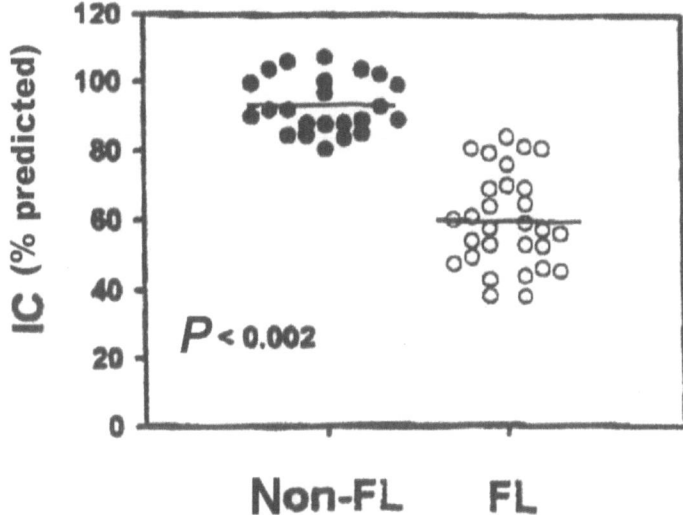

Fig. 2 IC, expressed as percentage predicted, in 23 chronic obstructive pulmonary disease (COPD) patients without (*non-FL*) and 29 COPD patients with (*FL*) tidal expiratory flow limitation at rest. Note that in most FL patients, IC was decreased while in the non-FL patients IC was within normal limits (modified from reference [8], with permission)

below FRC are insufficient to sustain even resting ventilation, as shown in Fig. 1 (right), and thus, tidal volume during exercise can increase only at the expense of the inspiratory reserve volume. Since in such patients IC is decreased because of dynamic hyperinflation at rest, the exertional increment of tidal volume is limited. As a result, in COPD patients with FL at rest the maximal tidal volume during exercise (VTmax), and hence exercise tolerance, should be reduced. In fact, recent studies have shown that in COPD patients there is a much stronger correlation of maximal O_2 uptake (O_2max) with IC than with FEV_1 and FVC [3, 8].

The coefficient of determination (r^2) of O_2max to IC is 0.56 (Fig. 3), indicating that IC can explain 56% of the variance in O_2max. Diaz et al. [8], however, also showed that FEV_1/FVC plays a significant role in predicting O_2max. In fact, using stepwise multiple regression analysis they showed that, taken together, IC and FEV_1/FVC account for 72% of the variance of O_2max (r^2=0.72). However, when stepwise multiple regression analysis was performed separately for FL and non-FL patients, for FL only IC was selected as a significant contributor, while for non-FL only FEV_1/FVC was selected. The latter is probably due to the fact that a high FEV_1/FVC ratio reflects a maximal expiratory flow-volume curve with an upper convexity (Fig. 1, left), with a concurrent high flow-reserve over the resting tidal volume range, while a low

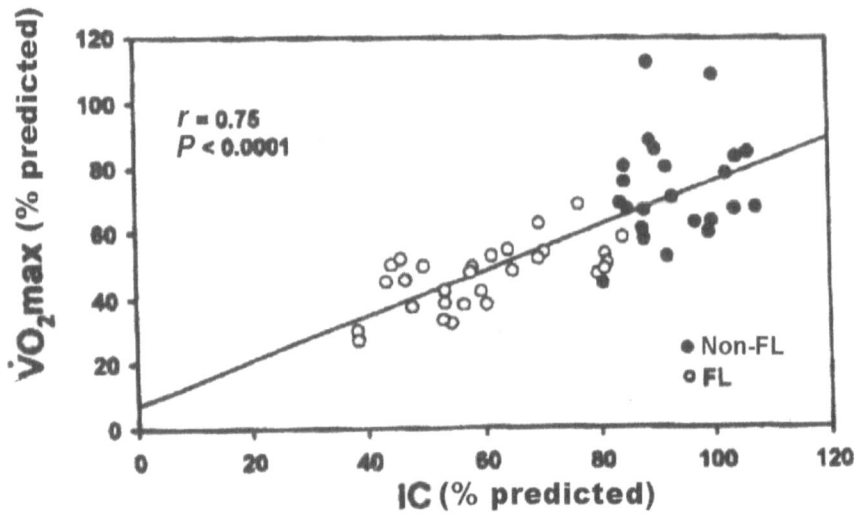

Fig. 3 Relationship of maximal O_2 uptake during exercise (O_2max) with resting IC in 52 COPD patients with (*FL*) and without (*non-FL*) tidal expiratory FL at rest. Same patients from Fig. 2 (modified from reference [8], with permission)

FEV_1/FVC ratio reflects a curve with an upper concavity (Fig. 1, right), with low flow-reserve over the resting tidal volume range. Thus, patients who are non-FL at rest but have a low FEV_1/FVC ratio are more prone to become FL with increasing ventilation during exercise than patients in whom this ratio is high. Accordingly, in the COPD patients who are not FL at rest, O_2max decreases with decreasing FEV_1/FVC ratio [8].

Since in COPD patients reduced exercise capacity shows only a weak link to lung function impairment measured in terms of FEV_1 and FVC [2,8,12,15], it has been suggested that factors other than lung function impairment (e.g., deconditioning and peripheral muscle dysfunction) are the predominant contributors to reduced exercise tolerance [16-18]. The recent studies based on assessment of IC and FEV_1/FVC, however, have shown that lung function impairment is the major contributor to reduced exercise tolerance [8,12]. In fact, since in COPD patients the IC and FEV_1/FVC taken together account for 72% of the O_2max variance, only the remaining 28% can be ascribed to other factors, such as deconditioning and peripheral muscle dysfunction [16], or decreased cardiac output as a result of intrinsic PEEP [19]. These considerations pertain to average values. In any given patient, however, the contribution of these factors may be entirely different.

In COPD patients who are FL at rest, the arterial PCO_2 is significantly higher than in non-FL patients ($P=0.04$) and correlates significantly ($r=0.62$) with IC (% predicted) [8]. Thus, hypercapnic COPD patients (the so called blue bloaters) are characterized by a reduction in IC due to dynamic hyperinflation elicited by tidal FL. These patients also exhibit a further significant ($P=0.002$) increase in arterial PCO_2 at peak exercise associated with a significant ($P=0.05$) reduction in arterial PO_2 relative to rest [19]. This essentially reflects reduced Emax due to a lower VTmax in FL than in non-FL patients. In fact, VTmax is significantly correlated with IC ($P=0.0001$) [19].

Assessment of severity of COPD

Assessment of the severity of COPD is commonly based on the value of FEV_1 expressed as percentage predicted [2]. To the extent that "severity" implies curtailment of exercise capacity and increased dyspnoea, the choice of FEV_1 does not seem to be appropriate, in view of the poor correlation of this parameter with both exercise capacity [8, 12] and dyspnoea [2]. Separation of COPD patients in two categories, namely FL and non-FL while sitting at rest, is more useful, since it reflects the arterial PCO_2 and PO_2 both at rest and during exercise [2, 3, 8, 10, 19]. However, a three- and a five-point FL scale has also been used to assess the severity of chronic dyspnoea in COPD patients [2].

Assessment of bronchodilator response

Measurement of IC also provides useful information in terms of bronchodilator treatment. The effect of bronchodilators in patients with obstructive lung disease is commonly assessed in terms of the change in FEV_1 seen after bronchodilator administration relative to the control values. According to the American Thoracic Society's recommended criteria, a change in FEV_1 of more than 12% and 200 ml compared with baseline represents a significant response [20]. Although most COPD patients do not exhibit a significant change in FEV_1 after bronchodilator administration, many nevertheless claim improvement in symptoms [21]. Since pulmonary hyperinflation plays a paramount role in determining the intensity of dyspnoea [2], it is likely that in such patients there should be a decrease in the degree of dynamic hyperinflation (decreased FRC and increased IC) after bronchodilator administration. Indeed, Belman et al. [22] have shown that the decrease in dynamic hyperinflation, with the concurrent improvement in inspiratory flow-reserve, inspiratory pressure reserve, and neuroventilatory coupling, was the key determinant of the reduced breathlessness claimed at peak exercise by COPD patients after bronchodilator administration. More recently it has also been shown that in COPD patients the increase in IC after anticholinergic therapy best reflected the improvement in exercise performance [23].

Recent studies [10,24] have shown that a significant reduction in IC after salbutamol occurs only in COPD patients who are FL at rest (and hence have a reduced baseline IC). This is associated with a significant reduction of dyspnea (Borg scale) both at rest and during light exercise [11]. Thus, in obstructive lung disease, the benefit of bronchodilator therapy should be assessed not only in terms of change of FEV_1 but, more importantly, also in terms of change in IC. Since performance of IC precedes the FVC manoeuvre, FEV_1 and IC are in fact commonly recorded together during bronchodilator testing. Although in the past bronchodilator testing has focused on changes in FEV_1 to assess the reversibility of airway obstruction, the scrutiny of changes in IC should be mandatory, because it provides useful information pertaining to dyspnea and exercise tolerance.

The fact that after bronchodilator administration there is a significant reduction of dynamic hyperinflation only in patients who are FL at rest in the sitting position further supports the usefulness of stratifying COPD patients into FL and non-FL subgroups [8, 10, 19]. Assessment of IC and FL has also provided useful information on the effects of surgical treatment in COPD patients [25]. Furthermore, a recent study (Soicher et al., unpublished observations) has shown that in COPD patients the IC but not FEV_1 was significantly correlated with health-related quality of life (HRQL) (St. George's Respiratory Questionnaire) and dyspnea (ATS scale).

In conclusion, measurement of the IC is useful for monitoring the status and progress of COPD patients, and for assessing the efficacy of their treatment. It is time for IC, the Cinderella of pulmonary function testing, to take pride of place with her two stepsisters, FEV_1 and FVC.

References

1. Agostoni E, Mead J (1964) Statics of the respiratory system. In: Macklem PT, Mead J (eds) Handbook of physiology. section 3. vol. I. The respiratory system: mechanics of breathing. American Physiological Society, Bethesda, pp 387-409
2. Eltayara L, Becklake MR, Volta CA, Milic-Emili J (1996) Relationship between chronic dyspnea and expiratory flow-limitation in patients with chronic obstructive pulmonary disease. Am J Respir Crit Care Med 154:1726-1734
3. Koulouris NG, Dimopoulou I, Valta P, et al (1997) Detection of expiratory flow limitation during exercise in COPD patients. J Appl Physiol 82:723-731

4. Castile R, Mead J, Jackson A, et al (1982) Effect of posture on flow-volume curve configuration in normal humans. J Appl Physiol 53:1175-1183
5. Hyatt RE (1961) The interrelationship of pressure, flow and volume during various respiratory maneuvers in normal and emphysematous patients. Am Rev Respir Dis 83:676-683
6. D'Angelo E, Prandi E, Marazzani L, Milic-Emili J (1994) Dependence of maximal flow-volume curves on time course of preceding inspiration in patients with chronic obstructive lung disease. Am J Respir Crit Care Med 150:1581-1586
7. Valta P, Corbeil C, Lavoie A, et al (1994) Detection of expiratory flow limitation during mechanical ventilation. Am J Respir Crit Care Med 150:1131-1317
8. Diaz O, Villafranca C, Ghezzo H, et al (2000) Exercise tolerance in COPD patients with and without tidal expiratory flow limitation a rest. Eur Respir J 16: 269-275
9. Shore SA, Milic-Emili J, Martin JG (1982) Reassessment of body plethysmographic technique for the measurement of thoracic gas volume in asthmatics. Am Rev Respir Dis 126:515-520
10. Tantucci C, Duguet A, Similowski T, et al (1998) Effect of solbutamol on dynamic hyperinflation in chronic obstructive pulmonary disease patients. Eur Respir J 12:799-804
11. Boni E, Corda L, Franchini D, et al (2002) Volume effect and exertional dyspnea after bronchodilator in COPD patients with and without expiratory flow limitation at rest. Thorax 57:528-531
12. Murariu C, Ghezzo H, Milic-Emili J, Gauthier H (1987) Exercise limitation in obstructive lung disease. Am Rev Respir Dis 135:1069-1074
13. Mota S, Casan P, Drobnic F, et al (1999) Expiratory flow limitation during exercise in competition. J Appl Physiol 86:611-616
14. Bates DV, Macklem PT, Christie RV (1971) Respiratory function in disease. Saunders p 35
15. Jones NG, Jones G, Edwards RHT (1971) Exercise tolerance in chronic airway obstruction. Am Rev Respir Dis 103:477-491
16. Maltais F (1996) Oxidative capacity of the skeletal muscle and lactic acid kinetics during exercise in normal subjects and in patients with COPD. Am J Respir Crit Care Med 153:228-293
17. Hamilton N, Killian KJ, Summers E, Jones NL (1995) Muscle strength symptom intensity, and exercise capacity in patients with cardiorespiratory disorders. Am J Respir Crit Care Med 152:2021-2031
18. Gosselink R, Troosters T, Decramer M (1996) Peripheral muscle weakness contributes to exercise limitation in COPD. Am J Respir Crit Care Med 153:976-980
19. Diaz O, Villafranca C, Ghezzo H, et al (2001) Breathing pattern and gas exchange at peak exercise in COPD patients with and without tidal flow limitation at rest. Eur Respir J 17:1120-1127
20. American Thoracic Society (1987) Standards for the diagnosis and care of patients with chronic obstructive pulmonary disease (COPD) and asthma. Am Rev Respir Dis 136:225-244
21. Guyatt GH, Townstead M, Pugsley SO, et al (1987) Bronchodilators in chronic air-flow limitation. Effects on airway function, exercise capacity, and quality of life. Am Rev Respir Dis 135:1069-1074
22. Belman, MJ, Botnick WC, Shin JW (1996) Inhaled bronchodilators reduce dynamic hyperinflation during exercise in patients with chronic obstructive pulmonary disease. Am J Respir Crit Care Med 153:967-975
23. O'Donnell DE, Lam M, Webb KA (1999) Spirometric correlates of improvement in exercise performance after anticholinergic therapy in chronic obstructive pulmonary disease. Am J Respir Crit Care Med 160:542-549
24. Pellegrino R, Brusasco V (1997) Lung hyperinflation and flow limitation in chronic airway obstruction. Eur Respir J 10:543-549
25. Murciano D, Pichot M, Boczkowki J, et al (1997) Expiratory flow limitation in COPD patients after single lung transplantation. Am J Respir Crit Care Med 155:1036-1041

Alveolar recruitment strategy improves arterial oxygenation in severe acute respiratory distress syndrome patients

A. GALLESIO, E. SAN ROMAN, S. GIANNASI

The morbidity and mortality of acute lung injury/acute respiratory distress syndrome (ALI/ARDS) patients remains high. Pulmonary damage results from the initial insult and the action of many inflammatory mediators, along with alterations in the coagulation cascade that leads to a procoagulation state. Pulmonary mechanics change dramatically in these conditions, characterized by a decrease in total lung aerated volume, alveolar collapse, mainly in dorsal areas, and a low lung compliance. Many mechanical ventilation therapeutic modalities have been proposed to improve the high mortality rate of these patients, but the final outcome remains a significant challenge for researchers and clinicians. The search for therapeutic modalities is a significant challenge. There is important information coming from animal and human experiments, indicating that either a high level of inspiratory pressure or high tidal volumes may cause lung lesions and poor clinical evolution. The current evidence [1] indicates that we should use in these patients a low tidal volume (Vt) around 4-6 ml/kg weight and low plateau pressure.

Some mechanical ventilation modalities based on these concepts emphasized maintenance of the patency of all potential recruitable airspace throughout the tidal cycle. The main aim is to increase lung volume, and so diminish shunt fraction and V/Q abnormalities, to improve arterial oxygenation and lung compliance. As high inspiratory level pressures and high volumes are deleterious for the alveolar-capillary membrane, open lung strategy must take into account these concepts, in order to avoid further damage to lung tissue. Reversal of alveolar collapse and avoidance of ventilator-induced lung injury are two important goals of lung-protective ventilation in ARDS.

A complication associated with the use of low tidal volume is the tendency for the collapse of the unstable alveolar units. Reversal of alveolar collapse and avoidance of ventilator-induced lung injury are two important goals of lung--protective ventilation in ALI/ARDS [2].

The main aim of this chapter is to review present knowledge of recruitment maneuvers, to analyze the physiopathological basis, and to report our own experience.

Pathogenesis and morphology of ALI/ARDS

ALI/ARDS is a heterogeneous condition, its macro- and microscopic histology change with etiology, time evolution, and mechanical ventilation. The inflammatory process begins with an abnormal thickening of the alveolar wall, incomplete filling of the alveolar space with inflammatory cells, cellular debris, and edema. This pattern, seen through computed tomography scan (CTs), is called ground-glass opacification [3]. If the inflammatory process continues, then consolidation appears; this may be due to either a complete filling of the alveolar spaces or to total collapse of potentially recruitable alveoli, atelectasic, or to a combination of both.

With CTs, in the early period of ALI/ARDS, we may consider the lung to comprise three compartments: normal or near-normal regions, located in non-dependent lung, ground-glass opacification in the middle lung, and consolidation in the most-dependent areas [4]. Furthermore, there is a vertical ventral–dorsal and cephalocaudal gradient, with density increasing from the lung apex to the lung base [5], following a gravitational distribution of densities.

Approximately a week after the initial injury, the exudative stage changes to a more-organized phase, in which fluid diminishes and the architecture undergoes extensive modification. Finally, parenchymal fibrosis causes distortion of the interstitial and bronchovascular structure. Beyond 1-2 weeks, there is a dramatic increase of subpleural cysts; these lesions may originate either from an infectious process or from "volutrauma/barotrauma", usually correlated with prolonged ventilation, and have been reported both in the dependent and in the nondependent lung [6]. When these lesions appear in the nondependent regions, they may be secondary to overdistention, if they are found in the mid-dependent lung regions, they could be due to shearing forces from airspace opening and closing in areas where lung is recruitable during inspiration. Finally, if the patient survives to a sufficiently severe process, fibrosis mainly occurs in the regions more exposed to mechanical ventilation, and consequently more exposed to "volutrauma/barotrauma."

Pulmonary mechanics of ALI/ARDS

Gattinoni et al. [7] described pathological and mechanical differences in ARDS, depending on whether it results from pulmonary or extrapulmonary causes. They showed that ALI/ARDS due to direct insult via the airway has a multifocal pattern involvement of the lung parenchyma, along with a low potential for recruitment maneuvers to be effective. However, with indirect insult to the lung, one should expect a more-diffuse and uniform parenchymal alteration, due to hematogenously distributed mediators. Moreover, as the indirect pulmonary insult is commonly due to abdominal diseases, basilar atelectasis increases due to the increased abdominal pressure from the cephalad shift of the diaphragm. Goodman et al. [8], prospectively comparing patients with early pulmonary ARDS (ARDSp) with patients with early extrapulmonary ARDS (ARDSexp), found that ARDSexp had predominantly symmetric ground-glass opacification and dorsal consolidation (atelectasis), whereas ARDSp tended to be asymmetric, with a mix of dense parenchymal opacification and ground-glass opacification. Other investigators reached similar conclusions [9, 10].

Pelosi et al. [11] found that the tissue mass, measured in each of the different lung levels along the sternovertebral axis, was almost double the normal mass at that level. This suggests that edema is homogeneously distributed throughout the lung parenchyma (no gravitational distribution). They also proposed that the antero-posterior lung size is similar both in ALI/ARDS patients and in normal subjects. They concluded that at least in this projection, the edema replaces an equal amount of gas space, maintaining lung volume (gas volume plus tissue volume). Puybasset et al. [5] found, as Pelosi et al. [11] did, an unmodified anteroposterior lung volume, but they observed a 15% decrease of the cephalocaudal dimensions of the lung in ALI/ARDS, possibly secondary to diaphragmatic pressure and the weight of the heart.

The apparent contradiction between the gravitational distribution of the tomographic densities and the nongravitational distribution of the edema would be explained by a decrease of the gas content along the sternovertebral axis [11]. This decrease in regional inflation in more-dependent areas is now attributed to the superimposed pressure determined by the increase in lung weight, which is doubled or tripled compared with normal parenchyma, increasing the pleural pressure along the vertical axis and decreasing the transpulmonary pressure that is the normal distending force of the lung [4]. The increased superimposed pressure decreases the transpulmonary pressure, causing a progressive deaeration along the ventrodorsal gradient principally in expiration. This concept was called a lung sponge model, where the increased interstitial edema and progressive deaeration along the ventrodorsal axis due to the superimposed pressure replace gas for edema, but the total lung volume, gas plus edematous tissue is not modified. Wilson et al. [12] proposed a different model, where the edema is predominantly in the alveoli, but similar to the sponge model the total lung volume is nearly normal. In contrast, Puybasset et al. [5] showed that there is a lung volume loss in ALI/ARDS, mainly close to the diaphragm area. They support the idea that there is a cranium-caudal gradient, as well as a ventrodorsal gradient of transpulmonary pressure. This suggests that the decrease of transpulmonary pressure at the lung base is probably due to the superimposed pressure added to the heart weight (more important in the supine than in the prone position) [13] and the increased abdominal pressure, as frequently found in ALI/ARDS of extrapulmonary origin [7].

The respiratory compliance in ALI/ARDS is not related to the amount of nonaerated or poorly aerated tissue, but it is closely associated with the amount of normally aerated tissue, which receives most of the inspiratory gas. Thus, the respiratory compliance in early ALI/ARDS appears to be a direct measure of normally aerated tissue [14], suggesting that in ALI/ARDS, the aerated lung was not "stiff," but rather it was small. This idea gave rise to the concept of "baby lung", for expressing the decrease in total lung aerated volume during ALI/ARDS. Much work in the experimental and clinical setting has demonstrated that the use of high pressures and large Vt during mechanical ventilation in these two conditions may further damage the normal areas of the lung. This damage was qualified as barotrauma and volutrauma. Finally, a randomized multicentric trial [1] comparing the utilization of low Vt (6 ml/kg) with conventional ventilation demonstrated the effectiveness of using low tidal volume and plateau pressures lower than 30 cmH_2O.

As consolidated, fully open and recruitable lung units co-exist in ALI/ARDS, a third approach in the ventilatory management of these conditions emerged besides the low pressure and low Vt techniques. One of the cornerstones of the lung protective strategy today is keeping the lung open, i.e., to establish and maintain the patency of all potentially recruitable airspaces throughout the tidal cycle, applying single or multiple recruitment maneuvers based on the use of short high-pressure cycle and the utilization of PEEP above the inspiratory inflexion point. The mechanical opening and closing of pulmonary units through the respiratory cycle may cause lung injury, "biotrauma," releasing inflammatory mediators that are potentially harmful to the lung [15]. The stresses at the junctions of closed and open airspaces (dynamic stress) may predominate in mid-zonal and dependent lung regions that are compressed by the superimposed pressure of the overlying lung they support [16].

PEEP counteracts the compressive forces, maintaining the opening of the alveolus obtained by the preceding high inspiratory pressure cycle. This process is called "alveolar recruitment." Alveolar recruitment is a pan-inspiratory phenomenon that occurs along the entire inspiratory time, well above the lower inflection point, and even above the upper inflection point of the volume–pressure curve [17]. This phenomena occurs with a definite spatial distribution: ventral to dorsal and cephal to caudal [5, 17, 18].

In ALI/ARDS lung, there are regions with different opening pressures, which range from a few cmH_2O to 45–70 cmH_2O [17, 18]. This range is likely due to differing types of atelectasis. In fact, the opening pressure for small airway collapse, typical of the compression atelectasis, is around 20 cmH_2O, whereas the opening pressure required to open alveolar collapse is considerably higher, 30–40 cm H_2O. Since the true opening pressure is the transpulmonary pressure, in patients with high chest wall elastance and high pleural pressure, such as ALI/ARDS originating from abdominal disease, the airway pressure required to reach a sufficient transpulmonary pressure may be higher than 40–45 cmH_2O. There are no data regarding the maintenance of recruitment over time.

Some remarkable factors related to the lung mechanics of ALI/ARDS lung are:

1. Derecruitment is also a continuous process, but is most prevalent over a pressure range lower than the lung recruitment process occurs.
2. There is an interaction between the extent of end-expiratory and end-inspiratory collapse.
3. Gravitational forces (i.e., the superimposed pressure) seem to play a substantial role in determining regional lung collapse

The end-expiratory collapse, at a given PEEP, depends on the previous inspiration. The end-expiratory collapse is greater when the previous inspiratory plateau pressure is lower. The computed tomographic (CT) scan provides evidence that the end-expiratory and end-inspiratory collapses are an interrelated phenomenon [17, 18]. Gattinoni et al. [19] found with CT scan that at plateau pressures of 21-46 cmH_2O, most of the recruitment is accomplished, and only 15-20 cmH_2O of PEEP were necessary to keep the acini already opened by the previous inspiratory recruitment maneuver open. Thus, after the recruitment maneuver causes complete opening, high plateau pressure is not necessary. Rather PEEP must be kept high enough to prevent end-expiratory collapse.

It is important to take into account that the lung will remain open only if the superimposed pressure is lower than the PEEP applied. If the superimposed pressure is greater than PEEP, whatever has been opened by the inspiratory plateau pressure would collapse at end expiration. These findings emphasize the concept that PEEP is an end-expiratory maneuver, which keeps the lung open at a given level, depending on the previous inspiratory opening and superimposed pressure. Recruitment maneuvers are intended to establish initial alveolar patency, and then this must be maintained at lower tidal pressures and PEEP levels than would otherwise be required. During inspiration, surface tension and adhesive forces must be overcome. These two forces are not operative during deflation. Although maximal distension is normally attained within a healthy lung by an alveolar to pleural pressure difference of approximately 30 cmH$_2$O, pressures more than twice that may be needed to open some refractory but potentially recruitable lung units [17]. Sustaining pressure helps to reopen the closed airway [20].

We should bear in mind that almost all experimental data favoring the use of recruitment maneuvers have been collected in models of ALI that are highly "recruitable": e.g., surfactant depletion and oleic acid injury. In these experimental conditions, more or less 50% of total lung tissue volume may be recruitable (defined by CT scan evaluations of tissue density) [17]. These same methods indicate that in the setting of pneumonia-caused ("primary") ARDS, only 5% -10% of consolidated lung tissue can be reopened [16].

Pulmonary recruitment

Pulmonary disturbances in ARDS mainly involve a collapse of lung tissue in dependent areas, as was initially observed by Goodman et al. [8] studying ARDS patients with computed tomography. The underlying lesions of this physiopathological process include alveolar and interstitial edema, alveolar collapse, atelectasic and cellular inflammatory infiltrations.

Hickling [21] has demonstrated, based on a mathematical model, that the lung is recruited during the whole inflation inspiratory phase, and that the main determinant of recruitment is peak inspiratory pressure. The pressure needed for lung recruitment is determined by the amount of collapsed pulmonary tissue, as a result of high surface tension of these units [20], lung fluid viscosity, and parenchymal tethering[16]. The application of a high level pf pressure is necessary for lung recruitment, and may result in alveolar overdistention of normal areas. Mead et al. [16] have calculated a pressure as high as 140 mmHg to be necessary to open collapsed alveolar units surrounded by normal tissue. This pressure is theoretically transmitted to these normal areas. The more severe the ARDS the greater the pressure necessary to apply to achieve lung recruitment.

There is no agreement in the literature about the ability of recruitment maneuver open the lung. Martynowicz et al. [22] described the application of high-level pressure to the oleic acid lung-injured model only distend normal parenchymal areas. Neumann et al. [23] using the same model in pigs observed that 25 and 50 cmH$_2$O applied during inspiration did not achieve significant opening of lung recumbent areas, as show by chest CT scan, but 25 cm H$_2$O of pressure applied during expiration maintained the lung open. They concluded that lung recruitment is a different process than keeping the lung open once recruited. Gattinoni et al. [19] observed that pressure to recruit lung areas and to increase total lung and residual expiratory capacity is higher than that necessary to maintained lung open. Perhaps this difference is a result of lung hysteresis determined by changes in the distribution of forces in lung parenchyma once it has been opened.

The approach most commonly used to carry out recruitment maneuvers is to apply sustained high pressure in the airway during inspiration. Greaves et al. found that 30 cmH$_2$O of transpulmonary pressure is enough to achieve total pulmonary volume (TPV) in atelectasic lungs. Similar values had been published for healthy individuals undergoing general anaesthesia. The scenario is different for recruiting the lung during ALI and ARDS. Gattinoni et al. [19] used 46 cmH$_2$O of peak airway pressure to open collapsed lung in ARDS. These authors also differentiated the effects of high inspiratory pressure to recruit closed alveolar space on the basis of whether the ARDS was pulmonary or extrapulmonary in origin. Marini and Amato [2] used a slightly different technique to achieve the same aim. They applied 35–40 cmH$_2$O of continuous airway pressure (CPAP) for 30–40 s before initiating a lung protective ventilatory strategy and whenever mechanical ventilation was disrupted.

Lapinsky et al. [24] made a substantial advance by demonstrating that patients are able to tolerate multiple recruitment maneuver without significant changes in their homodynamic status and development of barotrauma. The peak airway pressure used for the recruitment maneuver varied between 30 and 45 cmH$_2$O ventilating with a high tidal volume of 12 ml/kg. SpO$_2$ was maintained 20 s, 10 min, and 4 h after the procedure. If PEEP were not applied after recruitment maneuver was over, the improvement in arterial oxygenation was rapidly lost. It seems reasonable, based on clinical and experimental data, that a level of PEEP set up above the inflexion point value is necessary to keep the lung open after recruitment of closed alveolar areas. The level of PEEP to maintain the lung volume is generally lower than the inspiratory peak pressure used to recruit the lung. This effect has been hypothesized by Marini and Amato to be due to the shifting of the static pressure volume curve up and leftward, consequently the tidal volume loop will turn out to a better position in the pressure-volume (PV) curve in terms of respiratory mechanical load and work. If PEEP had been set higher and the ventilatory circuit was not disconnected allowing derecruitment, the oxygenation benefit could theoretically preserve in all patients [25].

There have been other approaches to single recruitment maneuvers to achieve a similar effect on oxygenation through recruiting the lung. These techniques have focused on periodic increases of peak inspiratory pressure. One of the best-known trials in this area was carried out by Pelosi et al. [25]. These authors investigated the periodic use of sighs in a small sample of ten patients with ARDS. The effect of 1 h of ventilation with sighs was compared with 1 h ventilation without; the patients were their own controls. Sighs were delivered at a frequency of three consecutive breaths every each minute at a Vt that results in a plateau pressure of 45 cmH_2O in volume ventilation during the 60-min sigh period. The PEEP level was set at 14.5±2.2 cmH_2O, this value was above the inflexion point established for the whole sample: 8.2±3.2 cmH_2O. The PaO_2 improved significantly to values above 120 mmHg in the sigh period; there was no statistical difference in the control period compared with the basal measurements. PCO_2 and shunt fraction decreased in the sigh period in the same fashion as did PaO_2.

Another study using intermittent recruitment maneuver has been published by Foti et al. [26]. These authors used three random approaches to recruit the lung during mechanical ventilation, the protocol was applied every 30 min: control mechanical ventilation (CMV) at a low PEEP level (9.4±3 cm H_2O), CMV at high PEEP level (16±2 cm H_2O) and CMV at the low PEEP level using mandatory cycles. Two breaths at the high PEEP level were delivered every 30 s. High values of PEEP increase PaO_2 sharply and decrease shunt fraction. Periodic high PEEP results in an increase in PaO_2 and decrease in shunt fraction intermediate between the other two branches

Both types of maneuvers sustained high inspiratory peak pressure, and periodic increases in pressure produce a benefit in term of oxygenation and decrease in shunt fraction and $PaCO_2$. Data in the literature do not provide information about the superiority of one of these two approaches. There is no evidence of hemodynamic deterioration or barotrauma if the maneuvers are properly applied. However the data available about the benefits of recruitment of the lung and the occurrence of complications are scarce because of the small size of the samples.

The use of sustained pressure recruitment maneuvers requires the use of a high level of PEEP above the inspiratory inflexion point, although the shape of the static PV curve is different during expiration, and the value of pressure to maintain the lung open is less than that needed to open the collapsed alveolus. On the other hand the use of periodic high inspiratory pressure seems less able to maintain the alveolar stability over time. The end-expiratory lung volume decreases progressively to its prerecruitment values between maneuvers and after a variable period. Disconnection from the ventilator accelerates the volume loss. It is not clear if these changes in lung volume determine alveolar injury; more work is necessary to elucidate these subjects.

Many studies have demonstrated in the last few years that mechanical ventilation in the prone position is useful for increasing the PaO_2 of patients with ALI and ARDS. This was first reported in the majority of patients with acute respiratory failure in the 1970s. Oxygenation improves from 50% to 78% depending on the series. Prone position has not only be used for ALI and ARDS but also for hydrostatic pulmonary edema that failed to increase PaO_2 after recruitment maneuvers. The small group of patients studied (n=8) increased their PaO_2/FiO_2 from 72±16 to 208±61 mm Hg after being ventilated in the prone position.

Gattinoni et al. [27] carried out a multicenter randomized trial that comprised 304 patients, comparing traditional ventilatory treatment in the supine position of patients with ALI or ARDS with a strategy of placing patients in prone position during 6 or more hours daily for 10 days. They found a mortality rate of 23% during the 10-day period, 49.3% at the time of discharge from the unit, and 60.5% at 6 months. The RR of death in the prone group compared with the supine group was 0.84 (CI 95%, 0.56-1.27). There was an improvement in PaO_2/FiO_2 ratio from 44.6±68.2 to 63±66.8. The authors concluded that although there was an improvement in oxygenation, the prone position does not change mortality rate in these very critically ill patients. The effects of the prone position on oxygenation are probably ascribed to the more-elastic and inflatable properties of the dorsal areas of the lung and the thorax, and decrease of the shunt fraction and virtual venous admission. The prone position works in this sense like a recruitment maneuver.

Recently Cakar et al. [28] demonstrated in oleic acid-injured dogs the benefit of carrying out recruitment maneuvers in the prone position. They performed recruitment maneuvers in the supine and prone position with two levels of PEEP, 8 cmH_2O and 15 cmH_2O. Recruitment was carried out by a single sustained inspiration at 60 cmH_2O for 20 s. The authors found that recruitment maneuvers were more effective in the prone than in the supine position in terms of blood oxygenation. Lower levels of PEEP were also needed to maintain the benefits at 15 min.

Alveolar recruitment strategy for improving arterial oxygenation

We investigated a new form of recruitment maneuver using PEEP from the baseline ventilator setting. PEEP was incremented in steps of 5 cmH_2O each every 60 s. The limit was to reach a PEEP of 35 cmH_2O and/or a peak airway pressure not exceeding 60 cmH_2O. Figure 1 shows a schematic representation

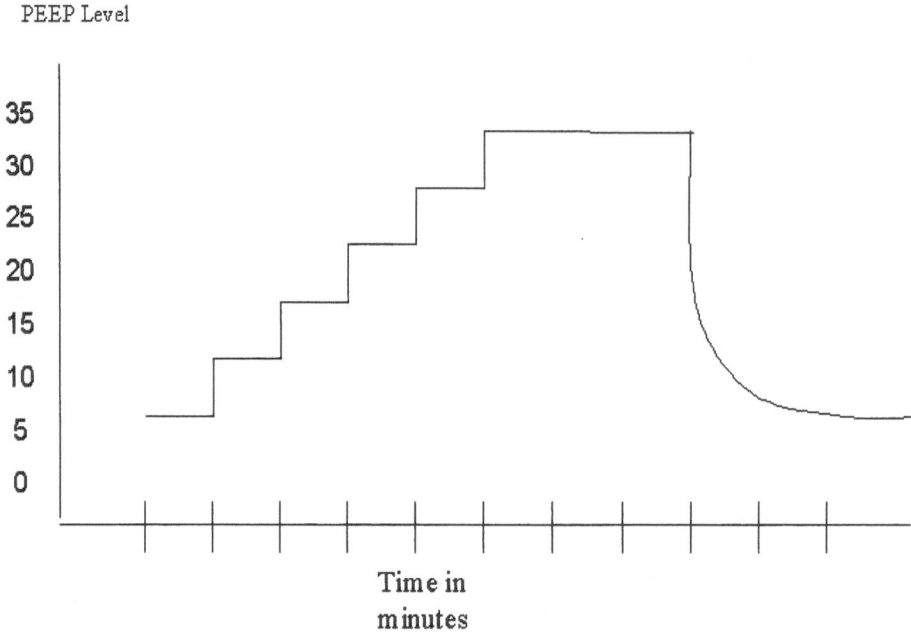

Fig. 1 Schematic representation of the recruitment maneuver. Design pattern of extended positive end-expiratory pressure (PEEP). It is considered in several steps. The objective was to obtain a maximum level of PEEP of 35 cmH$_2$O and/or a peak inspiratory pressure of 60 cmH$_2$O. When achieving the maximum level, ventilation was maintained for 3 min and after that a sudden PEEP reduction was set until the base level of 10 cmH$_2$O

of the recruitment plan. We recruited patients undergoing early severe ARDS, less than 3 days on mechanical ventilation and PaO$_2$/FiO$_2$ ratio less than 150 mmHg. ARDS was diagnosed according to the criteria of the American-European Consensus Conference [29].

We have tested the impact of alveolar recruitment strategy on arterial oxygenation and lung mechanics as well as the change of Vt after this procedure. Patients less than 18 years of age, intracranial hypertension, pregnancy, documented pneumothorax, or hypotension defined as systolic blood pressure < 100 mmHg were excluded. Eighteen consecutive patients diagnosed with ARDS were allocated to the recruitment protocol, 11 men and 7 women. Direct or indirect injury of the lung was assessed, 6 patients died (33.33%). Clinical characteristics, including lung injury score, are presented in Table 1.

Table 1. Subject's characteristics (*I* extrapulmonary ARDS, *D* pulmonary ARDS, *DIC* disseminated intravascular coagulation, *LIS* lung injury score, *S* survivor, *D* dead)

Patient	Age years	Gender	Apache II [a]	Primary disease	Direct/indirect injury	Day[b]	LIS	Out-come	PaO$_2$/FiO$_2$
1	40	F	15	DIC	I	2	3	S	151
2	54	F	16	Pneumonia	D	2	4	S	98
3	53	F	19	Abdominal sepsis	I	1	3	D	91
4	53	M	16	Trauma	I	2	2.75	S	136
5	34	F	16	Hypovolemic shock	I	2	3.25	S	37
6	86	F	15	Aspiration pneumonia	D	2	2.75	D	69
7	47	M	15	Postoperative esophageal cancer	I	3	2.5	D	149
8	65	M	14	Hypovolemic shock	I	3	2.5	S	100
9	30	M	12	Thorax injury	D	3	2.5	S	150
10	26	M	15	Trauma	I	1	3.25	S	150
11	34	F	22	Liver cirrhosis	I	3	2.75	D	42
12	74	M	17	Aspiration pneumonia	D	3	2.75	D	81
13	41	M	15	Peritonitis	I	1	2.5	S	153
14	25	M	12	Trauma	D	3	2.5	S	86
15	23	M	15	Trauma	I	1	3.25	S	66
16	21	M	17	Nosocomial pneumonia	D	3	3	S	150
17	27	F	12	Pneumonia	D	3	3	D	120
18	59	M	14	Hypovolemic shock	I	2	2.75	S	160

[a] Apache II score on admission to intensive care unit
[b] Days of ARDS

According to our protocol, baseline ventilator settings were as follows: ventilator mode setting, pressure control ventilation (Servo 300 Siemens Elema, Solna, Sweden), Vt < 8 ml/kg and > 4 ml/kg; PEEP 10 cmH$_2$O; respiratory rate 15-20 breaths/min, I:E ratio 1:1. To ensure patients safety during the application of high inflating pressure we use FiO$_2$=1. During the study period, midazolam and pancuronium were continuously administered intravenously to maintain sedation and prevent spontaneous respiratory movement. We compared measurements made before and at the end of the recruitment maneuver. Each patient served as its own control. Thoracopulmonary compliance was calculated as Vt/ (PIP – PEEP). DVt was calculated as Vt before versus Vt after recruitment maneuver at the same pressure control level of ventilation. The results showed an improvement in oxygenation (110.5±41.09 mmHg vs. 217.83±101.4, P<0.001), thoracopulmonary compliance (32.69±10.06 vs. 38.07±11.77 ml/cm H$_2$O), DVt (6.69±0.96 vs. 8.10±1.52 ml/kg, P<0.001). In

14 of 18 patients, hypotension was detected during maximal PEEP (125.78±25.08 vs.98.85±25.2 mmHg, P<0.001). Despite the decrease in systolic pressure level, no shock was detected. Physiological measurements before, during maximal PEEP, and 30 min after the recruitment maneuver are depicted in Tables 2 and 3. Changes in PO_2/FiO_2 ratio are shown in Table 4.

Table 2 Physiological variables before and during recruitment maneuver (maximal PEEP) (*PCV* pressure control ventilation, *PIP* peak inspiratory pressure, *MAP* mean airway pressure, *PEEP* positive end-expiratory pressure, *Vti* inspiratory tidal volume, *VtiMI-kg* inspiratory tidal volume oer kilogram, *Vte* expiratory tidal volume, *VteMI-kg* expiratory tidal volume per kilogram, *Cpt* total compliance of respiratory system)

	Basal	Maximal PEEP	P
PCV	17.22 ± 4.76	17.72 ± 4.53	0.3313
PIP	27.67 ± 4.86	50.39 ± 6.04	P<0.001
MAP	18.33 ± 2.83	40.11 ± 4.06	P<0.001
PEEP	10.06 ± 0.24	32.22 ± 3.49	P<0.001
Vti	533.00 ± 82.15	335.72 ± 67.24	P<0.001
VtiMI-kg	6.69 ± 0.96	4.23 ± 0.94	P<0.001
Vte	544.50 ± 90.73	328.50 ± 73.09	P<0.001
VteMI-kg	6.79 ± 0.79	4.12 ± 0.92	P<0.001
Cpt	32.5 ±10.06	19.66 ± 6.15	P<0.001

Table 3 Physiological variables before and 30 min after recruitment maneuver

	Basal	30 min after recruitment maneuver	P
PCV	17.22 ± 4.76	17.72 ± 4.76	NS
PIP	27.67 ± 4.86	28.67 ± 6.53	0.1075
MAP	18.33 ± 2.83	19.39 ± 4.59	0.1409
PEEP	10.06 ± 0.24	10.50 ± 2.38	0.3923
Vti	533.00 ± 82.15	642.28 ± 110.47	P<0.001
VtiMI-kg	6.69 ± 0.96	8.10 ± 1.52	P<0.001
Vte	544.50 ± 9073	662.28 ± 110.99	P<0.001
VteMI-kg	6.79 ± 0.79	8.32 ± 1.33	P<0.001
Cpt	32.5 ± 10.06	38.07 ± 11.75	P<0.001

Possibly, there are differences in lung dysfunction between ARDS resulting from pulmonary disease and that with an extrapulmonary etiology [14]. When the prevalent pathology is lung tissue consolidation, such as in pneumonia, application of PEEP should induce only a moderate lung recruitment, an increase of the respiratory system elastance, and possibly alveolar overdistention. On the other hand, when the prevalent pathology is interstitial edema and alveolar collapse, PEEP should induce significant lung recruitment, with a decrease of elastance of the respiratory system.

In our population there were no differences in blood oxygenation in patients with pulmonary or extrapulmonary disease. Sometime the distinction between pulmonary and extrapulmonary origin of ARDS seems to be controversial or difficult to evaluate. For instance, trauma and aspiration in the same patient may cause lung injury of pulmonary and extrapulmonary origin.

Table 4 PaO_2/FiO_2 ratio before, during maximal PEEP, and 30 min after recruitment maneuver in each patient

Patient	Basal	Maximal PEEP	30 min after recruitment maneuver
1	151	368	428
2	98	408	295
3	91	224	356
4	136	287	261
5	37	76	87
7	69	78	117
8	149	156	156
9	100	150	250
10	150	275	310
11	150	150	162
12	42	40	45
13	81	80	109
14	153	209	261
15	86	196	196
16	66	263	125
17	150	132	225
18	120	316	215
19	160	250	323
Average	110.5	203.22	217.83
SD	41.09	104.85	102.51

Our data suggest that recruitment maneuver is safe and improves oxygenation in pulmonary or extrapulmonary ARDS. Hypotension is a common finding, but is well tolerated in normovolemic patients over a short period. Although we documented overdistention, as shown by a drop in compliance during maximal PEEP, no barotrauma was detected during the next 24 h. This study suggested that in the refractory hypoxemic patient with early ARDS recruitment maneuver with PEEP could result in improvement in oxygenation and changes in DVt. A suitable level of PEEP applied after recruitment is a safe method of maintaining lung volume gained during the maneuver.

References

1. The Acute Respiratory Distress Syndrome Network (2000) Ventilation with lower tidal volumes as compared with traditional tidal volumes for acute lung injury and the acute respiratory distress syndrome. N Engl J Med 342:1301-1308
2. Marini JJ, Amato MB (2000) Lung recruitment during ARDS. Minerva Anestesiol 66: 314-319
3. Austin JH, Muller NL, Friedman PJ et al (1996) Glossary of terms for CT of the lungs: recommendations of the Nomenclature Committee of the Fleischner Society. Radiology. 200:327-331
4. Gattinoni L, Caironi P, Pelosi P, Goodman LR (2001) What has computed tomography taught us about the acute respiratory distress syndrome? Am J Respir Crit Care Med. 164:1701-1711
5. Puybasset L, Cluzel P, Chao N, et al (1998) A computed tomography scan assessment of regional lung volume in acute lung injury. The CT Scan ARDS Study Group. Am J Respir Crit Care Med 158:1644-1655
6. Rouby JJ, Lherm T, Martin de Lassale E, et al (1993) Histologic aspects of pulmonary barotrauma in critically ill patients with acute respiratory failure. Intensive Care Med 19:383-389
7. Gattinoni L, Pelosi P, Suter PM, et al (1998) Acute respiratory distress syndrome caused by pulmonary and extrapulmonary disease. Different syndromes? Am J Respir Crit Care Med 158:3-11
8. Goodman LR, Fumagalli R, Tagliabue P, et al (1999) Adult respiratory distress syndrome due to pulmonary and extrapulmonary causes: CT, clinical, and functional correlations. Radiology 213:545-552
9. Rouby JJ, Puybasset L, Cluzel P, et al (2000) Regional distribution of gas and tissue in acute respiratory distress syndrome. II. Physiological correlations and definition of an ARDS Severity Score. CT Scan ARDS Study Group. Intensive Care Med 26:1046-1056
10. Puybasset L, Cluzel P, Gusman P, et al (2000) Regional distribution of gas and tissue in acute respiratory distress syndrome. I. Consequences for lung morphology. CT Scan ARDS Study Group. Intensive Care Med 26:857-869
11. Pelosi P, D'Andrea L, Vitale G et al (1994) Vertical gradient of regional lung inflation in adult respiratory distress syndrome. Am J Respir Crit Care Med 149:8-13
12. Wilson TA, Anafi RC, Hubmayr RD (2001) Mechanics of edematous lungs. J Appl Physiol 90:2088-2093
13. Malbouisson LM, Busch CJ, Puybasset L, et al (2000) Role of the heart in the loss of aeration characterizing lower lobes in acute respiratory distress syndrome. CT Scan ARDS Study Group. Am J Respir Crit Care Med. 161:2005-2012
14. Gattinoni L, Pesenti A, Avalli L, et al (1987) Pressure-volume curve of total respiratory system in acute respiratory failure. Computed tomographic scan study. Am Rev Respir Dis 136:730-736
15. Tremblay L, Valenza F, Ribeiro SP, et al (1997) Slutsky, injurious ventilatory strategies increase cytokines and c-fos m-RNA expression in an isolated rat lung model. J Clin Invest. 99: 944-952
16. Mead J, Takishima T, Leith D (1970) Stress distribution in lungs: a model of pulmonary elasticity. J Appl Physiol 28:596-608
17. Crotti S, Mascheroni D, Caironi P, et al (2001) Recruitment and derecruitment during acute respiratory failure: a clinical study. Am J Respir Crit Care Med 164:131-140
18. Pelosi P, Goldner M, McKibben A, et al (2001) Recruitment and derecruitment during acute respiratory failure: an experimental study. Am J Respir Crit Care Med 164:122-130
19. Gattinoni L, Pelosi P, Crotti S, Valenza F (1995) Effects of positive end-expiratory pressure on regional distribution of tidal volume and recruitment in adult respiratory distress syndrome. Am J Respir Crit Care Med 151:1807-1814
20. Gaver DP 3rd, Samsel RW, Solway J (1990) Effects of surface tension and viscosity on airway reopening. J Appl Physiol 69:74-85
21. Hickling KG (1998) The pressure-volume curve is greatly modified by recruitment. A mathematical model of ARDS lungs. Am J Respir Crit Care Med 158:194-202

22. Martynowicz MA, Minor TA, Walters BJ, Hubmayr RD (1999) Regional expansion of oleic acid-injured lungs. Am J Respir Crit Care Med 160:250-258
23. Neumann P, Berglund JE, Mondejar EF, et al (1998) Effect of different pressure levels on the dynamics of lung collapse and recruitment in oleic-acid-induced lung injury. Am J Respir Crit Care Med 158:1636-1643
24. Lapinsky SE, Aubin M, Mehta S, et al (1999) Safety and efficacy of a sustained inflation for alveolar recruitment in adults with respiratory failure. Intensive Care Med 25:1297-1301
25. Pelosi P, Tubiolo D, Mascheroni D, et al (1998) Effects of the prone position on respiratory mechanics and gas exchange during acute lung injury. Am J Respir Crit Care Med 157:387-393
26. Foti G, Cereda M, Sparacino ME, et al (2000) Effects of periodic lung recruitment maneuvers on gas exchange and respiratory mechanics in mechanically ventilated acute respiratory distress syndrome (ARDS) patients. Intensive Care Med 26:501-507
27. Gattinoni L, Tognoni G, Pesenti A, et al (2001) Effect of prone positioning on the survival of patients with acute respiratory failure. N Engl J Med 345:568-573
28. Cakar N, Kloot TV der, Youngblood M, et al (2000) Oxygenation response to a recruitment maneuver during supine and prone positions in an oleic acid-induced lung injury model. Am J Respir Crit Care Med 161:1949-1956
29. Bernard GR, Artigas A, Brigham KL, et al (1994) The American-European Consensus Conference on ARDS. Definitions, mechanisms, relevant outcomes, and clinical trial coordination. Am J Respir Crit Care Med 149:818-824

Ventilator-associated pneumonia

V. Pavoni, G. Gritti, R. Alvisi

Nosocomial pneumonia represents the leading cause of death from hospital-acquired infections among patients requiring admission to the intensive care unit (ICU) [1]. Ventilator-associated pneumonia (VAP) typically refers to nosocomial pneumonia developing more than 24 h following endotracheal intubation and mechanical ventilation (MV). The EPIC and other studies demonstrate that 47% of all ICU-acquired infections are VAP and that VAP complicate the course of 7%-41% of patients treated with MV [1-3]. The mortality rate for VAP ranges from 25% to 50% and can be even higher when lung infection is caused by high-risk pathogens [4, 5].

Because VAP is associated with increased morbidity, longer ICU stay, increased health care costs, and higher mortality rate, prevention of this infection is a challenge for intensive care medicine [6].

Pathogenesis

The postulated mechanism is colonization with pathogenic bacteria of the upper airways and of the digestive tract (colonization of the stomach in the absence of gastric acid) and microaspiration of contaminated fluid in the lower airways [7]. The propensity for colonization of the upper airways is higher in serious illnesses. The dominant organisms in VAP are Gram-negative bacteria (50%--70%): the most-common bacteria within this category are *Enterobacteria* species and *Pseudomonas* species. *Staphylococcus aureus* is second to Gram--negative bacteria as a causative agent and accounts for 10%-20% of all VAP [8]. Finally, an ill-defined but increasing incidence of VAP caused by fungi should be considered.

Risk factors

Several studies have proposed as predictors of VAP, prolonged MV, decrease in level of consciousness, severity of illness, high-volume pulmonary aspiration, thoraco-abdominal surgery, chronic lung disease, immunosuppression, poor nutritional status [9,10], and inadequate airway management. The presence of endotracheal tubes and duration of this intervention are associated with the highest risk of developing VAP [9], and the procedure of intubation itself increases the risk significantly, as demonstrated in patients requiring re-intubation. There is an increased risk of tracheal aspiration of infected fluids during intubation manoeuvres in patients with respiratory tract colonization. Failure of extubation can cause a higher mortality rate [11]. However, a recent study that evaluated risk factors independently of the intubation procedure, showed that cardio-pulmonary resuscitation and continuous sedation are the most important risk factors for development of VAP [12]. This agrees with other reports suggesting that sedation has an adverse effect on local airway defences and increases the incidence of pneumonia in ventilated patients [13]. Randomized trials have shown that continuous infusion of sedatives, compared with intermittent infusion, prolongs MV and length of ICU stay [14].

Tracheostomy seems to be a risk factor for VAP in the community hospital [15]. The incidence of VAP increases when local infection is present at the time of tracheostomy [16]. A recent study demonstrated that the incidence of VAP is lower when the tracheostomy is performed early (within 5 days) than later (beyond 8 days) [17]. Early tracheostomy should be preferred when prolonged MV is needed (patient with neurological impairment).

Nasogastric and nasotracheal tubes increase the incidence of sinusitis. Some authors have supposed that sinusitis could determine a colonization of the oropharyngeal area and subsequently facilitate the insurgence of VAP [18]. However, we should consider that a diagnosis of sinusitis is more frequently a radiological finding rather than a real clinical diagnosis. Nasal-tracheal intubation is more comfortable for the patient who is awake, permits more easy oropharyngeal management, and therefore should be preferred.

Enteral nutrition seems to be a risk factor for VAP: it has been demonstrated that avoidance of large gastric volumes decreases the risk of VAP [19]. Small nasal-gastric tubes or post-pyloric tubes seem to lower gastric reflux [20]. The routine use of stress ulcer prophylaxis can favour the colonization of the digestive tract. Several studies have indicated lower rates of pneumonia for patients treated with a gastroprotective agent (sucralfate) rather than H_2 blocker agents [21].

Diagnosis

The usual presentation of VAP is a new, persistent pulmonary infiltrate on the chest radiograph combined with evidence of infection (fever, leukocytosis, or leukopenia, new onset of purulent sputum, or change in character of sputum) [22]. In relation to the start of MV, it is possible to distinguish early onset pneumonia, when it occurs within the first 4 days, and late onset pneumonia, after 4 or more days. A suspected diagnosis of VAP could be confirmed by isolation of a pathogenic organism from blood cultures (frequency of bacteraemia is 2%-6 %) or from respiratory secretions. In most cases, the only diagnostic specimens readily available are respiratory secretions obtained from the respiratory tract. The usefulness of fibreobtic bronchoscopy with quantitative culture of specimens from the protected brush or bronchoalveolar lavage is debatable [23, 24]. Quantitative cultures obtained with distal protected tracheal specimens seem to be an effective method for the early diagnosis of VAP but, as suggested in a recent study [25], endotracheal aspiration is comparable with other more--invasive methods and it is easily repeatable. A protocol for culture specimens should be available in every ICU.

Prevention

Evaluation of the efficacy of preventive measures is very complex and most published recommendations are empirical rather than based on controlled observations. Furthermore, there is an objective difficulty in precisely determining the impact of prophylactic measures on the pathogenic mechanism, i.e., tracheal colonization, and on the overall mortality in a general ICU population. However, data available about preventive measures can help the development of a program to prevent VAP:

1. *Hand washing and use of protective gowns and gloves.* Hand washing is widely recognized as an important but underused measure to prevent nosocomial infections [26]. The use of protective gowns and gloves appears to be most effective when directed at specific antibiotic-resistant pathogens, such as vancomycin-resistant enterococci.
2. *Non-invasive ventilation (NIV).* The use of NIV reduces the risk of VAP and nosocomial infection compared with endotracheal intubation, irrespective of the severity of the patient's illness [27]. Early extubation followed by NIV may prevent re-intubation and therefore reduces the risk of VAP [28].
3. *Airway management.* Daily interruption of sedative infusions, when necessary, and disconnection of patients from the ventilator allow an evaluation of breathing pattern and gas exchanges during spontaneous breathing. This

permits the removal of bronchial secretions spontaneously or with recruit-ment manoeuvres ("bagging") [29].

4. *Antibiotic use.* Intravenous prophylaxis reduces the incidence of VAP [30]. An appropriate initial antibiotic therapy, during the first days of the ICU stay, can reduce ICU mortality [31]. Scheduled changes of antibiotic classes used for empirical treatment of suspected Gram-negative bacterial infections seem to be useful for reduction of VAP and the growing of bacterial resistance [32].

5. *Selective digestive decontamination* (SDD). A significant reduction of VAP is demonstrated only in individual studies. No effect on length of MV and of ICU stay, as well as on hospital mortality, has been demonstrated. SDD performs insurgence of bacterial resistance; in a recent study the percentage of Gram-positive cocci increased during SDD [33]. However, SDD should be contra-indicated. Recently, oral topical antimicrobical prophylaxis (gentamicin/colistin/vancomycin) was proposed; despite a significant reduction of VAP in studied patients, this was not associated with shorter length of MV, ICU stay, and increased survival [34]. The efficacy of oral decontamination is still under debate [35]. Chlorhexidine has been shown to be effective in the control of ventilator-circuit coloni-zation and pneumonia caused by antibiotic-resistant bacteria. The use of preventive oral washes with chlorhexidine seems reasonable in selected high-risk patients (unconscious patients).

6. *Subglottic aspiration.* Aspiration of the secretion from lower airways is facilitated during manoeuvres, especially when cuff pressure is not con-trolled. All studies demonstrate a delay in the appearance of VAP when the cuff pressure is maintained at 20 cmH$_2$O. These prophylactic procedures are useful to prevent or at least to delay the insurgence of VAP [36, 37].

7. *Importance of biofilm.* Polyvinyl chloride is a substrate for colonization and should be avoided for prolonged tracheal intubation [38].

8. *Patient's position.* Semirecumbent body position can reduce gastro-oeso-phageal reflux and subsequent aspiration [39], and it is also preferable according to pulmonary mechanisms.

9. *Routine maintenance of ventilator circuits and humidification with heat and moisture exchangers.* Several clinical studies found no benefit from routinely changing ventilator circuit tubing [40]. A high concentration of pathogenic bacteria is found in condensed fluid, which may cause pneu-monia if aspirated. In theory, heat and moisture exchangers reduce the incidence of VAP by minimizing the development of condensation within the ventilator circuit [41]. In clinical practice heated-water humidification is preferred, in particular when copious or tenacious secretions are present

and when high minute volumes of ventilation are required (10 or more l/min).

10. *Physiotherapy*. There is no clear evidence that chest physiotherapy aimed at enhancing secretion clearance is useful in the prevention of VAP. Ntoumenopoulos et al. [42], in a small trial, suggested that chest physiotherapy was independently associated with a reduction in VAP but others studies concluded that routine use of physiotherapy manoeuvres should be avoided because of a lack of efficacy and the associated risks of arterial oxygen desaturation [43].

Treatment

Optimal therapy is based on isolation of a specific pathogen from cultures of uncontaminated fluids (i.e., positive blood cultures) or quantitative cultures of specimens obtained from distal respiratory secretions. Guidelines for empirical treatment based on recommendations of the American Thoracic Society are available. The authors distinguish likely pathogens in patients who have nosocomial pneumonia early in their ICU course (in the first 4 days); those who are not severely ill and lack specific risk factors usually receive a single-agent therapy, like third-generation cephalosporin, penicillin with beta-lactamase inhibitor, or a fluoroquinolone. Empirical treatment in patients who have late--onset nosocomial pneumonia or are seriously ill should include a combination of antibiotics with anti-*Pseudomonas* and/or anti-*Staphylococcus* activity. Empirical treatment can possibly lead to erroneous conclusions about bacteriological patterns.

An efficient infection control program is possible only when the epidemiology of microbial and antimicrobial agents is available, so that most frequent infection agents and their antibiotic resistance can help the choice of the antibiotic therapy.

To evaluate the influence of antibiotic strategies on prevention of VAP, we performed an observational study in a polyvalent ICU, in which we verified the incidence of VAP before and after scheduled antibiotic therapy change.

We considered two periods of observation: October 1999 to March 2000 (first period) and February 2001 to June 2001 (second period). We used two different antibiotic strategies: a prevalent use of cephalosporins in the first period and of penicillin/β-lactamase inhibitor combinations during the second period. The medical team and ventilated patient management were unchanged during the two study periods.

We evaluated only admitted patients in these periods in the ICU who had a length of ICU stay (LOS) > 48 h. In patients who received MV for 48 > h, the diagnosis of VAP was established when new pulmonary infiltrate appeared on the chest X-ray and at least one of the following clinical or biological findings [4]: (1) presence of purulent respiratory secretions; (2) body temperature > 38°C or < 35.5° C; (3) white blood cell count > 10,000/mm^3 or < 4,000/mm^3. The aetiological diagnosis of VAP was made using a quantitative endotracheal aspiration method. All cultures were incubated at 37°C under aerobic and anaerobic conditions. Cultures were evaluated for growth at 24 and 48 h and discarded if negative 5 days after. The threshold of 105 cfu/ml of bacterial cultures was used to distinguish colonization from true infection. All micro-organisms isolated were identified by standard laboratory methods.

We compared the following data: age, SAPS II, length of MV (VAM), LOS, ICU, and hospital mortality; moreover, we analysed the incidence and the microbiological characteristics of VAP. Comparison of parameters was performed using Student's t-test ($P<0.05$).

A total of 449 patients in the first period and 308 in the second period were admitted to the ICU. The patients who had a LOS > 48 h numbered 272 (60.5%) (158 men and 114 women) and 190 (61.6%) (136 men and 54 women), respectively. No differences were found regarding age (63.2± 14.5 vs. 66.5±16.4, NS), SAPS II (35.8±10.5 vs. 37.3±14.5, NS), and LOS (11.9±12.4 vs. 10.6±14.4 days, NS). Ventilated patients numbered 221 (81.2%) in the first period and 174 (91.5%) in the second period. The incidence of VAP in these patients was 7.2% versus 4%; length of VAM was similar between the two groups (8 ±10 vs. 7.1±15.1 days, NS). ICU and hospital mortality was 10.6% vs. 10% and 13.5% vs. 14%, respectively. The following bacterial pathogenic agents were identified: Gram-positive cocci (16.6% vs. 16%), *Pseudomonas aeruginosa* (27.7% vs. 50%), other non-fermenting Gram-negative bacilli (GNB) (11.1% vs. 0%), *Enterobacteriaceae* (27.7% vs. 16.6%), and fungi (16.6% vs. 16.6%).

The overall incidence of VAP was reduced during the observational periods, without any variation in the management of ventilated patients, except antibiotic therapy. We observed a reduction of GNB isolations, while Gram-positive cocci and fungi were unchanged. According to other studies, third-generation cephalosporins were associated with emergence of resistance to β-lactamases among *Enterobacter* and extended-spectrum β-lactamases among *Enterobacteriaceae*. These resistance trends could be curtailed by switching from cephalosporins to β-lactam/β-lactamase inhibitors [44]. The increase of VAP caused by typical Gram-negative bacteria with drug resistance such as *Pseudomonas aeruginosa* during second period of observation could be determined by the greater incidence of burned patients.

Conclusions

VAP is the most-common ICU-acquired infection. According to the literature, its prevalence varies from 6% to 52%, depending on the studied population. The mortality rate for VAP is still high, ranging from 25% to 50%, and even higher in specific settings or when caused by high-risk pathogens.

Independent risk factors and high-risk patients are identified by multivariate analysis. This may contribute to elaboration of effective preventive strategies, by indicating which patients might be most likely to benefit from prophylaxis against pneumonia. Based on efficacy and cost-effectiveness in clinical studies and local experience, we can conclude that avoidance of continuous sedation, correct airway management, and antibiotic therapy seem to be the most-important recommendations to prevent insurgence of VAP in ICU patients. VAP should be treated in accordance with guidelines that are customized according to local epidemiology, microbiology and pattern of resistance studies.

References

1. Vincent JL, Bihari D, Suter P (1995) The prevalence of nosocomial infection in intensive care units in Europe. EPIC study. JAMA 274:639-644
2. Chastre J, Fagon JY (1998) Ventilator-associated pneumonia. In: Hall JB, Schmidt GA, Wood LDH (eds) Principles of critical care. McGraw-Hill, New York, pp 617-652
3. Cook D (2000) Ventilator-associated pneumonia: perspectives on the burden of illness. Intensive Care Med 26:S31-S37
4. Rello J, Valles J (1998) Mortality as an outcome of hospital-acquired pneumonia. Infect Control Hosp Epidemiol 19:795-797
5. Fagon JY, Castre J, Vuagnat A, et al (1996) Nosocomial pneumonia and mortality among patients in intensive care units. JAMA 275:866-869
6. Heyland DK, Cook DJ, Griffith L, et al (1999) The attributable morbidity and mortality of ventilator-associated pneumonia in the critically ill patient: the Canadian Critical Trials Group. Am J Respir Crit Care 159:1249-1256
7. Craven DE, Steger KA (1995) Epidemiology of nosocomial pneumonia: new perspective on an old disease. Chest 108:S1-S16
8. Chastre J, Fagon JY (2002) Ventilator-associated pneumonia. State of the art. Am J Respir Crit Care Med 165:867-903
9. Cunnion KM, Weber DJ, Broadehad WE, et al (1996) Risk factors for nosocomial pneumonia: comparing adult critical care populations. Am J Respir Crit Care Med 153:158-162
10. Craven DE, Kunches LM, Killinsky V, et al (1986) Risk factors for nosocomial pneumonia and fatality in patients receiving continuous mechanical ventilation. Am Rev Respir Dis 133: 792-796
11. Torres A, Gatell JL, Aznar E, et al (1995) Re-intubation increases the risk of nosocomial pneumonia in patients needing mechanical ventilation. Am J Respir Crit Care Med 152:137-141
12. Rello J, Diaz E, Roque M, Valles J (1999) Risk factors for developing pneumonia within 48 hours of intubation. Am J Respir Crit Care Med 159:1742-1746
13. Nair P, Jani K, Sanderson PJ (1985) Transfer of oropharyngeal bacterial into the trachea during endotracheal intubation. J Hosp Infect 8:96-103

14. Kress JP, Anne SP, O'Connor MF, et al (2000) Daily interruption of sedative infusions in critically ill patients undergoing mechanical ventilation. N Engl J Med 342:1471-1477

15. Ibrahim EH, Tracy L, Hill C, et al (2001) The occurrence of ventilator associated pneumonia in the community hospital. Risk factors and clinical outcomes. Chest 120:555-561

16. Georges H, Leroy O, Guery B, et al (2000) Predisposing factors for nosocomial pneumonia in patients receiving mechanical ventilation and requiring tracheotomy. Chest 118:767-774

17. Ibrahim EH, Ward S, Sherman G, et al (2000) A comparative analysis of patients with early-onset vs late-onset nosocomial pneumonia in the ICU setting. Chest 117:1434-1442

18. Rouby JJ, Laurent P, Gosnach M, et al (1994) Risk factors and clinical relevance of nococomial maxillary sinusitis in the critically ill. Am J Respir Crit Care Med 150:776-783

19. Kollef MH (1999) The prevention of ventilator associated pneumonia. N Engl J Med 340: 627-634

20. Heyland DK, Drover JW, MacDonald S, et al (2001) Effect of postpyloric feeding on gastroesophageal regurgitation and pulmonary microaspiration: results of a randomised controlled trial. Crit Care Med 29:1495-1501

21. Tryba M (1991) Sucralfate versus antacids or H_2-antagonists for stress ulcer prophylaxis: a meta-analysis on efficacy and pneumonia rate. Crit Care Med 13:S44-S55

22. Dennesen PJW, Wan Der Ven A, Kessels GH, et al (2001) Resolution of infectious parameters after antimicrobial therapy in patients with ventilator associated pneumonia. Am J Respir Crit Care Med 163:1371-1375

23. Niederman MS, Torres A, Summer W, et al (1994) Invasive diagnostic testing is not needed routinely to manage suspected ventilator-associated pneumonia. Am J Respir Crit Care Med 150: 565-569

24. Chastre J, Fagon JY (1994) Invasive diagnostic testing should be routinely used to manage ventilated patients with suspected pneumonia. Am J Respir Crit Care Med 150:570-574

25. Chien LW, Dine IY, Nai YW, et al (2002) Quantitative culture of endotracheal aspirates in the diagnosis of ventilator associated pneumonia in patients with treatment failure. Chest 122: 662-668

26. Doebbeling BN, Stanley GL, Sheetz CT, et al (1992) Comparative efficacy of alternative hand-washing agents in reducing nosocomial infections in intensive care unit. N Engl J Med 327:88-93

27. Nourdine K, Combes P, Carlton MJ, et al (1999) Does noninvasive ventilation reduce the ICU nosocomial infection risk? A prospective clinical survey. Intensive Care Med 25:567-573

28. Girault C, Daudenthun I, Chevron V, et al (1999) Noninvasive ventilation as a systematic extubation and weaning technique in acute-on-chronic respiratory failure. A prospective, randomised controlled study. Am J Respir Crit Care Med 160:86-92

29. King D, Morrell A (1992) A survey of manual hyperinflation as a physiotherapy technique in intensive care units. Physiotherapy 78:747-750

30. Sirvent JM, Torres A, El-Ebiary M, et al (1997) Protective effect of intravenously administered cefuroxime against nosocomial in patients with structural coma. Am J Respir Crit Care Med 155: 1729-1734

31. Dupont H, Mentec H, Sollet JP, et al (2001) Impact of appropriateness of initial antibiotic therapy on the outcome of ventilator associated pneumonia. Intensive Care Med 27:355-362

32. Kollef MH, Vlasnik J, Sharless L et al (1997) Scheduled change of antibiotic classes. Am J Respir Crit Care Med 156:1040-1048

33. Zwalling JH, Maring JK, Klompmaker IJ, et al (2002) Selective decontamination of the digestive tract to prevent post-operative infection. A randomised placebo-controlled trial in liver transplant patients. Crit Care Med 30:1204-1209

34. Bergmans DCJJ, Bonten MJM, Gailard CA, et al (2001) Prevention of ventilator associated pneumonia by oral decontamination: a prospective, randomised double blind, placebo controlled study. Am J Respir Crit Care Med 164:382-388

35. Pittet D, Eggimann P, Rubinovitch B (2001) Prevention of ventilator associated pneumonia by

oral decontamination. Just another SDD study? Am J Respir Crit Care Med 164:338-339

36. Kollef MH, Nikolaos JS, Thoralf MS (1999) A randomised clinic trial of intermittent subglottic secretion drainage in cardiac surgery patients. Chest 116:1339-1346
37. Smulders K, Van Der Hoeven H, Weers-Pothoff I, et al (2002) A randomised clinic trial of intermittent subglottic secretion drainage in patients receiving mechanical ventilation. Chest 121: 858-862
38. Adair CG, Gorman SP, Feron BM, et al (1999) Implications of endotracheal tube biofilm for ventilator associated pneumonia. Intensive Care Med 25:1072-1076
39. Drakulovic MB, Torres A, Bauer T, et al (1999) Supine body position as a risk factor for nosocomial pneumonia in mechanically ventilated patients: a randomised trial. Lancet 354: 1851-1858
40. Kollef MH (1998) Prolonged use of ventilator circuits and ventilator-associated pneumonia: a model for identifying the optimal clinical practice. Chest 113:267-269
41. Kirton OC, deHaven B, Morgan J, et al (1997) A prospective randomised comparison of an in-line heat moisture exchange filter and heat wire humidifiers; rates of ventilator early-onset (community-acquired) or late-onset (hospital acquired) pneumonia and incidence of endotracheal tube occlusion. Chest 112:1055-1059
42. Ntoumenopoulos G, Presneill JJ, McElholum M, et al (2002) Chest physiotherapy for prevention of ventilator-associated pneumonia. Intensive Care Med 28:850-856
43. Hall JC, Tarala J, Tapper J, et al (1996) Prevention of respiratory complications after abdominal surgery: a randomised clinical trial. BMJ 312:148-152
44. Rice LB, Eckstein EC, DeVene J (1996) Ceftazidime-resistant *Klebsiella pneumonia* isolated recovered at the Cleveland Department of Veterans Affair medical Center. Clin Infect Dis 23: 118-124

Surgical treatment of end-stage emphysema

E. COHEN

Emphysematous changes are common in the general population, occasionally resulting in pneumothoraces; a significant number of these patients require surgical intervention. Many procedures have been performed to alleviate the dyspnoea in the severely emphysmatosy patient, some with beneficial effects but others without any proven beneficial outcome (Table 1). Recently, laser and videoscopic technology have been used to ablate small bullae [1-3].

Table 1 Procedure attempted to improve lung function in end-stage emphysema

Unproven efficacy	Proven efficacy
Costochondrectomy	Transtracheal oxygen catheter
Transverse sternotomy	Tracheostomy
Thoracoplasty	Needle aspiration of bullae
Phrenic nerve resection	Tube thoracostomy
Pneumoperitoneum	Bullectomy
Abdominal belting	Lung volume reduction
Talc pleurodesis	Lung transplant
Sympathectomy	
Vagotomy	

In 1959, Brantigan et al. [4], from the University of Maryland, reported on the surgical management of diffuse emphysema. "In patients with distended lungs caused by severe COPD, the normal outward circumferential pull on the bronchioles had been lost, causing their collapse during expiration. Reducing overall lung volume, by means of multiple wedge excisions or plications, would restore the elastic pull on the small airways and reduce expiratory airway obstruction" [4].

He suggested that in these patients with severe dyspnoea, a distended chest, and flattened diaphragms, surgical excision of functionless, but non-bullae area by multiple wedge resection can relief the dyspnoea.

Lung volume reduction surgery (LVRS) should not be confused with excision of bullus emphysema or with giant bullae. In these cases the presumed mechanism of improvement in lung function, exercise tolerance, and oxygenation is secondary to re-expansion of more-normal, underlying compressed lung [5].

The Brantigan procedure did not receive wide recognition. In the absence of an automated stapler, surgery was performed with a hand-sutured line of resection, which resulted in a high incidence of persistent airleak and a 18%--20% mortality. The procedure was resurrected by Cooper et al. [6], following their experience with lung transplantation in patients with severe emphysema. One issue was the optimal size of donor lungs for emphysematous recipients. The total lung capacity (TLC) of the recipient is much larger than the donor lung if the lung will not fill the recipient chest, complications such as prolonged air leak, pleural effusion will persist. To their surprise, "the distended thorax and the flattened diaphragms in the recipient immediately assumed a more--normal configuration postoperatively". This ability of the chronically distended chest to configure to a smaller volume gave credence to the notion that downsizing the lungs in an emphysematous patient might improve respiratory mechanics by alleviating the overdistension. At the same time, new technologies (lasers and thoracoscopes), and modern suturing, stapling, and buttressing materials have been developed. "We have developed a technique using strips of bovine pericardium to reinforce lung staple lines, prevent air leakage, which otherwise can occur at the staple holes when the lung is reinflated. This technique has significantly reduced the incidence and the duration of postoperative air leakage."

The NETT study

LVRS rapidly gained popularity [7-9]. Because of the possible dramatic increase in the numbers of such procedure without sufficient evidence of beneficial outcome, the US National Institutes Agency (HCFA) concluded in 1995 that, "although initial results were promising, LVRS was often being performed with insufficient evaluation and a randomized study should be undertaken to evaluate the procedure critically". [10] The National Emphysema Treatment Trial (NETT) was established as a randomized multicentre prospective clinical trial of medical versus surgical therapy plus LVRS for treatment of patients with severe bilateral emphysema. In addition, comparison of the surgical approach, sternal split versus bilateral video-assisted thoracoscopy, would be performed. Approximately 5,000 patients needed to be included in the trial with the primary outcome as survival [11]. The other parameters to be evaluated are the maximum exercise capacity, pulmonary function, and oxygen requirement /distance for walking for 6 min, quality of life, and costs. The main issues that need to be established are: which patients will benefit from the procedure, what is the best surgical approach, median sternotomy or bilateral video-assisted thoracoscopies, the cost effectiveness, and finally, the utility as an alternative or more likely as a bridge to lung transplantation.

The NETT study proposes following the patients for 5 years. Although the complete results of the NETT study are unknown yet; the research group published in the *New England Journal of Medicine* in October 2001 a preliminary report with the title "Patients at high risk of death after lung-volume – reduction surgery" [12]. That report recommended not performing surgery on very sick patients with emphysema. Of 1,033 patients enrolled so far, 69 patients have forced expiratory volume in 1 s (FVE1) less than 20% of their predicted, with homogeneous distribution of the emphysema, and the carbon dioxide diffusing capacity less than 20% of the predicted value. The 30-day mortality following surgery was 16% compared with 0% mortality among 70 medically treated patients (0.43 deaths per person-year vs. 0.11 deaths per year-person in the medical group). Figure 1 indicates that the operation harms some patients and does not benefit those who survive. Thus, patients who meet these criteria are no longer candidates for surgery in the NETT study.

In an editorial, Dr. Jeffry Drazen, the editor in chief of the *New England Journal of Medicine*, agrees "At this time, it does not make sense to use lung-volume – reduction surgery in patients whose emphysema is so severe that they meet these exclusion criteria." However, one questions whose answer must await the completion of the trial. It is possible that the patients with severe emphysema who survived the surgery will do better during long-term follow-up than short-term follow-up or patients who received medial therapy [13]. Unfortunately the final conclusion of the clinical trial and the outcome will not be available for several years.

Outcome of LVRS

Although the outcome of the randomized NETT study is not yet known, there is evidence of beneficial effects of LVRS, at least in the short term. It is beyond the scope of this chapter to review all the published data on LVRS and the reader can refer to several excellent reviews of the subject [11, 24, 25]. In brief,

Brenner et al. [14], in 256 consecutive LVRS cases reported 85% survival at 1
year and 81% at 2 years. There is evidence, however, that the initial improvement in FEV1, as an indicator of pulmonary function and improvement in
airflow, peaks at 6 months and than there is a subsequent deterioration.
However, Gelb et al. [15] found that 2 years after LVRS relief of dyspnoea
remained improved in 11 of 12 patients with reduction in TLC as a result of
reduction of residual volume and air trapping [15].

Tschernko et al. [16, 17] studied the changes in ventilatory mechanics in 12
patients after LVRS. Measurements of work of breathing (WOB), intrinsic
positive end-expiatory pressure (PEEPi), dynamic compliance (Cdyn), and
mean airway resistance (Rawm) were performed the day before surgery, early
postoperatively, and 1 and 3 months after surgery. All measurements were
performed on tracheally extubated patients, simultaneously assessing esophageal pressure via esophageal balloon catheter and air flow via tightly adjusted
mask. Standard spirometry was assessed preoperatively and 1 and 3 months
postoperatively. The patients presented with FEV1 of 670±50 ml and pathological values of WOB and PEEPi. Immediately thereafter, a marked and sustained decrease in WOB, PEEPi, and Rawm was noted, as well as an increase in
Cdyn (Fig. 2). Ventilatory mechanics improved immediately after LVRS,

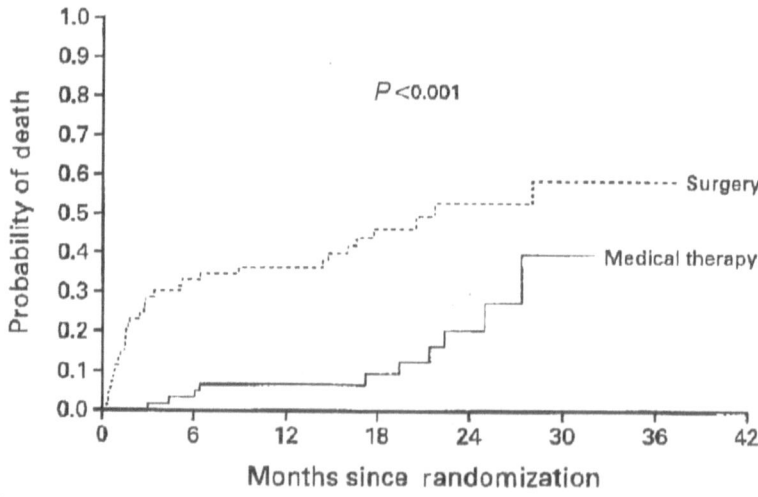

Fig. 1 Probability of death after lung volume reduction. Surgical group versus medically treated
group (modified from [12])

probably due to decompression of lung tissue, thereby enabling successful tracheal extubation.

Patient selection

The inclusion and exclusion criteria are summarized in Table 2. Indications for good outcome are age below 75 years, FEV1 greater that 0.5 l, PaO_2 above 55 mmHg, CO_2: 40-45 mmHg (greater than 50 is of concern).

FEV1 15%-20% is less useful as a predictor of postoperative respiratory support in lung volume reduction.

Body plethysmography (BP) versus inert gas technique (IG) will provide some information on the degree of trapped gas in the emphysematous lung with an index of: Trapped gas= IG/BP.

Ventilation/perfusion scan: The ideal candidate will present with 30-40% reduces perfusion (upper lobes). In case of Alpha1-antitrypsin deficiency: the reduce perfusion will be evident at the lower lobes. The least favourable

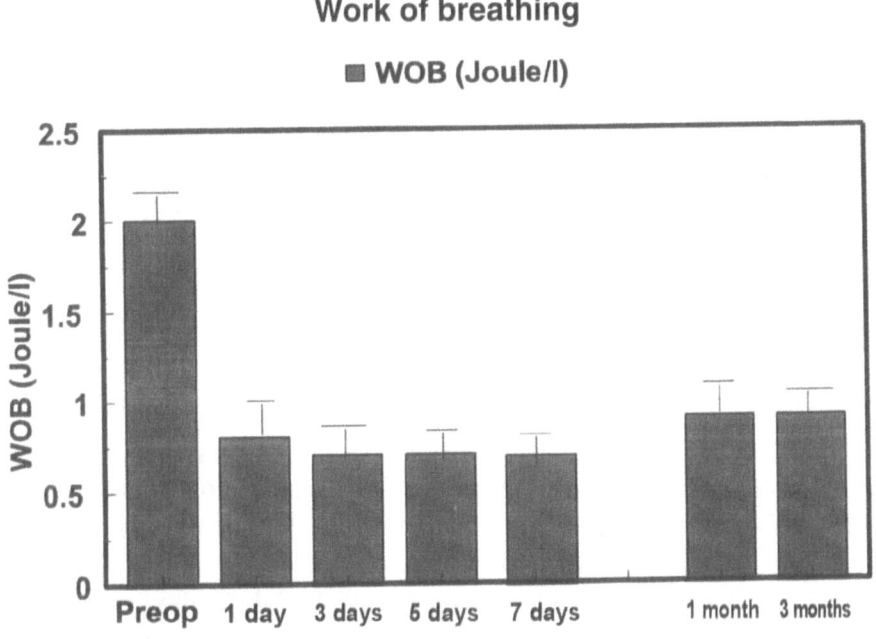

Fig. 2 Work of breathing (*WOB*) before and after surgery for lung volume reduction Tschernko et al. Analg Anaesth 83 990-1001 (1996)

Table 2. Criteria for patient selection

Patient selection
    Progressive emphysema
    Severe, symptomatic dyspnoea
    Radiographic evidence of diffuse emphysema
    Identifiable distention and hyperinflated lung tissue
    $FEV1 < 40\%$, $RV > 150\%$, $TLC > 120\%$ predicted
    No previous chest surgery
    Smoking cessation
    Acceptable cardiac function

Contraindication
    Age> 75 y
    Uniformly destroyed lungs
        $FEV1 < 15\%$
        $PaCO2 > 55mmHg$
        $O2 > 6\,L/min$
    Pulmonary Hypertension
    Sever kyphoscoliosis
    Predominance of chronic bronchitis, asthma
    Active infection
    Inability to complete preop rehabilitation program

---

candidates by scanning are those with patchy, mottled pattern, uniformly affecting the lung [18]. Finally, for the patients to maintain gas exchange they need considerable energy reserves. Adequate nutritional status is seen as an important part of the rehabilitation programs to which many institutions subject potential lung transplant recipients and those undergoing lung volume reduction. These patients have a reduced level of physical activity and muscular weakness (deconditioning). They should be placed on a reconditioning exercise program to build up their muscle mass with 6-10 weeks. The goal for acceptable physical activities is 30 min treadmill at 1 mile/h.

Anaesthetic management

Bronchodilator therapy should continue until the morning of surgery. Some will prefer morphine and atropine premedication, as the antisialogogue to facilitate insertion of bronchoscopes and tracheal intubation. Steroids and other bronchodilators have been commonly used.

Pain relief must be optimal as soon as possible, as it enables early tracheal extubation, and early mobilization is crucial to the recovery of patients undergoing lung volume reduction [19]. Thoracic epidural catheter is best placed prior to induction of anaesthesia in the sitting position at the T3–4 level. The most commonly used medications via the epidural catheter are opioid and low-dose bupivacaine combinations, often with a patient-controlled analgesia mode. In some cases of technical difficulty in placing the thoracic catheter, the doses of medication should be increased for effective analgesia [20].

During induction of anaesthesia an increase in an intrathoracic pressure following muscle relaxation should be avoided. These patients are intravascularly depleted, with a wasted muscle mass. The commonly present polycythaemia may give a false impression of adequate hydration. Therefore hydration and stable haemodynamic induction with agents such as etomidate, and gentle ventilation may attenuate the increase in intrathoracic pressure and the degree of hypotension. Patients who have undergone surgery for emphysematous conditions are safest breathing spontaneously as rapidly as possible after the procedure, and the trachea should be extubated as early as possible. Short-acting neuromuscular blocking agents are indicated. Rocuronuim, atracurium, vecuronium, fentanyl and remifentanyl infusion, and propofol are the current agents of choice [21, 22].

One lung ventilation is mandatory, whether the procedure is performed via sternal split or bilateral thoracoscopy [23]. The author (Cohen) prefers the use of a double-lumen tracheal tube to a Univent for complete reliable isolation and rapid lung deflation. However, whichever tube has been used, in these patients with a marginal respiratory reserve, perfect isolation and conformation with fiberoptic bronchoscopy is mandatory (Tables 3, 4). At the conclusion of the procedure, the trachea should be extubated in the operating room. Because these patients have marginal respiratory reserve, it is essential to use light anaesthesia, such as remifentanyl and propofol infusion. In the PACU it is important to recognize the early signs of tension pneumothorax and dynamic hyperinflation as possible complications. The most-important issues to bear in mind at the conclusion of the procedure are that the lungs are NOT being replaced. The anticipated improvement is NOT immediate, and the most-common complication is prolonged continuous airleak (Table 5). Adequate analgesia, chest physiotherapy, spirometry, and early ambulation are all important for a successful outcome.

Table 3 Anaesthetic management: induction (*CVP* central venous pressure)

Lung volume reduction

Premedication (light/none)
Thoracic epidural (optimally placed)
Monitoring (A-Line, CVP)

Induction

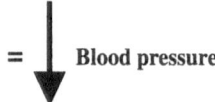 **Blood pressure**

Hydration prior to induction (CVP changes)
Ventilation: low peak airway pressure
Vasopressors (stable haemodynamic)
(avoid fluid overload)
Short induction to incision time
Etomidate/propofol induction
Rapid muscle relaxation
Chest tube available
Maintenance: remifentanyl /propofol

Table 4 Anaesthetic management: intubation and intraoperative management (*DLT* double-lumen tracheal tube, *OR* operating room)

Lung volume reduction
Intubation
DLT not Univent
Easy to switch ventilation between the two lungs
Frequent manipulation may cause desaturation
Easy to deflate the operative lung
Fiberoptic bronchoscopy is not absolutely necessary with a DLT

DLT or Univent MUST be optimally positioned!

Postoperative
Postoperative mechanical ventilation is undesirable

Patients should be extubated at the end of the surgery
Emergence should be smooth
Fluid overload or hypovolaemia may affect outcome
Long-lasting narcotics/anaesthetics may affect outcome
Pain management should start in the OR
            (bupivacaine 0.5% intraoperatively)
            (bupivacaine 0.25% postoperatively)

Table 5 Postoperative complications

Lung volume reduction

Conclusion

The lungs are NOT being replaced
The anticipated improvement is NOT immediate
Postoperative air leak is of prime concern
Postoperative mechanical ventilation is undesirable
Sensitive to increase intrathoracic pressure
Marginal respiratory reserve: intraoperative long-lasting narcotic should be avoided
Propofol, remifentany 1 for optimal maintenance

Hospital complications (100 patients)

Re-exploration	
Bleeding	3
Air leak	4
Space problems	1
Phrenic nerve palsy	2
Prolonged air leak (>7 days)	46
Reintubation	3
Tracheostomy	4
Pneumonia	9
Wound infection	1
Gastrointestinal perforation	2

References

1. Conacher D (1997) Lung volume reduction. Br J Anaesth 79:530-538
2. Mets B (2000) Current status of lung volume reduction. Curr Opin Anaesthesiol 13:61-64
3. Argenziano M, Moazami N, Thomashow B, et al (1996) Extended indications for lung volume reduction surgery in advanced emphysema. Ann Thorac Surg 62:1588-1597
4. Brantigan OC, Mueller E, Kress MB (1959) A surgical approach to pulmonary emphysema. Am Rev Respir Dis 80:194-202
5. Cohen E, Kirshner PA, Benumof JL (1990) Case conference. Anesthesia for bullectomy. J Cardiothorac Anesth 4:119-126
6. Cooper JD, Trulock EP, Triantifillou AN, et al (1995) Bilateral pneumonectomy (volume reduction) for chronic obstructive pulmonary disease. J Thorac Cardiovas Surg 109:106-119
7. Benfield JR, Cree E, Pellet JR, et al (1966) Current approach to the surgical management of emphysema. Arch Surg 93:59-70
8. Davies L, Calverley PMA (1996) Lung volume reduction surgery in chronic obstructive pulmonary disease. Thorax 51 [Suppl 2]:S29-S34
9. Deslauriers J (1996) History of surgery for emphysema. Semin Thorac Cardiovas Surg 8:43-51
10. The National Emphysema Treatment trail Research Group (1999) Rationale and design of The National Emphysema Treatment Trial: a prospective randomized trial of lung volume reduction surgery Chest 116:1750-1761
11. Fessler HE, Wiss RA (1999) Lung volume reduction surgery: is less really more? Am J Respir Criti Care Med 159:1031-1038
12. National Emphysema Treatment Trial Group (2001) Patients at high risk of death after lung-volume reduction surgery. N Engl J Med 345:1075-1083

13. Drazen MJ (2001) Surgery for emphysema - not for everyone (editorial). N Engl J Med 345:1075-1083

14. Brenner M, McKenna RJ, Chan K, et al (1999) Survival following bilateral staple lung volume reduction surgery for emphysema. Chest 118:390-396

15. Gelb AF, Brenner M, McKenna RJ, et al (1998) Serial lung function and elastic recoil 2 years after lung volume reduction surgery for emphysema. Chest 113:1497-1506

16. Tschernko EM, Wisser W, Hofer S, et al (1996) The influence of lung volume reduction surgery on ventilatory mechanics in patients suffering from severe chronic obstructive pulmonary disease. Anesth Analg 83:996-1001

17. Tschernko EM, Wisser W, Wanke T, et al (1997) Changes in ventilatory mechanics and diaphragmatic function after lung volume reduction surgery in patients with COPD. Thorax 52:545-550

18. Gaissert HA, Trulock EP, Cooper JD, et al (1996) Comparison of early functional results after volume reduction or lung transplantation for chronic obstructive pulmonary disease. J Thorac Cardiovas Surg 111:296-307

19. Triantafillou AN (1996) Anesthetic management for bilateral volume reduction surgery. Semin Thorac Cardiovas Surg 8:94-98

20. Hurford WE, Dutton RP, Alfille PH, et al (1993) Comparison of thoracic and lumbar epidural infusions of bupivacaine and fentanyl for post-thoracotomy analgesia. J Cardiothorac Vasc Anesth 5:521-525

21. Krucylak PE, Naunheim KS, Keller CA, Baudendistal LJ (1995) Anesthetic management of patients undergoing thoracoscopic lung reduction for treatment of end-stage emphysema. Anesth Analg 80:SCA80

22. Bussières JS (1995) Anesthesia for patients undergoing surgery for emphysema. Chest Surg Clin N Am 5:869-878

23. Wakabayashi A (1993) Thoracoscopic techniques for management of giant bullous disease. Ann Thorac Surg 56:708-712

Discontinuing mechanical ventilation: the role of a "respiratory acute care unit"

L.M. Bigatello, E. Gettings

The timing of discontinuing mechanical ventilation is important. Premature extubation of the trachea may lead to catastrophic complications such as the failure to re-establish an airway. More frequently, inability to sustain spontaneous ventilation manifests itself within 12 - 72 h and may be associated with hypoxemia, CO_2 narcosis, haemodynamic instability, and aspiration of gastric contents. Conversely, unnecessary prolongation of mechanical ventilation is associated with an increased chance of development of nosocomial pneumonia and of laryngeal damage. Hence, the appropriate timing of tracheal extubation is the subject of debate both at the patient's bedside and in a number of clinical investigations.

In the present review, we will first examine some of the studies looking at strategies of weaning from mechanical ventilation. We will then look at the problem of the patient with prolonged acute respiratory failure (ARF), its principal physiological issues, possible treatment approaches, and the use of a dedicated respiratory acute care unit.

Controlled studies of discontinuing mechanical ventilation

Only two clinical studies have compared different strategies of withdrawal of mechanical ventilation in a controlled fashion and with adequate numbers of patients [1, 2]. These studies have been discussed at a number of international meetings and in published reviews [3, 4]. We will use them as a springboard for discussion of the problem of the difficult-to-wean patient.

Esteban et al. [1] compared the efficacy of four different weaning strategies: (1) full support with assist-control ventilation (ACV) plus daily trials of spontaneous breathing (SBTs); (2) full support with ACV and multiple SBTs; (3) progressive withdrawal of pressure support ventilation (PSV); (4) progressive withdrawal of intermittent mandatory ventilation (IMV). They randomly assigned to these treatment groups 130 patients with ARF of mixed aetiology (of 546 patients enrolled) who failed an initial SBT. They found that full support with one or more SBTs was equally superior to progressive withdrawal of PSV and of IMV.

Brochard et al. [2] compared the efficacy of three weaning strategies: (1) full support with ACV and increasingly longer SBTs; (2) progressive withdrawal of PSV; and (3) progressive withdrawal of IMV. Similar to the previous study, they randomly assigned to these treatment groups 109 patients with ARF of mixed aetiology (of 456 patients enrolled) who failed an initial SBT. They found that progressive withdrawal of PSV was slightly superior to ACV with SBTs and to progressive withdrawal of IMV.

Table 1 Baseline patient characteristics of the two studies. Numbers represent approximate values, taken from the average values reported in the original papers (*MV* mechanical ventilation, *MIP* maximum inspiratory pressure, *COPD* chronic obstructive pulmonary disease)

	Esteban et al. [1]	Brochard et al. [2]
COPD	40%	30%
Days of MV prior to study	8	14
Days of MV during study	4	7
MIP (cmH$_2$O)	30	40
Tidal volume (ml)	450	370
Minute ventilation (l/min)	12	11.5

These two studies have to be commended because of their size and their controlled design. However, they have several shortcomings that limit their clinical utility. *First*, they examined **patient populations with good weaning potential**, as suggested by their relatively low prevalence of patients with chronic obstructive pulmonary disease (COPD), short duration of mechanical ventilation, and reasonably preserved respiratory mechanics (Table 1). *Second*, they provided surprisingly **scant physiological and clinical information** on their patients, two elements that clinicians would certainly want to consider when deciding which weaning strategy to apply. For example, basic respiratory mechanics such as compliance, resistance, and auto-positive end-expiratory pressure (PEEP) are important determinants of the patient's ability to sustain spontaneous breathing and can be measured at the bedside with reasonable accuracy [5]. Also, their interpretation of the results, albeit statistically correct, is somewhat "liberal." Both studies report the differences among study treatments in terms of "relative risk," which yields a "relative probability of successful weaning over time" [1, 2]. The abstract of Esteban's study states that "a once-daily SBT led to extubation about three times more quickly than IMV and about twice as quickly as PSV." This is not what one would think just by looking at the actual number of days spent on the ventilator: 3 (1 - 6) days by the two SBTs groups, 4 (2 - 12) by the PSV group, and 5 (3 - 11) by the IMV group, hardly "a threefold difference"! [1]

Clinical experience of discontinuing mechanical ventilation

As an addition to the results of these two trials, we propose the following approach. Most patients who receive mechanical ventilation for 24 h wean within a few days. For these patients, the weaning strategy may affect the duration of mechanical ventilation, although probably not in the way suggested by the two studies, which yielded opposite results [1, 2]. Esteban et al. [1] have long been promoters of the use of SBTs. In their experienced hands, SBTs with **ACV** [1] and also with PSV [6] have been the best weaning strategy. Brochard et al. [2] have been among the first to master the use of **PSV** [7]. In their hands, progressive withdrawal of PSV worked best [2]. Both studies agreed that progressive withdrawal of IMV was not effective, in line with earlier physiological studies [8]. It is probably fair to conclude that **multiple factors affect the ability to discontinue mechanical ventilation in short-term (a week to 10 days), relatively healthy mechanically ventilated patients, including the mode of ventilation used.**

A fraction of patients who receive mechanical ventilation for > 24 h remain ventilated for several weeks, generally because: (1) their lung injury is exceptionally severe; (2) they have debilitating chronic lung disease; (3) they have significant concomitant disease, most commonly cardiac and neurological. These patients are difficult to wean from mechanical ventilation. We propose that in these patients the mode of ventilation used is of secondary importance. **Rather, understanding of their physiology and treating their underlying diseases are key.** We present two cases that will illustrate these points.

Case 1

A 74-year-old woman underwent elective repair of a type-II thoraco-abdominal aneurysm in August 2001. She has a history of hypertension, coronary artery disease, and COPD. The extent of her pre-existent cardiovascular and respiratory compromise was likely underestimated preoperatively. Her intraoperative and immediate postoperative course were unremarkable, but she failed tracheal extubation from a combination of abundant bronchial secretions and general debilitation. She received a tracheostomy on postoperative day 10 and was thereafter sent to the general ward to complete withdrawal of ventilatory support. She continued to have the same problems and was eventually admitted to our respiratory acute care unit approximately 3 weeks following an otherwise successful surgery. She remained in our unit for an additional 2 months. Her prolonged ventilatory dependence was determined by several factors.

1. Repeated respiratory infections (nosocomial pneumonia, tracheo-bronchitis) and colonization with multiresistant Gram-negative flora.
2. Persistently increased airway resistance secondary to expiratory flow limitation and airway secretions, and associated with hyperinflation and frequent spells of acute bronchospasm.
3. Recurrent episodes of myocardial ischaemia, reproducibly associated with any increase of the heart rate above 70 - 80 beats per min, often triggered by attempts to decrease ventilatory support. A coronary angiogram confirmed the presence of severe coronary disease.
4. Severe systemic hypertension.
5. Generalized weakness, possibly left diaphragmatic dysfunction secondary to the surgical transection and repair of the diaphragm.
6. Recurrent episodes of acute tubular necrosis, precipitated by aminoglycoside antibiotics and by our attempts of diuresis.
7. Severe depression, delirium, agitation, and suicidal ideation.

Her pharmacopaeia was huge, requiring constant adjustments including courses of systemic corticosteroids, nebulized aminoglycoside antibiotics, multiple anti-hypertensives, aggressive β-blockade despite her bronchospasm, anti-delirium and anxiolysis to promote night rest, etc. She required frequent bronchoscopies to promote secretion clearance and lung re-expansion. Eventually, her respiratory infections cleared, her airway resistance decreased to tolerable levels, and her myocardial ischaemia became under control. She started to gain strength and mental lucidity. She was sent to a rehabilitation facility on hospital day 92 and remained free of mechanical ventilation. During her 3- -month postoperative course, she was ventilated with PSV, pressure and volume-limited ACV, with added "sighs" at times, and a variety of levels of PEEP. The ventilatory settings were always chosen on the basis of her current clinical situation, daily bedside measurements of respiratory mechanics, and subjective comfort.

Case 2

A 62-year-old woman underwent right thoracotomy and upper lobectomy for cancer in March 2002. She is a former smoker and has mild COPD. She also has hypothyroidism, hypertension, and non-bypassed coronary artery disease. She has tongue cancer, treated 1 year previously with chemo- and radiotherapy, which resulted in scarring of the floor of the mouth and inability to take solid food.

She was extubated at the end of surgery. Over the next 48-72 h her systemic blood pressure became difficult to control and she developed myocardial ischaemia. She was admitted to the coronary care unit, where she required tracheal intubation. Her ischaemia was eventually controlled and she never showed signs of infarction. However, she developed a nosocomial pneumonia of the right middle and lower lobe and she went on to require a tracheostomy and prolonged ventilatory support. She was admitted to the respiratory acute care unit at the beginning of May, ventilated with a moderate amount of PSV and PEEP. She failed a SBT on admission, probably from a combination of the following.

1. Poor nutritional status, likely pre-existing and related to her cancer of the mouth.
2. Hypothyroidism. Despite continuing her chronic thyroid replacement perioperatively, her thyroid-stimulating hormone was elevated and thyroxine was low. She appeared tired, somnolent, and very anxious.
3. Labile haemodynamics. Although she never developed obvious myocardial ischaemia in our unit, she frequently had labile haemodynamics, particularly at night, and her heart rate was low. She required frequent adjustment of her anti-hypertensives and of her β-blockade.
4. Her compliance of the respiratory system was 30 ml/cmH$_2$O and her resistance only slightly elevated. Her spontaneous minute ventilation was low, particularly at night, when she required a mandatory support as ACV or IMV.
5. Chest computed tomography (CT) was performed and is shown in Fig. 1. It showed massive consolidation of the two remaining right lobes and a substantial pleural effusion on the left, with collapse of the left lower lobe. It comes as no surprise that the patient was not weaning from the ventilator.

At this time, it was elected to continue a stable support without SBTs, using PSV with added "sighs" to promote recruitment of the collapsed lung and adding IMV at night to prevent hypoventilation, hypercapnia, and haemodynamic instability. Also, her thyroid replacement was increased despite her delicate coronary physiology.

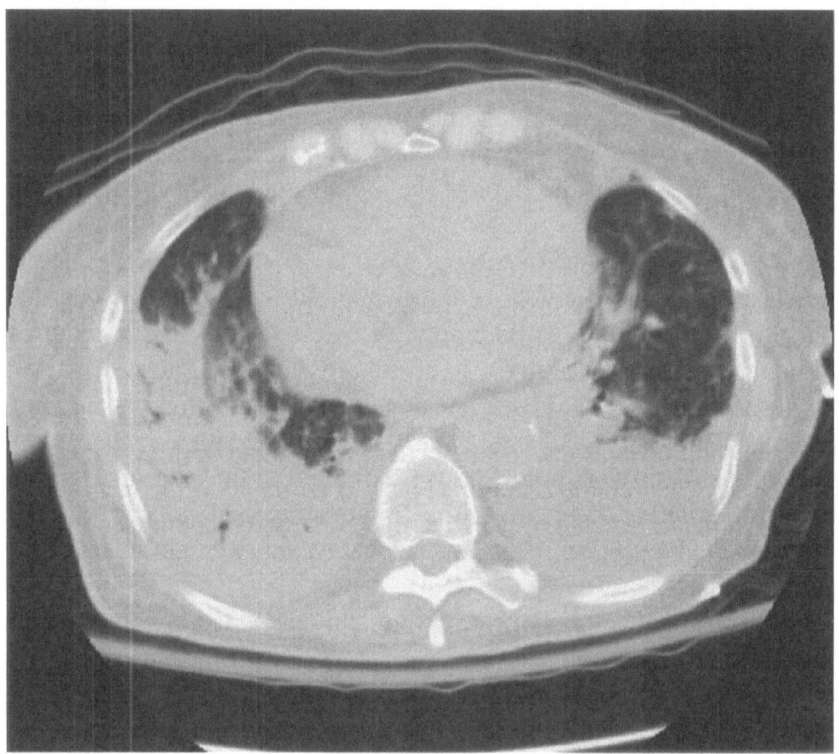

Fig. 1 Chest computed tomography of patient 2

After 2 weeks of this treatment, she was more awake and haemodynamically stable, and we started decreasing the level of PSV. At 3 weeks she could not tolerate more than a few minutes off ventilatory support, she still decreased her minute ventilation at night, and she developed an unusual breathing pattern, characterized by a fast respiratory rate and a "rocking" movement with each triggering of the ventilator. She attributed this pattern to "nerves." A repeat chest CT showed a significant improvement of the consolidation, but a persistent left pleural effusion and lower lobe collapse. Drainage of the effusion was associated with rapid respiratory improvement, including a progressive reversal of her abnormal ventilatory patterns, and eventual separation from mechanical ventilation.

These two cases illustrate several important points. *First*, **there is a patient population that may require mechanical ventilation for months, and yet**

eventually wean. The foremost priority in these patients is to diagnose and treat the respiratory and systemic determinants of their failure to progress. Multiple **respiratory abnormalities** may be present and often coexist.

1. **Abnormal gas exchange**. Persistent hypoxemia due to lung consolidation and collapse prolongs the need for positive pressure at the airway either through a tracheal tube or a face mask. Hypercapnia due to hypoventilation and/or alveolar dead space may result in obtundation and haemodynamic instability and requires ventilatory support.

2. **Increased ventilatory load**. Elastance and resistance are the two forces opposing the flow of air in and out of the respiratory system. An **elastic load** is due to pulmonary consolidation and pleural effusions, as in our patient 2. Persistent lung injury can be severe enough to be incompatible with unsupported breathing (Fig. 1). A **resistive load** is due to bronchospasm, collapsible airways, and increased tracheo-bronchial secretions. Lung surgery, asthma, and COPD all predispose to such an increased resistive load.

3. **Inadequate respiratory muscle function** can be due to weakness, fatigue, or an altered shape of the muscle fibres that decreases the efficiency of contraction. The latter occurs in COPD, where the radius of curvature of the diaphragm decreases and the intercostal muscles become more horizontal due to lung hyperinflation.

4. **Alterations of the control of breathing**. Hypoventilation, apnoea, and tachypnea often occur without an apparent physiological cause. The control of breathing is complex and difficult to investigate. Often, an abnormal breathing pattern prolongs the use of mechanical ventilation and, as in patient 2, seems to resolve as the overall patient condition improves.

Second, patients requiring prolonged mechanical ventilation are seldom suffering solely from a respiratory problem. More commonly, **other medical conditions** contribute to their persistent need for ventilatory support.

1. **Cardiovascular disease**. Both our patients had significant cardiovascular disease that affected their hospital course. The physiological changes associated with withdrawal of mechanical ventilation may bring about different cardiac complications. The increased venous return resulting from a lower intrathoracic pressure can overload both the right and the left ventricle (directly and from ventricular interaction) and, in patients at risk, precipitate myocardial ischaemia and chronic heart failure [9, 10]. Ischaemia and a catecholamine surge may also trigger arrhythmias.

2. **Endocrine, metabolic, and nutritional** abnormalities.

3. Management of **anxiety, delirium**, and **depression** may be important. Several studies have pointed out the negative effect of oversedation in

mechanically ventilated patients [11]. However, those studies were performed in the early phase of ARF, where patients are often kept heavily sedated with continuous infusions of hypnotics, opiates, or benzodiazepines to facilitate their complex care. In our patient population, awake and highly stressed by weeks of severe illness, anxiety, delirium, and depression are common and they should be appropriately treated [12].

Third, **the "weaning" strategy used is less relevant than in the patients studied by Esteban et al.** [1] **and by Brochard et al.** [2]. The most-important determinants of our ability to wean patients off mechanical ventilation are: (1) our understanding of their respiratory physiology and (2) correcting their co-existing medical problems. These challenges may be best met in a specialized unit.

Rationale for a respiratory acute care unit

Over the past 20 years, a new patient population has emerged in our intensive care units (ICUs), patients with "prolonged ARF." These are patients that have survived a complex ICU course due to aggressive medical and surgical therapy and are still dependent on mechanical ventilatory support. They may include as many as 20% of all ICU patients, particularly in medical ICUs, depending upon the individual characteristics of each institution [3, 13]. Clearly, better critical care practice over the past 2 decades has improved the outcome of many complex patients that would have not survived in earlier years. These patients (Table 2) may remain in the ICU for prolonged periods, despite being stable because of their need for mechanical ventilation. Economic pressure is now forcing movement of these patients to a less costly environment.

Table 2 Common characteristics of patients with prolonged acute respiratory failure (ARF)

Patients with prolonged ARF
Mechanically ventilated for > 3 weeks
Multiple medical issues
Potentially reversible respiratory disease
Haemodynamically stable
Nutritionally depleted, anxious and depressed

The salient clinical characteristics of the first 150 patients admitted to our respiratory acute care unit over the first 12 months of activity are summarized in Table 3. By comparing these data with those in Table 1, one can easily note that our patient population is more compromised from a respiratory standpoint.

Furthermore, their outcome is radically different, including an overall weaning rate of only 75% and a hospital mortality rate of 21%. Our data are in line with the available reports from acute care respiratory units similar to ours [3, 14], underscoring the fundamental difference between the patients in the two weaning trials and those who undergo mechanical ventilation for prolonged ARF. The term "acute care", used instead of "intensive care" to denominate these units, indicates the persistent acuity of their patients, who cannot be transferred to a regular ward because of ventilator dependency, high grade of nursing care, and the need for constant medical supervision due to their complex clinical status. However, they do not need the full "intensive" package of invasive monitoring, vasopressor infusion, intravenous metabolic control, etc. Hence, an "acute care" unit is less expensive than an "intensive care" unit. It is also important to distinguish this type of "acute care" unit from a "chronic care" unit.

Table 3 Baseline patient characteristics of the respiratory acute care unit (RACU) at the Massachusetts General Hospital, May 2001 to June 2002

	RACU
COPD	> 50%
Days of MV prior to admission	> 15
Days of MV in the RACU	16
MIP (cmH_2O)	≤ 20
Tidal volume (ml)	300
Minute ventilation (l/min)	7 - 20
Rate of discontinuing MV	75%
Mortality in the unit	11%
Hospital mortality of RACU patients	21%

We believe that concentrating these high-risk patients in a single unit may not only benefit the hospital budget, but may also improve their care. At the time of designing the structure of our respiratory acute care unit, we believed that the following characteristics would have a positive impact on patient care:

- A dedicated staff physician intensivist from both pulmonary medicine and anaesthesia.
- 24 h/day direct physician coverage
- A dedicated respiratory therapist
- Regular involvement of other ancillary services: physical therapy, occupational therapy, and speech pathology
- A 1:2 patient-to nurse ratio.

Management guidelines of patients with prolonged ARF

- It is critical to determine early on whether a patient with prolonged ARF has a reasonable chance of eventually breathing unassisted. Furthermore, it would be best to assess that at the time of the consult, avoiding unnecessary admissions to the acute care unit. A few conditions are highly predictive of the inability to discontinue mechanical ventilation, including those due to definitive or progressive neurological and muscular disease. In the absence of such clear-cut conditions, discontinuation of mechanical ventilation can occur several months after its initiation.
- The role of SBTs in the initial evaluation of these patients is unknown. While some clinicians like to carry out a SBT in all patients at the time of their initial evaluation as long as they are reasonably stable, others object that after weeks of mechanical ventilation it is unlikely to produce a surprising result, such as suddenly coming off the ventilator.
- After setting the ventilatory support to a level close to the minimum support without obvious distress, the patient's ventilatory progress is followed daily (sometimes twice daily) with basic measurements of respiratory mechanics, including:
- Unsupported tidal volume
- Spontaneous respiratory rate
- Semi-static compliance
- Airway resistance
- Auto-PEEP

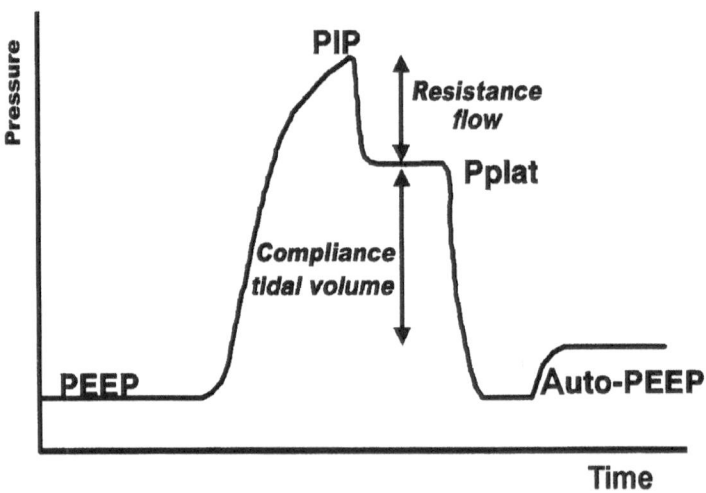

Fig. 2 End-inspiratory pause for the bedside measurement of respiratory mechanics

These basic respiratory mechanics can be easily measured at the bedside in patients with a reasonably slow respiratory rate by switching the ventilator to volume- limited ACV with a square-wave flow pattern of known flow rate. Once the patient is showing minimal spontaneous effort, an end-inspiratory hold can be obtained automatically in most currently available ventilators [5].

- Optimization of medical conditions is often the most challenging task.
- Discharge plans must be started as early as possible. Nearly all these patients will require a period of physical rehabilitation after discontinuation of ventilatory support. Rehabilitation facilities are precious and with limited bed availability. Early planning avoids unnecessary stay in the unit while simply waiting for placement.

References

1. Esteban A, Frutos F, Tobin M, et al (1995) A comparison of four methods of weaning patients from mechanical ventilation. N Engl J Med 332:345-50
2. Brochard L, Rauss A, Benito S, et al (1994) Comparison of three methods of withdrawal of ventilatory support during weaning from mechanical ventilation. Am J Respir Crit Care Med 150:896-903
3. ACCP, AARC, ASCCM (2001) Evidence-based guidelines for weaning and discontinuing ventilatory support. Chest 120:375S-396S
4. Tobin M (2001) Advances in mechanical ventilation. N Engl J Med 344:1986-1996
5. Hess D, Medoff B, Fessler M (1999) Pulmonary mechanics and graphics during positive pressure ventilation. Int Anesthesiol Clin 37:85-102
6. Esteban A, Alia I, Gordo F, et al (1997) Extubation outcome after spontaneous breathing trials with t-tube or pressure support ventilation. Am J Respir Crit Care Med 156:459-465
7. Brochard L, Pluskwa F, Lemaire F (1987) Improved efficacy of spontaneous breathing with inspiratory pressure support. Am Rev Respir Dis 138:411-418
8. Marini J, Smith T, Lamb V (1988) External work output and force generation during synchronized intermittent mandatory ventilation. Am Rev Respir Dis 138:1169-1179
9. Lemaire F, Teboul J-L, Cinotti L, et al (1988) Acute left ventricular dysfunction during unsuccessful weaning from mechanical ventilation. Anesthesiology 69:171-179
10. Hurford W, Lynch K, Strauss H, et al (1991) Myocardial perfusion as assessed by thallium-201 scintigraphy during the discontinuation of mechanical ventilation in ventilator-dependent patients. Anesthesiology 74:1007-1016
11. Kress J, Pohlman A, O'Connor M, Hall J (2000) Daily interruption of sedative infusions in critically ill patients undergoing mechanical ventilation. N Engl J Med 342:1471-1477
12. Inouye S, Bogardus S, Charpentier P, et al (1999) A multicomponent intervention to prevent delirium in hospitalized older patients. N Engl J Med 340:669-676
13. Seneff M, Zimmerman J, Knaus W, et al (1996) Predicting the duration of mechanical ventilation: the importance of disease and patient characteristics. Chest 110:469-479
14. Carson S, Bach P, Brzozowski L, Leff A (1999) Outcome after long-term acute care. An analysis of 133 mechanically ventilated patients. Am J Respir Crit Care Med 159:1568-1573

INDEX

A

abciximab, 748-750, 752, 756-757

abdominal pain, 186

acetylcholine, 121, 129-130, 133, 729-730, 734, 839, 871, 874

acidaemia, 24

activated protein C, 1062, 1064, 1084, 1160, 1165

acute cardiogenic pulmonary oedema, 67

acute coronary syndromes, 6, 9, 663, 722

acute lung injury, 360, 364, 477, 482, 542, 544, 551, 553, 556, 645

acute myocardial infarction, 3, 9, 60, 67, 270, 272, 663, 675, 720, 722, 731-732, 735, 737, 753-757

acute pancreatitis, 163, 523, 1047-1048,1062, 1064

acute respiratory distress syndrome, 421, 459, 466, 501, 510-511, 513, 525-526, 529, 531-532, 542, 544-545, 547, 556-557, 569, 582-583, 832, 1049, 1056, 1081, 1087

acute respiratory failure, 57, 67, 425, 446-447, 459, 556, 577, 582-583, 795

adenosine, 19, 27, 710, 713-715, 721-722, 873, 962, 982, 1151

adrenal insufficiency, 189

adrenaline, 14-17, 21, 23, 25, 94, 283-287, 289-290, 292-295, 306, 685

agitation, 105, 126, 130-132, 153, 156, 161, 305, 608

airway calibre, 441

airway closing pressure, 470-472

airway management, 23-24, 87, 309, 586-587, 591, 827, 829, 831

airway obstruction, 407, 504, 559-561, 566-567, 1015, 1030, 1033

airway occlusion, 417-420

airway opening pressure, 421, 472

airway pressure, 57, 59, 67, 367, 372, 412-413, 415, 417-418, 423, 442, 447, 459-466, 469, 505, 510-511, 573, 575, 577, 580, 625, 628

airway resistance, 418-419, 421, 424, 432-433, 435-436, 460, 511, 559, 561

alcohol intoxication, 132

aldosterone, 35, 201, 368, 370-371, 1109

alfentanil, 105, 311

allergic reactions, 51, 140, 144

almitrine, 554, 557

alveolar macrophages, 543, 1231

alveolar overdistention, 574

alveolar recruitment, 492, 553, 571, 573, 575, 577-579, 581, 583

amiodarone, 18-19, 23-24, 27, 31, 717-718, 720, 723

ammonia, 210-211

amnesia, 103, 105-106, 122, 127, 130, 843, 891

anaesthesia, 16, 52, 111, 121-122, 124-125, 127-129, 135, 137, 140, 142-144, 146, 154, 197-199, 201, 203, 205, 209, 211-215, 263-264, 297, 304, 313, 316-318, 322-324, 373, 376, 382, 437, 575, 613, 637, 640, 652, 655, 657-658, 675, 682-683, 685, 691, 706, 813, 819, 828-833, 835-842, 844, 850, 852, 870, 872, 874-875, 892, 908, 912, 916, 921, 925, 933, 955, 957-963, 965-969, 971, 973-978, 982-987, 996-997, 999, 1035, 1042, 1044, 1271

anaesthesiologist, 146, 318, 321-322, 635, 813, 829, 831, 833, 908, 912-915, 933, 966-968

anaesthetic drugs, 129, 870, 872, 1029

anaesthetic preconditioning, 713, 715

anaesthetic target sites, 837, 841

analgesia, 103-105, 107-109, 111, 123-125, 128, 137, 143-144, 161, 309, 317, 324, 831, 843, 864, 866, 870, 872-873, 903-909, 911-913, 916-917, 919-921, 923-935, 965-969, 982, 984-985, 987

angiotensin II, 368, 370-371, 375-376, 713

antibiotics, 126, 145, 184, 186, 589, 608, 1052, 1054-1055, 1098-1099, 1178, 1180, 1270

anticoagulation, 702, 1142, 1161

antidepressants, 130-131, 962

antidiuretic hormone, 35, 369, 1109

anti-inflammatory cytokines, 1164

anti-oxidant, 1183, 1188

antithrombin III, 201, 1157, 1159, 1164, 1184, 1188

anuria, 157, 1143

anxiolysis, 105-107, 608

aortic dissection, 6, 641, 701, 987

aortic stenosis, 6, 689, 705-706, 983

apnoea, 155, 210, 401-402, 406, 415-416, 429, 431, 611, 957

aprotonin, 1159

arrhythmias, 12, 15, 18, 59, 709-721, 723, 958, 982, 986, 1070, 1114

arterial oxygen content, 731

arterial oxygenation, 552, 569, 571, 573, 575, 577-579, 581, 583

artificial ventilation, 107, 109, 663-664, 674, 688, 772, 774, 794

aspiration, 130, 155, 320, 514, 518, 527, 579, 581, 586-588, 595, 942, 968, 1000-1001

pneumonia, 57-58, 60, 107, 166-167, 169, 179, 182-183, 314, 320, 484, 486, 489-490, 492, 495, 498, 514, 540, 547, 579, 581, 585-589, 591-593, 605, 608-609, 804, 1047-1048, 1055, 1073, 1095

asthma, 58, 60, 441, 445-448, 464, 537, 544, 567, 600, 611

asystole, 17, 21, 24-25, 709, 716, 719

atelectasis, 104, 154, 160-161, 437, 467, 475, 571, 573, 905

atrial fibrillation, 27-28, 159, 161, 688, 709, 720, 982, 984

atrial filling, 367

atrial flutter, 709

atrial myocardium, 714, 720

atrial natriuretic peptide, 204, 368, 370, 372

atrial receptors, 369

atropine, 14, 25, 135, 209, 307, 424, 719, 1114

auditing, 1251, 1254

autonomic nervous system, 407

auto-PEEP, 439-440, 446, 614, 663

awake craniotomy, 301-305, 307-312

B

baby lung, 572

bacteraemia, 1055, 1129, 1237

bacteria, 174, 182, 485, 516, 522, 585, 588, 590, 1052, 1076-1077, 1127, 1152, 1232-1235

bacterial pneumonia, 166, 169, 492

bacterial translocation, 45, 53-54

barbiturate coma, 889

barbiturates, 159, 882, 884-885, 1116

baroreceptors, 35, 368-371

barotrauma, 443, 570, 572, 575-576, 581-582

Bell's palsy, 971, 976, 978

belladonna-alkaloids, 130

benzodiazepines, 130, 211, 318-319, 884, 893-896, 898-899

Bernouilli equation, 667

beta-blockers, 6

bilevel positive airway pressure, 57

bioimpedance, 791, 794-795, 802, 807, 811-812

biotrauma, 572

bleeding, 20, 47-49, 98, 150, 158-161, 185, 198, 201-202, 204, 279, 302, 307-309, 313-314, 320, 322, 386, 554-555, 681-682, 684-686, 691, 702, 738, 745-750, 752, 940, 945-947, 949, 1032, 1034, 1155-1156, 1160-1163

blood coagulation, 1108

blood pressure, 48, 70, 91, 114, 134, 143-144, 146, 154-155, 159, 161, 199, 247-248, 259, 276-279, 370, 372, 391, 397, 407, 416, 445, 578, 691-692, 750, 813, 939, 942, 945-946, 951, 974, 992, 1014-1015, 1017, 1022, 1024, 1058, 1060

blood urea nitrogen, 701, 1094

blood viscosity, 43

body posture, 560

bradyarrhythmias, 132, 709, 719

bradycardia, 18-19, 25-26, 114-115, 133, 200, 206, 307, 401, 407, 416, 693, 719, 729, 733, 820, 943, 1000, 1114-1115

brain hypoxia, 253

brain ischaemia, 278

breathing, 58, 64, 154, 156, 163, 181, 306, 367, 371-372, 401-407, 409, 411, 413, 415-416, 429, 437, 467, 476, 502, 509-511, 550, 559-560, 562, 566-567, 587, 599, 637, 811, 995, 1017, 1021, 1028, 1030-1031, 1267, 1275

bretylium, 717-718, 723

Broadman's technique, 960

bronchodilation, 449, 455

bronchodilators, 548, 565, 567, 629

bronchoscopy, 358, 539, 587, 601-602, 831

bronchospasm, 134, 154

Brussels scale, 109

bupivacaine, 138, 306, 324, 849, 921, 930, 933, 962-963, 973

butyrophenones, 131-132

C

caesarean section, 141, 144, 906, 968-969, 974-976, 985-987, 996-997

carbamates, 116

cardiac arrest, 11-25, 27, 29, 31, 51, 131, 208, 263, 270, 272, 681, 693, 717-720, 722-723, 1017-1018, 1020, 1025, 1029, 1051, 1097, 1101

cardiac disease, 444, 812, 832, 979-983, 985, 987

cardiac effects, 117

cardiac function, 147, 200, 600, 636-637, 639-640, 655, 665, 670, 696, 721, 725, 727, 729, 731, 733, 735, 811

cardiac morbidity, 732

cardiac output, 41, 46-47, 64, 67, 139-140, 144, 146-150, 157-159, 270, 272, 329, 333-335, 368-369, 372, 445, 462-464, 501-503, 505, 510, 548, 550-551, 564, 624, 629, 650, 656-657, 659, 662, 670, 673, 676, 685-686, 707, 731, 791, 794-795, 803, 811-814, 817, 822, 995, 1058, 1113, 1139, 1188, 1232

cardiac rhythm, 12, 642

cardiac surgery, 54, 593, 636, 638, 640-641, 643-645, 663, 675-677, 679, 682, 690, 695-697, 702-704, 707, 720, 811-812, 1122

cardiac tamponade, 24, 624

cardiogenic shock, 50, 55, 162, 658, 679, 688, 692, 694-695, 700, 702-703, 707-708, 716, 738, 747, 751, 753, 816

cardiomyopathy, 676, 734, 979, 981-982, 986

cardiopulmonary bypass, 709, 711, 717, 722

cardiopulmonary resuscitation, 282, 722-723, 1051, 1055

caudal anaesthesia, 957, 961

central anticholinergic syndrome, 129-130, 134-136

central cholinergic transmission, 129-130, 132

central nervous system, 43, 49, 130, 135, 190, 835, 870, 872-873, 891, 972, 1033

central pontine myelinolysis, 49

central venous pressure, 37, 139, 141, 147, 203, 213, 548, 630, 655, 662, 675-676, 691, 1060

cerebral blood flow, 14-15, 160, 245, 253, 259-261, 877, 886-889

cerebral cortex, 885

cerebral hyperaemia, 276, 296

cerebral ischaemia, 151, 259

cerebral monitoring, 281

cerebral oedema, 38, 204, 209, 974

cerebral perfusion pressure, 254, 260-261

chemokines, 517, 519, 522, 535-536, 1076

chest pain, 3, 720, 739, 741, 746-747, 749, 751, 753, 981

chloride channel, 857

cholinesterase, 129, 131-134

cholinesterase inhibitor, 129, 132

chronic lung disease, 462-463, 586, 820

chronic obstructive pulmonary disease, 57, 464, 554, 559, 563, 566-567

clathrates, 836

clonidine, 128, 241, 315-317, 321, 323-324, 944

coagulation, 48, 158, 161, 320, 539, 569, 579, 682, 747, 916, 1049, 1061-1062, 1093-1094, 1101, 1107-1108, 1127, 1135, 1142, 1161, 1169, 1172, 1186, 1188

coarctation of the aorta, 987

compliance, 95, 154, 159, 427-432, 435, 437-438, 461, 471, 483, 532, 547-548, 569, 572, 579-581, 606, 609, 614, 663, 665-666, 668, 972, 986

confusion, 122, 130, 172, 396, 622-623, 867, 971-972, 1047, 1057, 1119

consumption coagulopathy, 1161

continuous positive airway pressure, 57, 67, 372, 412-413, 415, 511

continuous renal replacement therapy, 1119

convection, 461, 1128-1129, 1132, 1134

COPD patients, 405, 425, 559-567, 684

coronary artery bypass grafting, 681, 703-708, 981, 985

coronary artery disease, 8-10, 20, 133, 415, 667, 675, 679-682, 686-687, 690, 699, 701, 704-705, 720, 981, 1056, 1095

coronary artery reocclusion, 740

coronary blood flow, 681, 692, 700, 725-727, 730, 740, 742, 755

coroner, 1274, 1276-1279, 1282-1283

corticosteroids, 160, 181, 193, 480, 514-519, 521-523, 525-527, 529, 542

cortisol, 104, 170, 531, 536-538, 541, 543-544, 682, 1171, 1174-1176, 1187

cost of care, 1251

CRAMS Scale, 1038

critical care, 41, 58, 101, 115, 135, 145, 162, 169, 173, 175, 177, 185, 187, 189, 191, 193, 195, 299, 494, 591, 633, 635, 653, 827, 830-833, 886, 985, 987, 1013, 1015, 1017, 1041, 1043-1044, 1048, 1055, 1057, 1065, 1072-1073, 1090, 1101-1103, 1177, 1191, 1193-1199, 1201-1209, 1261, 1283

critically ill, 39, 46, 103-109, 111-112, 192, 439, 498, 577, 582, 591-592, 619, 633, 635-638, 645-646, 653, 655-656, 658-659, 674-677, 789-790, 794, 803, 810-811, 813-814, 816, 822, 1035, 1047, 1052-1055, 1062, 1070-1072, 1075, 1081, 1102-1103, 1120-1122, 1124-1125, 1139, 1143-1145, 1167, 1175, 1185-1190, 1195, 1199, 1263, 1270

Cushing reflex, 205

cyclopropane, 839

cytomegalovirus, 167, 171, 190-191, 193, 195

D

D-dimers, 996

death, 18, 20, 31, 39, 46, 49-50, 117, 119, 162, 182, 189, 200-203, 209, 217, 269, 271, 467, 493, 496, 542, 577, 585, 598, 649, 680, 709, 715, 720, 722, 727, 732, 735, 738, 746-747, 749-750, 752, 828, 907, 958-959, 971-973, 979, 985, 995, 1006, 1017, 1020-1022, 1025, 1027, 1039, 1075, 1079, 1084, 1089, 1093, 1119, 1127, 1147, 1156, 1158, 1161-1162, 1205, 1232-1233, 1235, 1263-1271, 1274, 1276-1277, 1279-1280, 1283

defibrillation, 11-14, 19, 23-24, 716-718, 720, 723

delirium tremens, 131-132

deoxyglucose, 886

desflurane, 714, 819, 897

dexmedetomidine, 315, 323

dialysis, 681, 1140-1141, 1144-1145, 1180

diaphragm, 444, 447, 459-460, 571-572

diethyl ether, 847

disseminated intravascular coagulation, 579, 1049

dobutamine, 152, 721, 727, 732-734, 1061, 1091, 1099-1100

dopamine, 152, 375, 503, 510, 695, 719, 794, 873, 986, 1061

dopexamine, 731

Doppler echocardiographic technique, 669

Doppler tissue imaging, 676

Drosophila, 845, 854, 1084-1085, 1135

drotrecogin alfa activated, 1062

dynamic hyperinflation, 427, 450, 559, 629

dynamic work of breathing, 429

dyspnoea, 561, 563, 565, 567

E

echocardiography, 6, 58, 65, 640, 663, 665-666, 668, 674-675, 688, 704, 706, 711, 721, 732-735, 743, 822, 827, 830-831, 833, 981

eclampsia, 972-973, 977, 999

education, 908, 911, 1191, 1203, 1206

Eisenmenger's Syndrome, 985

elderly, 36, 38-39, 49, 85, 213, 218-219, 268, 416, 684, 686, 703, 705, 712, 744, 764, 820, 937, 954, 1044, 1265

electromechanical dissociation, 25

emergency departments, 6, 1013, 1018

emergency personnel, 1014

emergency room, 10, 46, 48, 54, 69-70, 830, 1007-1008, 1010, 1012

emphysema, 446-447, 559, 562, 595

enalaprilat, 1183, 1189

enantiomer, 839-840

encephalitis, 131, 172

endocarditis, 641, 984

endocrine failure, 1167

endothelium, 43, 477-478, 485-486, 488, 729-730

endothelium-derived relaxing factor, 547, 556

endotoxin, 53, 485, 497, 516, 518-519, 522, 527-528, 538, 544, 659, 1052, 1055, 1082-1083, 1086-1087, 1120, 1124, 1129, 1134-1136, 1145, 1149, 1153, 1163, 1173

endotracheal intubation, 57-58, 60, 64-66, 301, 303, 585, 587, 591, 1029-1030, 1033

enflurane, 715, 722, 894, 898

enkephalins, 863

enoximone, 731

epidural anaesthesia, 137, 143-144, 212, 974-975

epilepsy, 898, 971-973

epinephrine, 143-144, 152, 297, 686, 693-695, 697, 706-707, 718-720, 1061, 1114

ergometrine, 982

Escherichia coli, 486, 488, 492, 495, 497, 1087, 1232, 1237

ethanol, 35, 203, 213-215, 219, 857, 862, 875, 892-895, 897-898

etomidate, 233, 714, 836, 839-841, 893

evidence-based medicine, 903, 1167

exercise tolerance, 10, 559, 561, 563-567

expiratory flow, 439-441, 446, 450

expiratory flow limitation, 450

expiratory tidal volume, 580

extracellular volume, 373

extracellular volume expansion, 373

extubation, 155, 159, 161, 313-317, 320-324, 586-587, 592, 605, 607, 615, 686

F

fentanyl, 311, 317, 319, 324, 720, 727, 734, 922, 925-926, 932, 934

fever, 71, 82, 132, 167, 175, 178, 183, 450, 540, 543, 587, 819-820, 944, 983, 1047, 1120, 1207

fibrin, 201, 485, 502, 539, 738, 996, 1097, 1108, 1116, 1147-1152, 1154-1155, 1157-1158, 1160, 1162

fibrinogen, 201-202, 996, 1097, 1149-1150, 1152, 1157-1159

fibrinolysis, 20-21, 31, 84, 202, 682, 737-748, 750-752, 1148-1152

fibroproliferation, 542

flow inflation, 419, 424

fluid challenge, 147, 636, 641, 646, 657, 665, 671-674, 676-677, 789

fluid loading, 636, 662, 665, 671-673

fluid overload, 214, 683, 1121, 1128

fluid responsiveness, 657, 659, 662, 664-665, 671-675, 677

flumazenil, 318, 324

fragment F1+2, 1157

Frank Starling relationship, 661, 664

Frank Starling curve, 664

functional residual capacity, 474

G

GABA Type A receptors, 891

gas exchange, 104, 203, 279-280, 323, 339, 460-461, 463, 501-505, 507, 509-511, 523, 532, 547-549, 551, 553-555, 557, 567, 583, 1033

gender, 189, 269, 579, 685, 943, 1042, 1044, 1241

gene knockout, 893-894, 897

gene targeting, 893

gene transcription, 516-517

general anaesthesia, 129, 135, 143, 199, 201, 212, 214-215, 263-264, 437, 575, 637, 652, 813, 819, 831, 835-841, 850, 852, 870, 872, 968, 983, 985

GISSI-I Trial, 738

Glasgow Coma Scale, 47, 49, 254, 260, 278

glucocorticoid receptor, 531, 535-536, 543-545

glucose, 70-71, 238, 256, 265, 276, 280, 282, 656-657, 659, 696, 877, 886-889

glycine, 203-204, 208-209, 839, 842-843, 871, 875, 892, 897

governance, 827, 829, 831, 833, 1252

GUSTO-I Angiographic Sub-study, 740-741

GUSTO-I Trial, 738, 743-744, 754

GUSTO-III Trial, 738, 749, 757

H

haematocrit, 140, 150-151, 154, 779, 995, 1000, 1091, 1098

haemodilution, 199, 229-230

haemodynamic monitoring, 635, 645, 759

haemodynamics, 27, 100, 375, 504, 549, 551, 553, 555, 557, 609, 629, 746, 807

haemofiltration, 715, 1129, 1131, 1133-1134, 1136

haemoglobin, 151-152, 224, 406, 554, 774

haemorrhage, 20-21, 129, 134, 157, 254, 263, 265, 279, 638, 674, 739, 746, 752, 788, 945, 985, 995-996, 998-1000, 1008-1009, 1020, 1022-1025, 1092, 1155-1156, 1159

haemorrhagic shock, 151, 997, 1022

half-life, 15, 118, 133, 210, 315, 318, 696, 779, 822, 921, 924

halothane, 233, 438, 714, 721-722, 734, 836, 841, 875, 897

hapten-dextran-1, 51

head injury, 44, 47, 254, 259-261, 266, 271-272, 275-276, 278-279, 281-282, 1009, 1012, 1029, 1031, 1033, 1044, 1116-1117

heart disease, 27, 60-61, 149, 213, 269, 675, 702-704, 707, 709, 720-722, 756, 781, 795, 979-985, 1020, 1025

heart rate, 27, 60-61, 139-140, 144, 146, 153-154, 288, 402, 407-412, 414, 416, 632, 638-640, 692-693, 706, 729, 771, 791-792, 807, 814, 816, 905, 914, 957, 987, 995, 997, 1048, 1058, 1060, 1093-1096, 1102

heart transplant, 702, 807, 987

heparin, 739, 930, 984, 1152, 1159-1161, 1165

herniation, 269

heroin intoxication, 132

hibernating myocardium, 710-711, 721, 727, 734

High Dependency Unit, 1017

high filling pressures, 694

high frequency oscillation, 465-466

hippocampus, 878-879, 881, 885-886, 1105

homeostasis, 146, 214

human immunodeficiency virus, 188-192, 194-196, 1095

hydraulic resistance, 43

hydrocortisone, 522, 1064

hydroxyethyl starch, 55, 656

hyperammonemia, 199, 210-211

hypercapnia, 129, 133, 306

hyperchloremic acidosis, 51

hyperglycemia, 280, 282

hyperinflation, 427, 450, 559, 592, 629

hyperkalaemia, 975

hyperosmolarity, 38-39, 49

hyperpolarization, 869

hyperpyrexia, 130-132, 135, 810

hypertension, 44, 61, 69, 104, 108, 133, 136,
    153, 199, 201, 205, 237, 240-243, 249-251,
    266-267, 269, 272, 345, 357, 404, 415-416,
    479-480, 513, 547-548, 550-551, 556, 578,
    676, 679-681, 763-764, 942, 951, 972, 974,
    982-983, 985-987, 992, 998, 1000, 1114

hyperthermia, 132, 263, 266-267, 271, 657, 944

hypertonic saline, 42, 45-47, 49-50, 52-55, 177,
    203, 279, 282

hypertonicity, 35-37, 39, 43-44, 50

hypnosis, 103, 106, 109, 920

hypocalcemia, 208

hypocapnia, 257

hyponatremia, 39, 49, 54, 199, 201, 203-205,
    209-210, 215, 658

hypoosmolality, 205

hypoperfusion, 38, 73, 93, 171, 211, 245-246,
    249, 252, 650

hypotension, 18-19, 44, 46, 48-55, 59-60, 107,
    131, 139, 153, 198-199, 201, 203, 214, 223,
    227, 229-231, 238-239, 244-247, 251, 268,
    275, 277-281, 369, 396, 406, 463, 465, 477,
    553, 578, 580-581, 674, 677, 697, 715, 719,
    813, 819-822, 942-943, 945, 982, 984, 986-
    987, 992, 995, 999, 1061, 1121, 1155-1156

hypothermia, 24, 51, 200, 263, 265-272, 280,
    282, 803, 944, 1008, 1022, 1024

hypoventilation, 314-315, 318, 609, 611

hypovolaemia, 24, 655, 925, 1156

hypoxaemia, 278-279, 401, 501, 547-548, 729-
    731, 735, 942, 985

hypoxia, 24, 31, 60, 129, 224, 227, 232, 253,
    259, 277-278, 281, 314, 320, 376, 407, 502,
    524, 731, 819, 1021, 1023-1024, 1156,
    1159, 1162

hysteresis, 469, 575

I

ibuprofen, 528, 920

IL-1 receptor antagonist, 517, 540, 1159

immunity, 166, 183, 527, 535, 1075-1076, 1080,
    1084, 1086, 1184

immunomodulation, 1185

immunosuppression, 53, 107, 166-167, 181-182,
    212, 527, 543, 586, 1136

infection, 71, 124-125, 132, 156, 165, 169-170,
    172, 174-176, 181-182, 184-196, 212, 465,
    477, 484, 522-523, 537, 539-540, 543-544,
    585-587, 589-592, 619, 686, 701-702, 820,
    832-834, 984, 1048, 1051, 1053, 1056-1057,
    1065-1066, 1068-1070, 1077, 1083-1084,
    1124, 1127, 1129, 1152, 1156, 1159-1160,
    1232, 1234, 1241-1242, 1244-1245, 1249

inflammatory mediators, 569, 572, 1051, 1053-
    1054, 1076

inflammatory response, 532, 534, 542, 655, 720,
    1048-1049, 1051, 1055-1056, 1066, 1072,
    1084, 1087, 1162-1163

inflexion point, 420-421, 423, 572, 575-576

informed consent, 80, 965-969, 1090, 1279,
    1283

inhalation injury, 484

injury severity, 1018, 1037-1040, 1044

innate immune response, 1080, 1085, 1087, 1127

inotropes, 58, 242-243, 249, 283, 463, 693, 986

inspiratory capacity, 559, 561-562

inspiratory inflexion point, 572, 576

inspiratory tidal volume, 580

intensive care, 20, 39, 46, 52, 57, 67, 103, 111,
129, 131, 133, 135, 145, 163, 169, 263, 268,
280, 284, 297-298, 367, 369, 401, 425, 438,
464, 466, 504, 510-511, 540, 542, 556, 579,
582-583, 585, 591-593, 619-620, 625, 627,
629, 633-635, 645-647, 653, 655-656, 658-
659, 663, 665, 672, 674-677, 681, 771-772,
774, 778-780, 789-790, 794, 803, 806, 810,
818, 821, 827, 830, 833, 903, 915-917, 930,
932, 934, 962, 975, 1016, 1018, 1038, 1044,
1049, 1055-1058, 1060, 1064-1065, 1072-
1073, 1084, 1087, 1089-1090, 1099-1103,
1117, 1119, 1121, 1124-1125, 1127, 1135-
1137, 1164, 1201, 1203-1205, 1207-1209,
1213, 1227, 1251, 1263, 1271, 1273

Intensive Care Units, 46, 401, 591-592, 619-620,
625, 645, 771, 827, 903, 1016, 1018, 1064,
1072, 1084, 1102, 1127, 1201, 1203, 1209

interleukin-1, 1077, 1085-1086

intermittent mandatory ventilation, 463

intracranial bleeding, 49, 308-309, 1155

intracranial haematoma, 320

intracranial haemorrhage, 265, 739, 746, 752

intracranial hypertension, 44, 266-267, 272, 578

intracranial pressure, 53, 107, 134, 159, 205,
266, 276, 282, 292-295, 975-976

intracranial hypertension, 44, 266-267, 272, 578

intraoperative echocardiography, 831

intrathoracic pressure, 159, 367-368, 370-371,
655, 663, 672

intravenous fibrinolysis, 737-738, 748

intravenous fluid therapy, 675

ipratropium, 134

ischaemia-reperfusion, 709

ischaemic neurological injury, 280

ischaemic stroke, 269

isoflurane, 690, 706, 713-715, 721-722, 819, 875

isoprenaline, 25

J

Jehovah's witness, 54

K

Kelvin body, 432

ketamine, 127, 130, 714, 850, 963

ketazocine, 863

kidney, 37, 39, 189, 204, 210-211, 291, 367-375,
390, 649, 685, 695, 846-848, 850, 854, 988,
1077, 1082, 1121, 1124-1125, 1156, 1160,
1163

L

labour, 965-969, 971, 974, 976, 1053, 1180

lactic acidosis, 160, 190, 281, 1048

laryngeal mask, 1029

left ventricular end-diastolic area, 636

left ventricular end-diastolic volume, 675

leukocytosis, 269, 587, 1120

lidocaine, 14, 18-19, 24, 27, 144, 315-316, 321-
323, 716-718, 722-723, 909

lipocortin-1, 517

lipopolysaccharide, 535, 1085-1086, 1232, 1238

long-term mortality, 47, 738, 740, 742, 1056, 1071

lorazepam, 303, 889

lung biopsy, 480-482

lung blood flow, 329-331, 333-337

lung function, 156, 360, 363, 456, 545, 553, 555, 559, 595-596, 604, 653

lung injury, 54, 339-340, 342, 344-346, 350-354, 358-364, 459, 461, 477-479, 482, 507, 532, 542, 544, 551, 553, 556, 645, 1056, 1182-1184, 1188, 1190

lung morphology, 349-350, 582

lung oedema, 554

lung parenchyma, 571

lung recruitment, 356, 360, 362, 462, 510, 573-575, 581-583

lung surgery, 810

lung volume, 343, 356, 359, 423, 450-451, 456, 462, 468-474, 559-561, 569, 571-572, 575-577, 581-582

LV stroke volume, 642-643, 645

M

magnesium, 19, 210, 999-1000

magnetic resonance, 7, 10, 145, 172, 743, 755, 831

mannitol, 159, 161, 199, 201-202, 204, 306, 974, 1178

maternal mortality, 971, 973, 981

mean airway pressure, 459-466, 580

mean arterial pressure, 46, 61, 152, 268, 277, 283-284, 286, 289-290, 295, 550-551, 1061, 1134

mechanical ventilation, 58, 67, 108-111, 123, 130-131, 156, 163, 301, 309, 314, 367, 369, 371, 373-376, 429, 435, 438, 459, 462-464, 466, 489, 493, 531, 538-539, 547, 553, 567, 569-570, 572, 575-576, 578, 585, 591-593,

605-615, 636-637, 642-643, 645, 652, 672, 789, 909, 1098-1099, 1206, 1264, 1270, 1273, 1280

Medical Emergency Team, 1017-1018

membrane stretch, 847

memory, 103, 105, 111, 409, 713, 721, 880, 899, 963

methaemoglobinaemia, 554-555

methylene blue, 398

methylprednisolone, 534, 539, 544-545

metoprolol, 241, 735

microcirculation, 43, 141-142, 743, 745

midazolam, 319-320, 324, 579, 714, 884, 889, 894

mitral stenosis, 663, 983-984

monitoring, 6, 8, 21, 51-52, 58-59, 70, 80, 83-84, 103, 110, 131, 137, 142-143, 146, 149-150, 159, 162, 198, 208, 211, 214, 221, 238-239, 244, 249, 251-252, 254, 271, 276, 279-281, 301-308, 310-311, 348, 355, 377, 380-381, 385, 387-391, 394-396, 398-401, 416, 554, 566, 602, 619, 635, 637-641, 643, 645-647, 657-659, 662, 665, 673-674, 677, 690, 712, 753, 759, 772, 776, 778, 780, 782, 786, 788-789, 791, 793-795, 797, 799, 801, 803, 805, 807, 809-812, 827, 829, 831-832, 903, 912-913, 923, 927, 929, 937-940, 948, 953, 982, 985, 987, 996-997, 1053-1054, 1090, 1093, 1103, 1204

morphine, 97, 105, 111, 268, 863-865, 872-873, 922-924, 932, 934-935, 961, 963, 991, 1264, 1269

mortality, 4, 6, 9, 18-19, 38, 45, 47-48, 61, 117, 119, 177, 185, 191, 193, 195, 197, 200, 204, 215, 268-270, 272, 275-276, 278-279, 281, 310, 401, 415, 462-465, 483, 493, 495-496, 498, 532, 537, 539-540, 543, 552-553, 555, 569, 577, 585-588, 590-591, 596-597, 619, 655, 684, 704-705, 715-716, 719, 725, 731-732, 735, 737-743, 746-747, 752-754, 829, 905-907, 971, 973, 981, 983, 985, 987, 1005, 1009-1012, 1018, 1020-1021, 1023, 1025, 1032, 1035, 1049-1050, 1055-1056, 1066-

1067, 1069-1073, 1075, 1081, 1087, 1089-1091, 1093, 1095, 1097, 1099-1103, 1139, 1142, 1147, 1152, 1158-1160, 1163, 1165, 1171-1172, 1175, 1177-1179, 1182-1183, 1185-1187, 1189-1190, 1195, 1232-1233, 1235, 1238

multicenter trial, 47-48, 54, 267, 282, 466, 1012

multiple organ failure, 106, 1048, 1124

multiple sclerosis, 971, 974-975, 977

mutation, 892, 895, 1078, 1083

myelitis, 172

myocardial hibernation, 725, 727-728, 734

myocardial infarct size, 272, 721, 737

myocardial infarction, 3, 5-6, 9, 18, 31, 60, 67, 270, 272, 641, 663, 675, 708, 720, 722, 725-726, 728, 731-732, 735, 737, 739, 741, 743-745, 747, 749, 751, 753-757, 981, 1187

myocardial injury, 5, 9, 271, 713, 715, 720

myocardial ischaemia, 213, 271, 751, 907, 943, 1114

myocardial preconditioning, 725, 728

myocardial reperfusion, 722, 737-738, 743, 746-748, 750-752, 754

myocardial reperfusion strategies, 737, 750

myocardial stunning, 6, 711, 713, 720, 726

myocarditis, 61, 979

myoglobin, 9, 652

N

nalorphine, 863, 872

naloxonazine, 864

naloxone, 135, 311, 318-319, 323, 863, 929

nausea, 130, 133, 166, 199, 203-204, 209-212, 319, 370, 906, 908, 914, 923, 929, 975

negative expiratory pressure, 505, 508, 561

neonatal respiratory failure, 459, 462-463

neostigmine, 124, 126, 133, 135, 318, 963

neuroleptic drugs, 132

neuroleptic malignant syndrome, 132, 135

neurological disease, 172

neuromuscular blockade, 155

neurosurgery, 82, 84, 250, 258, 260-261, 271-272, 281, 379-380, 389, 831

neurotransmitter receptors, 891

neurotrauma, 272, 275, 281-282

nimodipine, 250, 252

nitric oxide, 350, 357, 364-365, 491, 493-494, 499, 517, 527, 535-536, 547, 549, 551, 553-557, 699, 710, 721, 729, 1151, 1162

nitrogen dioxide, 358, 554

nitrous oxide, 839-841, 878, 882

nocturnal pulse oximetry, 405, 409, 414

non invasive positive pressure ventilation, 67

noradrenaline, 16, 729

norepinephrine, 94, 144, 694-695, 697, 706, 710, 820-821, 1061, 1114, 1134

normothermia, 263, 267, 834, 1032

nosocomial pneumonia, 585, 589, 591-593, 605, 608-609

nuclear factor-kB, 534, 1080

nurses, 255, 620, 633, 904, 911-912, 914-916, 932-933, 938-939, 948-949, 1090, 1203, 1206, 1213-1214, 1217-1218, 1220, 1222-1225, 1227, 1254, 1263

nutrition, 97, 158, 163, 239, 586, 611, 909, 1140, 1145, 1207, 1269

O

oedema, 38, 57, 63, 67, 126, 129, 151, 155, 161, 199-201, 204, 206-209, 228, 276, 303, 305-308, 314, 320, 485-487, 489-490, 501-502, 514, 518-519, 532, 547-548, 554, 625, 627, 637, 655, 658, 727, 806, 974, 983, 999, 1092, 1155

oesophageal pressure, 474

Ohm's Law, 288-289

oliguria, 95, 157, 1048, 1143

opioids, 130, 153-154, 254, 314, 316-319, 321, 324, 710, 863, 869-870, 872-873, 878, 880-881, 883-884, 941-944, 962, 991

organ dysfunction, 541, 553, 686, 1048, 1055, 1057-1060, 1062-1064, 1069, 1089, 1093-1094, 1102-1103, 1122, 1124, 1140, 1142, 1167, 1170-1171, 1175, 1184-1188

organophosphorus poisoning, 113

orphan receptor, 863, 867

osmometers, 34

osmotic concentration, 34

overdistention, 570, 574, 581

overdosage, 682, 958

oximes, 114, 116-118, 120

oximetry spectral analysis, 403, 405, 407, 409, 411, 413, 415-416

oxygen delivery, 46, 93, 95, 100, 276, 282, 288, 349, 351, 693-694, 814, 1089, 1102

oxygen uptake, 323

oxygenation, 24, 64, 107, 176, 224, 228-232, 234, 276, 280, 374, 401, 460-466, 483, 502-505, 513, 518, 527, 547-548, 551-552, 556, 569, 571, 573, 575-579, 581, 583, 771, 814, 1029, 1031, 1033, 1059

P

paediatric surgery, 831, 958, 962

palliative care, 1273

pancreatitis, 151, 163, 187, 523, 547, 1047-1048, 1062, 1064, 1066, 1125, 1147, 1207

papaver somniferum, 863

partial liquid ventilation, 553

patient-controlled analgesia, 916-917, 926, 984

peak inspiratory pressure, 574, 576, 578, 580

peer review, 1038

pendelluft, 428, 432, 461, 505

penetrating trauma victims, 48, 51

pentamidine, 171, 177-180

pentobarbital, 714, 874, 893-894, 897

percutaneous angioplasty, 737-738, 745, 748, 752

percutaneous coronary angioplasty, 756

perfusion, 7, 9-10, 64, 73-74, 79, 83, 87-88, 91, 93-95, 146-147, 150, 152, 155, 160, 208, 239, 241, 243, 245-249, 251-252, 254, 260-261, 264, 266, 273, 275, 339, 351, 353, 355, 363-364, 368-370, 372, 378, 380-382, 385-387, 390, 397-398, 467, 509-510, 548-549, 551, 555, 649-652, 655, 657, 681-683, 692-694, 699-700, 702, 704, 743-745, 747, 754-755, 760, 822, 995

perioperative medicine, 617, 827, 829-833

perioperative mortality, 197, 735

peripartum cardiomyopathy, 986

peripheral nerve blocks, 930, 933

peripheral neuropathy, 171

pethidine, 124-125, 922, 944, 991

phenothiazines, 131-132

phenylephrine, 242, 283, 286, 292, 294-295

phospholipase C, 713

physicians, 255, 296, 335, 620, 633, 662, 674, 979, 1057, 1065, 1072, 1103, 1222, 1227, 1264, 1273-1275, 1277-1278, 1281

physostigmine, 121-136, 316

piritramide, 304

plasma volume measurements, 42

plasminogen activator inhibitor 1, 1153

platelet count, 265, 1058-1059

platelet glycoprotein IIb/IIIa receptor inhibition, 748

pleural pressure, 444, 474, 571, 573-574, 626-629, 632, 634

pneumocystis, 167, 169-170, 179

Pneumocystis carinii pneumonia, 167

pneumonia, 57-58, 60, 107, 166-167, 169, 179, 182-183, 314, 320, 484, 486, 489-490, 492, 495, 498, 514, 540, 547, 579, 581, 585-589, 591-593, 605, 608-609, 804, 1047-1048, 1055, 1073, 1095

pneumothorax, 178-179, 191, 463, 578, 1252

poisonings, 126, 134

polymixin B, 1178

polymorphisms, 482, 1170, 1173, 1184, 1186

polyradiculopathy, 172

polysomnography, 415

positioning, 352, 355, 362, 364-365, 386, 390, 398, 553-555, 583, 805, 815, 930, 939-940, 948, 1189

positive end-expiratory pressure, 369, 461, 464, 502, 510-511, 532, 547, 578, 582, 627, 634

postoperative analgesia, 161, 317, 934

postoperative critical care, 827, 831

postoperative pain, 903, 934-935, 961, 963, 968

postoperative period, 50, 135, 308, 319, 1162

pralidoxime chloride, 118

pralidoxime iodide, 118

pralidoxime mesylate, 118

pregnancy, 578, 979-987, 1000-1001

preload, 93, 139-142, 147, 150, 152-154, 444, 632-633, 655, 657-658, 661-677, 691-692, 694, 696, 698, 711, 814, 822, 980, 986-987

premedication, 157, 303-304, 732

preoperative risk assessment, 827, 829

pressure amplitude, 459-461, 463-465

pressure control ventilation, 579-580

pressure volume, 362, 446, 456, 463, 467, 575, 664

primary angioplasty, 272, 745-747, 749, 751, 755, 757

primary ARDS, 486, 489-496, 524, 574

principle of Fick, 759

procainamide, 24, 717-719

pro-inflammatory cytokine, 538

prolactin, 1174, 1176

promethazine, 304

prone position, 350, 352-359, 363-365, 380, 481, 557, 572, 577, 583

propofol, 103, 106, 112, 304-306, 308-309, 311, 601-603, 714-715, 722, 882, 884-885, 887, 889, 940-941, 991

prostacyclin, 550, 557, 1142, 1151, 1160

prostaglandin, 45, 53, 542, 556, 1189-1190

prosthetic valves, 984

protein C, 1062, 1064, 1072, 1084, 1150-1151, 1154, 1157-1160, 1163-1165

protein kinase C, 266, 272, 713, 721, 869, 872, 875

protein S, 1150, 1154, 1164

Pseudomonas aeruginosa, 1235-1238

pulmonary artery catheter, 633-634, 662, 671, 674

pulmonary artery hypertension, 551

pulmonary artery pressure, 64, 547, 549-551, 553-555, 631, 668, 675

pulmonary blood flow, 337-338

pulmonary capillary wedge pressure, 93, 462, 661-662, 672, 674-676

pulmonary contusion, 1030

pulmonary damage, 88, 569

pulmonary hypertension, 547, 550, 556, 985

pulmonary infection, 176, 465

pulmonary oedema, 63, 67, 199-201, 207, 547-548, 625, 627, 727

pulmonary resistance, 418-419, 423

pulmonary shunt, 650, 652

pulmonary vascular resistance, 550-551

pulmonary vasodilator, 548, 550, 555-556

pulse oximetry, 59, 70, 280, 379, 381, 383, 385, 387, 389-391, 393, 395, 397-405, 409, 414-416, 673, 677, 942

pulse pressure, 657, 672, 674

pulse pressure variations, 672

pulseless electrical activity, 25, 719

pulseless ventricular tachycardia, 21

Q

quality of care, 828-829, 911, 1229

R

radiology, 582, 831

radionuclide ejection fraction, 637

raised ICP, 256, 1115

Raman scattering, 837

Ramsay scale, 109

ranitidine, 304-305

rapid adaptation, 37

rebound effects, 554

recanalization, 741-744, 752, 756

recombinant human activated protein C, 1084

recruitment, 343-344, 347-348, 350-351, 355-357, 359-360, 362, 364, 461-462, 472, 478, 480-481, 485-486, 491-492, 498, 503-507, 509-510, 523, 528, 553, 570-583, 628-630, 712

manoeuvres, 159, 381, 468, 504, 555, 560, 586, 588-589, 974

regional anaesthesia, 137, 140, 198-199, 201, 212, 912, 916, 921, 965, 967-968, 983-984, 986

relaxation volume, 559

relaxed expiration, 424, 427

remifentanil, 106, 111, 311, 317, 984

renal baroreceptors, 370

renal blood flow, 371-372, 694-695, 699, 1156

renal dysfunction, 9, 157, 701

renal effects, 44, 369-370

renal failure, 85, 95, 100, 157, 174, 199, 201, 204, 210, 283, 291, 553, 555, 682, 684, 702, 781, 795, 1048-1049, 1065, 1095, 1119, 1124-1125, 1127-1128, 1134-1137

renal nerve activity, 371

reperfusion injury burns, 477

rescue angioplasty, 746-747, 749, 756

resistance, 43-44, 104, 134, 138-140, 153-155, 182, 270, 288-290, 292-293, 417-421, 423-425, 427-433, 435-438, 460-461, 471, 475, 511, 522, 524, 526, 537-538, 541, 544-545, 548, 550-551, 559, 561, 588-591, 640, 651-652, 694, 771, 792, 806, 813-814, 819, 980, 983, 985, 1115

respiratory acidosis, 59

respiratory compliance, 430, 572

respiratory failure, 57, 67, 115, 117, 119, 424-425, 444, 446-447, 459, 462-463, 466, 531, 553, 556, 577, 582-583, 592, 795, 819-820, 975

respiratory mechanics, 438, 475, 490, 583

respiratory muscle fatigue, 439, 443, 447

respiratory muscles, 115, 444, 447

respiratory resistance, 417-418, 424, 437-438

respiratory system, 197, 418, 421-425, 427-433, 435-436, 438-440, 443-446, 475, 503-504, 510-511, 559, 566, 580-582

respiratory system elastance, 581

respiratory system resistance, 418, 429, 435

respiratory tract infections, 1231

resting lung volume, 469

resuscitation, 11, 39, 42-45, 47-49, 52-54, 145, 147, 149-151, 208, 263, 268, 270, 277-282, 586, 638, 658, 717, 719, 722-723, 997, 1000-1002, 1013, 1016, 1034-1035, 1048, 1051, 1055, 1082, 1089, 1093-1094, 1101-1102, 1207

reteplase, 738, 754, 756-757

rib cage, 429, 444, 447

right ventricular afterload, 725, 730-731

right ventricular end-diastolic volume, 646, 676

right ventricular stroke work, 771

risk assessment, 827, 829, 1038

risk management, 834, 1038, 1245

S

S. pneumoniae, 183

salbutamol, 566

sarcolemmal KATP channels, 713-714

scale, 47, 49, 98, 109, 111, 254, 260, 267, 269, 278, 565-566, 626, 908, 916, 932, 1018, 1038-1039

schistocytes, 1154

scoring system, 658, 941, 946-947, 1018, 1069, 1155

secondary ARDS, 485-487, 489, 491, 493, 495, 497, 499, 524

secondary brain damage, 253, 275, 278

secondary brain injuries, 277-278

sedation, 103, 107-109, 122, 129, 152, 155, 157, 161, 211, 213, 306, 309, 314-316, 319, 373, 579, 586, 591, 611, 629, 663, 831, 909, 912, 914

sedative drugs, 130

seizure, 70, 210, 239, 254, 881, 887, 944, 972, 974, 1000, 1092

selective vasodilator, 548

sepsis, 42-43, 53, 95-96, 125, 150, 154, 162, 171, 297, 465, 477-479, 514, 518, 522-523, 525-526, 528, 534, 537-538, 542, 544, 547, 553, 579, 634, 657-658, 701, 807, 810-812, 832,

988, 1020, 1047-1059, 1061-1073, 1075-
1077, 1079, 1081-1085, 1087, 1089, 1119-
1125, 1127-1129, 1131-1137, 1147-1148,
1152, 1157-1158, 1160-1165, 1178, 1207,
1232-1235, 1237-1238

sepsis syndrome, 465, 1055, 1163-1164

septic shock, 41, 43, 46, 53-54, 162, 479, 525-
526, 538, 542, 544, 675-677, 680, 764, 805,
812, 1048, 1053, 1064, 1067, 1070, 1072,
1075, 1083-1084, 1087, 1119-1120, 1122-
1125, 1127, 1134-1137, 1147, 1160, 1162-
1165, 1237-1238

serum albumin, 837-838, 841

severe sepsis, 537, 811-812, 1048-1050, 1052-
1053, 1055, 1064-1067, 1070, 1072, 1075,
1084, 1089, 1119, 1121-1122, 1124, 1127,
1131, 1134-1135, 1152, 1160, 1164-1165,
1238

severe trauma, 163, 907, 1005

sevoflurane, 819

shivering, 153-155, 158, 263, 271, 316, 944, 951

shock, 12-13, 15, 17-19, 21, 23, 25, 39, 41-47,
50, 52-55, 85, 93, 95, 100, 143, 151, 162,
282, 335, 464, 479, 518, 525-528, 536, 538,
542-544, 579-580, 633, 655, 658, 675-677,
679-680, 688, 692, 694-695, 700, 702-703,
707-708, 716-718, 738, 747, 751, 753, 763-
764, 781, 795, 805, 812, 816, 881, 995, 997-
999, 1022, 1025-1026, 1031-1033, 1048,
1053, 1064, 1067, 1069-1070, 1072, 1075,
1082-1087, 1089-1090, 1095, 1100-1103,
1119-1120, 1122-1125, 1127, 1134-1137,
1141-1142, 1145, 1147, 1155-1156, 1160,
1162-1165, 1169, 1171, 1173, 1175-1177,
1183-1190, 1234, 1237-1238

simulators, 832, 834

sleep, 103-105, 109, 111, 122, 394, 401-407,
409, 411, 413, 415-416, 832, 857, 863, 893-
894, 928

sleep disordered breathing, 402-403, 405, 407,
409, 411, 413, 415-416

sorbitol, 199, 201-203, 211

spinal anaesthesia, 144, 203, 212-213, 974-975,
982

staffing, 108, 924, 1206, 1208, 1227

static elastance of the respiratory system, 432

statics of normal lung, 469, 471, 473, 475

stereoselective, 839-841

steroids, 177, 181, 237, 239, 450, 515, 518, 523-
524, 526, 528, 537, 542, 898, 1235

streptokinase, 738, 754-755

stress adaptation, 433

stress echocardiography, 721, 830, 981

stretch receptors, 35

stroke, 36, 38, 69-84, 139-140, 156-157, 265,
268-270, 272, 415, 637-639, 641-643, 645,
657, 661, 664-665, 668, 670-674, 677, 738,
745-746, 748, 753, 762, 767, 771, 785, 791,
802, 811, 814, 971, 973, 987, 1049, 1274

stroke volume, 139-140, 637-639, 641-643, 645,
657, 661, 664-665, 668, 670-674, 677, 762,
767, 785, 791, 802, 811

stunned myocardium, 710, 720-721

subarachnoid haemorrhage, 254

substrate, 286, 588, 714, 853, 877, 898

successful fibrinolysis, 742, 748, 750, 752

supine position, 138, 340, 343, 353, 355-357,
380-381, 386, 474, 560, 577, 625

surfactant, 466, 523-524, 528-529, 553, 574

surgery, 47-48, 51-52, 54, 79-81, 84, 96, 104,
130, 201, 214, 216, 218-219, 247-248, 264,
271, 379-381, 386-390, 394, 418, 447, 527-
528, 586, 593, 635-636, 638, 640-641, 643-
645, 663, 671, 673, 675-677, 679, 681-692,
695-697, 699-709, 712, 720, 722, 735, 771,
788, 804, 807, 810-813, 818-819, 822, 827,
829-835, 903-907, 909, 913-914, 916-917,
919, 923, 925, 927, 929-933, 935, 937-939,
942-945, 949-951, 953, 958-962, 990, 996,

1023-1027, 1042-1043, 1055-1056, 1092, 1094, 1117, 1122, 1124, 1198

Swan-Ganz catheter, 149

syntocinon, 982

system, 19, 31, 38, 43, 49, 54, 59, 67, 108, 113, 115, 119, 121-123, 127, 130, 135, 190, 194, 197, 209-210, 217, 225, 244, 265, 277-278, 286, 288, 339, 343, 348, 352, 357, 360, 362, 373, 393, 407, 409, 418, 420-425, 427-433, 435-436, 438-440, 443-446, 450, 475, 477, 482, 503-504, 510-511, 516, 518, 521-522, 559, 566, 580-582, 609, 611, 621-624, 628, 630, 632-633, 635, 637, 650-652, 655-659, 670-671, 673, 742, 747, 759-760, 763, 765-766, 768, 789, 805, 811, 832-833, 835, 837, 843, 852-853, 855, 870, 872-873, 877, 879-881, 884-886, 888-889, 891, 897, 919, 931, 941, 945-947, 961, 972, 980, 982, 986, 988, 990, 1005, 1014-1019, 1021, 1023, 1033, 1037-1039, 1041-1044, 1047, 1055, 1059, 1066-1067, 1069, 1072, 1075-1076, 1084, 1087, 1089, 1103, 1114, 1147, 1149, 1155, 1162, 1174, 1197-1198, 1214, 1227, 1240, 1243, 1246, 1253, 1255-1256, 1258-1259, 1268

systemic inflammatory response syndrome, 1055-1056, 1087, 1162-1163

systemic vascular resistance, 134, 270, 288-290, 548, 771

systemic vasodilation, 549, 555

systemic vasodilators, 548

systolic fraction, 668

systolic pressure variation, 672, 674, 677

T

tachycardia, 11, 21, 27, 29-30, 115, 117, 130-131, 133, 284, 407, 663, 679, 695, 709, 718, 723, 729, 812, 821, 942, 982-983, 995, 1120, 1155

telemedicine, 832

temperature, 33, 117, 129, 140, 158, 175, 200, 214, 216, 263-266, 268-269, 271-272, 276,

280, 467, 590, 795, 803, 834, 836-837, 847, 925, 1048, 1052, 1066, 1092

tenecteplase, 738, 754

thalamus, 849, 851, 879-882, 884-886, 888

therapists, 1196

thermodilution, 635, 637, 639, 646, 670, 676, 759-761, 763-767, 769, 772, 781, 789, 794-796, 802-804, 806-807, 809, 811-812

thiopental, 159, 320, 714

thiopentone, 836, 940-941, 991

thromboembolism, 386, 748, 979, 986, 1155, 1157

thrombolysis, 31, 69, 74-77, 81, 83-84, 753-757, 1152

thrombosis, 82, 143, 150, 247, 719, 763, 905, 907, 972, 974, 1147, 1155-1156, 1159, 1162, 1164

thrombotic coronary occlusion, 737

tidal volume, 59, 155, 320, 373, 439, 441, 443, 445, 460-461, 464-465, 493, 498, 560, 562-564, 569, 572, 575, 580, 582, 606, 613-614, 642, 647, 775

tissue factor, 528, 1152, 1161

tissue resistance, 417, 524, 537, 541

toll-like receptors, 1077, 1080, 1084-1087, 1127

total pulmonary volume, 575

total respiratory resistance, 418

tracheal tubes, 447

transcranial Doppler, 258, 261

transesophageal echocardiography, 640, 665, 668, 675, 706, 833

transgenic, 857, 862, 893, 895, 898

transient paraesthesia, 958

transmembrane segments, 843-845

transmural myocardial infarction, 739, 741, 743, 745, 747, 749, 751, 753, 755, 757

transmural pressure, 626-627, 629-633

transport, 53-54, 146, 149-150, 162, 268, 275-277, 279-282, 465, 528, 537, 557, 649-653, 659, 683, 696, 874, 1013-1014, 1111, 1133

transpulmonary pressure, 468-469, 475, 571-573, 575

transthoracic defibrillation, 12-13

transthoracic electrical bioimpedance, 794-795, 802, 812

trauma centre, 1005-1007, 1012, 1043

trauma patients, 51, 54, 279, 282, 465, 677, 1001, 1038, 1040, 1044, 1205

trauma score, 1015

trauma scoring systems, 1014

trauma surgery, 830

traumatic brain injury, 53, 55, 237, 275, 281-283, 287, 294-296

triage, 3, 8, 145, 1006-1007, 1010, 1012-1018, 1038, 1040, 1042

tricyclic, 131

triggered arrhythmias, 710, 714

triggers, 201, 286, 523, 714, 1017

trimedoxime, 118

troponins, 5-6

U

ultrafiltration rate, 1122, 1133

ultrasonography, 216

V

value, 9-10, 37, 62-63, 93, 147-149, 162, 176, 205, 229, 232, 253, 277, 304, 310, 316, 405-406, 415-416, 419-421, 423, 471, 492-493, 565, 575-576, 622-623, 625, 627-628, 630-632, 639, 642-643, 645-646, 651, 657, 663-665, 667-669, 671-673, 686, 692, 733, 753, 775, 778-779, 782, 784-788, 795-796, 803-804, 807-809, 815, 834, 851, 911, 933, 935, 1010-1011, 1056, 1058, 1062, 1066, 1093, 1099, 1115, 1252, 1264

valvular heart disease, 61, 149, 707, 983

vasopressin, 15-17, 23, 31, 144, 371, 682

vasopressor agents, 1060

vasospasm, 224, 258, 314, 744

venous return, 144, 159, 264, 351, 367, 380, 386, 631, 633, 642, 661-662, 664-665, 672, 989, 992, 1001

ventilation, 23-24, 57-65, 67, 104, 107-111, 123, 130-131, 145-146, 154-156, 159-160, 163, 215, 224, 228-229, 234, 278, 301, 309, 314-315, 367, 369-377, 381, 386, 406, 416, 423, 425, 429, 431, 435, 438, 459-466, 473, 476, 489, 491, 493-494, 496, 498, 531, 538-539, 547-549, 553, 556, 563-564, 567, 569-570, 572, 575-576, 578-580, 582, 585, 587, 589, 591-593, 599, 605-615, 636-637, 642-643, 645, 647, 651-652, 662-664, 670, 672, 674, 677, 684, 686, 688, 772, 774, 777, 789, 794, 909, 912, 942, 973, 1009, 1029-1031, 1059, 1098-1099, 1206, 1264, 1266-1267, 1269-1270, 1273, 1280

ventilator associated pneumonia, 592-593

ventilatory patterns, 373

ventricular dysfunction and remodelling, 738

ventricular fibrillation, 709

ventricular function, 200, 637, 646, 662, 665, 671, 675-676, 680, 682-683, 687, 692-693, 697, 703-707, 725-728, 734-735, 740-743, 745, 754-755, 808

ventricular tachycardia, 21

ventricular tachydysrhythmias, 131

vigilance, 122-123, 125, 304, 308, 311, 314

viscosity, 43, 574, 582

vitamin C, 1178

vitamin K, 1159

volaemia, 638, 640, 642, 655, 657, 659, 779, 788

volatile anaesthetics, 720, 857-858, 862, 892-895, 897

volume expansion, 41-44, 50, 200-201, 373-374, 376, 672, 1110

volume loading, 93, 373, 662, 673, 677, 726, 782

volume receptors, 35

volutrauma, 435, 570, 572

W

weight, 51, 133, 149, 166-167, 175, 185, 200-201, 203, 205, 265, 340, 343, 372, 378, 395, 464-465, 480, 501, 569, 571-572, 720, 780-781, 793, 795, 806, 811, 875, 914, 930, 984, 1043, 1073, 1120, 1122, 1129, 1132-1133, 1159, 1161, 1224

work of breathing, 64, 154, 429, 511

X

xenon, 835, 839-842

x-ray crystallography, 835, 837

Z

zidovudine, 171, 174, 196

Zyvox, 1181

ALTRE

γ-aminobutyric acid, 891

δ-receptor subtypes, 865

κ-receptor subtypes, 866-867

μ-receptor subtypes, 864